Warning/Disclaimer

♦ The information contained within the *Vaccine Safety Manual* is for educational and informational purposes only, and is not to be construed as medical advice. Licensed health practitioners are available for this purpose.

♦ The author has endeavored to provide accurate information with credible citations. However, errors can occur. Therefore, readers are urged to verify all of the data and references in this book.

♦ Some of the information presented in the *Vaccine Safety Manual* may conflict with data presented elsewhere. Therefore, readers are encouraged to remain circumspect and use discretion when interpreting contradictory, complex or confusing concepts.

♦ The *Vaccine Safety Manual* is not endorsed by pharmaceutical companies, the American Academy of Pediatrics, the FDA, CDC or any other federal, state or "official" organization. For official information about vaccines, contact vaccine manufacturers, the FDA, CDC or World Health Organization.

♦ Vaccine recommendations change rapidly. Immunization schedules are periodically revised. Therefore, the FDA and CDC—not the *Vaccine Safety Manual*—should be consulted for the most up-to-date information regarding who should or should not receive vaccines, at what ages, and the number of doses.

♦ The *Vaccine Safety Manual* does not recommend for or against vaccines. Parents and other concerned people must make this decision on their own. Because the data in this manual tends to implicate vaccines (find fault with them), readers are advised to balance the data presented here with data presented by "official" sources of vaccine information, including pharmaceutical companies, the FDA, CDC and World Health Organization.

♦ The decision regarding whether or not to vaccinate is a personal one. The author is not a health practitioner nor legal advisor, and makes no claims in this regard. Nor does the author recommend for or against vaccines. All of the information in this book is taken from other sources and documented in the references listed in the back of the book. If you have questions, doubts, or concerns regarding any of the information in this book, go to the original source. Then research this topic even further so that you may make wise and informed choices.

Vaccine Safety Manual

For Concerned Families
and Health Practitioners

—2nd Edition—

By Neil Z. Miller

ISBN: 978-1881217374

Library of Congress Cataloging-in-Publication Data

Miller, Neil Z.
 Vaccine safety manual for concerned families and health practitioners /
by Neil Z. Miller. —2nd ed.
 p. ; cm.
Includes bibliographical references and index.
ISBN 978-1-881217-37-4 (alk. paper)
1. Vaccination—Handbooks, manuals, etc. 2. Immunization—Handbooks,
manuals, etc. 3. Vaccination of children—Handbooks, manuals, etc.
4. Immunization of children—Handbooks, manuals, etc. I. Title.
 [DNLM: 1. Vaccines—adverse effects. 2. Safety. 3. Vaccination—adverse
effects. QW 805 M649v 2008]
 RA638.M55 2010
 614.4'7--dc22

2 009036084

Cover photo: Fotosearch

Printed in the United States of America

Published by:
New Atlantean Press
PO Box 9638
Santa Fe, NM 87504
www.thinkchoice.com

Table of Contents

*This publication is dedicated to
vaccine-damaged children
and their families.*

Foreword

Russell Blaylock, MD

When I attended medical school more than 35years ago, vaccine reactions were rarely discussed. Like most people today, I was taught that vaccines saved mankind from mass death during sweeping epidemics and pandemics afflicting the world over the millennia. It was one of those foregone conclusions implanted in our brains. It was mentioned to us that, yes, sometimes, on rare occasions, adverse reactions do happen, but "the benefits far outweigh the negative effects."

In the course of my neurological training during my neurosurgical residency, I studied a number of cases of severe damage to the nervous system associated with vaccines, such as subacute sclerosing panencephalitis (SSPE), brachial plexitis, post-vaccinal encephalitis, transverse myelitis and peripheral neuropathies. The SSPE cases were especially depressing and laden with emotion because one witnessed the slow destruction of a child's mind to the point of coma and death. I never forgot these vaccine-related events and they flashed through my mind when it came time for my children to receive their vaccines. Like so many things in medicine, you have to see them and deal with them on a day-to-day basis to really understand the heartache and deep-seated pain associated with such an injury. Parents know this pain better than anyone.

Patients with chronic illnesses have a greater impact on the doctor's emotions than anything else, not only because he deals with all the numerous problems that will occur during the course of the illness, but because he becomes close to his patients, as well as their parents and other family members. In my experience, they become part of my family—you never forget them. At least that is the way it should be. Nowadays, I am seeing doctors who behave more like federal bureaucrats than humane men of healing.

As medicine becomes more regimented, collectivist physicians begin to lose their sense of humanity. In a collectivist system, it is the "plan" that matters, not individuals. In fact, individuals are to be sacrificed for the "plan." What you will be reading about in this monumental work is a description of the human effects of one of these "plans"—the vaccine program.

I was told by a researcher in the field of autism, that when he attended a conference in Italy on the genetic aspects of autism and mentioned the link between the vaccine program and autism incidence, one of the public officials in the Italian Health Department stood and told him in an angry tone that everyone knew that the vaccines were causing injury to children's brains, but the success of the vaccine "program" was more important. Further, he stated, these problems need to be downplayed so as not to endanger the vaccine "program."

I reported a similar conversation coming from the Simpsonwood conference held in Norcross, Georgia, attended by 53 specialists in vaccine effects—including members of the World Health Organization and major vaccine manufacturers—concerning data indicating that the vaccines were causing a statistically significant increase in childhood neurodevelopmental problems. One of the attendees stated that his main goal is to see that every child in this country receives his vaccines, today, tomorrow and forever. In other words, he could care less that the vaccines are significantly damaging children's brains and altering their brain development.

In this book, *Vaccine Safety Manual for Concerned Families and Health Practitioners,* you will learn of a great number of similar outrages and incidences of people in positions of power and influence who are purposefully putting your children at risk of serious disease and injury, often for little or no benefit. The collectivist mind-set asserts that for the "plan" to be successful it must override the wishes and even safety of the individual. You will see numerous examples of this cold, calculating mentality in this book.

A number of people will respond with incredulity. They cannot bring themselves to believe that men and women in positions of such important responsibility could do such a thing as destroy the health of tens of millions of people—young, old and yet unborn.

7

Yet, we witness similar events every day—CEOs of major corporations who lose the life savings and jobs of tens of thousands of workers who trusted them; corporations who taint foods with deadly poisons to increase profits; and government bureaucrats who destroy lives with the stroke of a pen. It has been said that lying asleep beneath all societies are monsters, red of tooth and claw, just waiting to burst forth and destroy society with their greed and avarice. History books are filled with such examples.

Those who move in the shadows of power often see the world differently than the rest of us. Where we see suffering and need, they see opportunity for profits. Where we see individuals, they see statistical tables and "masses"—people who are expendable and are to be moved around like chess pieces. The collectivists see individuals as mere cogs in a wheel of an all-embracing business-governmental coalition.

In this modern age, we are witnessing the absolute regimentation of man, where people are given instructions and expected to follow them without question. Physicians are more regimented than at any time in history, which is ironic because they were always considered the most independent thinking of the professionals. Today they do what they are told without question. I recently wrote a paper on this subject called "Regimentation in Medicine and the Death of Creativity," which I encourage you to read: www.russellblaylockmd.com. It will give you a better understanding as to why doctors react the way they do—with conventional denials—when confronted by the parents of vaccine-damaged children.

As a board-certified neurosurgeon with over 25 years of neurosurgical experience, I have a deep interest in the human brain and the diseases that affect it. Some 12 years ago I wrote a book called *Excitotoxins: The Taste That Kills,* in which I explained a mechanism by which certain food additives can cause damage to the brain. Of special interest to me was the effect on brain development. Over the years, I have researched the connection between vaccination and injuries to the brain, and have discovered that this excitotoxic mechanism is central to this process.

The vast majority of physicians have never heard of excitotoxicity, despite the fact that it is the most discussed mechanism in the field of neuroscience. Likewise, it is the major mechanism in virtually all brain disorders, including strokes, neurodegenerative diseases, viral, bacterial and mycoplasmal infections of the nervous system, seizures, brain trauma and multiple sclerosis.

As you read through this book, you will notice that some of the most devastating side effects of vaccines involve neurological damage, including encephalitis, transverse myelitis, peripheral nerve damage, autism, seizures, mental retardation, language delays, behavioral problems, multiple sclerosis and SSPE. Most physicians, especially pediatricians, think these events are "rare" and must be accepted to gain the benefit of vaccines. Most parents trust their pediatrician and feel that he or she knows the answers. In fact, these adverse vaccine reactions are not as rare as many believe. As you shall see, medical authorities are using clever ploys to hide and alter the data on vaccine injuries. They reclassify problems, deny a connection to the vaccines and more often than not, just brush such reactions off as "normal." For example, one deception is to classify cases of polio as "aseptic meningitis." By doing so, vaccine proponents can give the illusion that the polio vaccine policy was more successful than it actually was.

A more blatant example of this reclassification ploy is the label of sudden infant death syndrome (SIDS). As Neil Miller's book demonstrates, 70 percent of SIDS cases have been shown to follow pertussis vaccination within three weeks. A number of the new vaccines are also associated with sudden infant death. In order to avoid admitting that the sudden stoppage of breathing by a baby within hours to weeks of these vaccines was due to the vaccines, the vaccine defenders merely created a new disease and gave it the incredible name of sudden infant death syndrome (SIDS), which is like naming it the "Baby Mysteriously Dies of Anything but a Vaccine Injury Syndrome" (BMDAVIS).

As David Oshinsky details in his book, *Polio: An American Story,* both Jonas Salk and Albert Sabin, as well as other influential virologists, were aware that the early polio vaccines were contaminated with a number of other viruses, and that over 100 million people had been exposed to these viruses. They also knew that Dr. Bernice Eddy, a microbiologist at the National Institutes of Health (NIH), had proven that the SV-40 virus, present in both the killed and live vaccines, caused cancer in experimental animals. The public was not informed of this contamination until decades later. Worse, they continued to give the tainted vaccine to children assuming that it would not cause cancer. Modern science has proven them wrong.

Today we are facing a new problem of astronomical proportions. There is evidence that the great number of vaccines given to our children, and adults, is causing injury to their nervous systems and that it reduces the ability of people to think, learn, behave and function as normal adults. Sadly, we have understood for quite some time how this process works. It is well known and accepted that when you vaccinate someone, lets say by a shot in the arm, the body's immune system is thrown into high gear. What is less well known by doctors in practice, especially by pediatricians, is that it also activates the brain's special immune system. (Blaylock, RL. *JANA* 2003;6:21-35.) The central immune cells in the brain are called microglia (they also involve astrocytes). These normally sleeping immune cells become highly activated when a vaccination is given. Until activated they remain immobile, but after activation they can move around the brain like an amoeba, secreting very toxic amounts of inflammatory chemicals (called cytokines) and two forms of excitotoxins (glutamate and quinolinic acid). This puts the brain in a chronically inflamed state. When the brain is inflamed, it results in a physical change, something we call sickness behavior. You may recall how you feel when you have the flu, with difficulty thinking, being very sleepy and restless. Headaches are also common with an inflamed brain. As you will see in this book, many of the mothers noticed that their children had a high-pitched cry soon after their vaccination or vaccinations. This is called the encephalitic cry, meaning that it is caused by an inflamed, swollen brain. It also explains the difficulty many mothers have in waking their children, the vomiting, passing out and irritability following vaccinations. These are all signs of an inflamed brain.

The reason that pediatricians are telling these mothers that their children's reactions to these vaccines are normal is based on at least two factors. One, most pediatricians, in my experience, know absolutely nothing about a child's brain. When I was practicing, if anything happened to a pediatrician's patient that in any way indicated something was wrong with the child's brain, the doctor was on the phone with me in an instant. Most admitted they knew nothing about the brain. The second reason is that they are trying to avoid a lawsuit. If they can convince the mother that everything is well, they may avoid a trip to the courtroom. Most physicians are gun-shy about lawsuits. It can also hurt their reputation.

I made a special note while reading this book, of the number of cases of seizures being reported, which for some vaccines can increase over threefold. Multiple vaccines during a single office visit, or combination vaccines, raise the risk even higher. Seizures following a vaccination are due to two things happening in the brain. One is that many vaccines can cause a high fever, and this can trigger a seizure in seizure-prone babies, children and some adults (called febrile seizures in children). It is also known that overstimulation of the immune system, which can occur with certain types of vaccines and especially when multiple vaccines are given during one office visit, can cause seizures. The mechanism is the same as described above. The excess activation of the body's immune system leads to overactivation of the brain's microglia, and the subsequent release of the excitotoxins leads to the seizure. This mechanism has been carefully worked out in the laboratory—it is not theory.

When a vaccine or series of vaccines are given and a child develops a seizure minutes later or even several days later, there is no question that the vaccine triggered the seizure. Multiple seizures indicate a severely inflamed brain and emergency procedures need to be implemented. In many cases, the seizures can be silent, that is, they have other neurological or behavioral expressions, such as irritability or periods of confusion, rather than an obvious convulsion. (Blaylock, RL. *JANA* 2003;6:10-22.) Treatment means more than just prescribing anti-seizure medications, since this only masks the true process going on in the child's brain, that is, severe brain inflammation and excitotoxicity.

Parents and especially doctors should know that the human brain is different from the animal brain in that with humans the brain undergoes dramatic formation of its pathways long after birth. A great deal of the brain is formed in humans during the first two years after birth and continues until age 25 to 27. Excess vaccination disrupts this critical process and can result in a malformed brain, which manifests as either subtle impairment in thinking, concentration, attention, behavior or language, or serious problems with these processes. There are a number of factors that determine the severity of the damage.

It has also been shown that excess immune stimulation by vaccination can trigger an interaction between excitotoxicity and brain inflammatory cytokines that greatly magnifies the damage, and can do so for decades. A recent study of people with autism has shown that even in those 45 years of age, one sees continual activation of the brain's inflammatory systems (microglia and astrocytes).

As Neil Miller illustrates, vaccines are designed to powerfully stimulate the body's immune system using components called adjuvants. These include toxic metals such as aluminum and mercury, animal proteins (gelatin, hydrolyzed proteins and even MSG) and special lipids. Recent studies have shown that immune adjuvants can cause powerful stimulation of the immune system for as long as two years, which means the brain's immune system also remains overactive.

A growing body of research indicates that overactivity of the brain's immune cells (microglia) can lead to a gradual loss of brain connections (synapses and dendrites) and can even cause the brain to be miswired (abnormal pathways development). Once again, this is not theory—it is neuroscience fact. The problem is, most practicing physicians do not know this, primarily because they never read the scientific literature concerning these mechanisms.

It is unfortunate that most of the public are of the opinion that their physician has an in-depth knowledge of how the body works. For example, most parents assume that the pediatrician understands the immune system and therefore knows all about vaccine effects. Nothing could be further from the truth. In most medical schools, the basic sciences are taught during the first year. Medical students, in general, hate the basic sciences and see them as useless to the practice of medicine. Even worse, there are certain subjects that receive little or no coverage in medical education. Many people are aware that nutrition rarely receives any attention in the curriculum. Yet, of the basic sciences, it is immunology that gets little more than a footnote.

As you will discover in this book, even people making decisions concerning the vaccines your child will receive have admitted they know little or nothing concerning immunology. This is appalling. Anyone with even a basic understanding of immunology or having read the available research on the effects of excessive vaccination on the developing brain, would know that the present crowded vaccine schedule is extremely destructive to the child's brain. Likewise, there seems to be little concern as to the effects of multiple immunizations on the developing child's immune system. Pediatricians and public health authorities are of the opinion that they can give an unlimited number of vaccines to babies and small children without risk. Our neuroscience proves this is insane. Almost every year, these vaccine enthusiasts add another set of vaccines to the schedule, despite the growing list of neurological and other health disasters occurring in our children.

One of the principles of brain immunology is that priming the microglia can greatly aggravate the damage caused by subsequent vaccinations or even natural infections. For example, let's say a newborn is given the hepatitis B vaccine before leaving the hospital. The vaccine activates the baby's brain microglia (called priming). Then, shortly after this, let's say the child develops an ear infection (otitis media). The ear infection once again activates the baby's immune microglia, but this time the activation is greatly aggravated because of the previous vaccine-induced priming, resulting in a seizure or even sudden death. The pediatrician will blame it on the ear infection, not the previous vaccine.

Another scenario would be a baby who receives a hepatitis B vaccine at birth and then gets his or her DTaP vaccine within months of birth. Two weeks later, mom finds the baby dead in its crib. The doctor blames it on SIDS and never reports it to the CDC as a vaccine reaction. In this case the triple antigen exposure (diphtheria, tetanus and pertussis) triggers the baby's already primed microglia—this time in the brainstem, where the respiratory control neurons reside. When the baby is placed on its stomach, it cannot muster enough force to fill its lungs. Any fumes from the mattress only aggravate the problem. For the pediatrician, it is easier and safer to blame it on a mysterious disorder called SIDS, than to admit it was a sequential vaccine reaction.

In the case with live virus vaccines, such as the chickenpox vaccine and MMR (measles, mumps and rubella vaccines) studies have shown that these viruses frequently survive in the body and can enter the brain. A recent study of the elderly dying from non-infectious causes has shown that 20 percent of the brains contained live measles virus. They also found that 45 percent of the people autopsied had live measles virus in other tissues and that all these viruses were highly mutated. This means that the measles virus can persist in the body for a lifetime. In this book, you will read about a father whose son died after an MMR vaccine. The child's brain was examined and the live measles virus was cultured from the boy's frontal lobes. Immunological typing proved it was the same virus from the vaccine that he was given.

In this case, the measles virus in the child's brain (as well as adults') acts to prime the microglia, causing the brain's immune system to chronically secrete damaging inflammatory cytokines and excitotoxins. Any subsequent vaccinations or infections will greatly aggravate the immune/excitotoxic degeneration of the child's brain. This can result in developmental language problems, learning problems, behavioral problems (irritability, anxiety, depression, and violent episodes), in addition to seizures. It is instructive to note that a large percentage of autistic children have recurrent seizures deep within their brains, which are often missed by conventional EEG studies. It requires special MEG studies to uncover them.

Another thing that can prime microglia is vaccine adjuvants such as aluminum, mercury and protein additives. These products easily enter the brain, are stored for decades and can powerfully activate the brain's microglia, and do so for prolonged periods. Most pediatricians and family practice doctors have never heard of this.

Mercury tends to accumulate in the brain, especially in the brain's immune cells. This has been shown to not only result in priming, but also is a powerful stimulus for excitotoxicity within the brain. In fact, several studies have shown that mercury, even in extremely small concentrations, can powerfully activate microglia and cause the accumulation of toxic amounts of the excitotoxin glutamate within the brain. Again, this is not speculation, rather this is based on the work of some of the most respected experts in the field of brain mercury neurotoxicology. Yet, this important work is never reported in the media or among vaccine review studies conducted by government/pharmaceutical-selected panels. As I demonstrate in my review of the Simpsonwood panel, many of the so-called experts were not experts at all. In fact, one stated that he had to do a lot of review to catch up on mercury toxicity literature before he attended the conference.

Several studies have shown that many vaccines are contaminated by a number of bacteria, viruses, viral fragments and mycoplasma. When injected with the vaccines, these can easily enter the brain where they reside for a lifetime and thereby act to prime the brain's microglia. They cannot be removed. Proof of this mechanism has been shown in cases of herpes encephalitis in which the virus was killed in the brain by the immune system, yet degeneration of the brain continued. The evidence indicated that retained viral fragments acted as a source of continued microglia activation and that it was excitotoxicity that was causing the chronic brain destruction.

Another consideration is the ability of attenuated viruses to undergo mutation over time, eventually resulting in organisms that can cause new diseases. When live viruses are used to make vaccines, a process of repeated passage of the virus though growth media reduces its virulence, or the ability of the virus to cause disease. However, as occurs with measles, rubella and many other viruses used in vaccines, once in the body the attenuated viruses can be converted to quite virulent viruses. This is thought to explain the high incidence of Crohn's disease in people who were vaccinated as children with live measles viruses. (Broide, LA., et al. *Dig Liver Dis* 2001;33(6):472-6.)

The above referred to study found that the mutated measles viruses differed in each tissue, meaning that a variety of disorders could result. The risk of persistent viruses following vaccination with live viruses appears to be growing and may be secondary to a number of factors, which include the nutritional status of the person and the preexistence of immune suppression. Immunologists have voiced concern that the growing number of vaccines being given early in life may impair immune function for life. As this book demonstrates, the number of immune related disorders, such as lupus, rheumatoid arthritis and asthma, is growing substantially. All of these disorders have been linked by careful studies to vaccines.

Recent studies have also shown that when a person is generating high levels of free radicals, as seen with all chronic diseases (diabetes, heart disease and autoimmune ailments), the viruses retained in the body undergo rapid mutation, producing highly virulent organisms. These organisms can then spread through society causing epidemics of new diseases or atypical old diseases. To purposefully inject live viruses into millions of people is to invite disaster, as these viruses mutate in these unfortunate people and in those who come into contact with them. In essence, this could eventually produce deadly epidemics of whole new types of viruses. As you will discover, we are already seeing this. The age at which people are susceptible to certain viruses and bacteria is changing with the mass vaccination programs. For example, mass vaccination with Hib (haemophilus influenzae type B) shifted the disease from infants and small children to adults. The measles vaccine shifted the disease from normal at risk groups to very small babies and adults, who are more likely to suffer serious complications or death. We see the same thing with meningococcal and pneumococcal vaccines.

Vaccination programs can also cause the emergence of subtypes of viruses and bacteria that in the past rarely produced disease. This is a major worry with organisms that contain dozens or even hundreds of subtypes. For example, the human papilloma virus (HPV) contains more than a hundred subtypes. The vaccine protects against only four subtypes, and perhaps for only a relatively short period. If sexual promiscuity continues among the population, new subtypes will emerge and may be even more carcinogenic than the subtypes used in the vaccine.

Another major problem with vaccine programs is the lack of long-term protection, as occurs with natural infections. Natural immunization is now quite rare in younger people. For example, in the past most women were protected against these childhood infections by contracting them as children themselves. The protection was life-long. Most mothers were infected with wild-type viruses, such as measles, rubella, chickenpox, etc., early in life, which not only protected them, but also their newborn children. This transmaternal protection usually persists for 15 months after birth of the child. Vaccinated mothers do not offer this protection to their children. Thus, because of the mass vaccination programs, pregnant women and their babies are at increased risk.

Of great concern is the recent finding that immune activation in pregnant women can have dire consequences for the developing baby. At one time it was thought that viral infections in the mother endangered the baby because the virus was passed through the placenta into the baby's body. New research demonstrates that it is the mother's immune cytokines that are causing the damage, once they enter the baby's body, and is not caused by the virus itself. (Buka, S., et al. *Brain Behavior Immunol* 2001;15:411-420.) Researchers found that the eventual effect of maternal immune stimulation depended on the timing of the immune activation. Activation at mid-term could result in autism; stimulation late in the pregnancy could result in schizophrenia as the child grows into adulthood. What this means is that vaccinating a pregnant woman is associated with a high risk of autism, psychosis and other neurological problems as the baby reaches adolescence or adulthood. This is being completely ignored by those designing vaccines and making recommendations. At present, flu, chickenpox, hepatitis B and rubella vaccines are recommended for pregnant women. HPV was recommended for pregnant women at the beginning of the program, but a number of HPV-vaccinated women lost their babies or had babies born with deformities, resulting in a halt to such a dangerous practice.

One of the grand lies of the vaccine program is the concept of "herd immunity." It is based on the idea that if a certain percentage of the population is immunized against an infectious disease, epidemics can be prevented. The exact percentage changes, mainly, in my opinion, to suit the vaccine manufacturers. In the beginning it was 68 percent, but now some are calling for 95 to 100 percent immunization to reach these goals. We are constantly told, and many doctors believe, that herd immunity has prevented epidemics from occurring in modern America. Unfortunately, there is very little evidence of this for a number of reasons. For instance, it is assumed that high percentages of the population have been immunized through vaccine programs against diphtheria, smallpox, tetanus and pertussis, some of the older vaccines in the schedule. According to recent studies, the problem with this is that most of the protection afforded by these as childhood vaccines waned many decades ago, so that most baby boomers, the largest percentage of the population, have no protection. In fact, vaccines for most Americans declined to non-protective levels within 5 to 10 years of the vaccines. This means that for a majority of Americans, as well as others in the developed world, herd immunity doesn't exist and hasn't for over 60 years.

Aluminum is a very powerful inducer of brain microglia and macrophages. Its immune-enhancing effects led manufacturers to add aluminum to vaccines. However, until recently, most vaccine authorities ignored the possible toxicity of aluminum in vaccines, despite growing evidence that it is a significant neurotoxin (brain poison). Links to Alzheimer's disease have been made, but until recently the mechanism was poorly understood. We now know that aluminum causes significant abnormalities in neurotubules, microscopic tubes in neurons essential to their function, and these abnormal neurotubules are strongly associated with Alzheimer's disease.

Aluminum enters the brain by a number of mechanisms, for example by attaching to glutamate and fluoride. With the widespread use of the excitotoxin glutamate as a food additive and fluoride being added to drinking water supplies, aluminum absorption is common. In addition, injected aluminum can complex with fluoride within the body to produce a compound, fluoroaluminum, that has a number of harmful effects, including brain injury. There is some evidence that fluoride can trigger microglial activation and excitotoxicity, which in combination is particularly injurious to the brain. (Blaylock, RL. *Fluoride* 2004: 37(4);301-314.)

In 2001, Dr. R. K. Gherardi and co-workers described a new condition associated with retained aluminum in injected tissues from aluminum hydroxide vaccine adjuvants, which they called macrophagic myofasciitis. This infirmity was associated with intense, diffuse muscle pains, weakness and various neurological complaints. At the time of their first report there were 130 patients from France and a growing number of cases from Germany, USA, Portugal and Spain. In all cases, the problem was linked to hepatitis B (86%), hepatitis A (19%) or tetanus toxoid (58%) vaccines. A subsequent report found a number of patients with a multiple sclerosis-like illness. In 2004, a study reported in the journal *Neurology* (63:838-842) found that people exposed to the complete series of hepatitis B vaccines experienced a 300 percent higher risk of developing multiple sclerosis than the unvaccinated public. Others dispute this link.

One of the underhanded methods used by the promoters of vaccine schedule expansion is to resort to scare tactics. Many people have heard of the 36,000 deaths from flu each year ploy, which is unsupported by the data. Another way to scare the public is to use morbidity and mortality tables from previous historical eras or from Third World nations. In this way vaccine promoters can speak of deaths in the tens of thousands or millions infected. For example, if they send out warnings through the media that tens of thousands of infants may die of measles if children (and adults) are not vaccinated each year, it has a major impact on parental decisions to vaccinate. Vaccine promoters count on most of their audience being young parents, that is, those who do not remember when MMR vaccines didn't exist and when virtually all of us contracted measles. I cannot remember a single kid in any of my classes who was seriously injured or died by getting the measles. In fact, mothers used to purposefully expose their children to the measles to get it over with. Like nearly all of my classmates, I contracted most childhood infectious diseases—measles, rubella, mumps, chickenpox and pertussis. We all have life-long immunity as a result.

In my hometown of Monroe, Louisiana, during the peak of the polio epidemic in 1952, not a single child in any of my classes died of polio and only one girl had any paralysis (a weak lower leg). The incidence of polio at the time was 37 cases per 100,000 population. There were twice as many cases of muscular dystrophy in 1954, a very rare disease. Yet, modern vaccine proponents would have the present generation believe that the streets were piled high with dead and dying children, and that the rest were in varying states of paralysis. Polio was a terrifying and deadly disease for a small percentage of people, but the incidence is greatly overblown in present reports by vaccine scaremongers.

As you will learn, polio was a very mild disease in the majority of children who contracted it and extremely rare in adults. The most famous case was that of Franklin D. Roosevelt, who was stricken at the age of thirty-nine. His case is illustrative as to why some people developed paralysis and others didn't. According to Oshinsky, Roosevelt had been under enormous stress as a result of a government scandal. While vacationing at his home in Campobello Island, he engaged in regular drinking and a number of strenuous physical activities, one of which resembled an Ironman event. Exhausted, he spent much of the night drinking. The next day he experienced symptoms that were later diagnosed as polio.

Of great interest is the fact that Roosevelt had a carefully sheltered youth, which included a tutored education. Oshinski notes that he was protected from all childhood diseases until his teen years. At that point he caught virtually every infectious disease he was exposed to. It is critical for children to be exposed to these infectious organisms early in life, not only to protect them from later infections by these viruses, but because they strengthen the immune system and stimulate its proper development. This also explains the observation that polio was much less common as a paralytic disease among the poor and slum dwellers. It was the wealthier neighborhoods that were the focus of polio outbreaks. It was hypothesized that the poorer kids were exposed to the polio virus in large numbers, which gave them lifelong immunity. Because they had well-developed immune systems from being exposed to a number of bacterial and viral diseases early in life, they experienced mostly mild forms of the disease.

If this hypothesis is indeed true, then the mass vaccination programs are ruining the immune systems of our youth, in essence, setting them up for a lifetime of poor health and putting them at a greater risk of disease complications when they are exposed to infections. The evidence for this scenario is growing, with the rise in asthma, type-1 diabetes and other autoimmune diseases. With parents dragging their children to the pediatrician or medical clinic for a tetanus shot and antibiotics every time they have a cut or abrasion, the problem is compounded. As a child, I rarely went to the doctor. My parents, as most parents, knew a number of home remedies. Cuts and abrasions were treated with a little antiseptic or just warm water and soap.

When I worked in the emergency room, mothers would bring in their children with cuts so small they were difficult to see. My colleagues would dutifully give them all a tetanus booster. Children today are given multiple doses of antibiotics, often broad-spectrum, for virtually everything, even viral illnesses. This not only prevents them from developing immunity to the infection, but the antibiotics also destroy the probiotic (friendly) bacteria in the colon, which increasingly is being shown to play a vital role in immune system function and development.

Another important discovery being all but ignored by proponents of vaccination is that free radicals can cause previously benign viruses (attenuated viruses) to change their genetic expression, leading to a dramatic increase in their virulence. That is, they switch from benign viruses to powerful disease-causing viruses. This may explain the sudden appearance of the Spanish flu virus that killed millions in 1917-1918. This pandemic began during World War I. Preceding it, the soldiers experienced a mild flu epidemic. Then suddenly, the flu returned with a vengeance. Medical historians have been unable to provide an explanation for this. We know that the soldiers were living in crowded conditions, were under great stress, were extremely exhausted and were often suffering from malnutrition. Recent research has shown that when viruses of low virulence exist in the body (the first flu episode), the presence of large numbers of free radicals can convert these organisms into new "killer bugs." The soldiers were producing enormous amounts of free radicals and their poor diets provided few antioxidants for protection. This set the stage for the pandemic disaster.

The same process can work with any virus, including the measles, chickenpox, rubella, polio or mumps viruses. While they are of low virulence upon injection, over a lifetime the virus will be converted by free radicals produced in the body into viruses of varying virulence. This was proven in the previously mentioned case of the measles viruses isolated during autopsy of the elderly. The measles viruses in their organs were highly mutated. For this reason, live viruses should not be used in vaccines. A person with either a pre-existing inflammatory disease or who subsequently develops a chronic inflammatory disease (both of which are associated with the generation of enormous numbers of free radicals) will be at risk. Of even greater importance was the finding that this also put everyone else in danger, because these new mutated viruses could then spread the deadly infections throughout society—that is, the sick people would act as deadly virus generators.

Finally, a word needs to be said about vaccine contamination, which is much more common than the public or media understand. Studies have shown that 60 percent of vaccines examined from a number of manufacturers contained one or more contaminating organisms in the vaccines. The organisms included simian immunodeficiency virus (SIV—which resembles HIV, a precursor to AIDS), mycoplasma, pestivirus, SV-40 and cytomegalovirus. In addition, a number of vaccines contained viral fragments, which can trigger microglial activation and even become inserted in other viruses, creating dangerous chimeras. The finding of cytomegalovirus is especially important because of its link to strokes. One study found the virus in the carotid arteries of 70 percent of stroke victims examined.

The SV-40 virus is also of special concern because it contaminated millions of doses of the polio vaccine, both killed and live. Studies by Michele Carbone and co-workers proved conclusively that the SV-40 virus from the vaccines causes human brain tumors as well as mesotheliomas and osteosarcomas. He has linked this virus to a number of brain tumors, including medulloblastoma, ependymomas and choroid plexus papilloma. Despite a massive coverup, there exists absolute proof that this contaminating virus has caused, and continues to cause, thousands of cancers in this country and others.

It has been shown that people who were infected with the SV-40 virus from earlier vaccines (up until 1963) have passed the virus to their children (called vertical or transplacental transmission). This is why vaccine proponents continue to cover this disaster up—since knowledge of this mass contamination of tens of millions of unsuspecting people and future generations would devastate public trust in government health authorities and the sacrosanct vaccine program.

Virologists acknowledge that present vaccines may contain a great number of viruses and mycoplasma, many of which could be carcinogenic. It is known that when two weakly carcinogenic viruses are combined, sometimes they become powerfully carcinogenic through genetic recombination. It is also known that weak carcinogenic viruses in the presence of chemical carcinogens can greatly enhance the carcinogenicity of both. This may even be the case with fluoridated water, which appears to be a carcinogen.

When you consider the devastating effects of carcinogenic viruses contaminating vaccines and the effect of multiple vaccination on the immune system and brain, especially as regards autism, one can only speculate on how the perpetrators will be brought to justice. Decisions by parents to vaccinate their children, and the adult's decision to receive vaccinations, should depend on a careful study of the risks involved and an intelligent assessment of the real—not imagined—benefits. This book, *Vaccine Safety Manual for Concerned Families and Health Practitioners,* will go a long way toward helping people make those critical decisions.

Introduction

I have been investigating vaccines for more than 20 years. When my son was born, the matter became important to me. I began by studying medical and scientific journals. The data was disturbing. Evidence showed that vaccines are often unsafe and ineffective. In fact, some vaccines cause new diseases. I was even more shocked to learn that powerful individuals within the organized medical profession—including members of the American Medical Association (AMA), the American Academy of Pediatrics (AAP), the Food and Drug Administration (FDA), the Centers for Disease Control and Prevention (CDC), and the World Health Organization (WHO)—are aware of vaccine safety and protection deficiencies, but seem to have an implicit agreement to obscure facts, alter truth, and deceive the public. Vaccine manufacturers, health officials, lead authors of important studies, editors of major medical journals, hospital personnel, and even coroners, cooperate to minimize vaccine failings, exaggerate benefits and avert any negative publicity that might frighten concerned parents, threaten the vaccine program and lower vaccination rates. My first book, *Vaccines: Are They Really Safe and Effective?* was written to provide parents with a summary of my initial findings.

A few years later, I wrote *Immunization Theory vs. Reality* to document the shadowy underworld of vaccine production and corruption within the industry. For example, many people have no idea how vaccines are made or what they contain. Formaldehyde, aluminum and thimerosal—yes, some vaccines still contain this dangerous mercury derivative—are just a few of the ingredients used to manufacture vaccines. In addition, oral polio vaccines are incubated in monkey kidneys, the chickenpox vaccine is brewed in "human embryonic lung cell cultures," and the new HPV vaccine includes particles of sexually transmitted viruses which are now being injected into an entire generation of chaste, young girls.

I also wrote *Vaccines, Autism and Childhood Disorders*. My goal was to provide families with evidence of vaccine safety and efficacy defects—information that they are unlikely to hear from their doctors—so that truly informed decisions could be made. That book chronicled MMR studies, mercury damage, and congressional efforts to initiate positive change within the vaccine industry. I am opposed to bogus "proofs" of vaccine benefits—including studies funded by vaccine manufacturers—health mandates (forced immunizations), and other coercive tactics used to intimidate wavering parents into vaccinating against their will. Although generations of children are falling victim to medical "progress," autism and other developmental disorders are *not* childhood rites of passage.

I wrote this current book, *Vaccine Safety Manual for Concerned Families and Health Practitioners,* to counterbalance conventional dogma. There is extensive evidence of vaccine hazards and immunity limitations. I researched vaccine studies and articles from around the world, then summarized them for your benefit. All of the data is footnoted in the text and referenced in the back of the book. Keep in mind that I never intended to ratify traditional beliefs regarding vaccine safety and efficacy. The information I uncovered does not support the oft-heard claim that vaccine benefits outweigh their risks. In other words, if you'd like to read more about the benefits and less about the risks, there are plenty of "official" websites that you can visit (or speak to your doctor). In fact, I encourage this course of action. Of course, official vaccine websites are mainly promoted by the FDA, CDC, and vaccine manufacturers.

Each chapter in this book begins with a definition of the particular disease for which a vaccine has been developed, including data on who is most at risk, disease prevalence and severity. The vaccine for each disease is then analyzed according to its safety and efficacy profile. The safety sections include studies documenting vaccine-associated morbidity and mortality, as well as several personal stories from vaccine victims attesting to the real toll on human lives. Some chapters also include case histories from the U.S. government's own national database of vaccine damage—VAERS. The efficacy sections analyze data from multiple sources to reveal the prophylactic potential of each vaccine: how likely it is to protect against the disease and reduce its incidence throughout society. Excerpts from congressional hearings, and vaccine debacles of historical significance, are included in this book as well. Charts, graphs, tables and other illustrations supplement the text for added comprehension.

Many of the studies summarized in this book were published in reputable, peer-reviewed journals. Some of them originally appeared in distinguished foreign journals and were then translated into English. Newspaper articles, official reports, and unofficial sources of vaccine information are all referenced in this book as well. However, regarding proof of vaccine safety and efficacy, many "scientific" studies are literally nonsense. This is not a conspiracy theory. For example, the *Journal of the American Medical Association* recently published a paper showing that one-third of "highly cited original clinical research studies" were eventually contradicted by subsequent studies. The supposed effects of specific interventions either did not exist as the original studies concluded, or were exaggerated.[1]

Vaccine-related studies need to be read very closely, otherwise significant information that could affect their validity may be overlooked. For example, a small number of children who contract varicella naturally (wild chickenpox) experience serious complications. Many of these children have preexisting health problems, such as AIDS, leukemia or cancer. However, it's easier to convince parents to vaccinate their children against chickenpox, and to justify mandating this shot for all children, if a larger percentage of those who experience complications of varicella are *healthy,* rather than unhealthy, before the onset of the ailment. (It's frightening to imagine that your normal child could be devastated by a common disease.) Thus, after the chickenpox vaccine was licensed, several articles began to appear emphasizing that such complications occur "predominantly in children in whom one would not predict problems."[2] In one study, 73 percent of all children hospitalized for complications of varicella were healthy before the onset of varicella; just 27 percent had preexisting health problems. I was ready to include this data in the chickenpox chapter when I noticed that the study *excluded oncology patients!* In other words, this "study" omitted *unhealthy* children (with cancer) from analysis, then claimed that serious complications mainly occurred in *healthy* boys and girls.[3]

Vaccine studies are often funded by pharmaceutical companies with a financial interest in the outcome. Lead authors of important studies that are used to validate the safety or efficacy of a vaccine are often beholden to the manufacturer in some way. They may own stock in the company or are paid by the manufacturer to travel around the country promoting their vaccines. Lead authors may receive consultation fees, grants or other benefits from the drug maker that contravene ethical boundaries and compromise the integrity of the study. When studies of this magnitude are jeopardized, generations of people—and society itself—are placed at risk.

Sometimes study conclusions contradict core data in the study. I am always astounded when I read the abstract or summary of a major paper touting a vaccine's apparent safety or benefits, only to find that upon examining the actual paper, including important details, the vaccine is shown to be dangerous and may have poor efficacy as well. The media is loathe to publish anything that challenges the sacrosanct vaccine program. Newspaper articles about vaccines, and reviews of vaccine studies that are published, merely mimic the original spurious conclusions.

In some instances, study results may be preordained. For example, when the vaccine-autism link became a public concern, vaccine proponents moved into high gear to produce authentic-appearing studies that contradicted genuine data. I remember when tobacco companies used this very same ploy. They financed numerous bogus studies ostensibly "proving" that cigarettes didn't cause cancer. The real studies got lost in the muddle. Sadly, it's all too easy to obfuscate truth and deceive the public. At the infamous Simpsonwood conference held in Norcross, Georgia, experts knew that mercury in vaccines was damaging children. They had irrefutable proof—the very reason for convening the meeting. However, instead of making this important information public, they hatched a plan to produce additional "studies" that denied such a link. In fact, vaccine proponents had the audacity to claim in some of these papers that mercury in vaccines not only doesn't hurt children but that it actually benefits them! In the topsy-turvy world of overreaching vaccine authorities, the well-documented neurotoxic chemical mercury somehow makes children smarter and more functional, *improving* cognitive development and motor skills. Of course, this is absurd. Numerous real studies document mercury's destructive effects on brain development and behavior. Mercury in vaccines and the Simpsonwood debacle are thoroughly reviewed in the chapter on autism.

Another ploy used by vaccine proponents is to design studies comparing vaccinated people to other vaccinated people. Honest studies would compare them to an *un*vaccinated population. In addition, vaccine control groups rarely receive a true placebo, which should be a harmless substance. The scientific method has always been predicated upon removing all potentially confounding influences. However, many vaccine studies do not conform to this integral component of valid research. This is an important concept to grasp. For example, when the safety profile of a new vaccine is being tested, one group may receive the experimental vaccine made with aluminum while the "control" group receives an injection of aluminum as well (rather than water or another harmless substance). When vaccines are compared in this way, that is, to other substances that are capable of causing adverse reactions, the vaccine appears safer than it really is. Whenever this deceptive tactic is utilized, officially acknowledged adverse reactions to a vaccine may represent only a fraction of the true potential risks to the recipient.

It should also be noted that some clinical studies that are used to license vaccines exclude people in certain groups. For example, they may be too young, too old, pregnant, ill, or have other preexisting health ailments. However, once the vaccine is licensed, it may be recommended for people in these groups. Much like using false placebos, this unethical practice artificially inflates the vaccine's safety profile and places more children at risk of adverse reactions.

Although some studies are mere propaganda, part of a larger disinformation campaign designed to promote a vaccine agenda, other studies link vaccines to debilitating and fatal diseases. For example, the *British Medical Journal* published data correlating the haemophilus influenzae type b (Hib) vaccine to rising rates of type 1 diabetes. The hepatitis B vaccine has been linked to autoimmune and neurological disorders. Guillain-Barré syndrome—a serious paralytic disease—is a well-known adverse reaction to the flu vaccine. These are just a few of the many scientifically documented correlations between vaccines and incapacitating ailments that you will learn about in this book.

Vaccine adverse reaction rates have become unacceptably high. For example, according to the FDA, FluMist® (the live-virus nasal spray vaccine that is squirted up the nose) can cause "medically significant wheezing" and pneumonia. During pre-licensure clinical studies *3 percent* of all children six months to one year of age who received the vaccine ended up in the hospital with respiratory problems! Before this vaccine was approved, a large study conducted in 31 clinics showed that it caused "a statistically significant increase in asthma or reactive airways disease" in children under five years of age. Nevertheless, in September 2007 the FDA licensed this vaccine for children as young as two years old.

With some vaccines, the number of people who experience systemic reactions, such as fever, headache, respiratory infection, muscle aches, nausea, abdominal pain, diarrhea, chills and fatigue, is very high. For example, up to 10 percent of babies will vomit following their pneumococcal shots. In one study of the tetanus vaccine, 26 percent of the recipients had systemic reactions. A whopping 62 percent of 18-55 year-old recipients of the meningococcal vaccine had systemic reactions. (Common systemic reactions are separate from *severe* and *fatal* reactions, including neurological, immunological and paralytic disorders such as Guillain-Barré syndrome, demyelinating diseases, arthritis, anaphylactic shock, and other life-threatening conditions.) Doctors consider most systemic reactions "normal."

Some vaccines cause encephalitis (inflammation of the brain) and other nervous system disorders. Injuries caused by vaccines may be "disguised" under different names: learning disability, attention deficit, hyperactivity, epilepsy, and mental retardation, to name a few. Studies show that a disproportionate amount of violent crime is committed by individuals with neurological damage. The pertussis chapter (DPT and DTaP) investigates whether the rise in criminal activity and other pathological behaviors (e.g., school shootings) may be related to vaccinations.

Many parents are unaware that adverse reactions are even possible, so they fail to remain alert for neurological signs and other symptoms in their babies following their vaccinations. However, *Pediatrics* published a study in which parents were specifically asked to observe any change in their baby's behavior or physical condition after a shot; just 7 percent reported no reactions at all.

New vaccines may cause serious reactions, including death, yet still remain on the market. Although the FDA has removed defective toys and dog food from store shelves, once a vaccine is licensed, it is rarely recalled (the original rotavirus vaccine is a notable exception). The HPV vaccine illustrates this point very well. By May 2011, less than 5 years after Gardasil® was licensed in the United States, more than 21,000 adverse reaction reports were filed with the federal government. In the case reports submitted to the FDA, many of the vaccine recipients were stricken with serious and life-threatening disabilities, including Guillain-Barré syndrome, paralysis, paresthesia, loss of consciousness, seizures, convulsions, swollen body parts, chest pain, heart irregularities, kidney failure, visual disturbances, arthritis, difficulty breathing, severe rashes, persistent vomiting, miscarriages, menstrual irregularities, reproductive system complications, genital warts, vaginal lesions and HPV infection—the main reason to vaccinate. Hundreds of teenage girls and young women were rushed to the hospital for debilitating ailments following their HPV shots.

The general public is essentially unaware of the true number of people—mostly children—who have been permanently damaged or killed by one or more of the vaccines. *Every year more than 25,000 adverse reaction reports are filed with the federal government.* These include emergency hospitalizations, irreversible injuries, and deaths. Still, these numbers may be grossly underreported because the FDA estimates that 90 percent of doctors do not report reactions. A confidential study conducted by Connaught Laboratories, a vaccine manufacturer, indicated that "a *fifty-fold* underreporting of adverse events" is likely.[4] Yet, even this figure may be conservative. According to Dr. David Kessler, former director of the FDA, "only about one percent of serious events [adverse drug reactions] are reported."[5] (Multiply reported vaccine reactions by 100 for a more accurate sum.)

The federal government is aware that vaccines may permanently disable or kill your baby. In fact, Congress established a "hazard" tax on childhood vaccines. When parents pay the doctor for requested shots, some of that money goes into a special fund to compensate them when their children are seriously damaged or die. As of June 2011, $2.2 billion was granted for thousands of injuries and deaths caused by mandated vaccines. Numerous cases are still pending. Awards were issued for permanent injuries such as learning disabilities, seizure disorders, mental retardation, paralysis, and numerous deaths, including many that were initially misclassified as sudden infant death syndrome (SIDS).

The personal stories in this book are all unsolicited, meaning the vaccine victims were never asked to tell their stories; rather, they felt compelled to share them with anyone who would listen, often to warn others of the dire possibilities. These are included in this book because when we listen to vaccine victims tell their own stories we share in their pain. This cultivates empathy and helps us to understand the full cost of vaccine damage at both personal and societal levels.

Clearly, the damaged child is not the only victim. Parents undergo traumatic experiences when they discover that their child was seriously hurt by one or more vaccines. Families are often destroyed from the overwhelming emotional responsibility associated with caring for a vaccine-damaged child. There may be a large financial burden as well. Somebody has to pay for the medical bills and necessary treatments that might maintain, or hold the promise of improving, the health and well-being of the precious child they were entrusted to protect. Parents of vaccine-damaged children may also experience anger at the perpetrators, guilt for consenting to the vaccines, and sadness or grief for the child who will forever be missing his or her rightful wholeness in some manner. Brain impairments and immune system damage are difficult to reverse. Often, the child and family are stricken for life.

Relationships between husband and wife are greatly strained when a child is damaged by vaccines. Some marriages cannot withstand the stress. Grandparents often grieve as well, both for their damaged grandchild and the demanding family life their son or daughter is now destined to live. For example, autistic children require constant care. Dining out at a restaurant or going to the movies is either a horrendous chore or an impossibility. Undamaged siblings receive less time and attention from their parents due to the special needs of their handicapped brother or sister. Everyone suffers to some degree.

There is a great communal cost as well. Many permanently damaged children will never grow up and contribute to society in a meaningful capacity. There is a lost brain trust, so that future generations may not count on their creative gifts. Of course, some vaccine damaged children make wonderful contributions to society and provide the rest of humanity with several good reasons to open our hearts while expanding our grasp of the vaccine dilemma that confronts all of us, individually and collectively.

Parents need to understand that vaccines are drugs. Each one contains a proprietary blend of chemicals, pathogens and other foreign matter. That is the nature of a vaccine. Today, children receive one vaccine at birth, eight vaccines at two months, eight vaccines at four months, nine vaccines at six months, and twelve additional vaccines between 12 and 18 months (Figure 1). The pure and innocent baby is overdosed with 38 vaccine-drugs by the time he or she is 1½ years old! (DTaP and MMR are each given with a single injection but contain three vaccines. As an analogy, if you pour three separate glasses of whiskey, gin, and rum into one bottle, you're still ingesting *three* alcoholic drinks with all of the expected effects.) Imagine ingesting eight or nine drugs all at once. That's what babies receive. In fact, these babies are not ingesting the drugs; instead, the drugs are being injected directly into their tiny bloodstreams. When did *you* last take eight drugs all at the same time? Would you be more surprised if you *did* or *did not* have a serious reaction?

Some babies receive *more* than eight or nine vaccines at once. Since some shot dates are variable (due to "age range" flexibility built into the immunization schedule), it is permissible for babies to receive a cocktail of *13 vaccine-drugs* at their 12-month or 15-month doctor visits! (The vaccines recommended at these ages include DTaP, hepatitis B, Hib, PCV, polio, flu, MMR, chickenpox, and hepatitis A.) Up to seven vaccines (for DTaP, hepatitis B, polio, flu, and hepatitis A) can be administered to babies at 18 months.

In 2011, a study that I co-authored was published in *Human and Experimental Toxicology*.[6] Our study analyzed international immunization schedules and found that developed nations with higher (worse) infant mortality rates tend to give their infants more vaccine doses. For example, the United States requires infants to receive 26 vaccines (the most in the world) yet more than 6 U.S. infants die per every 1000 live births. In contrast, Sweden and Japan administer 12 vaccines to infants, the least amount, and report less than 3 deaths per 1000 live births. These findings provide evidence that multiple vaccines administered during early childhood may cause biochemical or synergistic toxicity.

If you choose not to vaccinate, there are risks involved. Your child could contract a disease for which a vaccine has been developed. Your child may also experience complications from this disease, which could be permanently debilitating or life-threatening, depending on the particular condition and other factors, such as the child's physical constitution and its ability to reestablish health. Of course, many people experience disease and then get well. There is evidence that when children are young and exposed to disease *naturally,* and then recover, the immune system is stimulated and strengthened. When sickness occurs, the innate intelligence of the body takes over and mounts a defense. The resourceful body usually wins the battle. This process is necessary and appropriate because it improves the immune system's memory and capability through its disease-fighting experiences. It may be able to detect future invaders more quickly and overtake them before any damage is done. The beneficial result is that you may be healthier in later life. For example, several studies show that women are less likely to develop ovarian cancer if they have had mumps in childhood.

Not vaccinating is just one risk; vaccinating is another. There are also risks every time you walk out of the house (and risks within your home as well). Your child could be stung by a bee, hurt in a car accident, or attacked by a shark while playing at the beach. These risks need to be weighed free of fear and bias. If you are afraid of bees, you may place more emphasis upon protecting your child from that threat, no matter how remote it may be. If you have nightmares about sharks, you may avoid the ocean. Likewise, when diseases are described in frightening detail and their risks exaggerated beyond reality,

Figure 1:

Multiple Vaccines Given Simultaneously: Overdosed Babies Receive 38 Vaccine-Drugs by 1½ Years of Age

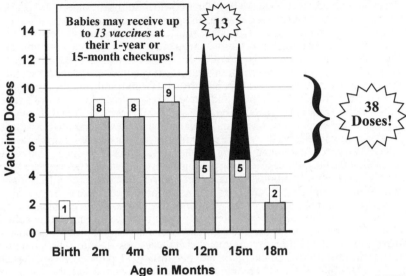

Today, children receive one vaccine at birth, eight vaccines at two months, eight vaccines at four months, nine vaccines at six months, and twelve additional vaccines between 12 and 18 months. The pure and innocent baby is injected with 38 vaccine-drugs by the time he or she is 1½ years old! Source: CDC, *Recommended Immunization Schedule 2011.* Note: Since some shot dates are variable, babies may receive up to *13 vaccines* at their 12-month or 15-month checkups! Read the immunization schedule for more information.

---

they must be avoided at all costs. Of course, there is a ready "solution" fabricated by the vaccine industry. Simply take a vaccine—and another and another—and you will be protected. If only life were so simple.

With vaccines (and many drugs as well) the "solution" is often developed prior to the marketing of fear. For example, *before* the chickenpox vaccine was licensed for general use in 1995, doctors would encourage parents to expose their children to the disease while they were young. Doctors recommended this course of action because they knew that chickenpox is relatively innocuous when contracted prior to the teenage years (but more dangerous in adolescents and adults). However, *after* the vaccine was licensed, the CDC began warning parents about the dangers of chickenpox. Doctors stopped encouraging parents to expose their children to this disease. Instead, they were told to get a chickenpox shot. The "solution"—a mandatory vaccine—preceded the apparent danger.

Vaccine efficacy is the most marketable aspect of preventive healthcare. Every manufacturer would like to claim that its product is effective—even when the evidence indicates otherwise. For example, every year authorities promote the flu vaccine. However, the *British Medical Journal* recently published a report that analyzed all pertinent influenza vaccine studies and concluded there is a large gap between evidence of the flu vaccine's efficacy and influenza policies established by health agencies. Flu vaccines were shown to have little or no effect on influenza campaign objectives, such as hospital stay, time off work, or death from influenza and its complications. Flu vaccines were found to be ineffective in children under two years of age, in healthy adults under 65 years of age, and in people aged 65 years and older. In addition, there is little evidence that flu vaccines are beneficial when administered to healthcare workers to protect their patients, when given to children to minimize transmission of the virus to family contacts, or when given to vulnerable people, such as those with asthma and cystic fibrosis.

Vaccine efficacy may be specious. For example, scientists presume that certain "surrogate markers" or "precancerous lesions" precede cervical cancer. With the HPV vaccine, they simply compared the number of these markers in women who received the vaccine to the number of these markers in women who received the placebo. However, *no actual cases of cervical cancer were prevented in any of the test subjects in any of the clinical studies of the HPV vaccine.* Besides, in more than 90 percent of cases HPV infections are harmless and go away without treatment. The body's own defense system eliminates the virus. Often, women experience no signs, symptoms or health problems.

Efficacy may also be deceptively marketed. When the new HPV vaccine was first introduced, it was promoted as 100 percent effective. Thus, most people innocently assumed that if females took the HPV vaccine, there would be *no* chance that they could ever be stricken with cervical cancer. Yet, numerous strains of HPV have been identified. The vaccine is only "100 percent effective" against two of these cancer-causing strains—not against cervical cancer itself. In fact, during pre-licensure studies, *361 women who received at least one shot of Gardasil went on to develop precancerous lesions on their cervixes within three years.*

Gardasil is not the only vaccine that targets some strains of the disease while excluding others. The Hib and pneumococcal vaccines were also constructed in this manner, and have become problematic due to "strain replacement." Scientists have discovered that when vaccines only attack some strains of a disease, other strains gain prominence. The disease becomes more virulent and people who are normally not susceptible to the ailment are infected. For example, there are several different types of haemophilus influenzae, including types a, b, c, d, e, and f. The "b" type is just one strain—the only one for which a vaccine was created—the Hib shot. Although this vaccine appears to have decreased cases of haemophilus influenzae type b in children, *the overall rate of invasive haemophilus influenzae disease in adults increased.* Ironically, researchers do not consider this a failing of the Hib vaccine; instead, "it raises the question whether a [new] vaccine will need to be developed."[7]

The pneumococcal vaccine—Prevnar 13®—is only designed to protect against 13 of the 90 different strains that can cause pneumococcal disease. Thus, when a child is vaccinated and is stricken with pneumococcus, the vaccine is still considered "effective" as long as one of the 13 vaccine strains did not cause the disease. However, in 2007, the *Journal of the American Medical Association* and the *Pediatric Infectious Disease Journal* published data showing that non-vaccine strains of pneumococcal disease are replacing strains targeted by Prevnar. The new strains are more dangerous and resistant to treatment. Current cases are more likely to be hospitalized and to be diagnosed with life-threatening infections.

Sometimes vaccines are given to one group of people mainly to protect another group. For example, mass rubella vaccination campaigns were never intended to protect vaccine recipients; the disease is usually harmless when contracted by children. Instead, the goal has always been to protect the unborn fetuses of rubella-susceptible pregnant women. Authorities reasoned that if all youngsters, male and female, are vaccinated, the wild virus should theoretically have fewer hosts to infect, and pregnant women would be less likely to contract the disease.

When the hepatitis B vaccine was originally introduced, this same rationale was employed. The groups at greatest risk of contracting hepatitis B are heterosexuals engaging in unprotected sex with multiple sex partners, prostitutes, sexually active homosexual men, and intravenous drug users. Children rarely develop this disease. In the United States, less than one percent of all cases occur in persons less than 15 years of age. The disease is even more uncommon in babies and toddlers. However, "because a vaccination strategy limited to high-risk individuals has failed," and since children are "accessible," they are compelled to receive the three-shot series beginning at birth. In other words, because high-risk groups are difficult to reach or have rejected this vaccine, authorities are targeting babies —even though babies are not likely to contract this disease. They are being subjected to all of the risks of this vaccine without the expected benefit. Although children are not likely to contract hepatitis B, many parents allow them to receive the vaccine because they believe it will protect them as adults when they may engage in risky behaviors. However, studies show that hepatitis B vaccine recipients lose protective antibodies after 5 to 10 years. The vaccine that babies receive shortly after birth at the hospital will not be effective a few years later. Thus, booster shots are required.

The necessity for multiple "booster" shots is disturbing. Initially, when a new vaccine is introduced, a single shot may be recommended. Later, when the artificial immunity wears off, vaccine manufacturers and the CDC recommend one or more additional shots—boosters (to increase or *boost* the waning antibodies). With natural immunity, which is acquired by being exposed to the actual disease, protection is not meager and temporary, but rather complete and lifelong. The child will rarely contract the disease again. This is not true with vaccines. Isn't it odd that the vaccine industry's answer to an ineffective vaccine is to compel more of it!

Unvaccinated children are often sent home from school during outbreaks of measles, mumps and other contagious diseases. For example, one mother writes: "My daughter was just removed from school for 21 days due to an outbreak of chickenpox. She is six years old and in the first grade. We are very upset."[8] Ironically, these children are not sent home for their own protection. On the contrary, doctors claim that unvaccinated children will spread disease. Of course, this does not make sense (unless we consider it a veiled confession of vaccine inefficacy). How is it possible for an unvaccinated child to imperil vaccinated children? If the shots are effective, then vaccinated children should be protected.

I include within the *Vaccine Safety Manual* brief excerpts from the congressional records to chronicle the gravity and magnitude of the vaccine dilemma. High-ranking members of the U.S. government are aware of shortcomings associated with the vaccine program. Sadly, our lawmakers are impotent to effect meaningful change. Hearings are regularly held to highlight problems with individual vaccines as well as to investigate the integrity of the vaccine program itself. For example, the chapter on the rotavirus vaccine contains a summary of a congressional hearing entitled Conflicts of Interest and Vaccine Development. Members of the exclusive FDA and CDC committees that are responsible for licensing and recommending vaccines for all children in the U.S. are permitted to have financial stakes in those vaccines.

I also include several historical accounts of documented vaccine travesties. Although these occurred in the past, there are many lessons still to be learned. For example, Edward Jenner, the British doctor who developed the smallpox vaccine, originally recommended a horrid concoction referred to as horsegrease cowpox. His vaccine consisted of pus taken from the open wounds of sick horses mixed with disease matter extracted from blisters that occasionally formed on the nipples of cows. Jenner's contemporaries were appalled by his recommendation and attempted to censor him. Later writings omitted information about Jenner's "horsegrease cowpox" smallpox vaccine.

The polio vaccine also has an interesting history. For example, it is well-known that Jonas Salk's "inactivated" polio vaccine was actually quite virulent. It paralyzed and killed many children. Perhaps less well-known is that polio vaccines are made by incubating polio viruses in monkey kidneys. Monkeys are naturally infected with several viruses and these infectious agents contaminated millions of doses of the polio vaccine. Studies from around the world appear to confirm that at least one of these viruses—SV-40—is a catalyst for many types of cancer. Moreover, SV-40 is spread from human to human and from mother to child.

The tetanus vaccine was also contaminated, but it appears to have been intentional. In the 1970s, the World Health Organization began working on an anti-fertility vaccine. Starting in 1991, pregnant women in Third World countries received several injections of a "neonatal tetanus" vaccine. In 1995, an international human rights organization, Human Life International (HLI), became suspicious of the WHO vaccination campaign. They had vials of the vaccine tested at an independent laboratory. According to HLI, millions of women "unknowingly received anti-fertility vaccinations under the guise of being inoculated against tetanus." HLI charged WHO with using women in several countries with high population growth rates "as uninformed, unwitting, unconsenting guinea pigs." Details of this outrage are included in the tetanus chapter.

Another catastrophe that should not be forgotten was perpetrated by measles vaccine researchers. In the 1980s, scientists traveled to Africa to test their new high-titer measles vaccine on babies. This experimental vaccine was up to 500 times more potent than standard measles vaccines. When it became clear that babies were dying after receiving this shot, researchers packed up their goods and returned to the United States. However, undeterred by the numerous baby deaths caused by this vaccine, the CDC decided to "test" it again on nearly 1,500 Black and Hispanic babies in California. The parents never knew that their babies were being injected with an experimental vaccine that had already killed other children. A complete account of this debacle may be found in the measles chapter.

Today, new vaccines are being introduced to counteract problems caused by old vaccines. For instance, a herpes zoster (shingles) vaccine was recently introduced to control a shingles epidemic that is expected to last for more than 50 years. Researchers have concluded that this epidemic was precipitated by the chickenpox vaccine. A complete explanation is provided in the shingles chapter.

The crowded childhood vaccination schedule, complete with a mandatory market, has proven to be a perpetual windfall for industry insiders. Yet, the real money may be in adolescent and adult vaccines. Preteens and teenagers are already being injected with vaccines for tetanus, diphtheria, pertussis, HPV, meningococcal, pneumococcal, flu, hepatitis A, B, polio, MMR and chickenpox. Other shots designed for this age group are in the pipeline. Authorities are "building a platform" for routinely vaccinating members of this lucrative market.

Future trends in the global vaccine market indicate that "at present, pediatric vaccines occupy a higher market share, but this trend will shift towards the adult vaccine segment."[9] Currently, U.S. adults are being injected with vaccines for 14 different diseases. The world vaccines market is expected to double by 2013, and will reach $40 billion annually by 2015. Cancer vaccines are expected to grow rapidly, while "addiction" vaccines will have a growth of over 100 percent after their launch. The market for vaccines required to travel overseas is expected to double by 2015, and the seasonal flu vaccine market is expected to yield more than $7 billion annually by 2016.[10] Of course, the United States is the largest market for vaccines which are "more profitable than generic pharmaceutical drugs."[11]

Several mothers have conveyed the following nearly identical story, which I paraphrase. It tells us a lot about the loss of maternal instinct:

> I took my child in for his 2-month vaccines. A short time later (this could be anywhere from one hour to two or three days) he had a horrible reaction (convulsions, seizures, loss of consciousness, etc.) and ended up in the emergency room. My child spent a lot of time (this could be anywhere from one day to two weeks) at the hospital while doctors performed numerous tests. I think the vaccines caused my child's serious reaction (because he was fine until he got his shots) but my doctor says that it was just a coincidence, that the many vaccines that my child received right before he had his reaction had nothing to do with it. It was caused by something else, although no one knows what this might be.

The story doesn't end here; it continues:

> When my child's 4-month vaccines were due I was afraid to take him back to the doctor. I was pretty sure that his 2-month vaccines caused his earlier hospitalization, but my doctor (or the nurse) told me horror stories about unvaccinated babies. I was afraid, so I let the doctor vaccinate my child a second time. Once again, he ended up at the hospital, this time fighting for his life. And once again, everyone told me the vaccines had nothing to do with it.

Now the story takes a twist:

> The reason I am telling this to you is because it's time for my child's 6-month vaccines. Of course I am terrified of the vaccines and very afraid that if I take my child in, he won't survive this time. However, the doctor says that he needs his shots. What do you think I should do?

Of course, I never give advice. Parents must make this decision on their own. What I want to tell them is: "Wake up! What happened to your protective impulse? Have you sold it out to these so-called experts? Do they live everyday with your precious child and know her more than you do? Yes, sometimes the world seems like a scary place, and confronting authority may be more than you wish to handle. But this is your child. When will you take a stand on her behalf?"

Many parents have awakened, but not always before some damage has accrued. I recently received the following letter: "I have four children. The first three were regularly vaccinated as required. A friend of mine lost a child hours after being vaccinated and alerted me to the hazards. Our fourth child was not vaccinated and is the only one who is not in special education like the rest of her siblings."[12]

Writing about vaccines is like traveling into the mythological underworld where Hades rules. It is a dark and dismal realm where innocent babies and their families are deeply traumatized. The call for a higher power is resounding. Vaccines may have some benefits in the minds of proponents but these have to be weighed against *true* safety and protection deficiencies. With this book, I have tried to provide parents and health practitioners with a good measure of this data.

I do not have an agenda other than to alert the populace to an existing and expanding problem. Much more needs to be done to awaken the masses and convince authorities that our current preventive healthcare paradigm is defective, requiring immediate attention. If you are aware and capable, please find your voice and speak out. I would prefer that people were free to choose for or against vaccines, and that they had a more well-rounded understanding—informed consent—before making their decisions. Parents are not getting complete information from their doctors. Moreover, the child's full "immunization schedule" is vehemently urged even after a serious reaction. Thus, multiple sources of information are required.

After reading this book, your sensibilities may be overwhelmed. The implications are immense. Some people will be outraged by what they discover. Something is very wrong with our vaccine industry, and now they'll know it. What can be done? Others will be incensed for different reasons, and will complain because this book does not emphasize vaccine benefits. Avid vaccine proponents do not want parents and health practitioners to have access to alternative sources of vaccine information. Instead, they want you and your family to rely upon "official" pronouncements regarding vaccine safety and protection, information that often conflicts with the studies and other data presented in the *Vaccine Safety Manual.*

Vaccines are not appropriate for everyone. Some people know this but are afraid to face their doctor, family and friends. However, the vaccination decision remains with the individual or parents of the child. Doctors cannot and will not take responsibility if you or your children are damaged from vaccines. Therefore, decisions should be made only after examining credible evidence from several sources. In addition, critical thinking should be exercised when interpreting information. I encourage readers to substantiate all of the references in this book and to research this topic even further if questions still remain. You are entitled to the facts about vaccines, and are responsible for obtaining as much information as possible with regard to the safety, efficacy, benefits and risks of vaccination.

Neil Z. Miller
Medical Research Journalist

Smallpox

What is smallpox?

Smallpox is a contagious disease caused by the *variola* virus. It is usually spread by inhaling droplets discharged from the nose and mouth of an infected person.[1] Smallpox can also be transmitted through infected blankets, linens and clothing.[2]

Symptoms begin 12 days after exposure to the virus: fever, nausea, vomiting, headache, back ache, and muscle pains. Two to five days later, the victim experiences severe abdominal pain. A rash develops on the face, inside the eyes, and subsequently covers the whole body. During the next six to ten days, the rash transforms into pus-filled sores (pustules) that could become secondarily infected by bacteria. As recovery begins, fever and other symptoms subside. The pustules crust over and may leave scars. The disease usually confers permanent immunity; the infected person will not contract it again.[3]

Antiviral medications and other drugs do not work to shorten the duration or alleviate the symptoms of smallpox. Treatment is focused on providing nutrition, increasing comfort, and reducing secondary infections. In addition, the patient is usually isolated from the public to prevent spread of the virus.[4]

Is smallpox dangerous?

Doctors sometimes differentiate between several clinical forms of the disease, including variola major, variola minor, fulminating, malignant, modified, and variola sine eruptione (without a rash).[5,6] Some forms are more serious than others. Secondary infections can cause hemorrhaging and gangrene. Corneal infections can lead to blindness. Death—caused by an infection of the lungs, heart, or brain—is a possibility as well.[7] The case-fatality rate can reach 20 percent or higher.[8]

How common is smallpox?

The disease is thought to be at least 3000 years old, spreading from Africa to India and China. Pock marks have been found on mummified skulls unearthed in Egypt. Epidemics of smallpox may have occurred in 1350 BC during the Egyptian-Hittite war, in 430 BC in Athens, and in the second century AD during the initial stages of the declining Roman Empire. In the 1500s, Spanish and Portuguese conquistadors brought smallpox to the New World, where it spread to Aztecs, Incas, and Native Americans.[9-18]

By the 18th century, smallpox was common throughout Europe. In Sweden between 1774 and 1798, the annual incidence rate ranged from 3 to 10 cases per 1,000 people (about ½ percent to 1 percent of the population). In London between 1685 and 1801, the number of smallpox cases ranged from 3 to 24 per 1,000 (about ½ percent to nearly 2½ percent of the population). In Copenhagen between 1750 and 1800, smallpox cases ranged from 9 to 18 per 1,000 (about 1 percent to 2 percent of the population). Smallpox deaths during this period ranged from 1 per 5000 cases of the disease to 4 per 1000 cases (Table 1).[19,20]

During the 19th and 20th centuries, smallpox continued to infect susceptible people. By 1967 (prior to an international campaign to eradicate the disease), smallpox remained endemic in 31 countries.[21] In 1972, the U.S. ended smallpox vaccinations.[22] By the mid-1970s, Pakistan, India, Nepal, Bangladesh and Ethiopia were declared free of the disease. On October 26, 1977, Ali Maow Maalin, a Somali cook, was the last person to officially contract a natural case of smallpox.[23] In 1980, the World Health Organization (WHO) announced that smallpox had been eradicated from the planet.[24]

How did smallpox disappear?

Variola had already stopped infecting people in more than 8 out of 10 countries throughout the world when WHO launched a worldwide vaccination campaign against smallpox in 1967.[25] At that time, only 131,000 cases were reported.[26] Yet, authorities credit their global initiative with eliminating the disease. Some medical historians question the validity

Table 1:

Smallpox in 18th Century Europe:
Annual Incidence Rates

Location	Years	Cases/1000	Population %
Sweden	1774-1798	3 to 10	.3 to 1.0
London	1685-1801	3 to 24	.3 to 2.4
Copenhagen	1750-1800	9 to 18	.9 to 1.8

Smallpox Deaths
Ranged from 1 death per 5000 cases (.0002)
to 4 deaths per 1000 cases (.004).

Every year in Europe during the latter half of the 18th century, between 3 and 24 people per 1,000 contracted smallpox (less than ½ percent to almost 2½ percent of the population). Smallpox deaths ranged from 1 per 5000 cases to 4 per 1000 cases. Source: *Annals of Internal Medicine* (October 15, 1997).

---

of this claim. Scarlet fever and the plague also infected millions of people. Vaccines were never developed for these diseases yet they disappeared as well.[27]

Several reputable historians credit *multiple* public health activities—sanitation and nutrition reforms—with reducing the incidence and severity of the early problematic diseases, including smallpox, plague, dysentery, scarlet fever, typhoid, and cholera. During the late 18th and early 19th centuries, "the etiology of disease was largely unrecognized and the breeding places of disease were undiscovered."[28] With the advent of the industrial revolution, droves of people left the countryside to seek employment in the cities. Unsanitary and crowded living conditions contributed to the spread of disease.[29] Protective measures were inconsistently applied before health authorities coordinated community efforts to: 1) clean streets, backyards, and stables, 2) remove trash, construct sewage systems, and properly dispose of human waste, 3) drain swamps, marshes, and stagnant pools, 4) purify the water supply, 5) improve the roads so that food could be rapidly transported to the cities and distributed while still fresh and nutritious.[30,31]

A Brief History of Smallpox Inoculations

By the 18th century, it was common knowledge that survivors of smallpox became immune to the disease. As a result, doctors intentionally infected healthy persons with smallpox organisms hoping to provoke a less severe infection than the naturally occurring illness. For example, children were often exposed to viral matter (pus) extracted from persons with "mild" cases of smallpox. This early preventive technique was named *variolation* (from variola).[32]

In China, variolation was practiced in one of two ways. Sometimes smallpox scabs were ground into a powder and blown into the nostrils of healthy persons through a tube.[33] Other times, dried matter of smallpox lesions was soaked into a moistened cotton swab and inserted directly into the nostrils of healthy persons.[34]

In 1715, Peter Kennedy, a Scottish physician, recommended collecting smallpox fluid on the 12th day of infection, keeping it warm, and introducing it to the patient through a scratch in the skin. This technique—inserting viral matter from a smallpox victim into a deliberate cut on a healthy person—became the model for future applications and research.[35] It quickly became customary for the upper and middle classes to submit to the procedure. But it was an uncertain and hazardous practice. Often, smallpox by variolation was indistinguishable from an attack of ordinary smallpox. Moreover, it rarely conferred permanent immunity; the variolated could contract the disease more than once. For some, it was followed by "malaise, disorders of the skin, and grave constitutional derangements."[36] The trouble and risks of variolation were disliked and feared but were accepted in the name of duty. Doting parents were grateful when the operation was accomplished without serious mishap. The variolated often died from the procedure, became the source of a new epidemic, or developed other illnesses from the lymph of the donor, such as syphilis, hepatitis or tuberculosis.[37-40] Before children were subjected to this practice, they were bled, purged, and deprived of food. Such preparation often lasted several weeks: "There was bleeding till the blood was thin, purging till the body was wasted to a skeleton, and starving on a vegetable diet to keep it so."[41]

Variolation spread throughout England, Europe, Canada, and the American colonies. However, the primary side effect of the procedure was smallpox itself.[42] This caused researchers to seek alternatives to the dangerous and uncertain medical technique.

During the late 18th century, English folklore and some dairymaids believed that if they caught cowpox, they would be immune to smallpox.[43] Cows are sometimes infected with a rash on their udders that can be transmitted to dairymaids when they milk the animals. The disease is relatively harmless in both cows and humans.[44] In 1774, an English farmer named Benjamin Jesty sought to prove that cowpox (caused by the *vaccinia* virus) protected against smallpox. He extracted diseased matter from infected cows and *vaccinated* (from vaccinia) his wife and sons. None of the Jestys developed smallpox during later epidemics. However, his wife nearly lost the arm in which she had been vaccinated because of severe inflammation, and Jesty was rebuked by his neighbors as an inhumane brute for experimenting on his own family.[45]

In 1796, Edward Jenner, an English doctor, also tried to prove that cowpox protected against smallpox (Figure 2). Jenner made a deliberate cut on James Phipps, a healthy 8-year-old boy, and inserted cowpox matter into the open wound. The boy caught cowpox. Seven weeks later, Jenner injected smallpox matter into the boy and claimed he was immune to the disease.[46] Jenner's medical colleagues disputed his claim that cowpox protected against smallpox: "We know that it is untrue, for we know dairymaids who have had cowpox and afterwards had smallpox."[47] Soon thereafter, even Jenner admitted: "There were not wanting instances to prove that when the cow pox broke out among the cattle at a dairy, a person who had milked an infected animal and had thereby apparently gone through the disease in common with others, was liable to receive the smallpox afterwards."[48]

Despite opposition to his efforts, Edward Jenner persisted. In 1798, he published *Inquiry into the Causes and Effects of the Variolae Vaccinae, a Disease Discovered in Some of the Western Counties of England, Particularly Gloucestershire, and Known by the Name of the Cow Pox*—a vulgar treatise on horsegrease cowpox (Figure 3).[49] He knew of men who milked cows soon after dressing the heels of horses afflicted with "the grease," an oily and detestable horse disease. Jenner now insisted that *these* men were immune to smallpox, and that children would forever be protected from the disease if they were injected with cowpox after the cow was infected with the rancid secretions from horses' heels. Jenner published *Inquiry* in order to recommend horsegrease cowpox. He carefully discriminated it from plain cowpox, which, he admitted, had no protective virtue:

Figure 2:

Edward Jenner

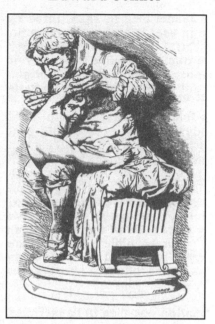

"There is a disease to which the horse, from his state of domestication, is frequently subject. The farriers have called it *the grease.* It is an inflammation and swelling in the heel, from which issues matter possessing properties of a very peculiar kind, which seems capable of generating a disease in the human body (after it has undergone the modification which I shall presently speak of), which bears so strong a resemblance to the smallpox that I think it highly probable it may be the source of the disease.

"In this dairy country a great number of cows are kept, and the office of milking is performed indiscriminately by men and maid servants. One of the former having been appointed to apply dressings to the heels of a horse affected with the grease, and not paying due attention to cleanliness, incautiously bears his part in milking the cows, with some particles of the infectious matter adhering to his fingers. When this is the case, it commonly happens that a disease is communicated to the cows, and from the cows to the dairymaids, which spreads through the farm until most of the cattle and domestics feel its unpleasant consequences. This disease has obtained the name of the cow-pox. It appears on the nipples of the cows in the form of irregular pustules.... Thus the disease makes its progress from the horse to the nipple of the cow, and from the cow to the human subject....

"It is necessary to observe that pustulous sores frequently appear *spontaneously* on the nipples of cows, and instances have occurred, though very rarely, of the hands of the servants employed in milking being affected with sores in consequence, and even of their feeling an indisposition from absorption. These pustules are of a much milder nature than those which arise from that contagion which constitutes the *true* cow-pox.... This disease [spontaneous or plain cowpox] is not to be considered as similar in any respect to that of which I am treating [horsegrease cowpox], as it is incapable of producing any specific effects on the human constitution. However, it is of the greatest consequence to point it out here, lest the want of discrimination should occasion an idea of security from the infection of the smallpox, which might prove delusive."[50]

The public was appalled by Jenner's recommendations. Horsegrease cowpox was disgusting and they wanted nothing to do with it. Still, many attempts were made to verify Jenner's prescription for protecting children; every experiment ended in failure. Jenner's peers were pleased to learn of his failures. One commented: "The very name of horsegrease was like to have damned the whole [practice of vaccinations]."[51] This may have been why, in 1806, when the esteemed Dr. Robert Willan published *On Vaccine Inoculation,* a treatise on the most recent developments in the field, Jenner was freely cited, yet neither horsegrease nor horsegrease cowpox was ever mentioned. Instead, plain cowpox was exalted as the true prophylactic.[52]

Although the public preferred the diseased secretions from cows' teats (cowpox) over the oozing pus from horses' heels (the grease), Edward Jenner continued to promote his nauseating remedy. Besides, the time was ripe to deliver people from "the inconveniences, uncertainties, disasters, and horrors of variolation."[53] Thus, in 1802 (and again in 1807), Jenner petitioned the House of Commons for monetary support to promote vaccinations. His formal request was persuasive: "Your petitioner has discovered that a disease which occasionally exists in a particular form among cattle, known by name of cow-pox, admits of being inoculated on the human frame with the most perfect ease and safety, and is attended with the singularly beneficial effect of rendering through life the person so inoculated perfectly secure from the infection of smallpox."[54]

Upon Jenner's bold declaration, Parliament granted his request, mass inoculation campaigns were launched, and soon thereafter cases of smallpox among the vaccinated were reported. At first they were denied. When denial was no longer possible—because the vaccinated were obviously afflicted with the disease—Jenner and his supporters claimed that if vaccination did not prevent smallpox, it at least provoked milder forms of the disease. But when the vaccinated caught the disease and *died*, new explanations became necessary. These deaths were attributed to "spurious" cowpox.[55] Jenner explained that "the disease

Figure 3:

Title Page of Edward Jenner's
1798 Treatise on Horsegrease Cowpox

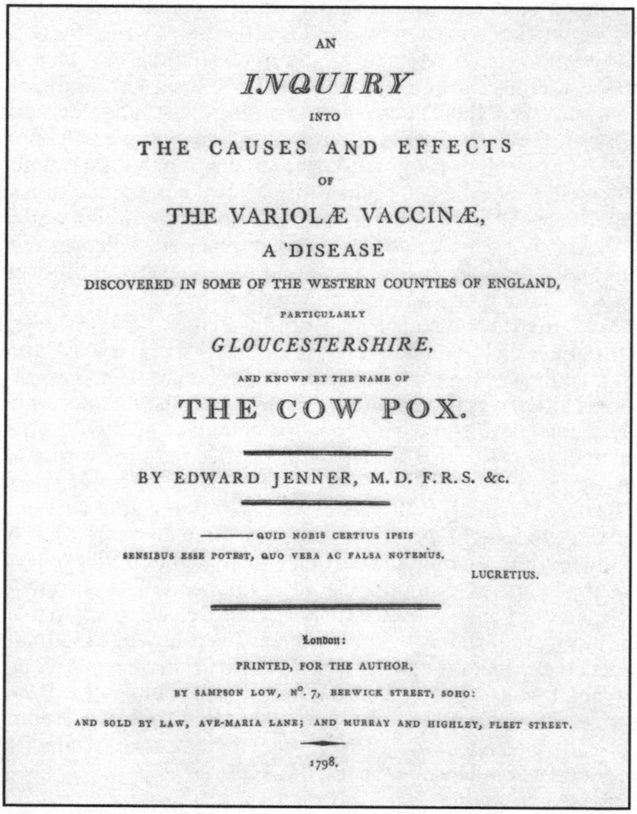

AN

INQUIRY

INTO

THE CAUSES AND EFFECTS

OF

THE VARIOLÆ VACCINÆ,

A 'DISEASE

DISCOVERED IN SOME OF THE WESTERN COUNTIES OF ENGLAND,

PARTICULARLY

GLOUCESTERSHIRE,

AND KNOWN BY THE NAME OF

THE COW POX.

BY EDWARD JENNER, M.D. F.R.S. &c.

————— QUID NOBIS CERTIUS IPSIS
SENSIBUS ESSE POTEST, QUO VERA AC FALSA NOTEMUS.

LUCRETIUS.

London:

PRINTED, FOR THE AUTHOR,

BY SAMPSON LOW, Nº. 7, BERWICK STREET, SOHO:

AND SOLD BY LAW, AVE-MARIA LANE; AND MURRAY AND HIGHLEY, FLEET STREET.

1798.

produced upon the cows by the colt and from thence conveyed to those who milked them was the *true* and not the *spurious* cow-pox."[56] According to Jenner, protection from smallpox is not possible "until a disease has been generated by the morbid matter from the horse on the nipple of the cow, and passed through that medium to the human subject."[57] However, it was virtually impossible to discriminate between the apparently different forms of cowpox. Thus, when the vaccinated recovered from the ordeal, Jenner claimed the cowpox was genuine; otherwise it was spurious![58]

Jenner admitted that his "gift" to the world often *caused* morbid disease and death: "The happy effects of inoculation, with all the improvements which the practice has received since its first introduction into this country, not very unfrequently produces deformity of the skin, and sometimes, under the best management, proves fatal."[59] He tried to blame some failures on improper inoculations: "A very respectable friend of mine, Dr. Hardwicke of Sodbury, inoculated great numbers of patients previous to the introduction of the more modern method by Sutton, and with such success that a fatal instance occurred as rarely as since that method has been adopted.... Is it not probable then that the success of the modern practice may depend more upon the method of invariably depositing the virus in or upon the skin, than on the subsequent treatment of the disease?"[60]

By the time Jenner died in 1823, three kinds of smallpox vaccination were in use: 1) cowpox—often promoted as "pure lymph from the calf," 2) horsepox, or horsegrease injections, promoted as "the true and genuine life-preserving fluid," and 3) horsegrease cowpox, the foul concoction originally promoted in Jenner's *Inquiry*. All were known to cause suffering and death.[61]

In the years following Jenner's death, vaccine failures were still being blamed on incorrectly administered inoculations. The usual practice of making one puncture for the injection was considered incomplete and ineffective. Two or more punctures were recommended. According to Dr. Marson, chief surgeon of Smallpox Hospital at Highgate, England, "A good vaccination is when persons have been vaccinated in four or more places."[62] Of course, "the mothers nearly always protest," he stated, especially since "some of the vaccinators use real instruments of torture," where multiple ivory points "are driven into the flesh."[63] But research has proved again and again that the number of puncture marks has no influence over the success or failure of the practice—the very reason *re-vaccination* was advocated. Contemporary medical authorities now asserted that "vaccine prophylaxy is only real and complete when periodically renewed."[64] People must be vaccinated again and again "until vesicles cease to respond to the insertion of virus."[65]

To bolster their claim that smallpox inoculations were safe and effective, vaccine proponents often resorted to medical ploys. Hospital records were consistently "doctored." For example, smallpox victims who were previously vaccinated and required hospital services were frequently registered as unvaccinated. According to Dr. Russell of the Glasgow Hospital, "Patients entered as unvaccinated showed excellent marks (vaccination scars) when detained for convalescence."[66] Vaccinated patients who died from either smallpox or the smallpox injection were often certified as unvaccinated as well, or had their death certificates falsified. For example, according to Dr. Herbert Snow, senior staff surgeon of the London Cancer Hospital, "Of recent years, many men and women in prime of life have dropped dead suddenly. I am convinced that some 80 percent of these deaths are caused by the inoculations or vaccinations they have earlier undergone. These are well known to cause grave and permanent disease of the heart. The coroner always hushes it up as 'natural causes.' I have been trying to get these cases referred to an independent commission of inquiry, but so far, in vain."[67] Even the renowned George Bernard Shaw (winner of a Nobel Prize in literature) was aware of the medical shenanigans used to hoodwink the public: "During the last epidemic at the turn of the century, I was a member of the Health Committee of London Borough Council. I learned how the credit of vaccination is kept up statistically by diagnosing all the re-vaccinated cases (of smallpox) as pustular eczema, varioloid or whatnot—except smallpox."[68]

How safe and effective was the smallpox vaccine?

Throughout the 1800s, several countries instituted compulsory vaccination laws. In 1807, vaccination was declared obligatory in Bavaria. In 1810, the shots were compulsory in Denmark.[69] England mandated smallpox vaccinations in 1853.[70] Prior to compulsory vaccine legislation, smallpox outbreaks were regional and self-limiting. The most severe epidemics occurred following mandatory shots. In England, from 1870 to 1872, after more than 15 years of forced immunizations —and a 98 percent vaccination rate[71]—the largest epidemic of smallpox ever recorded maimed and killed thousands of people. Most of the population had been vaccinated and re-vaccinated.[72] According to Dr. William Farr, Compiler of Statistics of the Registrar-General, London, "Smallpox attained its maximum mortality *after* vaccination was introduced. The mean annual mortality to 10,000 population from 1850 to 1869 was at the rate of 2.04, whereas in 1871 the death rate was 10.24 and in 1872 the death rate was 8.33, and this after the most laudable efforts to extend vaccination by legislative enactments."[73]

Further corroboration of vaccine failures comes from Sir Thomas Chambers, a London health official: "Of the 155 persons admitted to the Smallpox Hospital in the Parish of St. James, Piccadilly, 145 had been vaccinated." Records from Marylevore Hospital indicate

Table 2:

Smallpox Deaths Tumbled
After People Refused the Vaccine

Ten-Year Period Ending:	% of Babies Vaccinated:	Smallpox Deaths (Annual Average):
1881	96.5	3708
1891	82.1	933
1901	67.9	437
1911	67.6	395
1921	42.3	12
1931	43.1	25
1941	39.9	1

Source: Official statistics from England and Wales.

that 92 percent of the smallpox cases had been vaccinated. An official at Highgate Hospital confessed: "Of the 950 cases of smallpox [in 1871], 870 (92 percent) had been vaccinated." And records from the Hempstead Hospital show that up to May 13, 1884, out of 2,965 admissions for smallpox, 2,347 (79 percent) had been vaccinated.[74]

Figures were similar in many other countries where compulsory laws were established. For example, in 1870 and 1871 more than one million Germans contracted smallpox after Germany enforced mandatory shots; thousands died. Ninety-six percent of the victims were vaccinated.[75,76] According to the German Chancellor, "The hopes placed in the efficacy of the cowpox virus as a preventative of smallpox have proved entirely deceptive."[77] From 1887 to 1889, countless Italian citizens contracted smallpox after Italy enforced mandatory shots; thousands died.[78,79] According to Dr. Charles Rauta, Professor of Hygiene and Materia Medica at the University of Perugia, "Italy is one of the best vaccinated countries in the world.... For 20 years before 1885, our nation was vaccinated in the proportion of 98.5 percent.... The epidemics of smallpox that we have had [from 1887-1889] have been so frightful that nothing before the invention of vaccination could equal them."[80] From 1886 to 1908, hundreds of thousands of Japanese citizens contracted smallpox after Japan enforced mandatory shots every five years; thousands died.[81] And in 1918 and 1919, the worst epidemic of smallpox ever recorded in the Philippines occurred after the U.S. took control of the islands and enforced mandatory shots. The entire population was vaccinated; thousands died.[82,83] A 1920 Report of the Philippines Health Service, noted: "The 1918 epidemic looks prima facie as a flagrant failure of the classic immunization."[84]

Several countries outlawed vaccinations or enacted new legislation rescinding mandatory regulations. For example, according to the Secretary of the Governing Board in Dublin, Ireland, "Smallpox virus taken from the calf would communicate that disease to the human subject and be thereby a fertile source of propagating the disease, and would, moreover, render the operator liable to prosecution under the Act prohibiting inoculation with smallpox."[85] In the late 1800s, Australia abolished compulsory vaccination and reported only 3 cases of smallpox in 15 years.[86] Official statistics from England and Wales show an inverse correlation between the percentage of babies vaccinated and the number of smallpox deaths: the greater the number vaccinated, the greater the loss. Deaths from smallpox tumbled after people refused the vaccine (Table 2 and Figure 4).[87]

<u>Figure 4:</u>

Evolution of a Campaign
to Eradicate Smallpox

Begin with...
Unsanitary living conditions and poor nutritional awareness

This results in...
Regional and self-limiting outbreaks of smallpox

Conduct human experiments with...
Variolation—the practice of inserting viral matter
(infectious pus) from a smallpox victim
into a deliberate cut on a healthy person

When this fails...
Conduct human experiments with cowpox,
horsepox, and horsegrease cowpox

When this fails...
Deny it

When this fails...
Blame it on "spurious" cowpox, improperly administered
injections, or too few puncture marks

When this fails...
Recommend re-vaccination

When this fails...
Manipulate statistics by altering medical records
and falsifying death certificates

When this fails...
Mandate the smallpox vaccine

**When people refuse the shot, vaccination rates drop,
and cases of smallpox dwindle...**
Take full credit for eradicating the disease!

Source: See Notes 31-72.

Figure 5:

Title Page of Mary Catherine Hume's
1878 Treatise on Opposing British Vaccine Laws

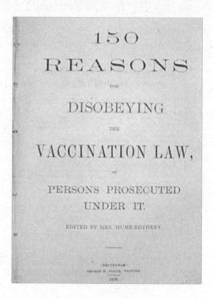

Early opponents of smallpox vaccinations:
Throughout the history of smallpox inoculations, intelligent people from all walks of life spoke out against the unscientific and perilous vaccine enterprise. For example, the great spiritual leader, Mahatma Gandhi, once stated: "I am, and have been for years, a confirmed anti-vaccinationist.... I have not the least doubt in my mind that vaccination is a filthy process that is harmful in the end."[88]

By the mid-1850s, a very large anti-vaccine movement had been established. After the 1870-1872 smallpox epidemic, thought to have been caused by mandatory shots, this movement gained credibility and became more organized in its efforts to resist compulsory laws and awaken others to the inherent dangers of smallpox vaccinations.[89] In 1878, Mary Catherine Hume published *150 Reasons for Disobeying the Vaccination Law by Persons Prosecuted Under It* (Figure 5).[90] Parents were being fined and jailed for refusing to submit their children to the shots. Before the Exemption Act was passed in 1907, every year thousands of parents were prosecuted for resisting vaccination. Many had their homes and property confiscated.[91,92] Hume's book advocated civil disobedience despite the punitive efforts of pro-vaccinators. It noted that "Vaccination is a poisoning of the blood... capable of sending inwards to the vital organs the blood-impurities which might otherwise have been safely got rid of by means of the natural eruptive process."

The consequences are often deadly. Furthermore, "The Vaccination Acts—for rendering compulsory (whether under pain of one fine or twenty) on the citizens of a so-called free country—are tyrannical, unconstitutional, and in the true sense illegal; Godless and insane; idolatrous, being acts for the continual offering up of human sacrifices; odious to all lovers of freedom; fraudulent, as evading and violating another existing Act of Parliament; demoralizing to the whole community; and, on the direct and indirect testimony of their own supporters and advocates, an utter and absolute failure." Such Acts make England "a nation not of freemen, but slaves."[93]

<u>Figure 6:</u>

Title Page of *The Vaccination Inquirer,* an Influential 19th Century Journal Opposing British Vaccine Laws

(Published by the *London Society for the Abolition of Compulsory Vaccination*)

```
                    ' THE

VACCINATION  INQUIRER
                    AND

         HEALTH  REVIEW.

    THE ORGAN OF THE LONDON SOCIETY FOR THE ABOLITION OF
              COMPULSORY VACCINATION.


    To a great extent the law is not obeyed.  It is disregarded, as every law is disregarded which does not
 agree with men's consciences.  It is a most mischievous thing that there should be a law in existence which
 good people are tempted to disobey.  It is a bad example to set, and it tends to bring laws into contempt
 which are of real importance.—LORD BRAMWELL.



              VOLUME THE FIFTH.




       APRIL, 1883, to MARCH, 1884.




                   LONDON:
    114, VICTORIA STREET, WESTMINSTER;
 AND EDWARD W. ALLEN, 4, AVE MARIA LANE.
                  1884.
```

In 1884, the London Society for the Abolition of Compulsory Vaccination published *The Vaccination Inquirer and Health Review,* a thick compendium of smallpox data containing unbiased vaccine statistics, newspaper stories about people who were damaged by the shot, and legal briefs regarding compulsory laws (Figure 6).[94] Vaccine objectors were often fined and jailed. Despite harsh laws, many people refused to be vaccinated and would not allow their children to receive the shots. According to Lord Bramwell, "To a great extent the law is not obeyed. It is disregarded, as every law is disregarded which does not agree with men's consciences. It is a most mischievous thing that there should be a law in existence which good people are tempted to disobey. It is a bad example to set, and it tends to bring laws into contempt which are of real importance."[95]

Doctors Oppose Vaccines

Numerous doctors and health officials of the late 19th and early 20th centuries were vocal opponents of mandatory vaccines. Here are a few of their comments on this topic:[96-99]

"I have been a regular practitioner of medicine in Boston for 33 years. I have studied the question of vaccination conscientiously for 45 years. As for vaccination as a preventative of disease, there is not a scrap of evidence in its favor. The injection of virus into the pure bloodstream of the people does not prevent smallpox; rather, it tends to increase its epidemics and it makes the disease more deadly. Of this we have indisputable proof. In our country (U.S.) cancer mortality has increased from 9 per 100,000 to 80 per 100,000 or fully 900 percent increase within the past 50 years, and no conceivable thing could have caused this increase but the universal blood poisoning now existing."
—Dr. Charles E. Page, Boston practitioner

"Vaccination does not stay the spread of smallpox, nor even modify it in those who get it after vaccination. It does introduce in the system contamination and, therefore, contributes to the spread of tuberculosis, cancer, and even leprosy. It tends to make more virulent epidemics and to make them more extensive. It did just what inoculation did—cause the spread of disease."
—Dr. Walter M. James, Philadelphia practitioner

"Cancer was practically unknown until cowpox vaccination began to be introduced. I have had to do with 200 cases of cancer and I never saw a case of cancer in an unvaccinated person."
—Dr. W. B. Clark, New York practitioner

"Many men and women in prime of life have dropped dead suddenly. I am convinced that some 80 percent of these deaths are caused by smallpox vaccinations. These are well known to cause grave and permanent disease of the heart."
—Dr. Herbert Snow, Senior surgeon, London Cancer Hospital

"Abolish vaccination and you will cut the cancer death rate in half."
—Dr. F. P. Millard, Toronto practitioner

"Vaccines are principally responsible for the increase of those two really dangerous diseases, cancer and heart disease."
—Dr. Benchetrit, practitioner

"In looking over the history of vaccination for smallpox, I am amazed to learn of the terrible deaths from vaccination which necessitated amputation of arms and legs and caused tetanus, foot-and-mouth disease, septicemia (blood poisoning), and cerebro-spinal meningitis."
—Dr. R. C. Carter, practitioner

"I am convinced that the increase of cancer is due to vaccination."
—Dr. F. Laurie, Medical Director of the Metropolitan Cancer Hospital, London

"It is my firm conviction that vaccination has been a curse instead of a blessing to the race. Every physician knows that cutaneous diseases (including cancer) have increased in frequency, severity, and variety to an alarming extent. To no medium of transmission is the widespread dissemination of this class of diseases so largely related as to vaccination."
—B. F. Cornell, M.D., practitioner

"I have removed cancers from vaccinated arms exactly where the poison was injected."
—Dr. E. J. Post, Michigan practitioner

"I have no hesitation in stating that in my judgment the most frequent disposing condition for cancerous development is infused into the blood by vaccination and re-vaccination."
—Dr. Dennis Turnbull, 30 year cancer researcher

"Never in the history of medicine has there been produced so false a theory, and such fraudulent assumptions, such disastrous and damning results as have followed the practice of vaccination; it is the ultima Thule (extremity) of learned quackery, and lacks, and has ever lacked, the faintest shadow of a scientific basis. The fears of the people have been played upon as to the dangers of smallpox, and the promise of sure prevention by vaccination, until nearly the whole civilized world has become physically corrupted by its practice."
—Dr. E. Ripley, Connecticut practitioner

"Vaccination is the infusion of contaminating elements into the system, and after such contamination you can never be sure of regaining the former purity of the body. Consumption (tuberculosis) follows in the wake of vaccination just as surely as effect follows cause."
—Dr. Alex Wilder, professor of pathology, Medical College of New York

"How is it that smallpox is five times as likely to be fatal in the vaccinated as unvaccinated? [Referring to data published in the *British Medical Journal,* January 14, 1928.] How is it that, as the number of people vaccinated has steadily fallen, the number of people attacked with variola has declined and the case mortality has progressively lessened? The years of least vaccination have been the years of least smallpox and least mortality. These are just a few points in connection with the subject which are puzzling me, and to which I want answers."
—Dr. L. A. Parry (summarizing Dr. R. P. Garrow), practitioners

"I now have very little faith in vaccination, even as to modifying the disease, and none at all as a protective in virulent epidemics. Personally, I contracted smallpox less than six months after a most severe vaccination."
—Dr. R. Hall Bakewell, Vaccinator General of Trinidad

"To affirm that there never has been any scientific warranty for a belief in the alleged protective virtues of vaccination and that its practice is backed by ignorance and indifference, is a sorry charge to make against the medical profession... but the charge, I regret to say, is only too true. I know whereof I affirm, for I, too, must plead guilty of the charge. Before discovering my mistake I had vaccinated more than 3,000 victims, ignorantly supposing the disease I was propagating to be a preventative of smallpox. Having taken for granted what my teachers had asserted, I was a staunch believer in the alleged efficacy of vaccination as a prophylactic against smallpox. I remained in this blind and blissful state of ignorance for several years. Not until I acquired a little experience in the school of observation and reflection did I discover that my faith was pinned to a shameful fraud."
—J. W. Hodge, M.D., practitioner

"I believed that vaccination prevented smallpox, or if it did not absolutely prevent it in every case, it modified the disease in some cases, and I believed that re-vaccination, if only frequently enough, gave absolute immunity. Experience has driven all that out of my head; I have seen vaccinated persons get smallpox, and persons who had been re-vaccinated get smallpox, and I have seen those who have had smallpox get it a second time and die of it."
—Dr. J. C. Ward, Royal College of Surgeons, England

"After collecting the particulars of 400,000 cases of smallpox, I am compelled to admit that my belief in vaccination is absolutely destroyed."
—Professor A. Vogt, chair of Vital Statistics and Hygiene at Berne University

Post-Vaccinal Ailments

Several studies and official declarations confirm that smallpox vaccines were dangerous and ineffective. For example, in 1915 the United States Department of Agriculture traced several epidemics of foot-and-mouth disease to the smallpox vaccine. Although this ailment primarily affects cattle, it may be communicated to man if the virus directly enters the blood through wounds of any kind, including smallpox injections.[100,101]

In 1923, Great Britain authorized the pro-vaccine Andrews Committee to investigate the smallpox vaccine. This small group of doctors documented 62 cases of post-vaccinal encephalitis and 36 deaths. In 1926, the Rolleston Committee was established to follow up on smallpox vaccine safety issues. This committee studied 30 new cases of post-vaccinal encephalitis with 16 fatalities.[102]

In May 1926, the *New York State Journal of Medicine* reported on several cases of encephalitis and meningitis that developed shortly after smallpox vaccinations.[103] In July of that year, the *Journal of the American Medical Association* found correlations between smallpox vaccinations and nervous disturbances. The authors noted: "In regions in which there is no organized vaccination of the population, general paralysis is rare. In patients with general paralysis...vaccination scars were always present."[104] In September 1926, *Lancet* published data confirming seven cases of encephalomyelitis following smallpox vaccinations. The authors declared: "There can be no doubt that vaccination was a definite causal factor."[105] In October 1926, *Lancet* reported on 35 cases of encephalitis following smallpox vaccinations. Fifteen of the victims died. The authors concluded: "Vaccination was a definite causal factor and no chance coincidence."[106]

In 1928, the *British Medical Journal* acknowledged that young adults vaccinated against smallpox were five times more likely to die from the disease than those who were not vaccinated.[107] That same year, the League of Nations in Geneva, Switzerland, issued the Report of the Commission on Smallpox and Vaccination, noting that "The post-vaccinal encephalitis with which we are dealing has become a problem in itself....The cases which have occurred have been sufficiently numerous and similar to require them to be considered collectively. Their occurrence has led to the realization that a new, or at least a previously unsuspected or unrecognized, risk attaches to the practice of vaccination."[108] The Report also noted 139 recent cases of post-vaccinal encephalitis and 41 deaths in one country alone, Holland. Compulsory smallpox vaccinations were discontinued as a result.[109]

In February 1930, Germany modified its compulsory vaccination law following numerous cases of post-vaccinal diseases: "Vaccinated people developed a cerebral inflammation which resulted in a number of deaths and several cases of mental derangement."[110] In April of that year, the *Journal of the American Medical Association* reported on several children with "encephalitic symptoms" following their smallpox vaccinations. Some were severe and ended fatally.[111]

From 1949 to 1951, in the United States, people died from complications of the smallpox vaccine—mainly from post-vaccinal encephalitis—at rates eight times greater than those who were not vaccinated.[112] In 1952, *Lancet* described the effects of smallpox vaccination given to a woman who was three months pregnant: "She developed a severe primary reaction and three months later she was spontaneously delivered of a feeble hydropic premature infant covered with a very severe generalized vaccinia. The child died 18 hours later."[113] In another study of pregnant women who were vaccinated during their first trimester, 47 percent failed to give birth to a normal child.[114]

During the late 1950s and 1960s, several medical and scientific publications, including the *British Medical Journal* and *Pediatrics,* documented numerous cases of post-vaccinal encephalomyelitis following smallpox vaccination. Neurological reactions ranged from encephalitis to epilepsy, polyneuritis, multiple sclerosis, and death. In some regions of the world, 1 of every 63 people vaccinated was damaged by the shot. Extreme sensitivity to multiple shots was also observed. Subsequent inoculations were responsible for many of the post-vaccinal ailments. In fact, the death rate from vaccination appeared greatest in those who were vaccinated early in life and then re-vaccinated in later years. The morbidity and mortality rates were extremely high in babies as well.[115-121]

Adverse Reaction Reports: Smallpox Vaccine

This section contains several reports of adverse reactions following smallpox vaccinations:[122-124]

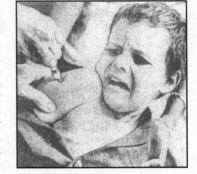

▸ "One day in the iron-dog year, in 1909, when I was five, a physician wearing a yellow hat came to Black Horse Village from Shigatse, saying he had medicine for smallpox. He gave each of the children vaccinations for the price of two coins. Strangely, as a result of this vaccination, nearly all of the children contracted the disease and many died, including 60 from families on the Shugu estate. I and three of my sisters and my young brother became ill, and the blisters on my eldest sister and my youngest brother never went away, and both died." —Tsipon Shuguba, a high official from the 14th Dalai Lama's original government

▸ "Our baby was vaccinated in the fall of 1921. Four days later the arm became very sore and swollen. Inflammation spread over the shoulder, up the neck to the back of the ear. It continued to get worse. The doctor said it was mastoiditis. The next day our baby went into convulsions and died."

▸ "My daughter, six years old, was in perfect health until December 3, 1921, when we were advised by our family physician to have her vaccinated. About the third day her arm began to hurt. On Saturday, she complained of a sore throat. She became sick at her stomach and vomited. Her condition grew worse. The doctors could do nothing to save her. She died on Tuesday, December 13."

▸ "My wife was vaccinated on October 27, 1922. She died a few hours after the vaccination in our home. The doctor pronounced it heart failure."

▸ "My wife was in good health until she was vaccinated November 1, 1922. In three days her arm was swollen. On the 9th of November, she broke out with a pronounced skin rash all over her body. On November 29, she became seriously ill. Sores appeared in place of the rash. The doctor said it was smallpox. She died on December 5."

▸ "Lafayette Hunt of Denver, Colorado was vaccinated November 6, 1922. He developed smallpox on November 18 and died of it November 28."

▸ "On November 13, 1922, my wife submitted to vaccination in order to hold her position with the telephone company. Up to the time of the vaccination she was in good health. On December 8, she became ill with enlarged lymphatic glands under her arms. She died on December 10."

▸ "Walter Call was vaccinated on November 20, 1922. He was able to work for a week after being vaccinated although he was ill during the time. He died on December 8 with black smallpox."

▸ "Mr. and Mrs. Alvord of South Cascade had a healthy, robust child. He was vaccinated. Nine days later he began to have convulsions. The child died. The cause of death was reported as colitis."

▸ "In the fall of 1922, we started our only child to school. She was in excellent health at the time, but after she had attended two months we were told that she must be vaccinated or leave school. Soon after she was vaccinated she broke out with sores and was not able to attend school for six weeks. She started again but was too sick to continue. Our family physician said she had erysipelas. She passed away nine days later."

▸ "Margaret Ann, the only daughter of Mr. and Mrs. Donald W. Gooding, was pronounced a perfect baby by the doctor when she was born. This beautiful and healthy infant was vaccinated at the age of four months. The first two injections didn't take, so a third vaccination was given, after which inflammation of the brain developed within five days. She was taken to the hospital where she remained for many weeks. At the age of 13 months she was blind and could not learn to walk. She also developed digestive disturbances and convulsions."

▸ "Horace Capewell was a fine, healthy baby with beautiful eyes. He was vaccinated when five weeks old. Nine days later his body was a mass of sores. His eyes became affected and at the age of five months he was totally blind."

▸ "Mona Stevenson was vaccinated at the age of five weeks with the official glycerinated calf-lymph. After five weeks of suffering in which the child's face and arm was partly eaten away by the vaccine disease, the child died."

▸ "Ethel Thompson, age seven months, was a beautiful, healthy infant until vaccinated. Soon after, ulcers began to develop that never healed. Her flesh decayed until the ribs were exposed. Festering sores formed on her body. After two months of untold suffering, the child died."

▸ "Ernest Cheeseman was vaccinated at the age of nine weeks with the standard glycerinated calf-lymph. Up to that time, he was healthy and normal. Five days after his vaccination a serious form of syphilitic skin disease developed. The body was covered with eczema-like eruptions and the feet were drawn up, all out of shape. The sores that broke out around the mouth looked like burnt meat and stood out at least an inch. Death relieved him of his suffering."

Smallpox and AIDS:

In 1987, the *New England Journal of Medicine* reported on a military recruit who contracted AIDS after being vaccinated against smallpox. Doctors who reviewed the case wrote: "Primary smallpox immunization of persons with subclinical HIV disease poses a risk of vaccine-induced disease [and] multiple immunizations may accelerate the progress of HIV disease. This case raises concern about the ultimate safety of vaccinia-based vaccine in developing countries where HIV infection is increasing."[125]

Two months later, the *London Times* published a compelling report indicating that "the AIDS epidemic may have been triggered by the mass vaccination campaign" conducted by the World Health Organization (WHO) against smallpox during the 1960s and 1970s, mainly in Africa.[126] The *Times* exposé was written in response to a tip from an advisor to the World Health Organization who was assigned by WHO to investigate the suspicion that its ambitious vaccination program in Africa had caused the AIDS epidemic. The WHO advisor did his study, concluded that the smallpox vaccine was a trigger for AIDS, and filed his report with WHO. When the report was buried, he contacted the *Times*.[127]

The greatest concentration of AIDS coincided with regions where the smallpox vaccination program was most intense—Zaire, Zambia, Tanzania, Uganda, Malawai, Ruanda, and Burundi. Brazil, the only South American country included in the vaccination campaign, had the highest incidence of AIDS on that continent. Haiti also had a high incidence of the disease. Several thousand Haitians were on a United Nations mission in Central Africa when WHO conducted its mass vaccination campaign; they received the smallpox shots.[128,129]

The WHO advisor told the *Times,* "I thought it was just a coincidence until we studied the latest findings about the reactions which can be caused by vaccinia. Now I believe the smallpox vaccination theory is the explanation of AIDS."[130] Dr. Robert Gallo, renowned authority on AIDS, commented on this possibility: "I have been saying for some years that the use of live vaccines such as that used for smallpox can activate a dormant infection such as HIV."[131] This has led some experts to fear that an attempt to control one disease, smallpox, transformed another disease, AIDS, "from a minor endemic illness of the Third World into the current pandemic."[132]

Monkeypox:

Some researchers question whether smallpox was ever truly exterminated. After WHO launched its global vaccination campaign against variola in 1967, suspected cases of smallpox were labeled as monkeypox.[133] In 1972, a report in *Lancet* noted that WHO's smallpox eradication program "can only be successful in the absence of a non-human reservoir for smallpox virus." However, the author of the report identified several poxviruses affecting both humans and animals, and conceded that the monkeypox virus can cause clinical smallpox in humans.[134] In 1976, researchers discovered monkeypox antibodies in humans. The monkeypox virus was indistinguishable by laboratory methods from the smallpox virus.[135]

Orthopoxviruses, the genera to which vaccinia, variola, cowpox, and monkeypox belong, have a high degree of similarity, with a "propensity for genetic recombination."[136] Monkeypox and smallpox produce exact clinical symptoms, with one insignificant difference: monkeypox also causes swelling of the cervical and inguinal (groin) lymph nodes.[137] In 1979, new research indicated that several animal species, including some rodents, may be carriers of variola-like viruses virtually identical to cowpox and monkeypox viruses.[138] In fact, several poxviruses from animal sources were tested and shown to behave like variola/smallpox viruses.[139] African squirrels and camels may also harbor the microbe.[140,141]

Scientists are "wondering whether the specter of smallpox might be rising from the dead, perhaps reincarnated in its close relative monkeypox, which is alive, well, and spreading in Central Africa."[142] From 1981 to 1986, investigators identified 338 monkeypox cases in Zaire (now the Congo). The person-to-person transmission rate was 30 percent; the case-fatality rate was 10 percent.[143] However, between February 1996 and October 1997, more than 500 cases were identified, the largest outbreak of monkeypox ever recorded.[144] The person-to-person transmission rate increased to 78 percent, while the case-fatality rate dropped to 2 percent, indicating that the disease is changing its pattern of infection.[145] According to Dr. Peter Jahrling of the U.S. Army Medical Research Institute of Infectious Diseases, for all practical purposes, smallpox is back.[146]

Smallpox and bioterrorism:
In 1978, two medical researchers in Birmingham, England were manipulating the smallpox virus, became infected and died.[147] This incident emphasized the need for close supervision and protection of all smallpox virus stocks in laboratories. To reduce the risk of future accidents and lessen the likelihood that vials of the virus might be stolen by terrorists, all remaining known samples were moved to secure facilities at the U.S. CDC in Atlanta, Georgia, and at the State Research Center of Virology and Biotechnology in Novosibirsk, Siberia. Authorities planned to destroy all strains of the disease but scientists argued that this safety measure would simply hamper future studies of the virus. Thus, smallpox has gained several reprieves from destruction. Deadlines of December, 31, 1993; June 30, 1995; June 30, 1999; and 2002, all came and passed without accord among members of WHO's executive board.[148-157] In fact, on November 15, 2001, the Bush administration postponed indefinitely any decision to eliminate seed stocks of the microbe—at least until scientists develop new vaccines and treatments for the disease.[158]

In 1972, the Soviet Union initiated an extensive biological warfare (BW) program. In 1980, variola was added to the schedule. Smallpox viruses were manipulated and mutated into weapons of war. In 1992, the program was terminated; scientists with BW experience became unemployed and may have sold information. Authorities believe that North Korea and other countries also secretly possess multiple strains of the contagious organism.[159]

On September 11, 2001, 19 terrorists hijacked four American commercial jets and flew them into occupied buildings killing nearly 3,000 people. A few weeks later, deadly anthrax was mailed to U.S. politicians and media personnel. Hundreds of people were exposed to the germ; several died.[160-162] These actions raised immediate concerns regarding how to protect innocent people from biological threats. However, even though health officials have identified several diseases that would wreak havoc if terrorists successfully circulated the germs, including botulism, ebola, tularemia, and plague,[163] authorities chose to concentrate their resources on developing a "new and improved" smallpox vaccine.

A "New and Improved" Smallpox Vaccine

Smallpox hasn't occurred in the United States since 1949, yet the government stockpiled 15 million doses of the aging and archaic vaccine.[164] Shortly after the September 2001 terrorist attacks, scientists conducted studies to see whether the existing inventory could be diluted to increase the number of doses to 150 million.[165] However, the current vaccine was developed by infecting calves with vaccinia and harvesting the pus.[166,167] This vaccine causes inflammation of the brain and other adverse effects, including smallpox and death.[168-179] (Officially, for every million people vaccinated, about 250 will be damaged and several will die.[180] However, in 1967 there were 131,000 *reported* cases of smallpox worldwide yet the CDC and WHO *estimated* that there were 15 million cases of the disease—a hundredfold increase over actual reports.[181] Thus, the true number of people likely to be damaged from the smallpox vaccine may be closer to 25,000 per million, with countless fatalities.) Infants, pregnant women, and people with weak immune systems, such as those with HIV, are especially susceptible to being injured or killed from the smallpox vaccine.[182-185]

In 1997, four years before the 2001 terrorist attacks, the Department of Defense contracted with DynPort Vaccine Company to produce a new smallpox vaccine. In September of 2000, one year before the terrorist attacks, the CDC contracted with OraVax (which changed its name to Acambis) to produce a new smallpox vaccine. Some researchers were puzzled by these actions since smallpox was supposedly eradicated and authorities were debating whether to destroy all of the remaining seed stocks of the virus. According to Dr. Margaret Hamburg, of the Department of Health and Human Services, "A lot of people thought this was a crazy idea, to make a new vaccine when the disease didn't exist."[186]

Dark Winter:
In June of 2001, a team of bioterrorism specialists, led by the Johns Hopkins University Center for Civilian Biodefense Studies, conducted an exercise code-named Dark Winter that simulated an outbreak of smallpox in the United States. Within two months after the hypothetical epidemic started, three million people were infected. Dark Winter ended with the collapse of interstate commerce, crowds rioting in the streets, and the nation moving toward martial law.[187] However, like any theoretical exercise, conclusions are predicated on the underlying assumptions. One key assumption was that each person with smallpox would infect at least 10 other people and that those 10 people would each infect at least 10 more people and so on.[188] But a recent CDC study published in *Emerging Infectious Diseases* regards those infection rates as grossly unrealistic. The authors of the study looked at data from numerous smallpox outbreaks and reported that on average less than one person was infected per infectious person. In all outbreaks, some infected persons did not transmit a single case of smallpox to another person. The researchers even cited evidence of 12 unvaccinated persons who had face-to-face contact with an infected person; none of the 12 became ill with clinical cases of smallpox. The CDC researchers concluded "the probability that the average transmission rate will be greater than two cannot be demonstrated...."[189,190] Thus, the Dark Winter simulation was seriously flawed. Yet, team leader Dr. Henderson, who also led WHO's global effort to eradicate smallpox, concluded that the threat is real, more vaccine is needed, and recommended 100 to 135 million doses.[191]

On September 20, 2001, just one week after terrorists flew hijacked planes into the World Trade Center buildings and the Pentagon, Vice President Dick Cheney was shown a video of the Dark Winter simulation and was urged to support an immediate increase in the production of smallpox vaccine.[192] On October 24, 2001, President Bush asked Congress for $509 million to develop and produce a new smallpox vaccine. He solicited bids for the job from several pharmaceutical companies, insisting on 300 million doses—one dose for every American—within the shortest possible time, not to exceed one year.[193]

Will the new smallpox vaccine be safe and effective?
The new smallpox vaccine was expected to be made from a "diploid cell substrate" (human embryo) or from animal tissue cell cultures, including those with "tumorigenic potential."[194,195] Ideally, it would not cause adverse reactions, would not be dangerous to people with immune system deficiencies, and would have the capacity to defeat genetically altered strains of variola. But researchers provided no evidence that the new vaccine would cause fewer adverse reactions than the old vaccine. Furthermore, experts were very concerned about "the transmissibility of vaccinia virus from a recently vaccinated person to a susceptible host."[196] In other words, some people—no one knows how many—will develop smallpox by coming into contact with a recently vaccinated person.

According to Franklin Top, a biotechnology expert who previously served as the commander of the Walter Reed Army Institute of Research, "reactogenicity" is going to be a problem.[197] According to Dr. Frank Fenner, one of the world's leading authorities on smallpox, "the risk of vaccination with ordinary smallpox vaccine [in countries with high levels of HIV] would be dangerous."[198] He does not believe that reintroducing vaccination will provide a simple solution. Dr. Mark Buller, a virologist who is investigating safer smallpox treatments at St. Louis University is even more candid: "I would not even consider having my family vaccinated. I'm more likely to be hit riding my bike to work than to be hit by a smallpox episode in my own life."[199]

Potential vaccine recipients must also understand that scientists may never be able to create a vaccine that can protect against mutated strains of the virus. Dozens of strains already exist.[200] New permutations of the variola microbe could be developed by bioterrorists rendering a new vaccine worthless, thus subjecting recipients of the shot to the inherent risk of serious adverse reactions without the expected benefit.[201]

In 2002, the U.S. government tested their existing smallpox vaccine on 200 "fit and healthy" college students. Following vaccination, 75 had high fevers, one-third missed at least one day of work or school, and several were put on antibiotics because their blisters resembled a bacterial infection. Common symptoms included a red, itchy bump that developed within three to four days, followed by a large blister filled with pus. In the second week, the blister dried and turned into a scab that fell off in the third week. During the three weeks, many of the students experienced flu-like symptoms, including lethargy, aches, fever and terrible itchiness."I just wanted to go to bed," exclaimed one student. Her arm was heavy and itchy: "I just thought, 'Can you just chop off my arm?'" Another student complained, "You can't scratch it; it's all bandaged up. All I could do was smack it." This student was miserable the whole weekend, suffering from a fever, an arm that was hot to the touch, and swollen lymph nodes in her armpit. Dr. Kathy Edwards, the physician overseeing the study, commented on the side effects: "I can read all day about it, but seeing it is quite impressive. The reactions we saw were really quite remarkable."[202]

In late 2002, smallpox vaccination was reinstated for U.S. military personnel. In early 2003, the program was expanded to include civilians considered at high risk during a smallpox outbreak (mostly healthcare and emergency service workers).[203] Shortly thereafter, several vaccinated people experienced serious adverse reactions, including heart problems. For example, a Maryland woman died from a heart attack after being injected with the smallpox vaccine, and several others developed grave heart complications after receiving the shot.[204-206] Authorities insisted that the smallpox vaccine has never been associated with heart problems before, that this was a new phenomenon, but doctors, researchers and laymen have known about this correlation for decades.[207] The seriousness of these reactions induced the CDC to issue a fact sheet on "new developments involving smallpox vaccination and heart problems." The CDC elaborated: "There is evidence suggesting that smallpox vaccination may cause cases of heart inflammation (myocarditis), inflammation of the membrane covering the heart (pericarditis), and a combination of these two problems.... Heart pain (angina) and heart attack have also been reported after smallpox vaccination."[208]

On December 7, 2005, the *Journal of the American Medical Association* published two studies that assessed the safety of the government's expanded smallpox vaccination program after analyzing adverse events associated with the shot. In the first study, there were 822 documented adverse events; 100 of these were labeled "serious." There were 85 hospitalizations including 21 complications of the heart (myocarditis or pericarditis). Three people died.[209] In the second study, researchers focused on neurologic side effects. More than half of the adverse events occurred within one week of smallpox vaccination. Serious events included cases of meningitis, encephalitis, myelitis, Bell's palsy, Guillain-Barré syndrome, seizures and death.[210] Despite these disturbing outcomes, researchers concluded that smallpox vaccination was associated with "few serious adverse events" and that if widespread smallpox vaccination is considered in the future, "these data will be reassuring."[211]

In March of 2007, a two-year-old boy was infected with a life-threatening disease that he contracted from his father, a U.S. army soldier who was recently vaccinated against smallpox. In addition, the boy passed the infection on to his mother. The boy developed vaccinia lesions over 80 percent of his body and went into sepsis, a devastating, systemwide infection. He was taking powerful pain medication and needed a ventilator to breathe. Doctors treating the boy said he will probably lose 20 percent of his outer skin layer.[212]

On May 17, 2007, an experimental smallpox vaccine called ACAM2000 made by Acambis received positive recommendations from the FDA following its declaration that ACAM2000 is safe and effective[213]—despite the fact that clinical trials of this vaccine were halted three years earlier when several recipients of the shot developed myopericarditis, inflammation of the heart and surrounding tissues.[214] Apparently ACAM2000 is "nearly as effective" as the older smallpox vaccine, Dryvax, and poses "similar risks of serious side effects."[215] According to the FDA, adverse reactions associated with Dryvax include autoinoculation (transfer of the vaccine virus to other parts of the body) affecting the face, nose, mouth, genitalia and rectum; accidental infection of the eye resulting in blindness; post-vaccinal encephalitis, encephalomyelitis, encephalopathy, progressive vaccinia, eczema vaccinatum, Stevens-Johnson syndrome, neurological sequelae, and death.[216]

Will the new smallpox vaccine be mandatory?

According to Tom Ridge, former secretary of U.S. Homeland Security, "It is the intention to determine, after we have sufficient supplies available to commence inoculation, to make the decision [whether to mandate the smallpox vaccine] at that time."[217] However, Tommy Thompson, former secretary of Health and Human Services, said that his department had no plans to implement a mandatory vaccination program. He cited horrendous side effects as the principal reason.[218] Dr. Anthony S. Fauci, director of the National Institute of Allergy and Infectious Diseases also believes that a mass vaccination program against smallpox, without evidence of an outbreak, would be unwise. He confirmed that complications related to the smallpox vaccine were greater than problems with shots children are receiving today.[219] Yet, if the past is any indication of the future, authorities will want to mandate the smallpox vaccine just as soon as it becomes available and passes the FDA's minimal standards for safety and efficacy.

"National Emergency" Enforced Vaccinations

Despite pervasive concerns about smallpox vaccine safety and the threat of mandatory shots with an accompanying loss of civil liberties, on October 23, 2001, the CDC unveiled new legislation—*The Model State Emergency Health Powers Act*[220]—giving public health officials and state governors the authority to arrest, vaccinate, medicate, and quarantine anyone they deem either unprotected from, or a threat to spread, infectious disease. (See Section 504a— Vaccination and treatment: To compel a person to be vaccinated and/or treated for an infectious disease.)[221] Local police and the U.S. military, by way of the National Guard, would enforce the law.[222,223] Previous laws permitting medical, religious, or philosophical exemptions would be repealed.[224]

Lawrence Gostin, the chief author of the newly proposed draconian edicts, has a long history of advocating the loss of civil liberties in exchange for theoretical health benefits derived from an expanded medical police state. According to Dawn Richardson, who operates PROVE, a Texas-based vaccine awareness organization, "Gostin is a threat to the freedoms our country was built upon. Now his ideas are codified in legislation that will be pushed around the country ostensibly offering security from microbes in exchange for your freedom to make your own medical decisions. Everyone who values our freedoms and rights in this country needs to commit to educating family and friends about the dangers of such an unchecked medical dictatorship. Because there has been no research into the biological mechanisms that predispose people to vaccine reactions and there has been no effort to screen out these individuals, this type of action should be condemned; it will create unfathomable human suffering and sacrifice."[225]

The proposed bill also threatens to seize private property for use by the state, to control access to communications, and to limit legal recourse. In fact, once a "public health emergency" is declared, the U.S. Constitution, Bill of Rights, and civil liberties will be suspended. Furthermore, this "model legislation" exempts the State, the police, the militia, and public health authorities from any liability due to their actions; if an individual opposes vaccines, is force-inoculated and dies, the perpetrators cannot be prosecuted.[226]

Figure 7:

Smallpox or Chickenpox:
Can Doctors Tell the Difference?

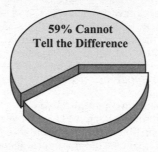

Fifty-nine percent of pediatricians cannot differentiate between smallpox and chickenpox.
Source: *Clinical Pediatrics* 2006; 45(2):165-72.

More recent developments:
The March 2006 issue of *Clinical Pediatrics* published the results of a recent survey indicating that 59 percent of pediatricians could not tell the difference between smallpox and chickenpox (Figure 7). In addition, "the majority would not accept smallpox vaccination in the absence of an outbreak and would not recommend smallpox vaccine to their patients."[227] The March 2006 issue of the *American Journal of Preventive Medicine* published the results of another recent survey, this one on healthcare workers and "first responders" who refused smallpox vaccination. The leading reasons for non-vaccination were concern about adverse reactions and believing a smallpox outbreak is unlikely. In addition, more than 80 percent would not be financially compensated if they developed side effects from the vaccine, although 40 percent reported that they could acquire liability coverage in case they transmitted vaccinia (smallpox) to a patient.[228] (In other words, legal protection is available if they are sued for spreading smallpox.)
State health departments, unions and hospitals representing "first responders" have long argued that without a compensation program to cover treatment of side effects and lost work time, it will be difficult to recruit volunteers to receive the smallpox vaccine. According to Congressman Henry Waxman, "The president has asked healthcare workers to volunteer to be immunized so that they can serve society. In turn, society should help them if they are hurt when they volunteer."[229] To remedy this situation, on May 24, 2006, the U.S. government published "final rules for the Smallpox Vaccine Injury Compensation Program," which "provides benefits to public health and medical response team members and others who are injured as a result of receiving the smallpox vaccine." In addition, "unvaccinated individuals injured after coming into contact with a vaccinated member of an emergency response plan, or with a person with whom the vaccinated person had contact, or their survivors may be eligible for the same program benefits."[230]
As of May 2007, the United States had already stockpiled 192.5 million doses of a new smallpox vaccine, ACAM2000, produced by the British pharmaceutical company, Acambis. This vaccine is mainly intended for use in persons considered high risk for contracting smallpox.[231] In June of 2007, the federal government announced that it will also purchase 20 million doses of Imvamune, a new vaccine manufactured by Bavarian Nordic, a Danish pharmaceutical company. Imvamune is produced with a weaker form of the vaccinia virus and is therefore expected to cause fewer side effects. In the event of a smallpox outbreak, this vaccine is mainly intended for people with compromised immune systems.[232]

Polio

What is polio?
Polio is a contagious disease caused by an intestinal virus that may attack nerve cells of the brain and spinal cord. Symptoms include fever, headache, sore throat, and vomiting. Some victims develop neurological complications, including stiffness of the neck and back, weak muscles, pain in the joints, and paralysis of one or more limbs or respiratory muscles. In severe cases it may be fatal, due to respiratory paralysis.

How is polio contracted?
Polio can be spread through contact with contaminated feces (for example, by changing an infected baby's diapers) or through airborne droplets, in food, or in water. The virus enters the body by nose or mouth, then travels to the intestines where it incubates. Next, it enters the bloodstream where "anti-polio" antibodies are produced. In most cases, this stops the progression of the virus and the individual gains permanent immunity against the disease.[1]

Many people mistakenly believe that anyone who contracts polio will become paralyzed or die. However, in most infections caused by polio there are few distinctive symptoms.[2] In fact, 95 percent of everyone who is exposed to the natural polio virus won't exhibit any symptoms, even under epidemic conditions.[3,4] About 5 percent of infected people will experience mild symptoms, such as a sore throat, stiff neck, headache, and fever—often diagnosed as a cold or flu.[5,6] Muscular paralysis has been estimated to occur in about one of every 1,000 people who contract the disease.[7,8] This has lead some scientific researchers to conclude that the small percentage of people who do develop paralytic polio may be anatomically susceptible to the disease. The vast remainder of the population may be naturally immune to the polio virus.[9]

Injections: Several studies have shown that injections (for antibiotics or other vaccines) increase susceptibility to polio. In fact, researchers have known since the early 1900s that paralytic poliomyelitis often started at the site of an injection.[10,11] When diphtheria and pertussis vaccines were introduced in the 1940s, cases of paralytic poliomyelitis skyrocketed (Figure 8).[12] This was documented in *Lancet* and other medical journals.[13-15] In 1949, the Medical Research Council in Great Britain set up a committee to investigate the matter and ultimately concluded that individuals are at increased risk of paralysis for 30 days following injections; injections alter the distribution of paralysis; and it did not matter whether the injections were subcutaneous or intramuscular.[16,17]

A 1992 study, published in the *Journal of Infectious Diseases,* validated earlier findings. Children who received DPT (diphtheria, tetanus, and pertussis) injections were significantly more likely than controls to suffer paralytic poliomyelitis within the next 30 days.[18] According to the authors, "this study confirms that injections are an important cause of provocative poliomyelitis."[19]

In 1995, the *New England Journal of Medicine* published a study showing that children who received a single injection within one month after receiving a polio vaccine were 8 times more likely to contract polio than children who received no injections. The risk jumped 27-fold when children received up to nine injections within one month after receiving the polio vaccine. And with ten or more injections, the likelihood of developing polio was 182 times greater than expected.[20]

Why injections increase the risk of polio is unclear.[21] Nevertheless, these studies and others[22-27] indicate that "injections must be avoided in countries with endemic poliomyelitis."[28] Health authorities believe that all "unnecessary" injections should be avoided as well.[29]

Nutritional deficiencies: A poor diet has also been shown to raise susceptibility to polio.[30] In 1948, during the height of the polio epidemics, Dr. Benjamin Sandler, a nutritional expert at the Oteen Veterans' Hospital, documented a link between polio and an excessive use of sugars and starches. He compiled records showing that countries with the highest

Figure 8:

Polio Cases Skyrocketed After Diphtheria and Pertussis Vaccines Were Introduced

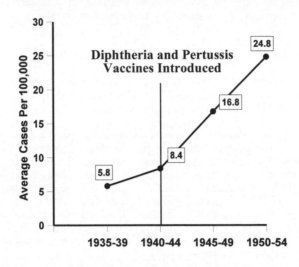

Studies show that injections increase susceptibility to polio. When diphtheria and pertussis vaccines were introduced in the 1940s, cases of paralytic poliomyelitis skyrocketed. This chart shows the average number of polio cases per 100,000 people during five-year periods before and after the vaccines were introduced. Source: National Morbidity Reports taken from U.S. Public Health surveillance reports; *Lancet* (April 18, 1950), pp. 659-63.

---

per capita consumption of sugar, such as the United States, Britain, Australia, Canada, and Sweden (with over 100 pounds per person per year) had the greatest incidence of polio.[31] In contrast, polio was practically unheard of in China (with its sugar use of only 3 pounds per person per year).[32]

Dr. Sandler claimed that sugars and starches lower blood sugar levels causing hypoglycemia, and that phosphoric acid in soft drinks strips the nerves of proper nourishment. Such foods dehydrate the cells and leech calcium from the body. A serious calcium deficiency precedes polio.[33-36] Weakened nerve trunks are then more likely to malfunction and the victim loses the use of one or more limbs.[37]

Researchers have always known that polio strikes with its greatest intensity during the hot summer months. Dr. Sandler observed that children consume greater amounts of ice cream, soft drinks, and artificially sweetened products in hot weather. In 1949, before the polio season began, he warned the residents of North Carolina, through the newspapers and radio, to decrease their consumption of these products. That summer, North Carolinians reduced their intake of sugar by 90 percent; polio decreased by the same amount! The North Carolina State Health Department reported 2,498 cases of polio in 1948 and 229 cases in 1949.[38]

One manufacturer shipped one million less gallons of ice cream during the first week alone following the publication of Dr. Sandler's anti-polio diet. Soft drink sales were down as well. But the powerful Rockefeller Milk Trust, which sold frozen products to North Carolinians, combined forces with soft drink business leaders and convinced the public that Sandler's findings were a myth and the polio figures a fluke. By the summer of 1950 sales were back to previous levels and polio cases returned to "normal."[39]

Can polio be treated?

Paralytic polio is rarely permanent. Usually there is a full recovery.[40-44] Muscle power begins to return after several days and continues to improve during the next 12-24 months.[45] A small percentage of cases will experience residual paralysis. In rare cases, paralysis of the muscles used to breathe can lead to death.[46]

Treatment mainly consists of putting the patient to bed and allowing the affected limbs to be completely relaxed. If breathing is affected, a respirator or iron lung can be used. Physical therapy may be required.

Does a polio vaccine exist?

In 1947, Jonas Salk, an American physician and microbiologist, became head of the Virus Research Laboratory at the University of Pittsburgh. He was interested in developing a polio vaccine. In 1952, Salk combined three types of polio virus grown in cultures made from monkey kidneys. Using formaldehyde, he was able to "kill" or inactivate the viral matter so that it would trigger an antibody response without causing the disease. That year he began his initial experiments on human subjects. In 1953, his findings were published in the *Journal of the American Medical Association.* In April 1955, the nation's first polio immunization campaign was launched. Shortly thereafter, 70,000 school children became seriously ill from Salk's vaccine—the infamous "Cutter Incident." Many of these children contracted polio from the vaccine, were paralyzed and died. Apparently, Salk's "killed-virus" vaccine was not completely inactivated.[47-50] The vaccine was redeveloped, and by August 1955 over 4 million doses were administered in the United States. By 1959, nearly 100 other countries were using Salk's vaccine.[51]

In 1957, Albert Sabin, another American physician and microbiologist, developed a live-virus (oral) vaccine against polio. He didn't think Salk's killed-virus vaccine would be effective at preventing epidemics. He wanted his vaccine to simulate a real-life infection. This meant using an attenuated or weakened form of the live virus. He experimented with thousands of monkeys and chimpanzees before isolating a rare type of polio virus that would reproduce in the intestinal tract without penetrating the central nervous system. The initial human trials were conducted in foreign countries. In 1958, it was tested in the U.S. In 1963, Sabin's oral "sugar-cube" vaccine became available for general use.[52]

Which vaccine is in use today?

In 1963, Sabin's oral vaccine quickly replaced Salk's injectable shot. It is cheaper to make, easier to take, and appears to provide greater protection, including "herd immunity" in unvaccinated people. However, it cannot be given to people with compromised immune systems.[53] Plus, it is capable of causing polio in some recipients of the vaccine, and in individuals with compromised immune systems who come into close contact with recently vaccinated children.[54-57] As a result, in 2000, the CDC "updated" its U.S. polio vaccine recommendations, reverting back to policies first implemented during the 1950s: children should only be given the killed-virus shot. The oral polio vaccine should only be used in "special circumstances."[58-60] (Several countries still use the live-virus, oral vaccine.)

Are polio vaccines safe?

When national immunization campaigns were initiated in the 1950s, the number of reported cases of polio following mass inoculations with the killed-virus vaccine was significantly greater than before mass inoculations, and may have more than doubled in the U.S. as a whole. For example, Vermont reported 15 cases of polio during the one-year report period ending August 30, 1954 (before mass inoculations), compared to 55 cases of polio during the one-year period ending August 30, 1955 (after mass inoculations)—a 266% increase. Rhode Island reported 22 cases during the before inoculations period as compared to 122 cases during the after inoculations period—a 454% increase. In New Hampshire the figures increased from 38 to 129; in Connecticut they rose from 144 to 276; and in Massachusetts they swelled from 273 to 2027—a whopping 642% increase (Figure 9).[61,62]

Figure 9:

Cases of Polio *Increased* in the U.S. After Mass Inoculations

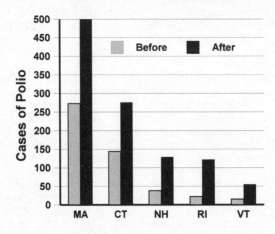

When national immunization campaigns were initiated in the 1950s, the number of reported cases of polio following mass inoculations with the killed-virus vaccine was significantly greater than before mass inoculations, and may have more than doubled in the U.S. as a whole. Source: U.S. government statistics.

Doctors and scientists on the staff of the National Institutes of Health during the 1950s were well aware that the Salk vaccine was causing polio. Some frankly stated that it was "worthless as a preventive and dangerous to take."[63] They refused to vaccinate their own children.[64] Health departments banned the inoculations.[65]

The Idaho State Health Director angrily declared: "I hold the Salk vaccine and its manufacturers responsible" for a polio outbreak that killed several Idahoans and hospitalized dozens more.[66] Even Salk himself was quoted as saying: "When you inoculate children with a polio vaccine you don't sleep well for two or three weeks."[67] But the National Foundation for Infantile Paralysis, and drug companies with large investments in the vaccine coerced the U.S. Public Health Service into falsely proclaiming the vaccine was safe and effective.[68]

In 1976, Dr. Jonas Salk, creator of the killed-virus vaccine used in the 1950s, testified that the live-virus vaccine (used almost exclusively in the U.S. from the early 1960s to 2000) was the "principal if not sole cause" of all reported polio cases in the U.S. since 1961.[69] (The virus remains in the throat for one to two weeks and in the feces for up to two months. Thus, vaccine recipients are at risk and can potentially spread the disease as long as fecal excretion of the virus continues.)[70] In 1992, the federal Centers for Disease Control and Prevention (CDC) published an admission that the live-virus vaccine had become the dominant cause of polio in the United States.[71] In fact, according to CDC figures, every case of polio in the U.S. since 1979 (not counting "imported" and "indeterminate" cases) was caused by the oral polio vaccine.[72,73] Authorities claim the vaccine was responsible for about eight cases of polio every year.[74] However, an independent study that analyzed the government's own vaccine database during a recent period of less than five years uncovered 13,641 reports of adverse events following use of the oral polio vaccine. These reports included 6,364 hospital/emergency room visits and 540 deaths (Figure 10).[75,76] Public outrage at these tragedies became the impetus for removing the oral polio vaccine from immunization schedules.[77,78]

Figure 10:

Polio Vaccine: Adverse Reactions

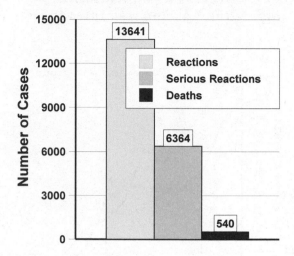

In the mid-1990s, during a period of less than five years, there were 13,641 *documented* adverse reactions to the oral polio vaccine: 6,364 of these were serious enough to require hospital emergency room visits; 540 people died. Source: Vaccine Adverse Event Reporting System (VAERS); OPV Vaccine Report—Document #14.

The following story is typical of the potential damage that is possible with oral polio vaccines: "Four months ago my son was taken to a local clinic for his polio vaccine. I wasn't aware that he was going to have one and would have prevented it if I had known. Unfortunately, he changed from that day—high-pitched screaming, smelly stools, non-stop crying, difficulty in breathing, high temperature, and lethargy. He also lost weight. Weeks of sleepless nights for all of us followed. His development ceased. He had been able to stand and move around, but he went back to remaining in basically whatever position we left him in. My wife was six months pregnant at the time, and about a week after our son's polio vaccine, she began to have headaches, loss of balance, muscular weakness, and frequent tiredness. I panicked because everything seemed to be pointing to polio infection. Then, a week after her continuous headaches began, she had to go to the hospital because there was something wrong with the pregnancy; she lost our daughter. I tried to get a polio test, and to find the cause of this tragic series of events, but the medical profession was extremely unhelpful. They laughed at me. I will never know why our son suddenly stopped growing or why his development regressed. I will never know why we lost our daughter. The only thing I am sure about is that the precursor to these events was the polio vaccine."[79]

How safe is the current inactivated polio vaccine?
A fact sheet on polio published by the U.S. Department of Health and Human Services warns parents that the inactivated polio vaccine (IPV) can cause "serious problems *or even death*."[80] Product information published by Aventis Pasteur, the IPV manufacturer, notes that "deaths have been reported in temporal association with the administration of IPV."[81] The IPV manufacturer further acknowledges that "deaths have occurred in temporal association after vaccination of infants with IPV."[82] However, apparently "no causal relationship has been established."[83] The IPV manufacturer also warns that Guillain-

Figure 11:

The Polio Death Rate was Decreasing on its Own *Before* the Vaccine was Introduced

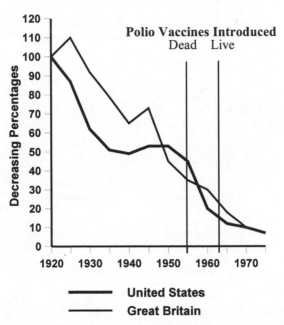

Polio Vaccines Introduced
Dead   Live

——— United States
——— Great Britain

From 1923 to 1953, before the Salk killed-virus vaccine was introduced, the polio death rate in the USA and England had already declined on its own by 47 percent and 55 percent, respectively. Source: *International Mortality Statistics* (1981) by Michael Alderson.

Barré Syndrome (a debilitating ailment characterized by muscular incapacitation and nervous system damage—symptoms that are virtually indistinguishable from polio) "has been temporally related to administration of another inactivated poliovirus vaccine."[84] Yet, despite these "danger alerts," medical authorities continue to assure parents that the currently available inactivated polio vaccine is both safe and effective.

How effective are polio vaccines?
Polio is virtually nonexistent in the United States today. However, according to Dr. Robert Mendelsohn, medical researcher and pediatrician, there is no credible scientific evidence that the vaccine caused polio to disappear.[85] From 1923 to 1953, *before* the Salk killed-virus vaccine was introduced, the polio death rate in the United States and England had already declined on its own by 47 percent and 55 percent, respectively (Figure 11).[86] Statistics show a similar decline in other European countries as well.[87] And when the vaccine did become available, many European countries questioned its effectiveness and refused to systematically inoculate their citizens. Yet, polio epidemics also ended in these countries.[88]
The standards for defining polio were changed when the polio vaccine was introduced. The new definition of a polio epidemic required more cases to be reported. Paralytic polio

Table 3:

Polio or Aseptic Meningitis?

Sample Months	Reported Cases of Polio	Reported Cases of Aseptic Meningitis
July 1955 (*Before* the new polio definition was introduced.)	273	50
July 1961 (*After* the new polio definition was introduced.)	65	161
September 1966 (*After* the new polio definition was introduced)	5	256

Cases of polio were more often reported as aseptic meningitis *after* the vaccine was introduced, skewing efficacy rates. Source: Los Angeles County Health Index: Morbidity and Mortality, Reportable Diseases.

was redefined as well, making it more difficult to confirm—and therefore tally—cases. Prior to the introduction of the vaccine the patient only had to exhibit paralytic symptoms for 24 hours. Laboratory confirmation and tests to determine residual paralysis were not required. The new definition required the patient to exhibit paralytic symptoms for at least 60 days, and residual paralysis had to be confirmed twice during the course of the disease. Also, after the vaccine was introduced cases of aseptic meningitis (an infectious disease often difficult to distinguish from polio) and coxsackie virus infections were more often reported as separate diseases from polio. But such cases were counted as polio before the vaccine was introduced. The vaccine's reported effectiveness was therefore skewed (Table 3 and Figure 12).[89,90]

The fact that dubious tactics were used to fabricate efficacy rates was corroborated by Dr. Bernard Greenberg, chairman of the Committee on Evaluation and Standards of the American Public Health Association during the 1950s. His expert testimony was used as evidence during congressional hearings in 1962. He credited the "decline" of polio cases not to the vaccine, but rather to a change in the way doctors were required to report cases: "Prior to 1954 any physician who reported paralytic poliomyelitis was doing his patient a service by way of subsidizing the cost of hospitalization.... Two examinations at least 24 hours apart was all that was required.... In 1955 the criteria were changed...residual paralysis was determined 10 to 20 days after onset of illness and again 50 to 70 days after onset.... This change in definition meant that in 1955 we started reporting a new disease.... Furthermore, diagnostic procedures have continued to be refined. Coxsackie virus infections and aseptic meningitis have been distinguished from poliomyelitis.... Thus, simply by changes in diagnostic criteria, the number of paralytic cases was predetermined to decrease."[91]

Polio vaccines and cancer:

In 1959, Bernice Eddy, a brilliant government scientist working in Biologics at the National Institutes of Health, discovered that polio vaccines being administered throughout the world contained an infectious agent capable of causing cancer. When Eddy attempted to report her findings and halt production of these contaminated polio vaccines, her government superiors barred her from publicly revealing the problem. Instead, her lab and equipment were taken away and she was demoted.[92,93]

Figure 12:

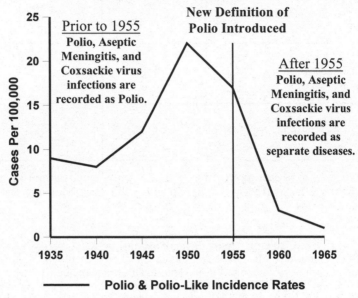

Polio Cases were Predetermined to Decrease when the Medical Definition of Polio was Changed

Prior to 1955
Polio, Aseptic Meningitis, and Coxsackie virus infections are recorded as Polio.

New Definition of Polio Introduced

After 1955
Polio, Aseptic Meningitis, and Coxsackie virus infections are recorded as separate diseases.

Cases Per 100,000

1935 1940 1945 1950 1955 1960 1965

—— **Polio & Polio-Like Incidence Rates**

Source: Congressional Hearings, May 1962; National morbidity reports taken from U.S. Public Health surveillance reports.

In 1960, Drs. Ben Sweet and M.R. Hilleman, pharmaceutical researchers for the Merck Institute for Therapeutic Research, were credited with discovering this infectious agent—SV-40, a monkey virus that infected nearly all rhesus monkeys, whose kidneys were used to produce polio vaccines. Hilleman and Sweet found SV-40 in all three types of Albert Sabin's live oral polio vaccine, and noted the possibility that it might cause cancer, "especially when administered to human babies."[94,95] According to Sweet, "It was a frightening discovery because, back then, it was not possible to detect the virus with the testing procedures we had.... We had no idea of what this virus would do." Sweet elaborated: "First, we knew that SV-40 had oncogenic (cancer-causing) properties in hamsters, which was bad news. Secondly, we found out that it hybridized with certain DNA viruses...such that [they] would then have SV-40 genes attached [to them].... When we started growing the vaccines, we just couldn't get rid of the SV-40-contaminated virus. We tried to neutralize it, but couldn't.... Now, with the theoretical links to HIV and cancer, it just blows my mind."[96]

Further research into SV-40 uncovered even more disturbing information. This cancer-causing virus was not only ingested via Sabin's contaminated oral sugar-cube vaccine, but was directly injected into people's bloodstreams as well. Apparently, SV-40 survived the formaldehyde Salk used to kill microbes that defiled his injectable vaccine.[97,98] Experts estimate that between 1954 and 1963, 30 million to 100 million Americans and perhaps another 100 million or more people throughout the world were exposed to SV-40 through ill-conceived polio eradication campaigns (Figure 13).[99,100]

Figure 13:

Polio Vaccines and Simian Virus #40

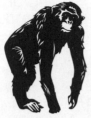 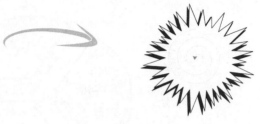

1. Monkey kidneys are used
to develop polio vaccines.

2. SV-40, a cancer-causing
virus, thrived in monkey kidneys.

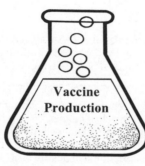

Vaccine
Production

3. Polio vaccines were
contaminated.

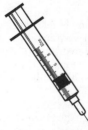

4. Millions of people in the USA
and throughout the world
were infected.

5. Cancer rates have increased.
SV-40 is found in brain tumors, bone
cancers, lung cancers, and leukemia.

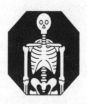

Figure 14:

SV-40-Tainted Polio Vaccines:
Zones of Contamination

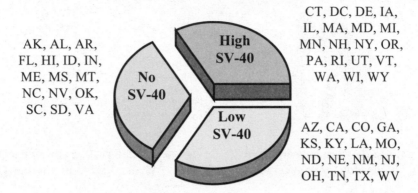

AK, AL, AR,
FL, HI, ID, IN,
ME, MS, MT,
NC, NV, OK,
SC, SD, VA

No SV-40

High SV-40

Low SV-40

CT, DC, DE, IA,
IL, MA, MD, MI,
MN, NH, NY, OR,
PA, RI, UT, VT,
WA, WI, WY

AZ, CA, CO, GA,
KS, KY, LA, MO,
ND, NE, NM, NJ,
OH, TN, TX, WV

100 million Americans were inoculated with SV-40-contaminated polio vaccines. This chart shows areas of the country in 1955 where 10 million people received polio vaccines with either no, low, or high amounts of SV-40 in them. Source: National Inst. of Health.

Numerous studies published in eminent journals throughout the world appear to confirm that SV-40 is a catalyst for many types of cancer.[101-120] It has been found in brain tumors and leukemia.[121] Michele Carbone, a molecular pathologist at Chicago's Loyola University Medical Center, was able to detect SV-40 in 38 percent of patients with bone cancer and in 58 percent of those with mesothelioma, a deadly type of lung cancer.[122-124] Carbone's research indicates that SV-40 blocks an important protein that normally protects cells from becoming malignant.[125]

In 1998, a national cancer database was analyzed: 17 percent more bone cancers, 20 percent more brain cancers, and 178 percent more mesotheliomas were found in people who were exposed to SV-40-tainted polio vaccines.[126] The National Institutes of Health created a map showing the geographic distribution of contaminated stock.[127] Using this map, researchers found osteosarcoma bone tumor rates to be 10 times higher than normal in some regions where this tainted vaccine was used (Figure 14).[128,129]

Perhaps the most alarming aspect of this ongoing simian virus debacle can be found in other studies suggesting that SV-40, introduced to humans through the polio vaccine, can be passed from human to human and from mother to child. A study of nearly 59,000 women found that children of mothers who received the Salk vaccine between 1959 and 1965 had brain tumors at a rate 13 times greater than mothers who did not receive those polio shots.[130-132]

Another study published in the U.S. medical journal *Cancer Research* found SV-40 present in 23 percent of blood samples and 45 percent of semen taken from healthy subjects.[133,134] Apparently, the virus is being spread sexually and from mother to child in the womb. According to biology and genetics professor Mauro Tognon, one of the study's authors, this would explain why brain, bone, and lung cancers are on the rise—a 30 percent increase in U.S. brain tumors alone during a recent 25-year period[135]—and why SV-40 was detected in brain tumors of children born after 1965 who probably did not receive polio vaccines containing the virus.[136]

Despite official denials of any correlation between SV-40-contaminated polio vaccines and increased cancer rates,[137] by April 2001, 62 papers from 30 laboratories around the world had reported SV-40 in human tissues and tumors.[138] The virus was also discovered in pituitary and thyroid tumors, and in patients with kidney disease.[139] Even the National Cancer Institute issued a statement that SV-40 "may be associated with human cancer."[140]

Studies yet to be conducted may provide additional clues about the link between contaminated polio vaccines, SV-40, and new diseases. But scientists have their hands full. The latest research has uncovered correlations between polio vaccines, *another* monkey virus, and AIDS.

Polio vaccines and AIDS:

SV-40, the cancer-causing monkey virus found in polio vaccines and administered to millions of unsuspecting people throughout the world, was just one of numerous simian viruses known to have contaminated polio vaccines.[141-143] "As monkey kidney culture is host to innumerable simian viruses, the number found varying in relation to the amount of work expended to find them, the problem presented to the manufacturer is considerable, if not insuperable," one early vaccine researcher wrote to a congressional panel studying the safety of growing live polio-virus vaccine in monkey kidneys.[144] "As our technical methods improve we may find fewer and fewer lots of vaccine which can be called free from simian virus."[145]

According to Harvard Medical School professor Ronald Desrosier, the practice of growing polio vaccines in monkey kidneys is "a ticking time bomb."[146] Evidently, some viruses can live inside monkeys without causing harm. But if these viruses were to somehow cross species and enter the human population, new diseases could occur. Desrosier continued: "The danger in using monkey tissue to produce human vaccines is that some viruses produced by monkeys may be transferred to humans in the vaccine, with very bad health consequences."[147] Desrosier also warns that testing can only be done for known viruses, and that our knowledge is limited to about "2 percent of existing monkey viruses."[148] Craig Engesser, a spokesman for Lederle Laboratories, a large vaccine manufacturing company, acknowledged that "you can't test for something if you don't know it's there."[149]

Virus detection techniques were crude and unreliable during the 1950s, 60s, and 70s when polio vaccines were initially produced and dispensed. It wasn't until the mid 1980s that new and more sophisticated testing procedures were developed.[150] That was when researchers discovered that about 50 percent of all African green monkeys—the primate of choice for making polio vaccines—were infected with simian immunodeficiency virus (SIV), a virus closely related to human immunodeficiency virus (HIV), the infectious agent thought to precede AIDS.[151-154] This caused some researchers to wonder whether HIVs may simply be SIVs "residing in and adapting to a human host."[155] It caused others to suspect that SIV may have mutated into HIV once it was introduced into the human population by way of contaminated polio vaccines.[156-160]

Vaccine authorities were so concerned about the possibility that SIV was a precursor to HIV, and that polio vaccines were the means of transmission from monkey to human, that the World Health Organization (WHO) convened two meetings of experts in 1985 to explore the data and consider their options.[161,162] After all, SIV was very similar to HIV and occurred naturally in the monkey species predominantly used by vaccine manufacturers.[163] Nevertheless, WHO concluded that the vaccines were safe and insisted that vaccination campaigns should continue unabated.[164]

Shortly thereafter, Japanese researchers conducted their own investigation and found that African green monkeys used to produce polio vaccines had antibodies against SIV.[165] The implication was clear: monkeys used to produce polio vaccines were natural carriers of a virus that looked and acted like HIV, the infectious agent linked to AIDS. In 1989, they recommended that monkeys infected with SIV not be used to make polio vaccines.[166]

In 1990, wild chimpanzees in Africa were found to be infected with a strain of SIV that was nearly identical to HIV.[167] Some researchers called it "the missing link" to the origins of human immunodeficiency virus.[168] And since chimpanzees were used to test viruses for potential use in vaccines, and were kept in captivity by research laboratories, they could have been a source of vaccine contamination.[169,170] Scientific concerns were also heightened when researchers found some West Africans who were infected with an SIV-like virus that was a fundamental twin to HIV. They called it HIV-2, and like the initial HIV subtype, it was implicated in the development of AIDS.[171] According to Robert Gallo, an expert on the AIDS virus, some versions of the SIV monkey virus are virtually indistinguishable from some human variants of HIV: "The monkey virus is the human virus. There are monkey viruses as close to isolates of HIV-2 as HIV-2 isolates are to each other."[172]

In May 1991, virus-detection techniques were improved once again, and researchers found SIV DNA in the kidneys of infected monkeys.[173] Minced monkey kidneys were (and still are) used to produce the live polio vaccine.[174] SIV was also found in the cancer cells of an AIDS victim, and in other people as well.[175-177] To many researchers, this trail of evidence had become too persuasive to deny. Apparently, millions of people were infected with monkey viruses capable of causing AIDS,[178] and this cross-species transfer very likely occurred by way of SIV-contaminated polio vaccines.[179-183]

Didn't AIDS originate in Africa?

Most historians agree that AIDS originated in Africa.[184] But Salk tested his vaccine in the United States, and Sabin's trials were conducted in Eastern Europe and the former Soviet Union.[185] If tainted polio vaccines were responsible for introducing SIV and HIV into humans, why did the initial cases of AIDS show up on this remote continent?

In March 1951, several years before Drs. Jonas Salk and Albert Sabin would scuffle over whose vaccine was the true prophylactic, Dr. Hilary Koprowski announced at a medical conference that he had become the first doctor in history to test a polio vaccine on humans. His "volunteers" included several institutionalized children with mental handicaps. They drank the vaccine in chocolate milk.[186]

From 1957 to 1960, after years of tinkering with monkey kidneys and polio germs, Koprowski tested his own experimental polio vaccine on 325,000 equatorial Africans, including 75,000 citizens of Leopoldville, Belgian Congo (now Kinshasa, Zaire).[187,188] Called by drums, rural natives traveled to local villages where they had a liquid vaccine squirted into their mouths.[189] Ninety-eight percent of the vaccine recipients were infants and toddlers.[190] The youngest children received 15 times the adult dosage.[191] Though Koprowski claimed he had the backing of the World Health Organization, WHO denied sanctioning the large-scale trials.[192]

In 1959, Dr. Albert Sabin reported in the *British Medical Journal* that Koprowski's polio vaccine used in the African trials contained an "unidentified" cell-killing virus.[193] It was never identified. However, in 1986 the earliest known blood sample containing antibodies against HIV was traced back to 1959. The serum came from a patient visiting a clinic in Leopoldville.[194] Until recently, there was no evidence that HIV infected humans before 1959.[195,196] Gerald Myers, a genetic sequencing expert with Los Alamos National Laboratories in New Mexico, tracked the evolution of HIV and confirmed that today's major subtypes of the AIDS virus in humans appear to have arisen as recently as 1960.[197] (Although this time period is widely accepted by medical researchers,[198] more recent conflicting reports suggest that the first HIV infection may have occurred years earlier.)[199-200]

Koprowski's vaccine was not approved for human use, so it was discontinued in 1960 following the African trials.[201] Thus, it was only administered to inhabitants of the Belgian Congo, Rwanda and Burundi[202]—the precise area where high levels of HIV infection were identified by researchers 30 years later.[203] Furthermore, the AIDS virus is known to infect mucous cells, prevalent in the mouth.[204] The African vaccines were squirted into people's mouths. Could squirting an HIV-contaminated polio vaccine into people's mouths cause AIDS? According to Tom Folks, chief retrovirologist at the CDC, "Any time a person has a lesion in his mouth, then there could be transmission" of the virus.[205] Dr. Robert Bohannon of Baylor College of Medicine maintains that the process of squirting the polio vaccine into people's mouths would tend to aerosolize some of the liquid. Tiny drops could then go directly into the lungs, and from there to the blood cells susceptible to infection.[206] This would have been an efficient mode of HIV transmission.[207]

Disease experts believe that the average time between HIV infection and the development of AIDS is 8-10 years.[208] If the African polio vaccine was indeed contaminated with SIV/HIV, initial outbreaks of AIDS would have occurred from the mid-1960s to early 1970s. This period accurately coincides with the emergence of AIDS in equatorial Africa.[209]

Test the polio vaccines:
Authorities are reluctant to acknowledge the possibility that medical scientists, preoccupied with growing polio vaccines in virus-laden monkey kidneys, may have been responsible for bringing about the AIDS pandemic. For example, Dr. David Heymann, who heads the World Health Organization's Global Program on AIDS, flatly stated that "the origin of the AIDS virus is of no importance to science today."[210] William Haseltine, a Harvard pathology professor and AIDS researcher also believes that any discussion about the origin of AIDS is distracting and nonproductive. "It's not relevant," and "I'm not interested in discussing it."[211] Jonas Salk wouldn't discuss the subject either. He was busy working on an AIDS vaccine.[212] Albert Sabin believes "you can't hang Koprowski with that."[213] And Koprowski dismissed the idea with a laugh, then later claimed "this is a highly theoretical situation."[214] However, samples of the polio vaccines used in Africa are kept in freezers at the Wistar Institute where Koprowski did much of his research. They could be tested.

Tom Folks of the CDC thinks it's a good idea to test the seed stocks of polio because "any time we can learn more about the natural history [of AIDS], it helps us understand the pathogenesis and…the transmission."[215] Robert Gallo also thinks it's important to determine whether a monkey virus sparked AIDS. Questions like this "are of more than academic interest because answering them may help avoid future zoonotic catastrophes—that is, transmission of disease from lower animals to humans."[216] Responding to these concerns, some AIDS researchers formally requested samples of the original polio vaccine seed stocks. But the government would neither release nor test them because there are "only a small number of vials" of the material, and tests "might use it all up."[217,218]

AIDS within the gay community:
If AIDS originated in Africa via contaminated polio vaccines, how did this disease spread to male homosexuals in America? In 1974, clinics in New York and California began experimental treatments for gay men afflicted with herpes. Therapy consisted of multiple doses of the live polio vaccine.[219] As noted earlier, this vaccine was produced in the kidneys of the African Green monkey, a known reservoir for simian immunodeficiency virus (SIV), a likely precursor to HIV.[220] Beginning in the early 1980s, simultaneous outbreaks of Kaposi sarcoma and serious opportunistic infections (later associated with AIDS) were reported among homosexual men, especially in New York City, San Francisco, and Los Angeles.[221] This time span coincides with the average incubation period between HIV infection and the development of AIDS.[222]

In 1982, the CDC concluded that such outbreaks "strongly suggests the occurrence of a single epidemic of underlying immunosuppression...."[223] The next year, HIV was identified as the causative agent.[224] In 1992, *Lancet* published the first scientific explanation showing how repeated doses of SIV-contaminated polio vaccines may have seeded HIV among American homosexual men.[225]

AIDS with no identified risk factor (NIR):
Another unusual event occurred in the 1980s. Hundreds of people diagnosed with AIDS had no identified risk factor (NIR).[226] They did not engage in risky behaviors related to AIDS infection. The CDC also listed numerous children as NIR.[227] Some parents believe that HIV-contaminated polio vaccines infected their loved ones.[228]

On February 12, 1994, Bruce Williams filed a civil suit against the American Cyanamid Company, claiming its polio vaccine caused his daughter's illness. The suit alleges that "the live oral poliovirus vaccine was produced, tested, and approved by the United States Food and Drug Administration pursuant to measures inconsistent with accepted standards of medical practice." The lawsuit also asserts that "the product was FDA approved despite the known presence of contaminants, including retroviruses such as HIV."[229]

Walter Kyle, the Williams' lawyer, identified the specific lots of vaccine the child received, but the CDC and federal health officials refused to test them.[230] Kyle believes "The CDC could disprove my entire hypothesis by testing the vaccines they have in their possession. The fact that they haven't done so is evidence there's something wrong with the vaccine."[231]

Some researchers believe the true number of NIR cases could be in the thousands.[232,233] When health officials examine people with AIDS, they try to identify a risk factor. If a patient admits he once had unprotected sex, that becomes his factor, even though there's no proof that is how he was infected.[234]

The evidence implicating polio vaccines grown in monkey kidneys with our current epidemics of cancer and AIDS continues to grow. But what if polio vaccines were produced in cow serum? Would that make a difference?

Polio vaccines and Mad Cow disease:

Mad cow disease, or bovine spongiform encephalopathy (BSE) is a progressive nerve disorder of cattle. Infected cows lose weight, drool, arch their backs, wave their heads, teeter back and forth, threaten other cows, act crazy, and eventually die. The first case of the disease was noticed in 1984. Since then, BSE has killed more than 200,000 cows.[235]

Mad cow disease is related to scrapie, a similar disease afflicting sheep.[236] In fact, authorities believe it spread to cows from sheep when they were fed scrapie-infected bone meal.[237] Creutzfeldt-Jakob disease (CJD) and vCJD (a newly discovered variant) are the human equivalents of mad cow disease.[238] They cause a comparable wasting of the brain leading to muscle incoordination, sensory loss, and mental confusion.[239] It is always fatal. There is no known cure.[240]

There is very strong evidence that mad cow disease and the newly discovered variant of Creutzfeldt-Jakob disease are caused by the same infectious agent. For example, a recent study showed that monkeys injected with BSE developed symptoms remarkably similar to vCJD.[241] Another study showed that BSE and vCJD had similar molecular characteristics—unlike "classical" CJD.[242] Two later studies appear to confirm that BSE from cattle causes vCreutzfeldt-Jakob disease in humans.[243,244] Researchers think that mad cow disease can be passed from cows to humans if they ingest BSE-infected beef,[245-247] or if they receive vaccines contaminated with BSE.[248-251]

BSE-associated infectious agents are capable of contaminating polio vaccines because polio vaccines are not only grown in monkey kidneys, but in calf serum as well.[252] In fact, many parts of the cow are used in vaccine production. Glycerol is derived from cow fat; gelatin and amino acids come from cow bones; and the growth medium for viruses and other microorganisms may require cow skeletal muscle, enzymes, and blood.[253]

Authorities knew that vaccines could be infected with BSE-associated transmissible agents as early as 1988. Yet, in England, vaccine manufacturers waited months before switching to cows less likely to be infected and refused to remove current stock off the shelves and out of doctor's offices until it was all sold, or expired five years later toward the end of 1993.[254] One outraged legislator declared that "the Department of Health was potentially criminally negligent in not requiring the immediate withdrawal or cessation of use of vaccines from potentially contaminated sources."[255] Despite nationwide apprehension, manufacturers continued to disregard European guidelines.[256] Finally, in October 2000, the Department of Health became so concerned about the likelihood of children being infected with BSE-contaminated vaccines and falling prey to vCreutzfeldt-Jakob disease—dozens of people, including children, had already contracted it[257] —that they issued a recall of hundreds of thousands of polio vaccines made using fetal bovine serum extracted from British cows.[258-260]

In the United States, authorities waited until December 1993 before issuing a "recommendation" that U.S. manufacturers not use bovine material from countries reporting BSE.[261] The FDA issued a second warning to manufacturers in 1996 informing them to "take whatever steps are necessary to reduce potential risk of transmission of BSE agent."[262,263] But in March 2000, the FDA discovered that its "recommendations" were ignored. Vaccines were still being made in bovine materials obtained from countries reporting BSE.[264]

Americans have something else to be concerned about as well. Although U.S. cows do not exhibit "mad cow symptoms," every year in the United States tens of thousands of cattle are severely incapacitated; they cannot stand and walk on their own. Farm Sanctuary, a national non-profit organization dedicated to halting irresponsible agricultural practices, believes that these "downed" animals may harbor a new variant of BSE, and is critical of the Food and Drug Administration's BSE surveillance efforts.[265] Despite early warning signs, downed cows are not examined for a new variant of BSE, and have not been ruled out of vaccine production.[266]

Dr. Richard Marsh of the Department of Animal Health and Biomedical Sciences at the University of Wisconsin, Madison, conducted research providing evidence that downed cattle in the U.S. may harbor a new variant of mad cow disease. He inoculated cows with TME, a variant of BSE. They became "downed" instead of "mad."[267] Other scientists inoculated cows with scrapie from U.S. sheep. They, too, became "downed" instead of "mad."[268]

Responding to the FDA's apparent indifference, Farm Sanctuary issued the following statement: "We are distressed that economic priorities have tended to take precedence over the health of consumers. We are also concerned that, like in Britain, there is a powerful economic incentive to ignore evidence that BSE, or a variant of BSE, exists in the U.S. We urge the FDA to examine the scientific evidence regarding BSE carefully and to act in the interest of American consumers."[269] Regardless, the FDA did not modify its BSE surveillance policies, and vaccines made in bovine material obtained from countries reporting BSE were not going to be removed from the market for at least another year, until 2002—after all existing stock had been purchased and consumed.[270,271]

More animal viruses:
Thousands of viruses and other potentially infectious microorganisms thrive in monkeys and cows, the preferred animals for making polio vaccines.[272] SV-40, SIV, and BSE-associated transmissible agents are just three of the disease-causing agents researchers have isolated. For example, scientists have known since 1955 that monkeys host the "B" virus, foamy agent virus, haemadsorption viruses, the LCM virus, arboviruses, and more.[273] Bovine immunodeficiency virus (BIV), similar in genetic structure to HIV, was recently found in some cows.[274]

In 1956, respiratory syncytial virus (RSV) was discovered in chimpanzees.[275] According to Dr. Viera Scheibner, who studied more than 30,000 pages of medical papers on vaccines, RSV viruses "formed prominent contaminants in polio vaccines, and were soon detected in children."[276] They caused serious cold-like symptoms in small infants and babies who received the polio vaccine.[277] In 1961, the *Journal of the American Medical Association* published two studies confirming a causal relationship between RSV and "relatively severe lower respiratory tract illness."[278] The virus was found in 57 percent of infants with bronchiolitis or pneumonia, and in 12 percent of babies with a milder febrile respiratory disease.[279] Infected babies remained ill for three to five months.[280] RSV was also found to be contagious, and soon spread to adults where it has been linked to the common cold.[281]

Today, RSV infects virtually all infants by the age of two years, and is the most common cause of bronchiolitis and pneumonia among infants and children under one year of age.[282] It also causes severe respiratory disease in the elderly.[283] RSV remains highly contagious and results in thousands of hospitalizations every year; many people die from it.[284] Ironically, scientists are developing a vaccine to combat RSV[285]—the infectious agent that very likely entered the human population by way of a vaccine.[286]

Dr. John Martin, a professor of pathology at the University of Southern California, has been warning authorities since 1978 that other dangerous monkey viruses could be contaminating polio vaccines. In particular, Martin sought to investigate simian cytomegalovirus (SCMV), a "stealth virus" capable of causing neurological disorders in the human brain. The virus was found in monkeys used for making polio vaccines. The government rebuffed his efforts to study the risks.[287] However, in 1995, Martin published his findings implicating the African green monkey as the probable source of SCMV isolated from a patient with chronic fatigue syndrome.[288]

In 1996, Dr. Howard B. Urnovitz, a microbiologist, founder and chief science officer of Calypte Biomedical in Berkeley, California spoke at a national AIDS conference where he revealed that up to 26 monkey viruses may have been in the original Salk vaccines. These included the simian equivalents of human echo virus, coxsackie, herpes (HHV-6, HHV-7, and HHV-8), adenoviruses, Epstein-Barr, and cytomegalovirus.[289-291] Urnovitz believes that contaminated Salk vaccines given to U.S. children between 1955 and 1961 may have set this generation up for immune system damage and neurological disorders. He sees correlations between early polio vaccine campaigns and the sudden emergence of human T-cell leukemia, epidemic Kaposi's sarcoma, Burkitt's lymphoma, herpes, Epstein-Barr and chronic fatigue syndrome.[292]

Urnovitz also discussed "jumping genes"—normal genes that may recombine with viral fragments to form new hybrid viruses called chimeras. He believes that this is exactly what happened when monkey viruses and human genes were brought together during early polio vaccine campaigns. And because the chimera "has the envelope of a normal human gene," typical cures won't work. How do you develop a vaccine or other antidote against the body's own DNA?[293,294]

Mutated polio strains:

Several years ago, the World Health Organization launched the Global Polio Eradication Initiative, with 2000 as its target date for eliminating the disease. However, by 2000 it became clear that not only was polio still around, but new strains of the disease—derived from the vaccine itself—were emerging.[295] Researchers first noticed something unusual in 1983. Outbreaks of polio in Egypt were being caused by a "vaccine-derived" polio virus.[296] In 1993, Dr. Radu Crainic of the Pasteur Institute, discovered that strains of the polio virus have the ability to spontaneously recombine with themselves and create new strains. Crainic showed that if you vaccinate a child with polio strains 1, 2, and 3, you can produce a new strain, strain 4, out of the child's stool. Crainic concluded that the polio vaccine creates favorable conditions contributing to the evolution of viral "recombinations."[297]

In October 2000, virologist Hiromu Yoshida of Japan's National Institute of Infectious Diseases in Tokyo reported finding a new infectious polio virus in Japanese rivers and sewage. Genetic sequencing confirmed that the virus had mutated from the polio vaccine and regained much of its original virulence.[298] According to Yoshida, it poses a "persistent environmental threat."[299]

In December 2000, researchers reported on a polio outbreak in Haiti and the Dominican Republic that resulted in numerous cases of flaccid paralysis.[300] Laboratory examinations confirmed health authorities' worst suspicions: the disease was caused by "an unusual viral derivative" of the polio vaccine. The virus demonstrates genetic similarity to the parent vaccine strain, "but it has assumed the neuro-virulence and transmissibility" of the wild polio virus.[301] Health officials are obviously concerned, "because a wild poliovirus has not circulated in the Western Hemisphere since 1991," and if the newly mutated polio virus spreads, it could cause new epidemics of the disease (Figure 15).[302]

People all over the world continue to be stricken with vaccine-derived polio viruses (VDPVs) because under certain circumstances polio viruses within the vaccine "regain both neuro-virulence and the capacity to circulate and cause outbreaks."[303] For example, from 2001 to 2005, there were several vaccine-derived polio outbreaks in the Phillippines, Madagascar, China and Indonesia. On the island of Madura in Indonesia, at least 46 people were stricken with paralytic polio caused by viruses that originated from the polio vaccine. In 2006, additional cases of vaccine-derived polio were recorded in Cambodia.[304]

Worldwide polio eradication:

By 2007, worldwide polio eradication remained an elusive goal. Cases were recorded in at least 16 countries, most notably in Nigeria, India, Pakistan, Somalia and Afghanistan.[305] It should also be noted that some children in foreign regions of the world are receiving "more than 12 doses of [polio] vaccine before their second birthday," yet they are still susceptible to the disease. For example, in India "a median of 10 reported vaccine doses

Figure 15:

Polio Eradication with Vaccines:
A Vicious Cycle?

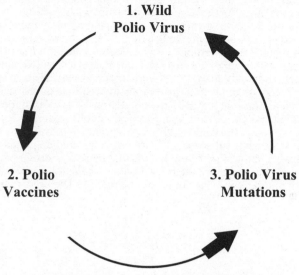

1. Wild
Polio Virus

2. Polio
Vaccines

3. Polio Virus
Mutations

Copyright © NZM

1) The wild polio virus brought about 2) the development of polio vaccines, which spawned 3) mutations of the polio virus, resulting in 1) new "vaccine-derived" wild polio viruses. Source: *Virolgy* 1993; 196:199-208; *Lancet* (October 28, 2000); *Reuters Medical News* (December 4, 2000).

---

have been received by persons who have contracted poliomyelitis; this has raised questions about the efficacy of the vaccine."[306] Poor nutrition has been proposed as one possible reason many children are not developing immunity to polio after receiving multiple doses of the vaccine. At any rate, a precise timeline for polio eradication "remains unpredictable."[307]

How is today's polio vaccine produced?
Despite the polio vaccine's long history of causing polio, and the manufacturer's inability to protect the public from dangerous microorganisms that perpetually contaminate an ever expanding repertoire of "new and improved" products, the currently available inactivated, or "killed-virus" polio vaccine continues to be manufactured in much the same way as earlier versions. Animal matter and questionable drugs are still used. In the United States, today's polio vaccine is a sterile suspension of three types of poliovirus. The viruses are grown in cultures of "a continuous line of monkey kidney cells...supplemented with newborn calf serum..." The vaccine also contains two antibiotics (neomycin and streptomycin), in addition to formaldehyde as a preservative.[308]

In Canada, the inactivated polio vaccine is made in "human diploid cells" (see *Appendix III*) instead of monkey kidneys.[309] Some researchers believe this is a safer alternative. According to Barbara Loe Fisher, president of the National Vaccine Information Center in Virginia, "With mounting evidence that cross-species transfer of viruses can occur, the United States should no longer be using animal tissues to produce vaccines."[310] However, Dr. Arthur Levine of the National Institutes of Health believes that making polio vaccines using human cells isn't risk-free either, "because they must be tested for human infections."[311]

Are positive changes possible?

Government officials worry that even debating the issue will frighten parents. Levine probably speaks for many people within the vaccine industry when he declares: "We do a grave disservice to the public if we were now to question the safety of the current polio vaccines...."[312] But Barbara Loe Fisher would like to see changes in the way vaccine safety is governed. She believes that agencies like the FDA have an inherent conflict of interest because of their mandate to promote universal vaccination on the one hand and regulate vaccine safety on the other. "Who's minding the store when the FDA has allowed drug companies to produce vaccines grown on contaminated monkey kidneys?" Fisher asks. "What happened to protecting the public health?"[313] Dr. John Martin agrees. He believes that we need to immediately determine the prevalence of stealth viruses of simian origin in the United States, and whether they may be contributing to chronic immune system and brain disorders in children and adults.[314] Dr. Urnovitz is even more resolute in his convictions. He thinks that an extensive study of human exposure to simian microbes is long overdue. "Half of the people in this country are baby boomers who were born between 1941 and 1961 and are at high risk for having been exposed to polio vaccines contaminated with monkey viruses. Are we just a time bomb waiting to happen, waiting to develop lupus, Alzheimer's and Parkinson's disease?"[315] Urnovitz also challenged medical science to prove him wrong. "What we are saying here is that there is a strong probability that no human retroviruses existed before the polio vaccines.... You have to realize that if you mess around with nature, you're going to pay the price.... The objective here is a better, healthier world."[316]

Influenza (Flu)

What is influenza?

Influenza, or the flu, is a contagious respiratory infection caused by a virus. It usually strikes during winter. Symptoms include fever, chills, runny nose, sore throat, cough, headache, muscle aches, fatigue, and decreased appetite. Conditions usually improve in two to three days. Treatment mainly consists of allowing the disease to run its course. Antibiotics will not subdue the flu virus. Bed rest and drinking lots of fluids are often recommended.[1]

How dangerous is the flu?

The flu can lead to complications, such as pneumonia, in high risk groups. People who are at greater risk of complications from the flu mainly include the elderly and other people with preexisting medical problems, such as heart, lung, or kidney dysfunctions. People with diabetes, anemia, or compromised immune systems are also at greater risk of complications from influenza. In some instances, severe complications in high risk groups can lead to death.[2,3]

How prevalent is the flu?

Every year, thousands of people contract the flu. It is a common ailment because there are three main types of flu virus, and each type can mutate, or change, from year to year. This makes it difficult to develop immunity to the disease.[4-6]

Does a flu vaccine exist?

In the United States, five inactivated, injectable flu vaccines produced by separate manufacturers are currently licensed for use: Fluzone, Fluvirin, Fluarix, Afluria, and FluLaval.[7] In addition, the FDA approved FluMist, a live-virus nasal spray vaccine that is squirted up the nose.[8] Although each vaccine is indicated for different age groups, they contain the same attenuated flu viruses.

How is the flu vaccine made?

Each year, in January or February, authorities travel overseas to assess the composition of currently circulating flu viruses. They assume that these same viruses will arrive in the United States several months later, in October or November (at the beginning of the flu season), causing many people to catch the flu. Thus, as soon as the authorities determine which flu viruses "are anticipated to circulate in the United States" later that year, they instruct flu vaccine manufacturers to include those particular strains in their products. For example, during the 2016-2017 flu season, flu vaccines were required to contain A/California/7/2009 (H1N1); A/Hong Kong/4801/2014 (H3N2); and B/Brisbane/60/2008.[9] During the 2007-2008 flu season, flu shots contained completely different strains: A/Solomon Islands/3/2006 (H1N1); A/Wisconsin/67/2005 (H3N2); and B/Malaysia/2506/2004.[10] (Because the flu is caused by several influenza viruses, they have been classified into types A, B, and C, and further classified into subtypes with names of cities, states or countries.)

Flu strains used in vaccine production are also chosen for their "favorable growth properties in eggs."[11] This is crucial because to develop a flu vaccine, chick embryos must first be inoculated with influenza viruses. This mixture is cultivated for several weeks. Each flu strain is then inactivated with formaldehyde[12] and preserved with thimerosal,[13] a mercury derivative. Mercury is a neurological toxin. Although it has been removed from several pediatric vaccines, *many flu vaccines still contain 25mcg of mercury per dose*[14-16] (see *Appendix I* on page 307 for more information). Flu vaccines may also contain polyethylene glycol, polysorbate 80, hydrocortisone, neomycin and polymyxin (antibiotics), sodium deoxycholate, MSG, and "porcine" (pig) gelatin.[17] The three viral strains are blended into a single vaccine, licensed by the FDA, then distributed by manufacturers. Scientific control-group testing for safety and efficacy is not required.[18]

Can the flu vaccine cause the flu?

Common reactions to the flu vaccine include flu-like symptoms which can last several days: fever, chills, sore throat, runny nose, nasal congestion, headache, muscle aches, abdominal pain, and fatigue.[19] Doctors often claim that it's not possible to contract the flu from the flu vaccine.[20] However, this contradicts the real-life experiences of many people. Besides, vaccines are designed to stimulate the immune system by mimicking disease. This has been openly acknowledged by some authorities. For example, according to Chris Anna Mink, MD, a medical officer with the FDA, "because [FluMist] is live, it can grow in the nose and some people get flu symptoms..."[21] Other authorities concede that in people with weak immune systems, "the vaccine virus can reproduce and create live virus which can cause flu symptoms and even the flu."[22] The following comments are typical of people who were vaccinated against flu yet still caught the disease:

"I've had the flu vaccine twice, and on both occasions I had the worst case of flu in my entire life. Never, ever again. Waste of time and money."[23]

"I was required to take a flu shot when I was in the army and I woke up the next morning sick as a dog. As a result, I didn't take a flu shot until recently when my doctor recommended it after I got pneumonia. I still caught the flu."[24]

How safe is the flu vaccine?

Serious reactions to the flu vaccine include life-threatening allergies to vaccine components, and Guillain-Barré syndrome (GBS), a severe paralytic disease.[25] GBS can occur several weeks following a flu vaccine and is fatal in about one of every 20 victims.[26] The most well-publicized link between the flu vaccine and GBS occurred in 1976 when the CDC concocted a frightening tale of deadly swine flu epidemics sweeping the nation if mass vaccinations were not instituted. President Ford authorized millions of tax dollars toward this goal. American adults were systematically vaccinated, and several weeks later hundreds were stricken with this crippling disease; many died. More than 4,000 lawsuits were filed and nearly $3 billion was paid in compensation. A moratorium was placed on all influenza vaccines, but this prudent response was ended just two months later. Hundreds of new cases of GBS were tallied following mass flu vaccination campaigns.[27-29] (For additional information about the swine flu vaccine, turn to page 303.)

In addition to GBS, numerous studies have investigated and/or documented other serious adverse reactions to the flu vaccine, including encephalopathy, brainstem encephalitis, polyneuritis, optic neuritis, myelitis, vasculitis, myelopathy, facial paralysis, brachial plexus neuropathy, reactive arthritis, bullous pemphigoid, polymyalgia rheumatica, uveitis, Gianotti-Crosti syndrome, erythromelalgia, pericarditis, polyangitis, thrombocytopenia, cellulitis, myositis, and "asthmatic exacerbations" in persons with a history of asthma.[30-66]

Influenza vaccine safety in children: In February 2005, *Lancet* published a review of all pertinent influenza vaccine studies in children. The authors of this review concluded that *the safety of influenza vaccines given to babies and children is unknown.* Most of the studies conducted on children were not designed to assess serious adverse reactions. Furthermore, the researchers "found clear evidence of systematic suppression of safety data." For example, authors of the original studies were denied access to safety data from their own clinical trials. In one influenza vaccine study, vaccinated children had nearly twice as many "medical adverse events" as unvaccinated children. However, these "events" were not adequately identified. When the vaccine manufacturer was contacted for the missing data, researchers were denied access to it because it is considered proprietary information. The CDC refuses to warn parents that safety data is lacking.[67,68]

The American drug maker MedImmune (which is being bought by AstraZeneca, a British drug manufacturer), recently submitted a confidential briefing document to the FDA containing safety data from studies that it conducted on its own vaccine. MedImmune was seeking permission to vaccinate children under 5 years of age with its live-virus nasal spray FluMist® vaccine (the one that is squirted up the nose). When this vaccine was originally licensed in 2003, the FDA only permitted it to be given to children 5 years of age and older because a large study conducted in 31 clinics showed that it caused "a statistically significant increase in asthma or reactive airways disease" in children under 5 years of age.[69] In addition to this confidential briefing document, the FDA also had access to data from studies that were not conducted by the manufacturer. According to the FDA, FluMist can cause "medically significant wheezing" and pneumonia. In fact, *3 percent* of all children 6 months to 1 year of age who received the vaccine ended up in the hospital with respiratory problems! (With the inactivated flu shot, 1 of every 100 vaccinated children in this age group had to be rushed to the hospital.)[70,71] In addition, of all children between 6 months and 1 year of age who developed "protocol-defined wheezing" after their FluMist vaccinations, *9 percent* required hospitalization. This figure was *7 percent* for children between 1 and 2 years of age. The median duration of hospitalization in children 6 months to 2 years of age was nearly 5 days with most requiring bronchodilators and steroids. Many of these children had multiple wheezing episodes.[72] Nevertheless, in September 2007, the FDA licensed this vaccine for children as young as two years of age.[73]

The flu vaccine is potentially dangerous in older children as well. For example, Maurice Lamkin, a healthy 5-year-old boy, recently received a flu shot. He ran a fever that evening and two days later had his first seizure. He was rushed to the hospital where he remained for the next 40 days fighting for his life with brain swelling. Dr. Kenneth Mack, a Mayo Clinic pediatric neurologist who consulted on the case, said an adverse reaction to the flu vaccine can cause encephalitis: "The body's immune system can get overactive and attack the brain." Maurice's doctor thinks the flu shot was "the most likely culprit." Maurice is now home but has to wear diapers and can no longer speak. His distraught mother said, "He was a healthy little boy. He was running around. He was so proud because he had just learned to read and write. He was living his life, singing, dancing, wrestling with his brother. He was perfectly fine before the flu shot."[74]

Adverse Reaction Reports

This section contains unsolicited adverse reaction reports associated with the flu vaccine, typical of the daily emails received by the *Thinktwice Global Vaccine Institute*.[75]

▸ "My 6-month-old daughter was just starting solids, so the doctor recommended giving her egg yolk before she received her flu shot to make sure that she's not allergic. I did that, she had no reaction, so she got the flu shot. However, the two times that I have given her egg yolk after the vaccination, she has had severe vomiting and diarrhea. Can vaccinations make a kid allergic to food?"

▸ "My 2½ year-old daughter received a flu shot on a Thursday in November. The following Monday, I brought her back to the doctor because her eyes were suddenly crossed. The doctor sent her to ER where she was diagnosed with GBS (Guillain-Barré syndrome) from the flu shot. She was transferred to one of the best hospitals in the area. The doctors did not think it was GBS but thought that it was caused by the flu shot. Basically, fluid built up around her brain causing her eyes to turn in, one more than the other. She now has to wear glasses and hopefully it will reverse the damage, but they can't tell us for sure. We are still in the process of seeing different specialists. She has already had a spinal tap, MRI, CT scan, and tons of blood work. My husband and I are worried about future problems. I am just so angry that this happened to her."

▸ "In October, my 9-year-old daughter got her flu vaccine (nose spray type). Two days later, she got a terrible cold, bad headache and sick stomach. That night, she woke up with a seizure. Six days later, she had another seizure. She is now on seizure medication."

▸ "I received a flu shot for the first time. The school's nurse made arrangements for someone to come in and inject us. I signed the little pink release form, didn't even bother to read it first, trusting it would do no harm. Super mistake! After getting it, I became ill, not really bad but sort of a nagging, lingering feeling of not being well for about 4 weeks. One day at school I just didn't feel well, but passed it off as probably coming down with something. I woke up next morning with my left arm paralyzed. I went to the ER (emergency room), they checked me for a stroke and some other things, and told me to come back if I got worse. By that evening my feet didn't work too well and they tingled, as did my fingers. Next day, I tried to walk and fell down. I somehow made it back to

ER; again they had no idea what was wrong with me. Things were getting worse, losing movement and ability to walk. My son carried me to bed that night. Went to my regular doctor; as soon as he saw me he knew what it was, and asked if I had received a flu shot recently. He said I had Guillain-Barré syndrome and explained to my horror what was going to happen to me—probably get much worse and I might need a tracheotomy tube. He sent me straight to the hospital. In 8 days I was totally paralyzed and on life support. I don't remember anything of the first year of hospitalization. After 16 months, I was moved to a skilled nursing facility, still totally paralyzed and with a trach tube and feeding tube. Somehow they got me to breathe on my own, but I still had a trach and feeding tube, and I went home after 22 months in a power wheelchair. I regained some motion through physical therapy, but nothing great. After a few months, my trach was removed and surgically closed. My stay at home was short lived; I relapsed in about 5 or 6 months. Totally paralyzed again, 8 months in hospital with physical therapy. Third relapse was of 6 month's duration, but another stomach tube had to be inserted. Fourth relapse was for 4 months at the hospital. My last relapse was for one month. The chronic inflammatory demyelinating polyneuropathy (CIDP) I had developed was and has been stopped by taking an immunosuppressant, and infusions of IVIG. I'm still in a wheelchair. My left arm has suffered the most, being the first to be paralyzed and has permanent nerve damage. I am able to walk using things to hold onto. On my last visit to my neurologist I was able to walk about 6 feet holding his hand, not much but it took years to be able to do that. I scratch my head when I hear them promoting flu shots. If I had only read that little pink paper and asked what GBS was. Most people that I talk to—in the hospital and out (nurses, doctors and regular people) —after hearing my story, feel that it is better to chance the flu and not get the shot."

▸ "I had a flu shot in November, and by December I became weak and continued to get weaker until I collapsed in my bedroom and was taken to the hospital. I was surrounded with intravenous lines, a feeding tube, bladder catheter, and tracheotomy for the ventilator. I was helpless, totally paralyzed with Guillain-Barré syndrome. I had a blood infection, pneumonia, a fever of 107.9 degrees, and blood pressure of 44 over zero. My wife was told to make arrangements for a post-mortem. I was in ICU for three weeks and then transferred to a rehabilitation center. Three months later I was released to come home because I could ambulate approximately 100 feet with a walker. I continued rehabilitation as an outpatient for the next three months until I could walk with hand crutches. Today, I need a cane. I was not warned of any possible hazard when they gave me the flu shot."

▸ "I have a friend, now in a wheelchair, who took the flu shot, got Guillain-Barré, and now cannot walk."

▸ "Ten weeks ago, on a Friday, my mother-in-law received a flu shot. On Saturday, she started feeling ill. By Monday, she was admitted to the hospital, diagnosed with pneumonia, and was in septic shock. She was put on a ventilator, given antibiotics, and read her last rites tonight; we don't expect her to make it through the evening. When I mentioned the flu shot to her doctor, it was dismissed. Has this happened to other people?"

▸ "When I was seven months pregnant with my 4th child, my doctor told me that he was requiring all of his patients to get the flu shot. I am 29 and very healthy. I rarely get sick. Within a week after getting the shot I got flu-like symptoms with a high fever, chills, body ache, headache—the whole deal. The symptoms lasted almost an entire month. There were many days that I couldn't even get out of bed. My husband took as long as he could off work and then it was pretty much up to my 9-year-old to run the house. I was that sick. It took several months to regain my energy and get back to normal. Strangely enough, nobody in my entire family got the flu but me. Coincidence? I think not."

▸ "For five days after my wife had a flu injection, she had flu-like symptoms. She then felt better, and for two days was back to normal. The next day, she was in bed complaining about me trying to wake her. She was agitated and vociferous—most unusual. Within one hour, her condition worsened. I called the doctor who immediately hospitalized her. She died there three weeks later. Although the doctors had not found out the cause, a post mortem stated that she had died as a result of an adverse reaction to the flu injection."

▸ "After my husband had a flu shot, he became weak and chilled all the time, with a dry cough. By the end of the second month he was vomiting. His doctor did several tests until one showed acute kidney failure. He was diagnosed with Goodpasture's syndrome. The treatment is immune suppressive therapy. Isn't that ironic. The flu shot that is supposed to build up immunity caused his to work too hard and didn't know when to shut down."

▶ "Three years ago, I was given one of only four flu shots I ever had. A [dangerous] strain was included in the vaccine. I believe it was this strain that infected me and almost killed me. The next year, unaware and never warned by doctors, I took the flu shot again. This time it contained a deadly strain that put me in ICU fighting for my life."

▶ "I'm a 67-year-old man who has had a flu shot annually for many years. Only once was I chilled, but yesterday I had a flu shot and from 11:30 p.m. until 4:30 this morning I had the most severe headache of my life. Today, I feel weak."

▶ "I received a flu shot in November, and in January I started to get a body rash. I am achy in my arm and neck. I believe the shot caused my misery."

▶ "I had the flu shot in October. Within days, I was seriously ill. I spent 24 days in the hospital and 11 days in rehab learning to walk again. I have muscle and nerve damage in my legs and feet. I go to physical therapy three times a week, and will go indefinitely. It will take at least a year for the nerves to heal, if they ever will. The neurologist agrees that my illness was caused by the flu shot."

▶ "My wife was diagnosed with subcutaneous T-cell lymphoma after receiving a flu shot. Two weeks after receiving the flu shot, lumps started appearing on her legs."

▶ "My father got myelitis from a flu shot."

▶ "I have a friend who received a flu vaccine on Monday and by Tuesday she was very sick. The doctors said it was not a reaction to the flu shot. Their diagnosis was "reactivated mono"—despite the fact that she never had mono. I have heard many people swear that they'll never get another flu vaccine. Now I understand."

▶ "The sister of an acquaintance died suddenly two nights ago. She was in her 40s and otherwise healthy. She got a flu shot that day, came home complaining about not feeling well, and died that night. She died at home, rather suddenly, without warning."

▶ "A friend who received the flu shot five weeks ago is having extreme pain in the arms, legs, and neck, with paralyzation. The doctors won't help."

▶ "My grandmother was given a flu injection and immediately contracted the worst case of pneumonia she had ever had. She was so sick that she nearly died. Now she has severe joint pain that has lasted ever since her shot."

▶ "My husband's aunt, who was very healthy before she got a flu shot, became ill after the shot for about four weeks, never improving until she died."

▶ "One of our patients died three days after her flu shot. The day after her shot, her daughter came into our clinic to apologize that her mother couldn't keep her appointment, because she had a bad reaction to her flu shot. That was on a Friday. The following Monday we were reading her obituary. Her death was not reported as a reaction to the flu shot."

Flu Scare Tactics

Every year, just prior to the impending "flu season," the CDC and their acquiescent media pawns terrorize the American public with false claims regarding annual flu deaths. The CDC boldly asserts that 36,000 people die *every year* from the flu—an odd claim since the CDC also maintains that the rare, once-in-a-lifetime 1968-1969 "Hong Kong flu pandemic" killed 33,000 Americans.[76,77] Such scare tactics are calculated to increase flu vaccine sales. However, according to the CDC's own official records documented in *National Vital Statistics Reports,* only a few hundred people die from influenza (flu) on an average year. Furthermore, many of these deaths occur in people with preexisting medical conditions, weakened immune systems, and the elderly.[78] For example, in 2003, 1,792 people died from the flu.[79] (Eighty-five percent of these deaths occurred in people 55 years or older.)[80] In 2002, 727 people died from the flu.[81] The year before that, in 2001, just 257 people died from the flu.[82] To put these numbers in perspective, 3,454 Americans died from malnutrition in 2001—more than 13 times the number of flu deaths![83] That same year, there were 4,269 deaths attributed to asthma,[84] a condition some studies have linked to vaccines[85-90] (Figure 16).[91-94]

Figure 16:

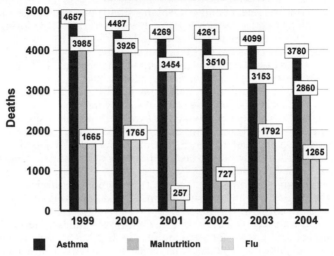

Annual Deaths from Asthma, Malnutrition and Flu

Copyright © NZM

Each year, in the United States more Americans die from asthma and malnutrition than from influenza. Source: CDC, National Vital Statistics Reports.

To rationalize this discrepancy between the true number of deaths caused by influenza every year (as documented in the CDC's own *National Vital Statistics Reports*) and the outrageously exaggerated bogus number of flu deaths promoted by the CDC, officials claim that the flu often leads to pneumonia and that many deaths from pneumonia are really deaths caused by flu. Apparently the CDC has a secret formula[95] for estimating how many pneumonia deaths (officially listed in the CDC's own *National Vital Statistics Reports* as deaths from pneumonia, not flu) are really deaths caused by flu. Adding to the confusion, influenza is caused by a virus; pneumonia is caused by bacteria. The CDC's own literature takes great pains to emphasize their differences. More importantly, the CDC has a pneumonia vaccine.[96] So why doesn't the CDC promote their pneumonia vaccine? In 2003, 63,371 people died from pneumonia; in 2002, 64,954 people died from this ailment.[97] If everyone took a pneumonia vaccine, especially the elderly and others most susceptible to the disease, wouldn't they be protected? Why is the CDC promoting a flu vaccine to protect against pneumonia, especially when one disease is caused by a virus and the other by bacteria? Also, how many people who died from pneumonia received a flu vaccine? How many received a pneumonia vaccine?

In 2004, flu vaccine manufacturers were unable to produce enough flu shots for everyone who wanted a flu vaccine. (Several batches were contaminated and had to be destroyed.)[98,99] Thus, only half of the population that is normally vaccinated against influenza (approximately 45 million people versus 90 million during an average year) received the vaccine.[100] If influenza is truly a deadly disease, as officials claim, the 2004-2005 flu season should have been catastrophic. If, as the CDC claims, 36,000 people die every year from the flu when *90 million people* are vaccinated against the disease, how many more should have died when only *45 million people* were "protected"? According to one influenza vaccine expert, Lone Simonsen, of the National Institute of Allergy and Infectious Diseases, who was questioned *before* that season's final flu numbers were calculated, "the shortage will have little impact [on mortality]."[101] In fact, in 2004, just 1,265 people died from the flu—527 fewer deaths than during the previous year, a 30 percent reduction![102]

Clandestine flu vaccine marketing strategies:
In April 2004, the CDC and the American Medical Association (AMA) co-sponsored a National Influenza Vaccine Summit in Atlanta, Georgia. The list of by-invitation-only participants included leaders of major health departments, medical organizations, media outlets, and drug companies.[103] Glen Nowak, Associate Director for Communications with the National Immunization Program gave a shrewd presentation that included a "Recipe that Fosters Higher Interest and Demand for Influenza Vaccine."[104] He provided several bullet-point strategies designed to achieve this goal. For example:

- Medical experts and public health authorities [should] publicly (e.g., via media) state concern and alarm (and predict dire outcomes)—and urge influenza vaccination.
- The flu season should be framed in terms that motivate behavior (e.g., as "very severe," "more severe than last year," "deadly.")
- Continued reports (e.g., from health officials and media) that influenza is causing severe illness and/or affecting lots of people—help to foster the perception that many people are susceptible to a bad case of influenza.
- Vaccination demand...is related to heightened concern, anxiety, and worry. For example: A perception or sense that many people are falling ill...or are vulnerable to contracting and experiencing bad illness.
- Success (i.e., higher demand for flu vaccine) stems from media stories and information that create motivating (i.e., high) levels of concern and anxiety about influenza.

Clearly, the goal is to frighten the public into obtaining flu vaccine at any cost. Nowak's presentation included several graphs that measured the precise number of daily news stories, week-by-week, that utilized the industry's most effective key phrases. These desirable phrases included: Influenza Outbreaks are Widespread; This Could be a Bad/Serious Flu Season; Flu Season Arrived Early; Doctors Recommend/ Urge Flu Vaccine; Pediatric Influenza Deaths; Elderly Influenza Deaths; Flu Kills 36,000 People Per Year.[105]

Eighteen months later, in October 2005, the *British Medical Journal (BMJ),* usually well-known for its unwavering support of the medical industry, broke rank and expressed deep cynicism at the CDC's marketing campaign of fear in which medical experts are taught to "predict dire outcomes" if people are not vaccinated against influenza. In this special report, data culled from the CDC's own official records was presented, confirming that the CDC intentionally hyper-inflates influenza mortality numbers to scare the public and sell more flu vaccine. *BMJ* acknowledged that CDC flu death figures are concocted for public relations rather than determined by science.[106]

How effective is the flu vaccine?
Precise flu vaccine efficacy rates are difficult to ascertain and unreliable because flu strains change all the time. According to the CDC, "Overall vaccine effectiveness varies from year to year, depending upon the degree of similarity between the influenza virus strains included in the vaccine and the strain or strains that circulate during the influenza season."[107] To clarify why flu vaccine efficacy rates are so problematic, it is important to understand how authorities attempt to manage and control this unpredictable virus: Each year, in January or February, authorities travel to the Far East to determine which strains of the flu virus are currently active. They assume that these same strains will circulate and infect people in the United States around October or November (the beginning of the flu season). Flu vaccine manufacturers are instructed to include those particular strains in their products. Thus, officials must guess nearly one year in advance which mutated strains of the flu virus will circulate throughout society.[108] If they guess right, the vaccine may provide temporary immunity to some recipients. If they guess wrong, as often occurs, or the circulating flu strains mutate again between January and the end of the year, which is quite likely, the vaccine may be worthless.[109,110] For example, in 1994 "flu experts" predicted that Shangdong, Texas, and Panama strains would be prevalent that year, thus millions of people were vaccinated with a flu shot that contained these viruses. However, when winter arrived, the Johannesburg and Beijing strains of influenza circulated through society.[111,112] In 1995, health officials modified their predictions and created a flu vaccine

containing Texas, Johannesburg, and Beijing strains of influenza. Again, millions of people were vaccinated. However, that winter the Wuhan strain of influenza circulated about.[113] Regarding the 1997-1998 flu season, officials once more had to admit that "the flu shot did not make a dent in flu cases because the strains included in the vaccine did not match the strains that actually circulated that year."[114] The vaccine was not effective. More recently, the 2003-2004 flu shot contained strains that did not circulate through society that year.[115,116] According to Barbara Loe Fisher, president of the National Vaccine Information Center, "Public health officials knew [in the spring of 2003] that it was highly likely that the A/Panama strain [included in the 2003/2004 flu shot] was not going to protect against the [circulating] A/Fujian strain of flu. If there is solid new evidence that the vaccine is protective against Fujian, then it should be released. If there is no such evidence, then it is not right to lead people to believe that if they get vaccinated, they will be protected against it."[117,118]

Even when there is a good match between the viral strains comprising a flu vaccine and that year's circulating flu virus, immunity from the shot is short-lived because antibody levels begin to decline within months, and are often low one year after vaccination.[119] Permanent immunity to a particular strain of flu is only possible by contracting the disease naturally. When natural infection is suppressed by force-vaccinating the whole population, healthy children and adults—who rarely suffer complications from flu—will not be able to develop natural antibodies and permanent immunity to that flu strain.

Respiratory ailments that are not caused by influenza, intestinal disorders and ear infections caused by bacteria, and disease conditions caused by flu viruses not included in the vaccine or by microorganisms associated with different diseases, such as colds, will not be alleviated by getting an annual flu shot. Each flu vaccine is only designed to protect against the three viral strains which are included in that year's flu vaccine.

Efficacy in Children: The United States and Canada recently recommended influenza vaccines for healthy children as young as six months old. To assess the merits of this policy, researchers combed the planet for all significant influenza vaccine studies up to June 2004. In February 2005, *Lancet* published the results of their analysis.[120] Researchers found no evidence that influenza vaccines prevent flu in children younger than 2 years old. In addition, there was "no convincing evidence that [flu] vaccines can reduce mortality, hospital admissions, serious complications and community transmission of influenza."[121,122] There was also little evidence that flu vaccines could reduce secondary cases, lower respiratory tract disease or acute otitis media. According to the lead researcher, "immunization of very young children is not lent support by our findings."[123]

In 2006, researchers working for *The Cochrane Collaboration*—an objective, independent well-respected source of scientific evidence—analyzed all relevant influenza vaccine trials conducted on children worldwide, totaling 51 studies involving more than 260,000 children. They determined that in healthy children older than two years of age, the live flu vaccine was just 33 percent effective; the inactivated influenza vaccine was just 36 percent effective. In healthy children under two years of age, the efficacy of the inactivated flu vaccine "was similar to placebo" (Figure 17).[124] The lead author of the review, Dr. Tom Jefferson, expressed his concern regarding American influenza vaccine policies: "We just cannot understand how you can vaccinate millions of small children in the absence of convincing scientific evidence that the vaccines make any difference."[125]

In October 2008, *Archives of Pediatrics and Adolescent Medicine* published a study that analyzed influenza vaccine effectiveness in children aged 6 months to 5 years. The study was conducted over two consecutive flu seasons. Authors of the study "could not demonstrate vaccine effectiveness" at reducing influenza-related doctor or hospital visits.[126]

Efficacy in Healthy Adults: Researchers working for the independent *Cochrane Collaboration* reviewed the evidence of influenza vaccine efficacy in healthy adults. They analyzed 25 studies involving thousands of people and discovered that in healthy adults under 65 years of age, influenza vaccination "did not affect hospital stay, time off from work, or death from influenza and its complications." Authors of the study concluded that "universal immunization of healthy adults is not supported" by the data.[127]

Figure 17:

Effectiveness of the Influenza Vaccine in Healthy Children

a) Older Than 2 Years of Age

Live Influenza Vaccine   **Inactivated Influenza Vaccine**

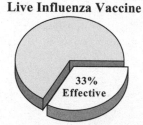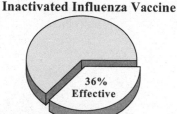

b) Under 2 Years of Age

Inactivated Influenza Vaccine

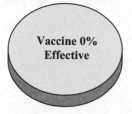

Researchers analyzed 51 studies involving more than 260,000 children. They determined that in healthy children older than two years of age, the live influenza vaccine was just 33 percent effective; the inactivated influenza vaccine was just 36 percent effective. In healthy children under two years of age, the efficacy of the inactivated influenza vaccine "was similar to placebo." Source: *The Cochrane Collaboration: Cochrane Database of Systematic Reviews* (John Wiley & Sons, Ltd.), 2006(1). Art. No. CD004879.

Efficacy in the Elderly: Influenza vaccination of elderly individuals is recommended worldwide. To assess the merits of this universal policy, researchers working for *The Cochrane Collaboration* reviewed the evidence of influenza vaccine efficacy in people aged 65 years or older. They conducted a thorough, systematic review of 64 studies carried out over 40 years of influenza vaccination. Their results showed that for elderly people living in the community, influenza vaccines "were not significantly effective against influenza or pneumonia." For elderly people living in group homes—*in years when the vaccine is a good match with the circulating influenza virus*—the influenza vaccine is merely 23 percent effective against "influenza-like illness," 46 percent effective against pneumonia, and "non-significant against influenza" (Figure 18).[128] Researchers found no correlation between the percentage of people vaccinated and the overall rate of influenza-like illness.[129]

Vaccine failures in the elderly are typical—even when there is a precise match between the influenza vaccine strain and the circulating flu virus. For example, in one influenza outbreak in a Minnesota nursing home, 95 percent of the residents, and 72 percent of the staff members with direct patient contact had been vaccinated 4 to 8 weeks prior to the outbreak. Authorities were especially baffled when they discovered that the viral strain isolated from the outbreak was "antigenically identical" to the one contained in the vaccine. In other words, the vaccine was a "perfect" match for that year's circulating flu virus and yet it was a complete failure.[130] The authors of the study concluded that "despite widespread vaccination...influenza outbreaks continue to occur."[131]

Figure 18:

Effectiveness of the Influenza Vaccine in the Elderly

a) Elderly Living in the Community

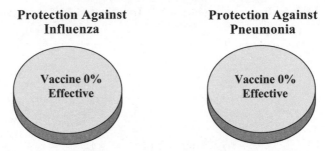

Protection Against Influenza	Protection Against Pneumonia
Vaccine 0% Effective	Vaccine 0% Effective

b) Elderly Living in a Group Home

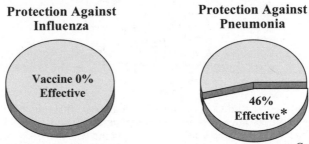

Protection Against Influenza	Protection Against Pneumonia
Vaccine 0% Effective	46% Effective*

Researchers conducted a thorough, systematic review of all significant data (64 studies) carried out over 40 years of influenza vaccination. Their results showed that for elderly people living in the community, influenza vaccines "were not significantly effective against influenza or pneumonia." For elderly people living in group homes, the influenza vaccine is "non-significant against influenza" and 46 percent effective against pneumonia. (*The 46% efficacy rate is based on years in which the vaccine is a good match with the circulating influenza virus. The vaccine has little or no efficacy in years when it is not well-matched with the circulating influenza virus.) Source: *The Cochrane Collaboration: Cochrane Database of Systematic Reviews* (John Wiley & Sons, Ltd.), 2006(3). Art. No. CD004876.

Efficacy in Healthcare Workers: Healthcare workers (nurses, hospital workers, etc.) are often required to receive annual flu vaccines because authorities are concerned that they might transmit influenza to those in their care, especially the elderly. To assess the merits of this policy, researchers working for *The Cochrane Collaboration* reviewed all pertinent studies and discovered that staff vaccinations "have no efficacy against influenza."[132] They concluded "there is no...evidence that vaccinating healthcare workers reduces the incidence of influenza or its complications in the elderly in institutions.... An incremental benefit of vaccinating healthcare workers for the benefit of the elderly cannot be proven."[133]

"[How can you] vaccinate millions of small children in the absence of convincing evidence that the vaccines make any difference?" —Dr. T. Jefferson, flu vaccine expert

Additional influenza vaccine efficacy studies:

In February 2005, the *Archives of Internal Medicine* published a comprehensive study that analyzed immunization data from 33 influenza seasons, from 1968 through 2001. In the United States, just 15 percent of elderly persons were vaccinated before 1980. By 2001, 65 percent were vaccinated, *yet mortality rates remained constant.* In other words, although immunization rates in people 65 years or older increased by 50 percent during a 20-year period, there has not been a corresponding decline in flu (or pneumonia) related deaths. "We could not correlate increasing vaccination coverage after 1980 with declining mortality rates in any age group," authors of the study noted. In fact, "observational studies substantially overestimate vaccination benefit."[134,135]

In 2006, the *Journal of American Physicians and Surgeons* published a study showing that influenza vaccination has "little or no effectiveness over the U.S. population for preventing influenza cases, deaths, or hospital admissions."[136] That same year, the *British Medical Journal* published a paper that analyzed all pertinent flu vaccine studies and concluded there is a large gap between evidence of the flu vaccine's efficacy and the influenza policies established by health agencies. According to the paper's author, Dr. Tom Jefferson, "Every year enormous effort goes into producing influenza vaccines for that specific year and delivering them to appropriate sections of the population. Is this effort justified?"[137] Apparently not. Flu vaccines had little or no effect on influenza campaign objectives, such as hospital stay, time off work, or death from influenza and its complications. Flu vaccines were found to be ineffective in children under 2 years of age, in healthy adults under 65 years of age, and in people aged 65 years and older. In addition, there is little evidence that flu vaccines are beneficial when administered to healthcare workers to protect their patients, when given to children to minimize transmission of the virus to family contacts, or when given to vulnerable people, such as those with asthma and cystic fibrosis.[138-141] Jefferson found little proof of the flu vaccine's merit: "There is a misfit between the evidence and policy, and taxpayers ought to ask why."[142]

Jefferson provided possible reasons for the large gap between influenza vaccine policies and the actual data: 1) There is a lot of confusion between influenza and influenza-like illness. Often, "any case of illness resembling influenza is seen as real influenza, especially during peak periods of activity. Some surveillance systems report cases of influenza-like illness as influenza without further explanation. This confusion leads to gross overestimation of the impact of influenza, unrealistic expectations of the performance of vaccines, and spurious certainty of our ability to predict viral circulation and impact." 2) Authorities want to be seen as resolute decision makers, which often results in "optimism bias"—an unwarranted belief in the efficacy of interventions. They may recommend using currently available flu vaccines when they are not necessarily appropriate for the current flu season. They may also fail to wait for pertinent flu data prior to making important decisions. 3) Conflicts of interest also affect flu vaccine policies, irrespective of the actual data.[143]

In December 2006, the *New England Journal of Medicine* published a study looking at the viability of vaccinating all school children to reduce the spread of influenza in households and communities. Researchers wanted to determine whether vaccinating one group of people—children—would provide "herd immunity" for, or protect, another group of people—their families and neighbors. Thus, they vaccinated children in some schools (the intervention schools) but not in others (the control-group schools), then tallied the rates of absenteeism, illness and hospitalizations. The results surprised the investigators: Although there were fewer "influenza-like symptoms" in households with children in the intervention schools than in households with children in the control-group schools, *intervention school households (both children and adults) had significantly higher rates of hospitalization.* There were no differences in missed days of school. In addition, children who received the influenza vaccine had a "statistically significant increase in influenza-like symptoms" after vaccination. They also took more drugs to control the undesirable side effects. Four of the children had serious adverse events after vaccination.[144]

In December 2009, *The Lancet* published a study showing that annual flu shots prevent immunity to future strains of the disease. Children who are vaccinated every year against seasonal flu may be *more* susceptible to dangerous pandemic strains than are children that contract seasonal flu.[145] In a study of mice vaccinated against seasonal flu strains, they developed severe disease and died when exposed to alternate strains. Unvaccinated mice became less ill and did not die when exposed to more lethal strains.[146]

How cost-effective is the flu vaccine?

Authorities often claim the flu vaccine saves money. However, in a double-blind controlled study conducted by the National Center for Infectious Diseases at the CDC, thousands of employees over a two year period were either vaccinated with a flu shot or received a placebo. Researchers then calculated how many employees got the flu and what their illnesses cost. Lost wages were included in their computations. When everything was tallied, the authors of the study concluded that vaccination is *not* a cost-effective choice. Furthermore, employers who encourage their employees to get the flu vaccine, or who pay for their employees' shots, should not expect to save money. In fact, an employer could expect to pay more than $6,500 for every 100 employees vaccinated.[147,148]

Is the flu vaccine mandatory?

The CDC and vaccine industry have become fanatical in their zeal to vaccinate more and more people against influenza. Initially, the CDC strongly encouraged the elderly—people over 65 years of age—to receive annual flu shots. Then authorities lowered the recommended age to 50. The CDC's Advisory Committee on Immunization Practices (ACIP) recommends that all nursing home residents and staff members receive annual flu vaccinations.[148] Healthcare workers are now expected to receive annual flu shots as well.[149] In practical terms, official "recommendations" generally result in medical coercion and compulsory vaccinations. For example, one healthcare worker had this to say: "The hospital where I have worked for the past 15 years is now forcing all employees to take an influenza vaccine. We have no choice but to take the shot or be disallowed to work. My rights and freedoms are being trampled on."[150] Another healthcare worker is upset with this policy as well: "Help! I work for the Veteran's Administration (VA) as part of a joint venture hospital run by the military and VA. I am a civilian, not military. Yet, we just received notification that we must get an annual influenza vaccine. I am not alone as far as employees not wanting to take the flu vaccine every year. They are giving us one week to comply."[151]

Even though healthcare workers and nursing home residents are being forced to receive annual flu vaccines, studies have shown that mass vaccinations of staff members and nursing home residents does not reduce the institutional risk of contracting the flu nor of developing complications from the disease.[152-155] Although many elderly residents do not like being forced-injected, this is exactly what authorities are requiring. Many long-term nursing home residents must now choose between receiving an annual flu vaccine or finding a new place to live and be cared for. Yet, in one recent survey nearly 4 million elderly people refused *free* influenza shots.[156]

The CDC and vaccine industry were not satisfied with their goal to market annual flu vaccines to the elderly, adults over 50 years of age, and healthcare workers. They added pregnant women to the list—even though flu vaccines contain mercury and the CDC admits that pregnant women and their fetuses are highly vulnerable to mercury.[157] Before the CDC altered its own recommendations, pregnancy was a contraindication to the flu vaccine.[158]

Encourage, recommend and mandate: The vaccine industry implements a three-step strategy toward compulsory inoculations. Before the ACIP "recommends" a vaccine, it often "encourages" or advocates its use. At this time, distribution channels are established, marketing strategies are initiated, and doctors begin vaccinating the targeted group of people. If everything runs smoothly, the vaccine is fully recommended. With the ACIP's stamp of approval, the pharmaceutical companies now begin lobbying states to mandate their lucrative product. For example, in 2002 the ACIP "encouraged that, when feasible, all children aged 6 to 23 months...receive influenza vaccinations each influenza season."[159,160] In 2004, the ACIP strengthened the encouragement to a full recommendation.[161]

In February 2006, the ACIP gratified influenza vaccine manufacturers once again when their recommendation was expanded to include children up to 59 months of age.[162,163]

Figure 19:

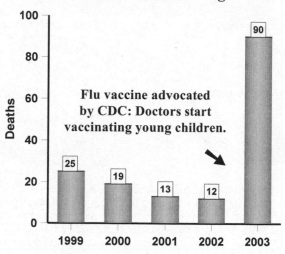

Influenza Deaths in Children
Under 5 Years of Age

In 1999, before flu vaccines were recommended and administered to small boys and girls, just 25 children in the United States under 5 years of age died from influenza. In 2000, 2001 and 2002, there were just 19, 13 and 12 influenza deaths, respectively, in this age group. However, in the latter half of 2002 the CDC began advocating that all young children receive influenza vaccines. Thus, doctors started vaccinating as many young children as possible against the flu. The following year, in 2003, influenza deaths in children under 5 years of age skyrocketed to 90 cases—a sevenfold increase over previous years. Source: CDC, National Vital Statistics Reports.

The CDC also added household contacts of children and caregivers of young children to the list of people expected to receive the flu vaccine.[164] In February 2008, the flu vaccine recommendation was expanded again to include children and teenagers up to age 18.[165] Today, an annual influenza vaccine is recommended for other groups of people as well.

In 1999, before flu vaccines were recommended and given to small boys and girls, just 25 children in the U.S. under 5 years of age died from influenza.[166] In 2000, 2001 and 2002, there were just 19, 13 and 12 influenza deaths, respectively, in this age group.[167] However, in the latter half of 2002 the CDC began advocating that all young children receive flu vaccines. Thus, doctors started vaccinating as many young children as possible against the flu.[168] The following year, in 2003, influenza deaths in children under 5 years of age skyrocketed to 90 cases—a sevenfold increase over previous years (Figure 19).[169]

In the Fall of 2005, Johns Hopkins' senior epidemiologist, Trish Perl, initiated a campaign to mandate influenza vaccination for all healthcare workers. Despite free and easy access to the vaccine, only 40 percent voluntarily get one; 30 percent are afraid of catching the flu from the vaccine itself.[170] In a nationally representative study of 1,651 U.S. healthcare workers (e.g., nurses aides and medical assistants), researchers at Harvard University and the University of Southern California discovered that 62 percent were *not* vaccinated against the flu.[171] A survey reported by the *Associated Press* found that doctors and nurses are among the *least* likely to be vaccinated. More than two-thirds (about 70 percent) of doctors and nurses do *not* get annual flu shots (Figure 20).[172]

Although current federal workers' rights prevent employers from making vaccinations a requirement, Perl wants to make influenza vaccination "as mandatory for workers as

Figure 20:

Annual Flu Shots: Do Doctors, Nurses & Healthcare Workers Get Them?

Doctors and Nurses

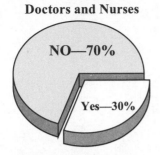

Healthcare Workers

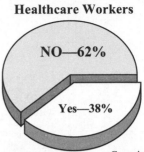

Although doctors want *you* to receive an annual flu shot, a survey shows that doctors and nurses are among the *least* likely to be vaccinated. In fact, about 70 percent of doctors and nurses do NOT get annual flu shots. In a nationally representative study of healthcare workers (e.g., nurses aides and medical assistants), 62 percent did not get a flu vaccine. Source: *Journal of General Internal Medicine* (February 6, 2006); *Associated Press.*

---

the law allows."[173] She believes a new marketing strategy is required, one that shifts the message "from self-interest to altruism in protecting patients."[174] However, the American College of Occupational and Environmental Medicine, an international medical society of more than 5,000 health professionals, opposes mandatory flu shots for healthcare workers. They believe that a compulsory influenza vaccine policy is not justified for several reasons, including studies showing the vaccine itself is variably effective. In addition, the College notes that "given the ubiquitous nature of influenza in the community, patients will continue to be exposed to influenza through family members and friends regardless of the vaccination status of their healthcare workers, with whom they have much less intimate contact."[175]

Although flu vaccines for children and other groups of people are now recommended, in most states they are not yet mandated. (New Jersey became the first state to require all children attending preschool or licensed daycare centers to get an annual flu shot —mandated as of December 31, 2008.)[176] However, in states where the flu vaccine is not required, some parents are reporting that school nurses are vaccinating their children without consent! For example, in Santa Fe, New Mexico, one young boy came home from César Chávez elementary with a runny nose and headache. He told his mother that "someone at the school had sprayed something up his nose." Apparently, state officials left it up to school districts to decide how parents were informed (or not) about a new flu vaccine pilot project.[177] If flu vaccines are eventually mandated where you live, exemptions may be possible. Be sure to read your state vaccine laws for details.

Vitamin D and Influenza:
Researchers have known for many years that influenza mainly occurs in the winter when there is less sun, and is less prevalent near the equator where there is lots of sun. Today, we also know that when people are exposed to ultraviolet radiation (from sunlight or artificial sources) they produce vitamin D. Vitamin D deficiency is common, especially among the elderly in the winter. In a landmark study published in *Epidemiology and Infection,* researchers linked these pieces of the puzzle together and showed that vitamin D deficiency weakens the immune system creating susceptibility to influenza. Vitamin D supplements (2000-4000 i.u. daily) —especially in the winter—may provide protective benefits against the flu.[178-180]

Tetanus

What is tetanus?

Tetanus is a non-contagious bacterial disease that causes severe muscular contractions. It is also called *lockjaw* because some victims are unable to open their mouths or swallow. Other symptoms include depression, headaches, and spasms that interfere with breathing.[1,2]

Tetanus is caused by toxins produced by a bacterium called *Clostridium tetani*. The dormant spores live in soil, dust, and manure. They can enter the body through cuts and puncture wounds, but will only multiply in an anaerobic (oxygen-free) environment. The incubation period, from the time of the injury until the first symptoms appear, ranges from a few days to three weeks. However, careful attention to wound hygiene will eliminate the possibility of tetanus in most cases. Deep puncture wounds and wounds with a lot of dead tissue should be thoroughly cleaned and not allowed to close until healing has occurred beneath the skin.[3]

Is tetanus a common and dangerous disease?

During the mid-1800s, there were 205 cases of tetanus per 100,000 wounds among U.S. military personnel. By the early 1900s, this rate had declined to 16 cases per 100,000 wounds—a 92 percent reduction. During the mid-1940s, the incidence of tetanus dropped even further to .44 cases per 100,000 wounds.[4] Some researchers attribute this decline to an increased attention to wound hygiene.[5,6]

Today, authorities claim that tetanus infects about 500,000 people each year worldwide, primarily in developing countries.[7] However, in the United States, from 1995 to 2005 (an 11-year period), there were just 386 total cases of tetanus—an average of 35 cases per year. Of this total, 43 people died—about four persons per year. The case-fatality rate was 11 percent (Figure 21).[8] In Australia, there are about 10 cases of tetanus per year with a case-fatality rate of 10 percent.[9] In Canada, there have been about five cases of tetanus annually in recent years, with no deaths recorded since 1991.[10]

During the 1970s and 1980s, approximately 70 percent of all cases of tetanus in the United States, and 80 percent of all cases in Australia, occurred in adults over the age of 50 years.[11-14] About 95 percent of all tetanus fatalities occurred in this age group. Only five percent of tetanus cases in the U.S. were in persons less than 20 years of age, and these were rarely fatal.[15]

During the 1990s, the percentage of cases among persons aged 25-59 years increased. For example, in 1999 there were 40 cases of tetanus in the United States; 22 of these (55%) were in this age group. Seven of the 22 cases in this age group (32%) occurred in intravenous drug users; two of these cases were fatal. Thirteen of the 40 cases (32.5%) were in persons older than 59; Just five cases (12.5%) were in persons younger than 25 years of age.[16]

Does a tetanus vaccine exist?

A tetanus toxoid vaccine became available in 1933. During the 1940s it was combined with diphtheria toxoid and pertussis vaccines. This became known as the DPT vaccine. Today, the tetanus toxoid vaccine is available from several different manufacturers. It can be given individually,[17] in conjunction with the diphtheria vaccine (DT and Td),[18] or in combination with both diphtheria and acellular pertussis vaccines (DTaP).[19] In addition, one manufacturer combines tetanus with diphtheria, pertussis and haemophilus influenzae type B—four vaccines in one shot.[20] Another manufacturer produces tetanus in combination with diphtheria, pertussis, hepatitis B and inactivated polio—five vaccines in one shot.[21]

A *tetanus immune globulin* (TIG) injection—an antitoxin—is also available. This shot may be administered to persons with low tetanus antibody levels (including unvaccinated individuals) shortly after a serious wound occurs or if tetanus symptoms appear. This injection introduces tetanus-fighting antibodies directly into the body. The antibody levels achieved with TIG are often adequate to defend against the disease until your body can produce its own antibodies against tetanus.[22,23]

How is the tetanus vaccine made?

The current tetanus vaccine developed for infants 6 weeks to 7 years of age is usually combined with diphtheria and pertussis as DTaP. *Clostridium tetani* cultures are grown in "a peptone-based medium containing a bovine extract." This combination vaccine also contains diphtheria toxoid, pertussis antigens, aluminum, "a trace amount of thimerosal" (which is a mercury derivative), gelatin, polysorbate 80, and "residual formaldehyde."[24,25]

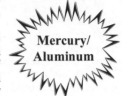

The current tetanus vaccine developed for children 7 years of age and older, and adults, is "a sterile suspension of aluminum potassium sulfate toxoid in an isotonic sodium chloride solution." *Clostridium tetani* culture "is grown in a peptone-based medium and detoxified with formaldehyde." Thimerosal (25mcg mercury per dose) is added to the final product.[26,27] When the tetanus vaccine is combined with diphtheria toxoid (Td), the tetanus culture is grown in a medium containing "an extract of bovine muscle tissue" detoxified with formaldehyde. The final product also contains aluminum and "a trace amount of thimerosal."[28,29] (For more information about mercury and aluminum in vaccines, see *Appendices I* and *II* on pages 307-308.)

Tetanus immune globulin (TIG) is prepared "from the plasma of donors immunized with tetanus toxoid." Tri-n-butyl phosphate (a solvent) and sodium cholate (a detergent) are added. The solution is then heated for up to six hours to kill potentially infectious agents. After "viral inactivation"—a crucial step because human plasma may contain viruses—the mixture is formulated as a protein solution in glycine, incubated for 3 to 4 weeks, then standardized for use.[30]

How safe is the tetanus vaccine?

Several studies have documented a link between the tetanus vaccine and adverse reactions. Local reactions include erythema (abnormal inflammation at the injection site), induration (abnormal hardening at the injection site), pain and tenderness, abscess or nodule formation, and subcutaneous atrophy. Systemic reactions include fever, headache, muscle aches, chills, and malaise.[31-38] In one study of the combined tetanus and diphtheria vaccine, local reactions occurred in 80 percent of the subjects; 26 percent experienced systemic reactions.[39]

Numerous studies and case reports have linked the tetanus vaccine to *severe* and even *fatal* reactions, including neurological and paralytic disorders such as Guillain-Barré syndrome (GBS), demyelinating diseases, arthritis, joint inflammation, anaphylactic shock, and other life-threatening reactions. For example, as early as 1966 the *Journal of the American Medical Association* documented peripheral neuropathy following a tetanus toxoid vaccine.[40] In 1967 and 1972, researchers confirmed correlations between this vaccine and post-vaccinal neuritis, including "paralysis of the recurrent nerve" and brachial plexus neuropathy.[41,42]

In 1977, the *Journal of Neurology* reported on a 36-year-old woman who developed neurological complications, including slurred speech, lethargy, and a loss of sensation, five days following a tetanus vaccine.[43] In 1978, the *Journal of Neurological Sciences* described a 42-year-old man who developed acute polyneuropathy diagnosed as Guillain-Barré syndrome after receiving a tetanus vaccine.[44] The following year, researchers published data confirming a link between the tetanus vaccine and various neuropathies.[45]

In 1981, the *New England Journal of Medicine* published a study showing that tetanus booster vaccinations cause T-lymphocyte blood count ratios to drop below normal. The greatest decrease occurred up to two weeks later. The authors of the study noted that these altered ratios are similar to those found in victims of HIV/AIDS.[46] Even a brief suppression of normal T-lymphocyte ratios is undesirable, and may be the underlying cause of at least one immunological disorder found in infants.[47]

From the early to mid-1980s, several medical and scientific periodicals, including the *Archives of Neurology* and the *Journal of Pediatrics,* published data showing correlations between the tetanus toxoid vaccine, peripheral neuropathy, poly-radiculoneuritis, and other serious neurological disorders.[48-51] The CDC documented encephalopathy and convulsions following the shot, and reported that overly frequent injections of the tetanus vaccine may lead to "arthus-type" allergic and hypersensitive reactions due to very high

Figure 21:

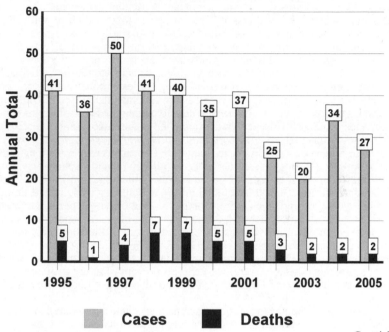

Tetanus Cases and Deaths:
United States, 1995-2005

Cases **Deaths**

In the United States, from 1995 to 2005 (an 11-year period), there were 386 total cases of tetanus—an average of 35 cases per year. Of this total, 43 people died—about four persons per year. The case-fatality rate was 11 percent. Source: CDC. Figures extracted from several *Morbidity and Mortality Weekly Reports (MMWR)*.

---

serum antitoxin antibodies.[52,53] Several years later, the CDC published updated information on vaccine side effects and confirmed that too frequent injections of tetanus toxoid can lead to high fever and hypersensitive reactions.[54]

In 1986, German researchers published a review of adverse reactions to the tetanus vaccine. They documented several cases of swelling and "inflammatory changes of joints."[55] In 1987, scientists confirmed "Guillain-Barré syndrome after vaccination" with tetanus toxoid.[56] In 1988, researchers reported on a 21-year-old man who developed acute midbrain syndrome and went into a coma after receiving a tetanus toxoid vaccine.[57] In 1989, the *Annals of Rheumatic Disease* found correlations between tetanus toxoid and chronic joint inflammation. Laboratory tests were able to show that this vaccine can lead to rheumatoid arthritis.[58]

In 1992, *Lancet* reported on a case of acute transverse myelitis in a 50-year-old man after receiving a tetanus vaccine. He developed a headache, muscle aches, and fatigue. Two days later he was admitted to the hospital with flaccid paralysis of the legs, no reflexes, loss of sensation, back pain, and inability to urinate.[59] *Lancet* also reported on an 11-year-old girl who developed optic neuritis and myelitis after she received a routine tetanus booster shot. She became blind from the vaccine, partially paralyzed in her legs, and lost control of her bladder.[60]

In 1994, The U.S. Institute of Medicine (IOM) corroborated a causal relationship between tetanus toxoid and brachial neuritis and Guillain-Barré syndrome.[61] The IOM also reported on several cases of anaphylactic reactions—severe, life-threatening allergic responses resulting in swelling of the mouth, inability to breathe, shock, collapse, or death—within four hours of tetanus vaccine injections.[62] Earlier studies by German scientists already documented deaths resulting from anaphylactic reactions to the tetanus vaccine.[63,64] The IOM also chronicled several dozen cases of severe joint inflammation following tetanus vaccines. When investigators conducted follow-up studies, it became evident that many of the victims had not recovered and were suffering long-term effects.[65]

In 1997, *Epidemiology* published a study comparing asthma and allergy rates in unvaccinated children versus children who received a vaccine containing tetanus. None of the unvaccinated children had recorded asthma episodes or consultations for asthma or other allergic illnesses before age 10 years. In the vaccinated children, 23 percent had asthma episodes and asthma consultations, while 30 percent had consultations for other allergic illnesses. Similar differences were observed at 5 and 16 years of age.[66]

In 2000, a new study in the *Journal of Manipulative and Physiological Therapeutics* confirmed earlier findings that children who receive DPT or tetanus vaccines are significantly more likely to develop a "history of asthma" or other "allergy-related respiratory symptoms" than those who remain unvaccinated. The study was conducted from 1988 to 1994 and included data from nearly 14,000 infants, children, and adolescents, aged 2 months to 16 years. A child who received the DPT or tetanus vaccination was 50 percent more likely to experience severe allergic reactions, 80 percent more likely to experience sinusitis, and twice as likely to develop asthma. In fact, the authors of the study calculated that "fifty percent of diagnosed asthma cases (2.93 million) in U.S. children and adolescents would be prevented if the DPT or tetanus vaccination was not administered. Similarly, 45 percent of sinusitis cases (4.94 million) and 54 percent of allergy-related episodes of nose and eye symptoms (10.54 million) in a 12-month period would be prevented after discontinuation of the vaccine."[67]

Product inserts published by the tetanus vaccine manufacturer (updated in 1999, 2003 and 2005) describe officially acknowledged adverse reactions. For example, "malaise, transient fever, pain, hypotension, nausea and arthralgia may develop in some patients after the injection. Arthus-type hypersensitivity reactions, characterized by severe local reactions may occur, particularly in persons who have received multiple prior boosters."[68,69] The manufacturer also notes that "...an anaphylactic reaction (hives, swelling of the mouth, difficulty breathing, hypotension, or shock) and death have been reported after receiving preparations containing tetanus and diphtheria antigens."[70] In fact, "the Institute of Medicine concluded the evidence established a causal relationship between tetanus toxoid and anaphylaxis."[71] Once again, "death following vaccine-caused anaphylaxis has been reported."[72]

The tetanus vaccine manufacturer also acknowledges (with supportive scientific data) that "neurological illnesses have been reported as temporally associated with vaccine containing tetanus toxoid."[73] Many of these neurological complications are listed in the product inserts: "cochlear lesion, brachial plexus neuropathies, paralysis of the radial nerve, paralysis of the recurrent nerve, accommodation paresis, Guillain-Barré syndrome (GBS), and EEG disturbances with encephalopathy."[74] Product inserts also acknowledge that "cases of peripheral mononeuropathy and of cranial mononeuropathy have been reported following tetanus toxoid administration."[75] In addition, "cases of demyelinating diseases of the central nervous system have been reported following some tetanus toxoid-containing vaccines or tetanus and diphtheria toxoid-containing vaccines."[76] Regarding adverse reactions reported during post-approval of this vaccine, the manufacturer notes that "events were included in this list because of the seriousness or frequency of reporting."[77]

Adverse Reaction Reports

This section contains unsolicited adverse reaction reports associated with the tetanus vaccine.[78] More reaction reports possibly linked to the tetanus vaccine may be found in the chapter on DPT and DTaP.

▸ "I received a tetanus shot because the doctors said it was way overdue. That night my arm hurt so bad that I could not lay on it. My temperature was 104 degrees. The pain eventually spread to my upper back and neck."

▸ "My daughter had three tetanus shots within 1½ years, and my son had two within this period. She was diagnosed with lupus, and now he has asthma and an immune system disorder."

▸ "I developed reflex sympathetic dystrophy (RSD) following a tetanus toxoid vaccine. I have very little use of the entire left side of my body and the disease now appears to be moving into my right hip and leg."

▸ "I received a tetanus vaccine and started adverse effects eight days later. After many months of tests, I was informed that there is no antidote."

▸ "My 26-year-old friend was given a tetanus and diphtheria shot at work. Five hours later she developed neck pain. It was pulled to the left and she couldn't move it. Three days later she also developed swelling at the injection site."

▸ "I had the tetanus-diphtheria vaccine in July. I was 29 years old. Four weeks later, I developed a 'virus' and two days after that I had my first asthma attack. I went from never having any respiratory problems to having asthma. Of course, the doctors deny that it was caused by the shot. If I had that type of a reaction, I know my kids are at a greater risk for vaccine reactions too."

▸ "My boyfriend had a tetanus vaccine four days ago. He developed a fever. Then, on the third day he developed a very stiff neck and back, and his back molars were aching terribly. I took him back to the emergency room where he got the vaccine in the first place and they dosed him up with ibuprofen and IV bags. The whole experience has definitely made me think twice about the tetanus vaccine. They say it is a known fact that you cannot contract tetanus through a tetanus shot, however my boyfriend developed all the symptoms from the vaccination."

▸ "I received a tetanus shot. That evening, my arm swelled the size of a softball. It was hot and sore. My doctor won't report this reaction. I will definitely think twice before allowing myself to be subjected to this kind of medical abuse again."

▸ "I had a tetanus vaccine and the area turned red and swelled up about the size of a tomato. Was my reaction normal?"

▸ "I am 43 years old and had a tetanus booster six days ago. My neck is still swollen on both sides. I am miserable and in pain. Where do I report this reaction?"

▸ "I am a 47-year-old mother of two who had to have a tetanus shot to work in a public school. About a week after I received the shot, my shoulders and neck became so stiff that I could barely move. Pain killers didn't do much to help. It has taken about four days for the stiffness to subside."

▸ "I am 47 years old and went to my physician for a physical. He gave me a tetanus shot. I developed a rash on my arms that became very blotchy but would lessen and then flare up occasionally. I received steroid cream from more than one doctor but it still hasn't gone away. The rash has spread to my hips, buttocks, feet, and legs. I also started getting inflammation in my fingers, but not every day. It would subside in a day or two and then would crop up again without warning. I notice abnormal pain on the tips of my fingers when I play the guitar. On occasion, there has also been abnormal stiffness in my middle back (right below each scapula) and also in both sides of my neck. This would last for a few days and be very uncomfortable (restricting motion in my neck). Areas around my eyes have also had soreness and rash, and my eyes have been red. Yesterday, six months after receiving the shot, the muscle soreness flared up and the rash has been very itchy."

▸ "I am a 55 year old male, in excellent health. Recently, I cut my thumb camping. It was three days until I could get tended. It was beginning to heal, and because I couldn't recall when I last got a tetanus shot, I was given one. One week later, I developed head cold symptoms. It has been two weeks and I am still symptomatic: mild night fevers, night sweats, lots of nasal congestion, low energy and fatigue. There is no question in my mind that this is directly related to the vaccine."

▸ "My 78-year-old mother was given a tetanus shot in July in a hospital emergency room after a fall in her living room. She had scratched her nose with her eyeglasses, and they apparently give the shot routinely to anyone admitted with a scratch or cut. Within three hours, she was intubated, as her throat had closed and her tongue had swelled outside of her mouth. She also had some facial swelling. The ventilator was removed after four days. However, she wasn't able to swallow, eat, or breathe properly after that, and passed away seven days later."

▸ "I had a tetanus shot in September and have been sick ever since. Where can I get information from someone who knows this is possible? My doctor just acted like I was an idiot, so I went untreated for four months."

▸ "My friend has an immune disease and was given a tetanus shot, starting muscular degeneration. She and her mom attribute her rapid decline to the shot."

▸ "When I was three months pregnant I cut myself and was 'required' to get a tetanus shot. My son has been diagnosed with cerebral palsy and attention deficit disorder. He also has grand mal seizures, an enlarged liver and heart, and made no growth hormone at birth."

▸ "I went to a health clinic for a check-up and was told I needed a tetanus shot. I soon became pregnant and miscarried in my second month. My husband and I were distraught. I became pregnant a short time later and miscarried again. Since that time, I had another miscarriage—my third in my first year of marriage."

▸ "In October, I received a tetanus shot. In December, I became pregnant. Our beautiful son was born 9 months later quite suddenly by C-section after a severe bleeding episode. Unfortunately, he passed away two days later. He had a deformity that begins in the early days of pregnancy."

▸ "We think the tetanus toxoid vaccine is killing in-vitro babies among the Akha Hill Tribe in Thailand—deaths and deformities. Please help us."

How effective is the tetanus vaccine?
Authorities recommend five doses of the tetanus vaccine before a child enters school. A booster dose is expected at 11 to 12 years of age, and every 10 years thereafter.[79] However, according to the eminent pediatrician Dr. Robert Mendelsohn, there is no credible scientific evidence indicating how often tetanus boosters are required. During the 1970s and 1980s, 40 percent of the child population was not protected yet tetanus infection rates continued to decline.[80]

Several studies and reports indicate that tetanus can occur in fully vaccinated people, that is, despite having tetanus antitoxin levels that are substantially above officially established protective levels.[81-83] For example, during World War II, the tetanus toxoid vaccine was mandatory for all U.S. military personnel. Still, 12 cases of tetanus were recorded. Four of these cases (33 percent) occurred in persons who were "adequately" vaccinated.[84] This enigmatic phenomenon has led early researchers to euphemistically label such cases "modified tetanus."[85,86] More recently, the September 2000 issue of the *Canadian Medical Association Journal* documented a case of tetanus in a patient whose tetanus antitoxin titer "was more than 20 times higher than 'protective levels' reported by the Provincial Health Laboratory in Toronto."[87]

The geriatric population is especially susceptible to inadequate protection despite up-to-date vaccinations. In older persons, "the response to immunization with tetanus toxoid has been demonstrated to be slower, of lower magnitude, and decreased duration."[88] In one study, a group of geriatric patients (mean age 70.6 years) exhibited significantly lower antibody titers for up to 12 months after an injection of tetanus toxoid as compared to a group of younger subjects (mean age 31.3 years).[89,90] In another study, subjects between 65 and 84 years old who received tetanus toxoid showed decreased IgG antibody production as compared to adults between 25 and 34 years.[91] However, in 1997 the *Journal of the American Medical Association* published a study showing that vitamin E supplements "enhances certain clinically relevant in vivo indexes of T-cell-mediated function in healthy elderly persons. No adverse effects were observed." Healthy elderly subjects who received a tetanus vaccine after ingesting 200 milligrams of vitamin E daily for more than 6 months produced more tetanus-fighting antibodies when compared to a similar group of elderly subjects who did not receive the vitamin E supplements.[92]

Tetanus Vaccines and Population Control

Scientists allied with the World Health Organization (WHO) began working on an anti-fertility vaccine in the mid-1970s.[93] Several studies throughout the 1980s and 1990s documented their progress.[94-97] They knew that in early pregnancy women secrete hCG (human chorionic gonadotropin), a special hormone that halts menstruation and immunologically prepares the uterus to accept the fetus.[98] Thus, these scientists reasoned, if *anti-hCG* antibodies could be induced in women of childbearing age, fertilization would remain incomplete and pregnancies would spontaneously abort.[99]

Under normal circumstances, the body will not attack naturally occurring substances, including the hCG hormone produced by pregnant women. The body has to be fooled into treating hCG as a foreign enemy. To accomplish this goal, scientists linked hCG to a "carrier"—the tetanus toxoid. A tetanus toxoid vaccine laced with hCG tricks the woman's body into producing two types of antibodies: one against tetanus and the other against hCG.[100-103]

Neonatal tetanus: In 1991, with their new vaccine in hand, WHO announced a plan to eliminate neonatal tetanus (NT) by 1995.[104] NT is defined by normal feeding and crying for the first two days of life, then onset of illness between 3 and 28 days of life: an inability to suck, followed by stiffness and/or muscle spasms.[105] NT accounts for more than half of all tetanus cases worldwide.[106] Neonatal tetanus rarely occurs in the U.S. and other developed countries; NT presents the greatest problem in Third World regions because of unsanitary birthing practices. Attendants may not wash their hands, delivery tools are often unsterilized, and a dirty knife used to sever the umbilical cord can lead to infection.[107-109]

During the early 1990s, WHO took their "neonatal tetanus" vaccination campaign to the Philippines, Mexico, and Nicaragua.[110] Millions of women of childbearing age (between the ages of 15 and 45) were vaccinated with a tetanus toxoid vaccine. They were given multiple injections—three within three months, followed by two additional doses. These women were told that the vaccine would protect their babies from neonatal tetanus. No one had the slightest idea that a secret, hidden agenda was being implemented.[111]

Human guinea pigs: In 1995, an international pro-life and human rights organization, Human Life International (HLI), became suspicious of the WHO vaccination campaign. Affiliates of HLI in the Philippines acquired vials of the vaccine and had them tested at an independent laboratory. The test results were positive for hCG. According to HLI, millions of women "unknowingly received anti-fertility vaccinations under the guise of being inoculated against tetanus."[112] HLI charged WHO and UNICEF of using women in several countries with high population growth rates "as uninformed, unwitting, unconsenting guinea pigs."[113]

In the Philippines, the controversy led to a court injunction halting use of the vaccine. As noted in the court petition seeking a restraining order, "The tetanus vaccine being administered to women of childbearing age has been tested positive for human chorionic gonadotropin (hCG) which has no business being part of the tetanus toxoid. In a laboratory analysis conducted by the Nuclear Department of the Makati Medical Center, it was found to be an abortifacient."[114] In Mexico, the Secretary of Health was charged with genocide.[115]

When HLI initially made public its concern that the tetanus vaccine was laced with anti-fertility hormones, WHO and the Philippine Department of Health (DOH) immediately denied that the vaccine contained hCG. When confronted with the laboratory test results, WHO and DOH claimed the evidence was somehow tainted because HLI authorized the tests. New vials of the tetanus vaccine were then submitted by DOH to St. Luke's Medical Center in Manila; all of the vials tested positive for hCG. When confronted with the new evidence, WHO shifted its story from outright denial and claimed instead that the amount of hCG in the vaccine was "insignificant." More vials of the vaccine were tested in the U.S. at the National Institutes of Health and were shown to contain "negligible" traces of the hormone. Authorities now declared that hCG's apparent presence in the vaccine was due to other substances in the vaccine that were somehow confounding or tricking the laboratory tests into producing "false positives" for hCG. But new tests designed to detect the presence of hCG antibodies in blood serum showed that 26 of 30 Philippino women who received the tetanus toxoid vaccine tested positive for high levels of anti-hCG.[116]

According to Sr. Pilar Verzosa, the nun who headed the Philippine branch of HLI, and who initially raised the tetanus toxoid/hCG issue, the vaccinated women "started complaining of infected arms and then miscarriages or premature deliveries or even defective babies."[117] Many of the vaccinated women had painful experiences with this vaccine, and remain convinced that it can cause severe adverse reactions and unwanted abortions. One disillusioned Philippino was even more candid: "They are giving this immunization to control our population."[118]

According to James Miller, special correspondent to HLI, several clandestine groups collaborated with WHO, including the World Bank, the Population Council, the Rockefeller Foundation, and the U.S. National Institutes of Health (NIH).[119] The NIH supplied the hCG hormone in some of the anti-fertility experiments.[120] Moreover, the vaccine was never even licensed for sale and distribution.[121] Authorities violated several internationally recognized laws and ethical standards, including the 1947 Nuremberg Code prohibiting medical experiments on human subjects without their knowledge or consent. HLI has called for a congressional investigation. Yet, to date no public admission of wrongdoing or apology has been issued, and few details of this illicit, covert operation ever reached the general media.

Should pregnant women get a tetanus vaccine?
Although the current tetanus vaccine is unlikely to contain the hCG hormone, mistrust among potential recipients remains high. For example, in May of 2007, one concerned woman wrote the following: "I live in Tanzania. Recently, our house help said she was pregnant and the medical facility that she attends told her she must have three tetanus injections before the birth and two after, and then one every year. I'm terribly worried. My tetanus injection lasts 10 years. How can I check that her injections are just for tetanus?"[122]

The tetanus vaccine manufacturer warns pregnant women that "animal reproductive studies have not been conducted." Furthermore, "it is also not known whether [this vaccine] can cause fetal harm when administered to a pregnant woman or can affect reproductive capacity." Nursing mothers are warned as well: "It is not known whether [this vaccine] is excreted in human milk. Because many drugs are excreted in human milk, caution should be exercised when [this vaccine] is administered to a nursing woman."[123]

Is the tetanus vaccine necessary?
Vaccine production is a commercial enterprise. For example, Wyeth-Ayerst, a leading tetanus vaccine manufacturer, surprised authorities by abruptly ceasing to produce the shot. The company called it a "business decision." As a result, a nationwide shortage of the vaccine caused health authorities to ration supplies. To cope with the shortage, state health departments suspended school requirements for tetanus booster shots. However, this wasn't expected to make a difference because according to Dr. Suzanne Westman of the New Mexico Department of Health, "We do not anticipate that suspending this year's school requirement for the tetanus immunization will have a negative effect on children's health."[124]

Diphtheria

What is diphtheria

Diphtheria is a contagious bacterial disease of the upper respiratory system. It is mainly spread by the coughing and sneezing of infected persons. The first symptoms appear two to five days after infection. They include a sore throat, headache, coughing, fever, and swollen lymph nodes in the neck. As the disease progresses, a thick membrane forms on the surface of the tonsils and throat, and may extend into the windpipe and lungs. This membrane may interfere with breathing and swallowing. In severe cases, it can completely block the breathing passages and cause death if not treated. Other complications include inflammation of the heart muscle and respiratory paralysis.[1]

Diphtheria requires medical attention but is treatable with common antibiotics such as penicillin. Heart failure is treated with medication, while a respirator is used to aid in breathing. A diphtheria antitoxin may also be administered.[2]

Is diphtheria a common disease?

Diphtheria was a common disease during the late 19th century. For example, from 1891 to 1895, Massachusetts recorded an average of 2,700 cases per year. New York averaged 7,200 cases per year.[3,4] The case-fatality rate was about five percent.[5,6] In the United States during the 1940s, the number of diphtheria cases fluctuated between 15,000 and 30,000 annually.[7] However, in 1980 a new pattern emerged, with only a few cases occurring each year. In fact, from 1980 to 1989, there were just 24 cases in the entire country. Eighteen of these (75 percent) were in persons 20 years of age or older. Two of the cases were fatal.[8] From 1995 to 2005 (an 11-year period), there were just 14 cases of diphtheria—about one case per year. Four of these cases were fatal (Figure 22).[9-11]

Does a diphtheria vaccine exist?

A diphtheria antitoxin became available in 1895 and was used on a limited scale from the beginning of the 20th century through the early 1940s. It supplied the body with a quick infusion of diphtheria-fighting antibodies. This antitoxin was administered to persons with low diphtheria antibody levels or immediately after being exposed to the disease.[12] Today, a diphtheria antitoxin is still available. It is derived from the blood of horses after they are inoculated with diphtheria organisms.[13]

A diphtheria vaccine was introduced in the 1920s. However, widespread use of this modified toxoid did not occur until the 1940s when it was combined with the tetanus and pertussis vaccines. This became known as DPT. Today, the diphtheria toxoid is administered in conjunction with the tetanus vaccine (DT), or in combination with both tetanus and acellular pertussis vaccines (DTaP).[14,15]

How safe and effective is the diphtheria vaccine?

In England, from 1876 to 1880, years before the diphtheria antitoxin was introduced, the diphtheria death rate was 1.22 per 10,000. However, from 1896 to 1900, *after* the diphtheria antitoxin was introduced and mandated, the diphtheria death rate soared to 2.72 per 10,000—a 123 percent increase.[16] In New York, from 1875 to 1894, years before the antitoxin was introduced, the diphtheria death rate had declined on its own by 45 percent.[17] From 1891 to 1895, there were 36,000 cases of the disease. However, from 1896 to 1900, *after* the antitoxin was introduced, there were 62,000 cases of the disease—a 72 percent increase. Massachusetts jumped from 13,000 to 28,000 cases during these same years—a 115 percent increase.[18] According to J.T. Biggs, a public health officer who analyzed the data, "The most startling feature of the report of 1895 to 1901 is the higher fatality rate in those inoculated with antitoxin when compared with the untreated cases."[19]

The diphtheria death rate continued to plummet long before the vaccine was introduced. In the United States, from 1900 to 1930, diphtheria fatalities declined by more than 85 percent.[20] In fact, mortality from the disease decreased from 7.2 deaths per 10,000 in 1911 to .9 deaths per 10,000 in 1935—an 88 percent decline.[21]

In 1919, the *Journal of the American Medical Association* published the first of several admissions that diphtheria antitoxin can sensitize the inoculated person so that "after ten, fifteen or twenty years, a second dose of the serum may cause death."[22] That same year, scores of children in Dallas, Texas, had severe reactions to their shots. When 10 children died, their parents joined together and filed a lawsuit against the manufacturer. They told the court, "The diphtheria antitoxin...was unfit, poisonous, and deadly."[23-25] The drug company was found guilty, but it was allowed to continue making the vaccine. An article in the local newspaper noted that "city officials regret the result of the treatment which caused the deaths...but urged that the treatment with antitoxin be kept up."[26]

In 1922, Dr. John Hogan, head of the Bureau of Communicable Diseases, Baltimore Department of Health, wrote that "Performing Schick-tests (to determine diphtheria antibody levels) and inoculating school children with toxin-antitoxin is of little value in the control or eradication of diphtheria, nor is it lowering the death rate."[27] Shortly thereafter, Dr. William H. Park, director of New York City Laboratories, confirmed this assessment. He wrote: "Vital statistics reveal that diphtheria mortality and morbidity had not decreased during the last five years. In New York state (before antitoxin) the mortality (from diphtheria) was only 12.8, which in 1921 (after compulsory antitoxin) had increased to 16.8."[28]

In 1924, the *Journal of the American Medical Association* cited several cases of suffering and death following diphtheria antitoxin:

Case #1: Antitoxin was given, and immediately the patient felt a lump in her stomach. Five minutes later she had tingling, restlessness, followed by convulsions, cyanosis and respiratory failure. Three minutes later her heart stopped. Death occurred in eight minutes.

Case #2: Seven minutes after antitoxin injection, the patient had itching on the body and scalp, then suddenly broke out with large "confluent wheals." There was nausea and vomiting. A severe convulsion was followed by death 35 minutes from time of injection.

Case #3: A strong healthy child received diphtheria inoculation, had a sudden reaction and died in five minutes.

Case #4: A school boy was given a prophylactic injection of antitoxin; he reacted and died in 20 minutes.

Case #5: Five minutes after injection, the patient became apprehensive. The heart beat continued 15 minutes after respiration ceased; death occurred 20 minutes after injection.

Case #6: The patient was given antitoxin. Two minutes later, it had gone to his stomach. He began to choke, became cyanotic and collapsed. Death occurred in five minutes.

Case #7: The patient was given a prophylactic dose of serum, collapsed and fell from his chair. Death occurred in ten minutes.[29]

In 1925, after several Austrian children died from diphtheria antitoxin, it was outlawed by the Austrian government.[30] In 1928, the Australian government curtailed use of diphtheria antitoxin after 21 children became seriously ill from the serum and 11 died.[31]

In 1929, the *Journal of the American Medical Association* conducted a survey in which physicians were asked about the diphtheria vaccine and serum therapy. More than 1,200 doctors participated. "Over 90 percent of them stated that they do not favor or use it or consider the injection of vaccine a satisfactory method of treatment. The reactions were too severe and the deaths and permanent disability were too frequent to justify its use."[32]

In 1932, Dr. Joseph Winters, professor of Children's Diseases at Williard Parker Hospital, New York, made the following comments: "I am here tonight to speak in opposition to the antitoxin treatment of diphtheria. Of 154 cases of diphtheria treated, in not one single case has there been the least evidence that the formation of the false membrane (in the throat and mouth) was checked, or that the throat was free from membrane earlier than in cases which have not been treated by antitoxin. In not a single septic case has the antitoxin made the least impression on the symptoms. The toxemia (blood poisoning) has not in one instance been relieved or lessened. At the Williard Parker Hospital in the month of December 1894, the recoveries from laryngeal diphtheria *without toxin-antitoxin* were about 75 percent. This has never been equaled since then with the antitoxin treatment."[33]

In 1934, Dr. F. Temple Grey, a pathologist, made the following observation: "The death rate from diphtheria has been rising in spite of the fact that antitoxin has been given. Recent work in England has confirmed that a certain number of patients, even if antitoxin

Diphtheria Cases and Deaths:
United States, 1995-2005

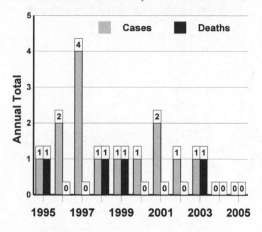

In the United States, from 1995 to 2005 (an 11-year period),there were 14 total cases of diphtheria—an average of about one case per year. Four of these cases were fatal. Source: CDC, *Pink Book* (December 13, 2006). *MMWR* 2001; 48(53) and 49(51).

---

is given in time, die nevertheless."[34] In 1935, the *British Medical Journal* reported 15 cases of "paralysis resulting from the use of diphtheria antitoxin. The onset is characterized by violent pain during the course of typical serum sickness 8 to 10 days after inoculation."[35]

In 1938, the renowned medical journal, *Lancet,* astounded the scientific community when it published a blunt admission by Dr. D.C. Okell: "Suppose we include in our propaganda a candid account of the various untoward 'accidents' which have accompanied (diphtheria vaccination). If we badly told the *whole* truth it is doubtful whether the public would submit to inoculation."[36]

At the beginning of World War II, Germany mandated the diphtheria vaccine. Shortly thereafter, epidemics of the disease swept across the country. In unvaccinated Norway, there were only 50 cases. When Germany occupied France, the people were compelled to receive diphtheria vaccinations. As a result, by 1941 there were nearly 14,000 cases of the disease. The shots were continued and by 1943 case numbers swelled to 47,000.[37]

In 1947, the *Vaccination Inquirer* reported that "No special prevention of diphtheria was practiced in Sweden before World War II, yet diphtheria almost disappeared. There are areas of London where only some 5 percent of the children were inoculated and there was a greater decline in diphtheria than 15 years earlier (when vaccination was compulsory)."[38] In 1949, American newspapers reported that 64 persons in Kyoto, Japan, died and 900 became seriously ill after receiving diphtheria antitoxin.[39]

In 1950, Dr. John Martin of City Hospital in Hobart Tasmania reported 80 cases where children developed infantile paralysis (polio) soon after being vaccinated for diphtheria.[40] Several studies published in medical journals have confirmed that "injections are an important cause of provocative poliomyelitis," and individuals are at increased risk of paralysis for 30 days following their shots.[41-52] [Read the chapter on polio for more information.]

In 1969, there was an outbreak of diphtheria in Chicago, Illinois. The city Board of Health reported that 38 percent of the cases had been fully vaccinated or showed serological evidence of full immunity. More than 50 percent of the cases had been partially or completely vaccinated prior to contracting the disease.[53] A report on another outbreak revealed that 14 of 23 infected persons (61 percent) had been fully vaccinated.[54]

Figure 23:
Diphtheria Cases were Predetermined to Decrease when the Medical Definition of Diphtheria was Changed

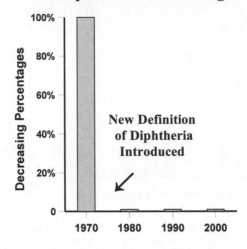

After 1979, a new method of calculating diphtheria was introduced. This caused an immediate decline in reportable cases. Source: CDC, *MMWR* (April 6, 2001); *PDR* 2001, p. 787.

In a 1975 official report, the Food and Drug Administration concluded that diphtheria toxoid "is not as effective an immunizing agent as might be anticipated." Authorities confessed that diphtheria may occur in vaccinated individuals, and noted that "the permanence of immunity induced by the toxoid...is open to question.[55]

In 1979, authorities changed the medical definition of diphtheria. Prior to the change, "cutaneous" and "inhalation" cases of the disease were counted. After the change, only inhalation cases were labeled as bona fide diphtheria. As a result, official statistics showed an immediate 95 percent drop in cases the following year (and a 99.3 percent drop from 1970 to 1980). The number of cases remained low every year thereafter (Figure 23).[56]

During the mid-1990s, there were outbreaks of diphtheria in eastern Europe and the newly formed states of the former Soviet Union. Many of the cases occurred in persons who were properly vaccinated. Thus, authorities questioned the merits of diphtheria vaccine programs.[57,58] Shortly thereafter, the *British Medical Journal* published a study showing that an adult diphtheria booster shot "is insufficient to obtain adequate protection."[59]

In 1999, the Food and Drug Administration (FDA) announced that diphtheria vaccines given to children during the previous year were "too weak to protect against diphtheria."[60] However, since diphtheria is very rare in the United States and other developed countries, officials did not recommend new vaccines for children who received the worthless ones. The FDA's decision may have been complicated by the fact that the manufacturer, Pasteur Merieux Connaught, refused to disclose how many doses were sold and who received them, calling that "proprietary information."[61]

The DT and DTaP vaccines:

Today, the diphtheria toxoid is administered in conjunction with the tetanus vaccine (DT), or in combination with both tetanus and acellular pertussis vaccines (DTaP). Thus, adverse reactions are difficult to attribute to any single component of the shot. For more information about the potential side effects of this vaccine, read the chapters on tetanus and pertussis (including DTaP).

Pertussis
(DPT and DTaP)

What is pertussis?
Pertussis is a contagious disease caused by a bacterium that affects the respiratory system. Sometimes called whooping cough, this disease got its name from the high-pitched whooping noise victims make when they try to catch their breath after severe coughing attacks. Symptoms progress through three stages. In the first stage, which usually lasts one to two weeks, victims have trouble breathing, and may develop a cough and fever. In the second stage, which usually lasts two to three weeks, severe coughing attacks occur during the night, and then later during the day and night. The attacks can lead to inadequate oxygen, which can cause convulsions. During this stage death can occur. In the final stage, coughing lessens and recovery begins. Full recovery may take two to three months.

How prevalent and serious is pertussis?
Pertussis epidemics were relatively common in Europe during the 16th, 17th and 18th centuries. Outbreaks were also common in America. By the 1930s, 73 percent of all U.S. children under 10 were exposed to the disease and a small percentage died.[1] Today, pertussis is rarely fatal.[2] However, when infants under six months contract the disease, it can be serious and life-threatening. There is no specific treatment for pertussis. Antibiotics and cough suppressants have been used, but with little effect, and are generally not recommended.

Does a pertussis vaccine exist?
The first "whole-cell" pertussis vaccine was developed in the early 1900s and put into general use during the mid-1930s and early 1940s. In 1946, the pertussis vaccine was mixed with vaccines for diphtheria and tetanus. (Read the separate chapters on these diseases.) This became known as DPT, the world's first "three-in-one" combination shot.[3] In 1981, Japan replaced DPT with DTaP because it contains a supposedly safer "acellular" form of pertussis.[4] The United States switched from DPT to DTaP in 1996.[5]

How is the DTaP vaccine made?
The current DTaP vaccine developed for infants 6 weeks to 7 years of age contains *Bordetella pertussis* antigens, *Corynebacterium diphtheriae* toxoid, plus *Clostridium tetani* cultures "grown in a peptone-based medium containing a bovine extract."[6] This combination vaccine also contains 170mcg of aluminum, "a trace amount of thimerosal" (a mercury derivative), gelatin, polysorbate 80, and "residual formaldehyde."[7] GlaxoSmithKline produces a DTaP vaccine with the inactivated polio virus and hepatitis B as well—a "five-in-one" shot! It also contains 850mcg(!) of aluminum, neomycin sulfate, polymyxin B, polysorbate 80, residual formaldehyde, and yeast protein.[8] (The DPT vaccine that was eventually removed from the market after 50 years of pediatric use contained 25mcg of thimerosal per dose.)[9] (For more information about mercury and aluminum in vaccines, see *Appendices I* and *II* on pages 307-308.)

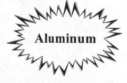

Aluminum

How safe is the pertussis vaccine?
In 1954, researchers at the U.S. Public Health Service developed the first test to determine whether the pertussis vaccine is safe for children: they injected the vaccine into the bellies of young mice to see if they would die. If the mice lived and gained weight, the vaccine was considered safe and was approved by the FDA.[10] The United States never conducted its own clinical tests in children to determine whether the pertussis vaccine is safe. Instead, it relied on data collected by Great Britain during the 1950s on children between six months and one-and-a-half years of age. Even though 42 of these children had convulsions within 28 days, 80 percent of the babies were 14 months of age or older, and the tests were designed to measure the efficacy—*not safety*—of the vaccine, U.S. health authorities used these

results as evidence that the vaccine is safe to give to babies as young as six weeks of age. In fact, a two month old baby weighing less than ten pounds receives the same dose of pertussis vaccine as a 50 pound child entering preschool.[11]

The pertussis vaccine may cause fever as high as 106 degrees, pain, swelling, diarrhea, projectile vomiting, excessive sleepiness, high-pitched screaming (not unlike the so-called cri encephalique, or encephalitic scream associated with central nervous system damage), inconsolable crying bouts, seizures, convulsions, collapse, shock, breathing problems, brain damage, and sudden infant death syndrome (SIDS).[12,13] In one report, serious reactions (including grand mal epilepsy and encephalopathy) were shown to be as high as one in 600.[14] In another study, approximately one out of every 200 children who received the full DPT series suffered severe reactions (shock-collapse or convulsions).[15]

The manufacturer lists several serious adverse reactions that have been reported after its DTaP vaccine was licensed and mass marketed. These include anaphylaxis, encephalopathy, grand mal convulsion, thrombocytopenia, hypotonia, neuropathy, autism, apnea and sudden infant death syndrome (SIDS).[16] Several other serious reactions were reported by DTaP manufacturers (including the maker of the five-in-one shot): swelling of the mouth, difficulty breathing, cranial mononeuropathy, brachial neuritis, Guillain-Barré syndrome, demyelinating diseases of the central nervous system, neuroblastoma, gastroenteritis, bronchiolitis, asthma, diabetes, chronic neutropenia, seizures, convulsions, bulging fontanelle, cyanosis, lymphadenopathy, arthralgia, myalgia, angioedema, alopecia, apnea, and death.[17-20]

Neurological disorders: As early as 1933, the *Journal of the American Medical Association* published data acknowledging neurological damage following pertussis vaccinations. For example, one child had convulsions, cyanosis, and died within 30 minutes of his injection.[21] In 1948, *Pediatrics* published data on 15 children who had severe reactions after their pertussis shots. Most of these children had persistent neurological damage, including coma, cerebral palsy, and mental retardation. Two of the children died.[22] In 1950, *Lancet* described severe neurological damage in a child after receiving a diphtheria-pertussis vaccine. The child became mentally retarded and was paralyzed.[23] In 1955, the *Journal of Pediatrics* described the case of a young girl who had severe convulsions 12 hours after her second DPT shot; she died a few hours later.[24] In 1957, the *Journal of Pediatrics* published another paper documenting infantile myoclonic seizures following DPT vaccination. Several children had normal development until they received their shots.[25] In 1958, the *British Medical Journal* analyzed 107 cases of neurological damage within 48 hours of pertussis vaccination.[26] A 1974 paper linked the pertussis vaccine with mental retardation. The authors reviewed dozens of cases and concluded that a clustering of neurological ailments in the first 24 hours after vaccination suggests a causal, not coincidental, link to the shot.[27] That same year, the Royal Society of Medicine held a conference in which authorities questioned whether the pertussis vaccine "outweighs the damage which it may be doing."[28] Also in 1974, German researchers documented 59 cases of convulsive reactions after pertussis vaccination.[29] In 1977, *Lancet* published a Scottish study analyzing 160 cases of DPT reactions, of which 65 were "followed by convulsions, hyperkinesis [attention deficit hyperactivity disorder] and severe mental defect."[30] The author of the study concluded that "most adverse reactions are unreported and...overlooked."[31] In 1979, a Belgian report linked the pertussis vaccine to several children who suffered persistent screaming, shock, seizures, and other neurological damage. Thirteen of the vaccinated babies died.[32] In 1981, the *British Medical Journal* published the results of the National Childhood Encephalopathy Study (NCES) conducted in England, Wales and Scotland from 1976 to 1979. During this period, nearly 1,200 children were hospitalized with neurological illness. Researchers concluded that DPT vaccination had occurred significantly more often within 72 hours, and within 7 days, prior to the damage, than in control subjects who did not exhibit neurological impairment.[33,34] Also in 1981, *Pediatrics* published data on a California study comparing DPT-vaccinated children to control subjects who only received the DT components of the shot. The DPT-vaccinated children had more inconsolable screaming episodes, excessive sleepiness, and 1 in 133 suffered from seizures.[35] In 1983, a large study published in *Lancet* confirmed a greater risk of seizures in DPT-vaccinated children compared to children who did not receive the pertussis component of the shot.[36] In 1993, the *British Medical Journal* published a follow-up study of the 1981 NCES research. This study located over 80 percent of a) the children who suffered neurological damage following their pertussis shots, and b) the control subjects. The authors concluded that the pertussis-vaccinated children "were significantly more likely than controls to have died or to have some form of educational, behavioral, neurological, or physical dysfunction" ten years after their initial adverse reaction.[37] Numerous other studies document neurological sequelae following DPT or pertussis vaccination.[38-50]

Anaphylaxis, bulging fontanelle and blood disorders: The pertussis vaccine was used in animal experiments to help produce anaphylactic shock, and to cause an acute autoimmune encephalomyelitis (allergic encephalitis).[51] A Spanish study investigated several children who went into shock and lost consciousness, or had their throats swelled shut, following their pertussis vaccines.[52] A *Lancet* study documented several children who suffered anaphylactic shock or collapse within 24 hours following pertussis vaccination.[53] Other reports have confirmed anaphylactic reactions following pertussis shots.[54-57] Several studies have also shown a link between the DPT vaccine and a bulging fontanelle (unnatural pressure in the skull)[58-62] and hemolytic anemia (the destruction of red blood cells).[63-65]

Asthma: In 1994, the *Journal of the American Medical Association* published data showing that children diagnosed with asthma were five times more likely than not to have received the pertussis vaccine.[66] In 1997, *Epidemiology* published a study that compared children who had been vaccinated with pertussis to children who did not receive the pertussis vaccine. More than 20 percent of the pertussis-vaccinated children developed asthma within 5 to 10 years, whereas none of the children in the control group acquired the ailment.[67] In 1998, a study published in *Thorax* showed a 1.4-fold increased risk of asthma associated with pertussis vaccination.[68] In 2000, a new study showed that children who received DPT or tetanus vaccines were significantly more likely to develop a "history of asthma" or other "allergy-related respiratory symptoms" than those who remained unvaccinated.[69] In 2008, the *Journal of Allergy and Clinical Immunology* published a study of 11,531 children who received DPT and found that babies vaccinated on schedule were twice as likely to develop asthma when compared to babies whose first DPT shots were delayed.[70] That same year, *Pediatric Allergy and Immunology* published a study showing that pertussis-vaccinated babies were more than twice as likely to develop atopic disorders—asthma, hay fever and food allergies—by 8-12 years of age, when compared to unvaccinated children.[71]

Autism: The first cases of autism in the U.S. occurred at a time shortly after the pertussis vaccine became available in the 1930s and 1940s. During the 1960s and 1970s, mass vaccination campaigns were instituted. The growing number of children suffering from this new illness directly coincided with the increasing popularity of the mandated immunization programs during these same years. Europe began promoting the pertussis vaccine in the 1950s; the first cases of autism began to appear on that continent in the same decade. In England, the pertussis vaccine wasn't promoted on a large scale until the late 1950s. Shortly thereafter, the first British autism support organization was established.[72]

Sudden infant death syndrome (SIDS): In the 1960s and 1970s, Aborigine infants began to mysteriously die at astonishing rates. In some regions of Australia, 1 of every 2 babies succumbed to an unexplained death—a fatality rate of 50 percent! Hospitalization and western medicine failed to save them. Eventually, Dr. Archie Kalokerinos solved the riddle when he realized the deaths were occurring after the babies were vaccinated against pertussis and other diseases. Health officials had recently initiated a mass vaccination campaign to "protect" Aborigine babies; their deaths corresponded with the program. Evidently, these babies were severely malnourished, especially deficient in vitamin C. When they were vaccinated, their undeveloped immune systems couldn't handle the additional stress. Dr. Kalokerinos was able to save other babies from the same fate by administering small quantities of vitamin C (100mg per month of age) prior to their shots.[73]

In Japan, from 1970 to 1974, there were 37 documented infant deaths following pertussis vaccinations.[74] Doctors boycotted the vaccine, and in 1975 Japanese authorities raised the age of vaccination from two months to two years. As a result, babies stopped dying unexpectedly. According to scientists writing in *Pediatrics,* "the category of 'sudden death' is instructive in that the entity disappeared following both whole-cell and acellular vaccines when immunization was delayed until a child was 24 months of age."[75] In fact, the Japanese infant mortality rate improved from 17th place to best in the world.[76]

In 1979, a cluster of SIDS deaths occurred in Tennessee within 24 hours after the babies' DPT shots. Researchers concluded that there was "an unusual temporal association between DPT vaccination...and SIDS."[77,78] In 1983, researchers analyzed 53 SIDS deaths following the babies' DPT shots and concluded the sudden deaths were "significantly more than expected were there no association between DPT immunization and SIDS."[79] In 1987, researchers wrote about twins who died abruptly after their pertussis shots.[80] That same year, the *American Journal of Public Health* published a study that found "the SIDS mortality rate in the period zero to three days following DPT to be 7.3 times that in the period beginning 30 days after immunization."[81] A 1992 study reported that babies die at a rate *8 times* greater than normal within 3 days after getting a DPT shot.[82]

A remarkable Australian study of SIDS (cot death) measured episodes of apnea (cessation of breathing) and hypopnea (abnormally shallow breathing) before and after pertussis shots. *Cotwatch* (a sophisticated microprocessor placed under the baby's mattress to measure precise breathing patterns) was used, and the computer printouts it generated (in integrals of the "weighted apnea-hypopnea density") were analyzed. The data clearly revealed that pertussis vaccination caused an inordinate increase in episodes where breathing either nearly ceased or stopped completely (Figure 24).[83-86] These episodes continued for months following vaccinations. Dr. Viera Scheibner, the main author of the study, concluded that "vaccination is the single most prevalent and most preventable cause of infant deaths."[87]

In another study of children who died of SIDS, Dr. William Torch found that two-thirds had been vaccinated with pertussis prior to death. Of these, 6.5 percent died within 12 hours of vaccination; 13 percent within 24 hours; 26 percent within three days; and 37, 61, and 70 percent within one, two, and three weeks, respectively (Figure 25).[88] Dr. Torch also found that unvaccinated babies who died of SIDS did so most often in the fall or winter while vaccinated babies died most often at 2 and 4 months—the same ages when initial doses of pertussis are given to infants. He concluded that pertussis shots "may be a generally unrecognized major cause of sudden infant and early childhood death, and that the risks of immunization may outweigh its potential benefits. A need for reevaluation and possible modification of current vaccination procedures is indicated by this study."[89]

Congressional Testimony of Donna Gary
Grandmother of a DPT-SIDS victim

The following excerpt is from a statement made by a distraught grandmother testifying before Congress:

My name is Donna Gary. Our family should have celebrated our very first granddaughter's first birthday last month. Instead, we will commemorate the anniversary of her death at the end of this month. Lee Ann was just eight weeks old when her mother took her to the doctor for her routine checkup. That included her first DPT inoculation and oral polio vaccine. In her entire eight weeks of life this lovable, extremely alert baby had never produced such a blood-curdling scream as she did at the moment the shot was given. Neither had her mother ever before seen her back arch as it did while she screamed. She was inconsolable. Even her daddy could not understand Lee Ann's uncharacteristic screaming and crying.

Four hours later Lee Ann was dead. 'Crib death,' the doctor said—'SIDS.' 'Could it be connected to the shot?' her parents implored. 'No.' 'But she just had her first DPT shot this afternoon. Could there possibly be any connection to it?' 'No, no connection at all,' the emergency room doctor said definitely.

My husband and I hurried to the hospital the following morning after Lee Ann's death to talk with the pathologist before the autopsy. We wanted to make sure he was alerted

<u>Figure 24:</u>

The Pertussis Vaccine, Stress-Induced Breathing Patterns and SIDS

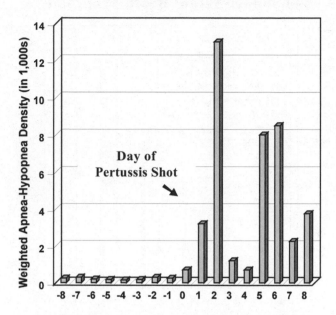

Days Before and After Pertussis Shot

This chart represents a 17-day record of one child's breathing patterns before and after receiving the pertussis vaccine. Values above 1000 indicate acute stress-induced breathing. The author of this study concluded that "vaccination is the single most prevalent and most preventable cause of infant deaths." Source: *Vaccination: 100 Years of Orthodox Research* by Dr. Viera Scheibner (Blackheath, Australia, 1993), pp. 59-71 and 225-235.

---

to her DPT inoculation such a short time before her death—just in case there was something else he could look for to make the connection. He was unavailable to talk with us. We waited two-and-a-half hours. Finally, we talked to another doctor after the autopsy had been completed. He said it was 'SIDS.'

In the months before Lee Ann was born I regularly checked with a friend as to the state of her grandchild's condition. He is nearly a year-and-a-half older than Lee Ann. On his first DPT shot he passed out cold for 15 minutes, right in the pediatrician's office. 'Normal reaction for some children,' the pediatrician reassured. The parents were scared, but they knew what a fine doctor they had. They trusted his judgment. When it was time for the second shot they asked, 'Are you sure it's all right? Is it really necessary?' Their pediatrician again reassured them. He told them how awful it was to experience, as he had, one of his infant patient's bout with whooping cough. That baby had died. They gave him his second DPT shot that day. He became brain-damaged.

This past week I had an opportunity to read through printed copies of the hearings of this committee. I am dismayed to learn that this same talk has been going on for years, and nothing has progressed to incorporate what seems so obvious and necessary to keep from destroying any more babies, and to compensate financially those who have already been damaged for life. How accurate are our statistics on adverse reactions to vaccines

Figure 25:

The Pertussis Vaccine and Sudden Infant Death Syndrome

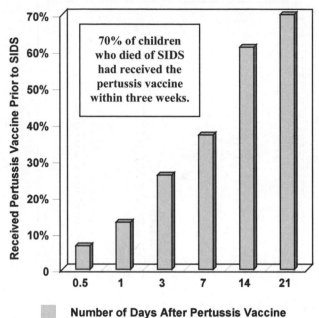

Number of Days After Pertussis Vaccine

In a study of children who died of SIDS, two-thirds had been vaccinated with pertussis prior to death. Of these, 6.5 percent died within 12 hours of vaccination; 13 percent within 24 hours; 26 percent within three days; and 37, 61, and 70 percent within one, two, and three weeks, respectively. Source: Torch, WC. *Neurology* 1982;32(4): pt.2.

---

when parents have been told, are still being told, 'No connection to the shot, no connection at all?'

What about the mother I have recently talked with who has a four-year-old brain-damaged son? On all three of his DPT shots he had a convulsion in the presence of the pediatrician. 'No connection,' the pediatrician assured. I talked with a father in a town adjoining ours whose son died at the age of nine weeks, several months before our own granddaughter's death. It was the day after his DPT inoculation. 'SIDS' is the statement on the death certificate.

Are the statistics that the medical world loves to quote to say, 'There is no connection,' really accurate, or are they based on poor diagnoses, poor record keeping? What is being done to provide a safer vaccine? Who is overseeing? Will it be the same scientists and doctors who have been overseeing in the past? How are physicians and clinics going to be held accountable to see that parents are informed of the possible reactions? And how are those children who should not receive the vaccine to be identified before they are damaged—or dead?

Today is the National Day of Prayer. My prayer is that this committee be instrumental in doing what needs to be done—and soon. May there not be yet another year pass by with more children afflicted, and some dead, because those who can do so refuse to 'make the right connection.'[90]

Adverse Reaction Reports:
The Pertussis Vaccine and SIDS

This section contains unsolicited adverse reaction reports linking the pertussis vaccine with SIDS. They are typical of the daily emails received by the *Thinktwice Global Vaccine Institute* (www.thinktwice.com).[91]

▶ "We lost our beautiful, precious and adored four-month-old son 26 hours after receiving the DPT vaccination and oral polio [vaccine] at his well-baby check-up. Our son's behavior patterns changed after the shot. He was staring, looked spacey, only took short naps, vomited his bottle. The doctor was insistent that this was a SIDS death."

▶ "My grandson had his 1st DPT shot and oral polio [vaccine] at his two month well-baby check-up. Within 21 hours he was dead. After the shot he started high-pitched screaming. My grandson began projectile vomiting and continued the high-pitched crying. At 7 a.m. my daughter awoke and found my grandson to have a purple color on one side of his face, clenched fists, blood coming from his nose and mouth, and not breathing. My grandson was dead. I promised my daughter that his death will not be in vain and just another statistic labeled SIDS."

▶ "I had a child die of SIDS. I dug out his shot records and baby book only to find that he had the DTaP just three weeks prior to his death, and during those three weeks, my records show that I had him to the pediatrician four times for respiratory infection and two times to the emergency room for respiratory distress. These symptoms began within two days after the administration of the shot! I am convinced after my research that the DTaP is responsible for his death. The three precious children I have left will not receive another vaccine!"

▶ "I gave birth to a beautiful baby girl after a normal pregnancy. She was very healthy. In November, I took her to the doctor for her second series of shots. The doctor said she was a very big, healthy girl, and that her mobility was that of a six-month-old. She screamed terribly. The DPT shot made her bleed so much that I had to change her diaper because the blood ran down her leg. I held her closely and got her calmed down. We then left. We had a 45-minute drive home. She went to sleep right after we got into the car. I watched her carefully because she had taken a few deep sighs in her sleep. There were a few times when I could not see her breath, so I put my hand on her chest and could feel her heart beating faintly. This concerned me, but I thought I was just being paranoid because of my concern about giving her these shots. I had always been worried when any of the kids had received their shots because I heard of some terrible reactions. After she had her first series of shots I questioned the doctor in depth about them. She informed me that babies run a much higher risk of complications and even death if they do not receive vaccinations than if they do. I asked her if she ever had anyone have problems after receiving these shots. She told me she had one case of SIDS pending; however, she did not see the connection between the SIDS and the shots. She said that the baby died seven days after receiving the shots and she didn't believe it was the shots that caused his death. When I got my daughter home that afternoon she just wanted to be held, and she slept a lot. That evening she was unusually fussy. She woke up in the middle of the night with an unusually loud cry. She always slept with my husband and I ever since she was born, and never woke up like that before. She was all sweaty, and she had urinated so much that I had to change all of her clothes. I nursed her and held her closely and she went back to sleep. I began noticing changes in her. She wasn't as determined as she used to be. She didn't like being in her walker anymore. She didn't try to sit straight up like she used to when you held her. She didn't want her pacifier anymore. When I did try to give it to her, she gagged. When I held her up on my shoulder and rocked her she would just lay her head on my shoulder and stare. This was really unusual because the only time she was still like that was when she was nursing or asleep. Six days later, I was at work when I received a call from my babysitter that our daughter had quit breathing, and to hurry up and get home. I was only a couple of minutes away, but it felt like it took hours to get there. I ran in the door and grabbed my limp baby from the arms of her babysitter and immediately laid her on the couch and gave her mouth-to-mouth. Within a few moments the emergency squad got there and transported her to the hospital. I followed in my car and called my husband from our car phone. I never stopped praying until they came out and told us there wasn't anything they could have done for her. They started to tell me about SIDS but I didn't want to hear anything they wanted to say. I just wanted to hold my baby girl one more time. There she was, lying there with just a blanket around her looking as if she were sleeping, other than her blue lips. I held her, sobbed, and prayed to God to please take good care of her until I come home to be with her. I had heard of SIDS before, but the only thing that kept going through my mind was the case of SIDS that our doctor told me about, which was one week after he received his shots. I couldn't accept that my beautiful healthy baby just quit breathing for no reason one day, no matter what rationalization was being told to me. I am so angry at the deception and lies concerning this. I feel like I need to do something to avoid this from happening to someone else, and for the precious memory of my beautiful baby girl. I just wish that the doctor would have painted an honest picture concerning the reality of vaccinations. It is so hard to live with the truth after it is too late, especially when you are the one who took her to the doctor in the faith that you were protecting the precious gift God gave you, and you find out later that you did just the opposite."

▸ "I spoke with a woman who held her screaming infant from the time it received its DPT shot until it breathed its last breath. The autopsy report read 'SIDS'! I can never be swayed from believing that many deaths reported as SIDS were really DPT reactions. As the former parents' group DPT (Dissatisfied Parents Together) used to state: 'When it happens to your child, the risks are 100 percent.'"

Developmental disabilities: According to the medical historian, Harris L. Coulter, Ph.D., "the family and society are both victims of vaccination programs forced on them by state legislatures that are entirely too responsive to medical opinion and medical organizations." The entire postwar American generation is suffering from "post-encephalitic syndrome"—the name he gives to define a variety of vaccine-induced disabilities.[92] To support his assertions, Coulter presented evidence showing that the long-term effects of pertussis shots may be more pervasive than suspected. However, injuries caused by the pertussis vaccine are often "disguised" under different names: autism, dyslexia, learning disability, epilepsy, mental retardation, hyperactivity, and minimal brain dysfunction, to name a few. Juvenile delinquency, an unprecedented rise in violent crime, drug abuse, and the collapse of the American school system unable to contend with the estimated 20 to 25 percent of students mentally and emotionally deficient, represent other conditions that may be attributed to the pertussis vaccine.[93]

The developmental disabilities and other conditions noted above are frequently caused by encephalitis, or inflammation of the brain. Medical practitioners know that encephalitis can be caused by a severe injury to the head, a severe burn, from an infectious disease, *or from the vaccines against these diseases*—post-vaccinal encephalitis.[94] According to Dr. Coulter, *the principal cause of encephalitis in the United States today, and in other industrialized countries as well, is childhood vaccination programs.*[95] The symptoms of post-vaccinal encephalitis are identical to the symptoms of encephalitis arising from any other cause.[96] Since any segment of the nervous system may be affected, every possible physical, intellectual, and personality deviation, and combinations of them, are possible.[97,98]

Autopsies after post-vaccinal encephalitis show a loss and destruction of myelin on the brainstem and spinal cord. Myelin covers and protects the nerves much like the insulation on an electric wire. Without myelin, nerve impulses are short-circuited and the nervous system remains undeveloped and immature.[99] An overt reaction to the pertussis vaccine is not required to confirm that post-vaccinal encephalitis, or damage to the central nervous system, occurred. In fact, there is no correlation between the degree of cerebral damage that may later ensue and the severity of the reaction that led to encephalitis in the first place.[100-104] In other words, subtle and often overlooked reactions to the vaccine (i.e., a fever, fussiness, drowsiness) can be, and often is, a case of encephalitis which is capable of causing severe neurological complications months or even years later.[105]

Hyperactivity/minimal brain dysfunction: In the 1950s, another disorder rapidly spread among school children and gained prominence in the medical science and health literature: hyperactivity (attention deficit hyperactivity disorder—ADHD). In 1963, the U.S. Public Health Service listed dozens of symptoms associated with hyperactivity and officially changed the name to "minimal brain dysfunction" (MBD). By the 1970s, some leading authorities noted that this disorder appeared to lie at the root of nearly every type of childhood behavior problem and had become the most commonly diagnosed illness among child guidance counselors.[106] In 1988, the *Journal of the American Medical Association* acknowledged that minimal brain damage had become the leading disability reported by elementary schools, and "one of the most common referral problems to child psychiatry outpatient clinics."[107] In some school districts, up to 13 percent of the children are now enrolled in "special education classes."[108] But minimally brain damaged children often go undetected, and some researchers believe that the actual figures for children with this disorder are closer to 15 to 20 percent.[109]

Although many children are not diagnosed as learning disabled or minimally brain damaged, teachers complain that nearly all of their students are cognitively inferior and have shorter attention spans when compared to kids they taught in the 1960s. One instructor notes that when she gives directions many forget them almost immediately, even after several repetitions. "They look around, fidget, and doodle."[110] Another teacher laments that "kids' brains must be different these days."[111] In fact, beginning in 1964 the average SAT verbal and math scores have continued to steadily decline.[112] In an attempt to appease school administrators, who are often blamed for declining scores, and to safeguard the truth, test-makers have been "dumbing down" their tests since the 1960s. Our children today are taking tests much more simple than those given decades ago.[113]

Like autism, minimal brain dysfunction was initially thought to have psychological origins. But these children usually exhibit symptoms associated with neurological damage: seizure disorders, tics, tremors, infantile spasms, EEG abnormalities, motor impairments, poor visual-motor coordination, and cranial nerve palsies (capable of causing visual defects, eye disturbances, and hearing and speech impediments).[114]

A few brief examples of the neurological basis for minimal brain dysfunction are given below:

- Harold reacted to his 2nd DPT shot with high-pitched screaming (the cri encephalique). Harold is now blind.[115]
- Kate was four months old when she received DPT. Within 72 hours she was shrieking in pain. Today she endures seizures and cannot speak.[116]
- Wesley reacted to his 2nd DPT shot with glazed eyes and seizures. Today he has up to 30 seizures daily and is permanently brain damaged.[117]
- Judy had her first grand mal seizure seven days after her 2nd DPT shot. Today she has a very low attention span and tends to reverse letters and write things backwards.[118]
- Ralph reacted to his first three DPT shots with persistent crying and a 104 degree fever. Today he has visual perception problems and cannot read or write correctly.[119]

Violent crime: A disproportionate amount of violent crime is committed by individuals with neurological damage.[120] As early as the 1920s researchers were aware that children who had "recovered" from encephalitis were more likely to engage in abusive, cruel, and harmful behavior. They were called "apaches."[121,122] Today we call these children juvenile delinquents (suffering from hyperactivity or conduct disorder), but their numbers are now epidemic and their crimes more violent (rape, shootings, etc.).[123] Dyslexia and other learning disabilities have been found in nearly 90 percent of delinquents.[124] Delinquent children with these disorders are often reclassified as sociopaths upon reaching adulthood.[125]

Perceptive parents may notice the onset of violent or antisocial behavior in their children following their vaccines. For example, a distraught mother describes her experience: "After my child received his shots at six months, he had high fever, screaming, and convulsions. The doctor said these reactions are normal side effects. From that day on my easygoing, happy, baby boy became what he is today. The last five years have been filled with life revolving around his moods. He goes from happy to outraged in seconds, has impulsive fits and hurts his siblings, argues with everything and everyone, can't focus or sit still. It was so confusing and scary to see this all start in a six-month-old baby."[126]

Another mother describes her experience: "My son was born perfectly healthy. He had a bad reaction after his first vaccines—inconsolable crying for 12 hours. The doctor told me to never give him another pertussis shot. And we didn't. As time went by we noticed that he didn't learn from discipline. Then, as he got older he couldn't tell the truth even if he wanted something that he was offered. We struggled, reached out for help, took him to a psychiatrist. He has no impulse control; he knows right from wrong but when put in a situation, he can't choose right if his life depended on it. I have believed for many years that this vaccine caused brain damage, but I can't get anyone to order a brain scan. He is almost 17 and is going to juvenile prison for the second time. Who is tracking these kids? How do we know that these vaccines aren't causing bipolar, antisocial disorder, mood disorders or ADHD? Certainly vaccines are what these children have in common. If a child has a seizure after a vaccine or dies, that is reported and tracked, but who is watching out for all these kids who have had 'milder' reactions?"[127]

Studies confirm that children with neurologically based disorders often engage in violent criminal behavior as adolescents and adults. In one study, hyperactive children were twenty times more likely than the rest of the population to end up in a reform school.[128] In another study, half of the incarcerated delinquents had an IQ below 85.[129] A report in the *Journal of the American Medical Association* acknowledged that a disproportionate number of felons suffered from hyperactivity disorder (ADHD) during their earlier years.[130]

Epilepsy and seizure disorders frequently occur following cases of post-vaccinal encephalitis. Studies indicate that epileptics find it significantly more difficult to control their impulses and aggressiveness.[131] In one study, the prevalence of prisoners with a history of seizures was found to be nearly ten times greater than the general population.[132] In another study of 321 mostly white, middle-class, extremely violent individuals, more than 90 percent showed evidence of brain damage, including a medical history implicating epilepsy.[133]

Drug abuse: Psychiatrists and pediatricians prescribe a variety of drugs to young children to control hyperactivity and MBD. In one study, it was estimated that six percent of U.S. children rely on these compounds to render them "manageable." In some regions, where doctors "specialize" in these disorders, the percentage is much greater.[134] Many of these drugs have adverse side effects that are considered by some researchers to be worse than the original symptoms. These new symptoms are sometimes irreversible.[135]

Many people who have studied these problems believe that the medical abuse of drugs in school children predisposes them to abuse "street drugs" later in life.[136] Adolescents suffering from minimal brain dysfunction are at risk for engaging in unusually early smoking, drinking, and substance abuse.[137] Adults with this disorder are also notably susceptible to alcoholism and the misuse of drugs.[138]

Adverse Reaction Reports: DPT

Sudden infant death syndrome (SIDS) is not the only risk associated with the DPT vaccine. The following true stories reveal the tragic realities:[139]

▶ "My daughter's episode began when she was given her first shot at two months of age. Prior to her first shot she was a normal and healthy baby. After her first DPT shot, her appetite greatly decreased, she cried excessively and would arch her back as if in pain. She was also constipated and less active. X-rays and an MRI on the mid-section of her body did not reflect anything unusual. She was given her second DPT shot when she was four months old. She immediately displayed distress and a lack of appetite. All of her previous health problems magnified. By the next day, she was crying excessively and was too weak to move her head. The pediatrician attributed this to the flu. That night as I was trying to rest after comforting her all day, her crying ceased. I called out to my husband who had been in the next room to check on her, and then there was complete silence. I asked my husband if there was anything wrong, yet there was still silence. I went into her room and found my husband giving her CPR. He yelled to call 911 which I immediately dialed. After completing the call, I watched in horror as my husband continued to give her CPR. She was bluish-gray and still not breathing on her own. Less than five minutes later, I watched as if in slow motion the paramedics pick up my daughter and carry her into the awaiting ambulance. The same pediatrician was in the emergency room with no answer to account for her grave condition. A team from another hospital arrived and transferred her to the nearest ICU unit. She was placed on a ventilator. For the next week, my daughter was put through every test imaginable, including numerous MRIs. Each test was inconclusive. My daughter remained on a ventilator as I painstakingly realized that medicine was indeed not a perfect science. An MRI the next week confirmed that my daughter had transverse myelitis, inflammation of the spinal cord including the brainstem. As the doctors told us this news, they informed us that her condition was grave. She remained on a ventilator for the next month. She was eventually taken off the ventilator, and two months after her being admitted, she was finally discharged. I thought this real life experience might make a difference in one child's life whose parents are still contemplating the decision to vaccinate their child."

▸ "My 2-month-old daughter had her recommended shots (DPT, polio, etc) and was non-responsive for 26 hours afterwards. She could not be woken up for feedings or anything else. The pediatrician blew me off, so I found a doctor who took the reaction seriously, and he told me not to give her the pertussis vaccine again. She is now 26 months old and has a speech and language delay of 10 months. My pediatrician did not report my daughter's reaction. Can parents report their child's reaction without the blessing of the pediatrician?"

▸ "Our son was born healthy. Two months later he got his first set of vaccinations. Within hours, he was irritable, he had lost the ability to hold his head upright, he lost his appetite, and was just not himself. Within a week, our son had a case of apnea, where he would stop breathing during sleep. We had him in the hospital overnight on an apnea monitor, and again we were told nothing was wrong. Finally, our doctor said it may be a reaction to the DPT shot, and that we could postpone any further shots."

▸ "My daughter had a reaction to her first immunizations at age two months. I am an RN and had been taught that they were just something that all children had to have. I never even realized one had a choice. My daughter had her injection at 3:30 pm. She fell asleep around 6:30. I let her sleep on my shoulder while I relaxed on the couch. Something made me pick her up so I could look at her. Her face was gray, she was not breathing, and when I checked she had no heartbeat. I immediately started CPR and called 911. By the time the paramedics had arrived she was conscious and making an effort to cry. We went to the hospital. Her heart rate stayed at 250 for the next few hours in a very strange arythmia. Neither the doctor nor I could figure it out. She also stayed mottled for the next three hours. When they felt her crisis had passed, they admitted her into the pediatric ward. This was one o'clock in the morning. The hardest part was when they told us to call our family members in. I knew then that they didn't expect her to live. But my little angel surprised us. Six days later we went home with her on heart and lung monitors, with us having a lot of unanswered questions. No one was willing to admit she'd had a DPT reaction. When I phoned public health, the reaction had never been reported. I looked everywhere for information and found little to none. I contacted every pediatrician I could network with. The result of that was being called into my family doctor's office and being reprimanded for doing this. A big conference was held, and somehow I got conned into re-immunizing her at four months. They admitted her to the hospital for this one, as it was the only way I would allow it. She turned gray around three hours after the injection, but otherwise being awake she pulled through it. She had what I felt were petit mal seizures and one grand mal seizure following this at home. Each time, I was discredited by the doctors. Being a nurse, I've seen enough to know what they were. She also suffered long bouts of crying, totally inconsolable. I finally went to see a chiropractor (out of sheer desperation because I really didn't think he could do anything) and he was able to work with her. Her manner and behavior changed so quickly it was amazing. He also gave me the information I needed to fight the doctors, and my daughter had no further immunizations. It was such a victory to finally be able to say No!"

▸ "My daughter was born three weeks early with an apgar score of 9. At her 2-month check-up she was fine, gained weight, good everything. She was to have her first DPT shot. Within hours, her fever went to 103 and she had severe muscle spasms which caused her not to be able to sleep. I videotaped it. I called the doctor fearing she was have seizures. He said she was fine. We were told it was probably indigestion and stomach upset. I called a neurologist and couldn't get an appointment for another two months. I returned to my doctor because I thought my daughter was more limp and less aware. Again, I was being overprotective and was assured she was fine. I questioned the DPT shot and asked if it could have caused her to have seizures. I was told that it was impossible that this shot would cause any problems like that. When my daughter was four months old we went to the neurologist. He went on and on about developmental delays and genetic testing. We were so unaware of what he was saying. I finally asked him to slow down and explain it to us in a language we could understand. He said very bluntly that our daughter was severely mentally retarded and brain damaged, and that we should have her institutionalized before we got attached to her, and never to have another child because it would only be worse than my daughter. My daughter went from a perfectly healthy child from her 2-month check-up to a severely handicapped child at four months. The only thing that was different in my child's life was the DPT shot and very poor medical care. I continued to question the shot and was constantly told that it was not the cause, that it was probably genetic. We had every test possible done and nothing genetic was found. It was not until I had my third child four years later that I firmly believed it was the DPT. After each shot, she went backwards. At six months, she started crawling, then a shot, no more crawling. Talking was okay until the 15-month-old shot, then no more new words, etc. I know that I harmed my child under the careful watch of her doctors. They say she has brain damage with no known cause. I was told that 80 percent of all mental retardation cases like my daughter's have no cause, it just happens. The happy part of my story is that she is very happy and knows no different. She will be like a child the rest of her life. We love her just the same."

▸ "After I left the doctor's office from giving my son DPT, he started wailing high-pitched shrieks as soon as I started driving. I was going to pull over because I wanted to get him out of his car seat and try and soothe him. While I was looking for a place to pull over, he stopped crying. I turned around to look at him, and he was limp. I immediately rushed back to the doctor's office in a hysterical panic. The waiting room was full of parents and I was screaming. The doctor came running out and the first thing he said was, 'It wasn't from the DPT shot. No, this can't be from the shot,' and he went on and on. I was livid. My baby was passed out and he didn't even take him from me. The nurse got so irritated with him that she said to me, 'Give me this baby now,' and threw the doctor a dirty look. She told me after that she was mad because instead of the doctor taking the baby from me to help him, he chose to try and cover himself. Matthew woke up as soon as the nurse took him. Thank God he was fine. I started a new doctor after that and I refused to let Matthew have another shot. I told the new doctor what happened and I will never forget what he said. He said, 'We can treat pertussis. We can't treat a baby who is no longer with us because of the DPT shot.'"

▸ "When I allowed our daughter to be vaccinated at four months, she got very sick that night. She screamed nonstop in a high-pitched scream. She wouldn't nurse and couldn't be comforted. Her temperature was quite high. I called the emergency number for my doctor and he told me it was very important to never let her receive the pertussis vaccine again, but that I should continue with the other vaccines. Our daughter's neurological problems were first noticed a few weeks later. She was behind in development and never did actually crawl. Her speech came in late. After several tests, I was told that her seizure problems make it difficult for her to concentrate and thus learn, although she is quite intelligent. No one ever told me about the risks associated with vaccines. I asked, but they still did not tell me of the dangers. Almost every warning about DPT fits our daughter: premature birth; low birth weight; family history of seizures; family member with severe allergies. Today, she has seizures all the time. Doctors say she has an 'attention deficit.' She is easily distracted and has difficulty concentrating. When she tries to express her thoughts and feelings, her eyes flutter and she stutters. It causes her deep frustration and anger. As a result, she is about two years behind in school because she has to learn in small increments. In spite of all this, she has a great attitude, a wonderful sense of humor, and is very athletic. We try to focus on the good things. I have great hopes for her, but I also have profound regret that somehow I could have protected her from this terrible violation of human life."

▶ "Our grandson received his 2-month DPT and had a small convulsion. He received his 4-month vaccination and again ran a fever and had a convulsion. My daughter and son-in-law have made the decision to discontinue all vaccinations. Their boy is a little slow for a 16-month-old. He did not sit up until about 11 months, and is just beginning to crawl and pull himself up. The doctor will begin testing at 18 months if he is not walking."

▶ "I was encouraged to take my daughter to the doctor to receive her DPT shots. Not having any information on the subject, I did so with the understanding that I was being a responsible parent. That night, when I was out of the room, my daughter stopped breathing. I was told that the nurse gave her oxygen. When I tried to get information on what actually took place it was as if nothing important happened. It was never recorded in her records and I was told it was purely temper—at eight weeks old! When we left this hospital, my daughter developed a skin rash which over the past two years has worsened and no doctors can give me an explanation for it. I am grateful that when my daughter stopped breathing she was with someone and could be helped, but what would have happened if she had been in bed at home? Would she have been another case of cot death?"

▶ "I took my healthy 5-month-old to the doctor for his well-baby check-up. He received his third set of vaccinations, including a DPT shot. Two hours later he began having severe diarrhea, vomiting and shortness of breath. His body was limp and he was going in and out of consciousness. I took him to the hospital where he was examined by a doctor who told us he was fine. They kept saying it was a stomach virus, but I know better."

▶ "I have a sister who, at six months, received her third DPT shot. My father noticed her having little seizures. My mother took her to a doctor and expressed concern that it was a reaction to the DPT. This inhumane man told her, 'It's just a spoiled reaction, take her home and start smacking her.' By the time a doctor finally did listen, it was way too late; the damage was done. She was my parents' fourth child, so who better to know that she was a normal healthy, developing child, than those who had three children already."

▶ "My brother was a normal, healthy 2-year-old when he got his 3rd DPT vaccination from our doctor. Within a few days, he had forgotten how to talk, walk, use the bathroom and use eating utensils. My mother confronted the doctor with what she thought were seizures. The doctor said they were tantrums, and that my mother should try more strict discipline! When she tried to enroll my brother in the local school for mentally and physically challenged people, they refused to admit him without a fourth DPT shot. Our new doctor said a fourth shot would almost definitely kill him or make him a vegetable."

▶ "My son was born healthy and full term. After his first DPT shot, he started screaming right away. He screamed and cried for the next few days, except when he fell into a deep sleep. When he was awake, he had a glassy, odd look in his eyes, as though he was looking right past us. He just wasn't right. I took him to the emergency room where I was told he was having 'a bad day.' I asked if the shot had anything to do with his behavior. I was told 'no.' I brought him home and knew something was wrong. I know now he suffered from encephalopathy and convulsions. I did not know that our son had a reaction to his first DPT shot. After his second shot he screamed, and when we got home he went to sleep. I checked him and he was stiff as a board with glaring eyes. He had no expression on his face and I got no response. However, when I picked him up his head was floppy. I held him for 30 minutes. Then, as if nothing happened, he sat up. After this episode, I noticed a lot of jerking movements. I now know these were seizures. About a week later I was holding him on my lap and his legs went out, and his tongue hung out; he had his first grand mal seizure. I took him to the doctor's office the next day, but before I got him ready to go he had several more grand mal seizures. The doctor told me it seemed like epilepsy to him and ordered EEGs and blood work. The next day, back home in his high chair, we thought he was choking on baby food. He was having another grand mal and we rushed him to the doctor. They took him to the hospital by ambulance. That is where we were confronted with what was wrong. The doctor asked when he had a DPT shot; she said don't get another. From that day on our lives were changed dramatically. We went from hospital to hospital hoping we could find something to help our son. He has been on every medication available and some that are experimental, all to no avail. When our son was six months old we noticed an uncommon type of reaction. He would look at our kitchen floor and have a seizure. He could not look at screens or anything with a weave, including grass, cement, jeans, and sweaters, to name a few. As he got older I tried dark glasses on him; it seemed to help. The medications and diets he has been on in his last eight years have been to no avail. He had brain surgery that helped with the patterned seizures. He continues to have grand mal clusters every two weeks. These last 12 to 15 hours; he has about 30 seizures in this time period. Our son is mentally retarded and has symptoms of cerebral palsy. He wears leg braces and a seizure helmet. His behavior is not good. Although he is 8 years old, he is a 1-year-old in many ways. He can't dress himself or color or write or print. He goes to a special class. We are with him 24 hours a day. He cannot be alone for 10 seconds. He is a danger to himself. For 5 years, he could not look at a TV screen because it was an instant grand mal. As I write this, he is unconscious from a bout of seizures. Our friends are few. Our son is our whole life. Our daughter has been showing signs of unhappiness. She misses out on a lot, but we feel she'll be a better adult for this."

▸ "My son was born a healthy baby boy, apgar 9. He ate well, slept well, was doing fine. He had his DPT shots then started doing mild jerks that increased each day. By the tenth day he was put into the hospital with infantile spasms. No one ever told me why this happened. The doctors said 'unknown.' Today, my son is almost seven, with global developmental delays and seizures. Still, no doctor can tell me why this happened. I know it had to do with the DPT shot."

▸ "My son was damaged by DPT. His condition has worsened over the years, and he has had another brain surgery. Things have gotten worse as far as his grand mal seizures. He used to have them either every 14 or 21 days and they would last for 15 hours. Now they are every 10 days and last for 22 hours, with as many as 85 grand mals in this time frame. I could write a book on all the things that go into raising a vaccine-damaged child."

▸ "My daughter was born with a near perfect apgar. She thrived on breast milk until her 2-month checkup. We had told the pediatrician [that her brother had a serious reaction to DPT, and we have a family history of seizure disorder, a contraindication to receiving vaccines]. He insisted she get the DPT shots anyway, and we were young and naive. I even trusted him. Within several hours of getting her first shot she screamed inconsolably for hours. After about 24 hours she stopped screaming and became apathetic. She was limp and disinterested in eating or smiling. She no longer turned over or kicked vigorously when placed on her back. She could no longer hold her head up when held on my shoulder. We called the doctor several times during the initial 24 hours and days that followed. They always assured us her reaction was normal and told us to keep giving her Tylenol. (Looking back now, I wonder how baby Tylenol heals damaged brain cells.) After a few days she developed her first definable illness, 'coincidentally' an upper respiratory infection. We took her to the doctor and he diagnosed her as 'failure to thrive' and 'complete loss of muscle tone.' He still would not admit it was the shot! In fact, even though we fought him, she still received her 4-month and 6-month doses of pertussis. He was the almighty doctor and therefore knew more than us. However, by her 18-month shot he told us that because we insisted, he would withhold the pertussis. Who knows, though, because years later when he retired and we transferred her records, his records show that she received DPT at 18 months. Our older son also reacted to the DPT. He began having night terrors and visual auras. The night terrors continue to this day whenever he has a fever. He is in college now. So what happened to our daughter? She is in special classes with a recorded IQ of 50. She is 16 years old now and struggles daily to complete a 2nd grade curriculum. Physically, she has very poor muscle tone, poor small and large motor coordination. The good news is that we just moved to another state and they are actually educating her rather than just babysitting. I am grateful my child is alive. I love her like she is, but I do hurt for her when I realize many of her dreams will not come true—and they are such easily attainable dreams for an average person. She wants to marry and be a mommy like me. Meanwhile, life does go on. Our third child is five years old and never had any shots! She is as healthy as a horse. The toughest part is that no one will admit the reactions were from the shot. We have been told, in fact, that it absolutely was NOT the shot. Duhh! I was there. It WAS the shot! I hate being patronized and told I am only a mother. I have researched a lot, am very bright, and can understand as much as the doctors we have seen."

▸ "I have a brother who is now 20 years old. When he was of age as an infant to receive his DPT shot, he shortly thereafter started to have violent seizures. He was a normal baby, very happy, until he had that shot. The doctors, of course, would not link the shot to his all-of-a-sudden abnormal actions, but what they do is protect the drug companies. Eleven years later, my mother ended up winning a lawsuit due to the 'P' in the DPT shot. No amount of money fixes a life that was taken. He is, and always will be, at the developmental stage of two years old. There are many things in life he will never experience. He still has seizures, some worse than others. He will never be able to read, write, talk, or do anything anyone else a 20-year-old can do. The only thing that keeps me from feeling sorry for him is that he is happier than anyone I know. The sad part is that doctors and drug companies cover the truth up all too well."

▸ "I am the mother of a 22-year-old daughter who was first immunized with DPT at three months of age. Today she is severely to profoundly mentally handicapped, and has irretractable seizures. She functions on about a two- to three-year-old level. Luckily we had a military doctor overseas who noted on her shot record that she could have had a possible reaction to the shot. We were to only give her DT from that point on. I had no idea what that meant or why, but I always reminded the airman who would give her the shot. I am sure that this saved my daughter from any further damage. The sad thing was that although someone very early had recognized that there could be a connection, NO ONE would say it was so. I agonized over what to call it for ten years! I could only say she was 'mentally retarded and had uncontrollable seizures.' That is, until ABC's '20/20' showed a program with many other families in our same nameless, hopeless situation. When I confronted the doctor, she said 'Yes, of course that is what happened to your daughter, but you'll never be able to prove it.' I thought that at least now I can go and look in a book to see what to expect. But there is no book that tells you what to expect when your vaccine-injured child begins different phases of life. Every day is a learning process. These children don't fit into the convenient little special education slots that most school systems offer. My beautiful daughter is a square peg and the only things available for her are round holes."

▸ "My 24-year-old son is mentally disabled. The problem started with his first shot at two months, which caused fever and lethargy. This happened again with the second shot at four months, and at six months he received the third shot. The next morning when I turned on the light he went spastic and started making strange staccato sounds. Each day got worse, and the seizures continued. This went on for months. The doctor diagnosed him as deaf, which I knew could not be correct, because until that time he reacted to noises. He did appear deaf for about six months, and then started reacting to sounds again. He no longer could roll over, sit up, or have eye contact with anyone. At almost a year, a friend called to tell me about a program on Phil Donahue; parents were attributing the problem to DPT. When I asked my doctor about it, he became very defensive and explained it away, but 'lost' all of Tim's records. My son could not walk until five years of age, was not potty trained until age six, on and on. Through the years, I have had him with neurologists who refused to believe it could have been the shot. My son has had seizures through most of his childhood. He is on meds for ADD and other issues and has the mentality of a 3-year-old in most areas. He has gone from a diagnosis of deaf to autistic, until today he is considered undiagnosed with autistic-like behavior. He started out as a very healthy, happy baby (an apgar score of 10). He has been in special education all through the years, and now lives in a residential home close by. He is a happy, pleasant, tall (6' 5") very attractive young man who has no idea what has happened to him. There were many struggles through the years because he did not understand what was wrong, and training him was an uphill battle at best. Unless you have lived through the problems I speak of, you cannot imagine what it does to the dynamics of the whole family. Through the years I have tried to get doctors to consider seriously this could have been caused by the shot so stats realistically represent what is happening. They always say there is no proof to support our claim."

▸ "My son, who is now 24, had a reaction to DPT. After the shot, he got a dark red band around his leg about 5 inches wide, with swelling and fever, and he was having seizures and limb jerking. His doctor gave him an EEG with a possible diagnosis of encephalitis. My son went through years of having such anger outbursts and seizures that he would pass out from exhaustion right afterwards. Learning disabilities, teasing at school, quit school—he cannot even keep part-time work. He is now living on disability but was born healthy and smart."

▸ "I am 29 years old. I suffered an adverse reaction to the DPT vaccine. I suffered grand mal seizures and mild ones also. My mother had to give me steroid shots to control my seizures. She was going to sue but our doctor and the hospital would not release my medical records. I have a 6-year-old son and cannot help him with homework. I have a second grade level in math. I am really bad when it comes to working with money. When I was young, my mother told me I lost my sucking motion so that is why still today I suck my thumb and I have some problems mentally. I feel like I am not myself. I feel real bad."

▸ "My 31-year-old daughter is a victim of her first DPT shot. She functions at the mental age of three, and has seizures. I have talked to many people during the years and educated them on the dangers of vaccines. Ironically, a few years ago my grandsons, who did NOT receive the pertussis shot, as well as their aunt, all contracted whooping cough. While it was a spooky ordeal, they all survived, yet sadly my daughter didn't 'survive' her first whooping cough shot, and lives today with the devastating aftereffects."

▸ "My husband is 39 years old. At the age of six months he was given his DPT and had a serious seizure. He had seizures ever since, all his life, sometimes every 7 to 10 days. He is on medication all the time. The medications slow him down. He suffered from learning disabilities, and now he lost many of his teeth too, due to taking seizure medications and during seizures grinding his teeth. Doctors regularly want to give him tetanus shots when he is taken in injured from a seizure."

DTaP

Is DTaP safer than DPT?

In 1981, Japan began giving their children a new "acellular" pertussis vaccine (DTaP). They claimed it was less toxic and more effective than the standard "whole-cell" vaccine (DPT) used in the United States. Many authorities in this country agreed, but claimed that the additional cost to produce the vaccine, and the logistics involved, did not justify making the switch.[140] Japan reported a significant drop in serious reactions following use of the acellular vaccine. However, in 1975, a few years before the new pertussis vaccine was introduced in Japan, authorities raised the age of vaccination to two years. In the U.S., pertussis shots are begun at two months, and are continued throughout the infant's early, high risk months. Thus it has been hard to ascertain whether the acellular vaccine is truly safer.[141-143]

In 1987, the *Journal of the American Medical Association* reported that the DTaP vaccine reduced "mild" vaccine reactions by 60 percent when compared to the DPT shot. However, the new acellular DTaP vaccine and the original whole-cell DPT shot had similar rates of severe reactions.[144] That same year, 66 victims of the Japanese acellular pertussis vaccine won huge awards from their government. The court recognized that the authorities were denying adverse reactions. The damaged plaintiffs were victimized so that the "public interest in preventing contagious diseases" wouldn't be undermined.[145]

In 1988, a Swedish study documented four fatalities in babies who received the acellular vaccine. Although there was no "proof" that the vaccine caused the infant deaths, Swedish authorities recommended withdrawing their application to license the shot.[146] In 1989, *Pediatrics* published the results of another Swedish study confirming fewer mild reactions with the DTaP vaccine, but children were still succumbing to unusual, prolonged crying (the cri encephalique), hypotonic reactions and encephalitis. In fact, 1 of every 106 DTaP-vaccinated babies had serious adverse reactions such as inflammation of the brain—a much higher rate than official figures for the whole-cell DPT vaccine.[147]

In 1992, the American Academy of Pediatrics (AAP) recommended replacing the standard whole-cell pertussis vaccine (DPT) with the acellular (DTaP) vaccine for the 4th and 5th doses only.[148] In 1996, U.S. authorities replaced DPT with the DTaP vaccine for all five doses—despite the contention by some researchers that "most of the mild and serious reactions which have been reported following DPT vaccination have also been reported following DTaP."[149] In fact, by 2007, updated product inserts published by DTaP vaccine manufacturers throughout the world included several dire warnings of irreversible risks and an extensive list of serious adverse reactions that have been reported following receipt of the shot. These include anaphylaxis, cyanosis, encephalitis, Guillain-Barré syndrome, convulsions, neurological disorders, autism, and sudden infant death syndrome.[150]

Adverse Reaction Reports: DTaP

This section contains a few unsolicited adverse reaction reports linking the acellular pertussis vaccine (DTaP) with serious adverse reactions:[151]

▸ "My son was given DTaP three days ago. He was very tired after the shot, but was otherwise fine. Yesterday he had a temperature of 102 with no appetite. He has been doing some jerking while he sleeps and has not been himself. I took him to the doctor this morning who told me that it has nothing to do with the DTaP vaccine. I know in my heart that the shot caused these problems. When he was two months old he had his first dose and some of the same symptoms. I called the doctor then and she said that because it was three days later it wasn't the vaccine. Now I am kicking myself for letting them convince me it was okay. I am worried sick about my son and the doctors will not admit that it could be the shot."

▸ "At eight weeks of age, the day after receiving his DTaP shots, my son displayed unequal pupil size when in dim light. I called the pediatrician right away and was told over the phone that he was fine and it was not possible that the vaccine could have caused this. After referring myself to a pedi-ophthalmologist, it was determined that he has acquired Horner's syndrome from damage to a nerve."

▸ "My son had a crying fit two weeks after the first round of shots, which included the DTaP. He was inconsolable for hours which was so unusual we were really scared. I called the doctor and she told me it was probably colic or something, and to cut garlic and dairy out of my diet, since he was nursing (still is). We were kind of unsure about getting the second round of shots, but the doctor kept telling me all of the benefits outweigh the risks and I shouldn't even think about it, so we went ahead and did them. Exactly two weeks later he had his first seizure. He was four months old then. We were in and out of the hospital for the next year and a half. The doctors performed the necessary tests, which were all negative, and kept pumping drugs into his tiny veins. We keep telling them that it was the DTaP, but they assure us that it is "acellular" and doesn't do the same damage as the DPT. But I made her sign a form making both of my kids exempt from any more shots (for school). My son is now two-and-a-half, and he still continues to have a seizure or two every few months, even on medication, and on top of it all he is developmentally delayed and speech delayed as well. I want parents out there to know it is also very possible for your baby to have a reaction to DTaP as well as DPT. My son has a life-threatening disorder. He has to take medication every day or he has 5-minute long grand mal seizures. He is only two now but I stay awake at night worrying about the future, with school, and especially going swimming at a friend's house, etc. No parent should have to experience the guilt I live with every day from giving him those poisonous shots."

▸ "My son is one year old. On his 9-month visit, he received the DTaP shot. The next two days he was doing a strange sort of jerking movement with his face that I'd never seen before. It looked like a mini-seizure. His body would tighten up when they would occur. I am now worried about getting the next DTaP shot."

▸ "My youngest daughter had a 'mild' reaction to the DPT. Her fever lasted three to four days, and she was cranky for a few weeks. My doctor suggested ½ dose for the next round; she had no reaction at all. Then we moved and her new pediatrician stated that ½ doses aren't recognized as a valid vaccination, but suggested the DTaP. Within hours she started to get a high fever, black diarrhea, and vomited. I called the doctor immediately, who stated this is a normal reaction. However, within a month her hair started falling out. I took her back to the doctor who told me to stop putting her hair into ponytails, that I was pulling her hair too tight! I am not going to get her vaccinated again."

▸ "They gave my daughter DTaP at three months after they told me there were no known side effects. I objected, but they threatened to call Child Protection Services if I refused. Being a teen parent, the fear of losing her loomed over me, so I let her have it. Within minutes of arriving home she began to scream like I had never heard before. It scared me. She screamed for 16 hours, with no break. The doctor swore that she was okay and just 'colicky.' After screaming, she became lethargic. She wouldn't even look up when I said her name, which she had always done before. She went into a seizure and ended up in the emergency room. My daughter now receives only the DT shot, and although the nurses get angry, I insist that I see the label of the shot bottle before any injections are given to her."

▸ "Two weeks ago, a lady called whose 8-year-old daughter is now paralyzed from the neck down after receiving her DTaP booster shot."

How effective is the pertussis vaccine?

The incidence and severity of whooping cough had begun to decline long before the pertussis vaccine was introduced.[152] From 1900 to 1935, the death rate from pertussis in the United States and England had already declined on its own by 79 percent and 82 percent, respectively (Figure 26).[153] A study published in the *Journal of Pediatrics* revealed that the whole-cell pertussis vaccine may be only 40 to 45 percent effective[154] —despite official claims of 63 to 91 percent efficacy.[155] Further evidence indicates immunity is not sustained. Susceptibility to pertussis just a few years after full vaccination may be as high as 95 percent.[156,157]

A 1988 Swedish study evaluated two different acellular pertussis vaccines and concluded they were 54 and 64 percent effective, respectively.[158] As a result, Swedish officials asserted that "the efficacy of the [DTaP] vaccine may be lower than that of whole-cell vaccines."[159] On this basis, along with some concerns about safety issues, they withdrew their application to license the shot.[160] However, a 1997 German study, embraced by U.S. DTaP manufacturers, claims greater efficacy—about 80 percent—but only after "adjusting" for sibling age, number of siblings in day care, well-baby visits, and father's employment status![161]

A 2006 Canadian study suggests that the current DTaP vaccine is not as effective as the older DPT shot, and may not protect young children.[162] A 2007 study published in *Clinical Infectious Diseases* found that five years after adolescents received an acellular pertussis booster shot (their 5th dose by 11-13 years of age!), pertussis toxin antibody levels were actually *lower* than they were before vaccination. In fact, they were *undetectable* in 28 percent of the subjects.[163]

Vaccine failures: In 1984, 2,187 cases of pertussis were reported to the CDC. Of the 560 patients aged 7 months to 6 years with known vaccination status, nearly half (46 percent) had received vaccine protection.[164] In 1986, 1030 cases of pertussis were reported in Kansas;[165] 90 percent of the patients were "adequately" vaccinated.[166] In 1993, during a pertussis outbreak in Ohio, 82 percent of younger children stricken with the disease had received multiple doses of the vaccine.[167] That same year, during a large pertussis outbreak in Alberta, Canada, 62 percent of the people who contracted the disease had received their "age-appropriate" shots.[168]

In 1996, there was a statewide outbreak of pertussis in Vermont, where vaccination rates were among the highest in the United States: nearly 97 percent of all children 19-35 months were properly vaccinated. Yet, their pertussis shots were not effective because 74 percent of all children 7-47 months who were stricken with the disease had received 3 to 5 doses of the vaccine (Figure 27).[169] In addition, 68 percent of all 7-18 year-olds who were stricken with the disease had received 4 or 5 doses of the pertussis vaccine.[170]

<u>Figure 26:</u>

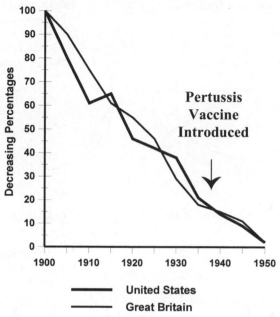

The Pertussis Death Rate
was Decreasing on its Own
Before the Vaccine was Introduced

**Pertussis
Vaccine
Introduced**

— United States
— Great Britain

From 1900 to 1935, *before* the pertussis vaccine was introduced, the death rate from pertussis in the United States and England had already declined on its own by 79 percent and 82 percent, respectively. Source: *International Mortality Statistics* (1981) by Michael Alderson.

Also in 1996, there was a large pertussis outbreak in the Netherlands. According to researchers, "our results clearly show that pertussis remained endemic with epidemic peaks in the Netherlands, *despite high vaccination coverage.*"[171] In fact, vaccine effectiveness had already begun to decline in 1994 and 1995 even though vaccination rates were as high as they've ever been. Researchers speculated that there might be "a mismatch between circulating strains and vaccine strains."[172]

In Cyprus, pertussis vaccination rates rose from 48 percent in 1980 to 98 percent by 1997. In 2003, the pertussis vaccination rate remained at 98 percent yet there was a large pertussis outbreak. According to researchers, "most cases in the outbreak had previously been vaccinated for pertussis."[173] In fact, 79 percent of everyone who contracted the disease had received 3 to 5 doses of the vaccine. Only 13 percent of all people stricken with pertussis were completely unvaccinated.[174]

In Israel, cases of pertussis rose 16-fold between 1998 and 2004, even though "national pertussis immunization coverage by age 2 years was stable during the last ten years."[175] Official figures show that every year, for the past ten years, nearly 93 percent of all 2-year-olds had received 4 doses of the pertussis vaccine and 95 percent had received at least 3 doses. In Israel, the acellular pertussis vaccine was introduced in 2002. From 2003 through 2005, compliance to pertussis vaccination actually *increased,* but pertussis incidence continued to climb.[176] Similar trends have been occurring in many other countries with high pertussis vaccination rates, including the United States, Canada, the Netherlands and France.[177]

Figure 27:

Pertussis Outbreaks Often Occur in
Highly Vaccinated Populations

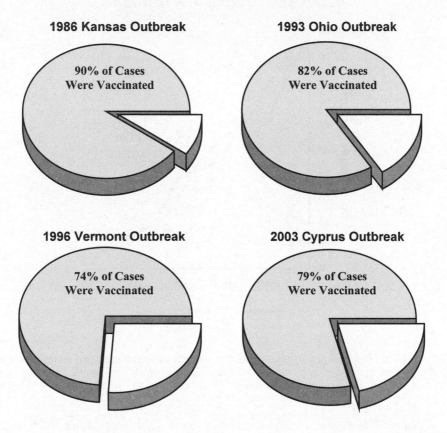

1986 Kansas Outbreak

90% of Cases
Were Vaccinated

1993 Ohio Outbreak

82% of Cases
Were Vaccinated

1996 Vermont Outbreak

74% of Cases
Were Vaccinated

2003 Cyprus Outbreak

79% of Cases
Were Vaccinated

During pertussis outbreaks in Kansas (1986), Ohio (1993), Vermont (1996), and Cyprus (2003), most of the people stricken with pertussis had been properly vaccinated against the disease. Source: The CDC and official data presented in surveillance studies.

Is the pertussis vaccine mandatory?

The CDC recommends 5 doses of DTaP for infants and children up to 7 years of age.[178] A DT shot may be a safer alternative for children at greater risk of damage from the pertussis component of the vaccine.[179] During the 1980s, 1990s and 2000s, the number of pertussis cases among adolescents and adults substantially *increased,* despite high vaccination rates.[180] Before the pertussis vaccine was introduced, more than 93 percent of all cases occurred in children. However, the vaccine shifted the epidemiological patterns of the disease. Today, the majority of cases are in adolescents and adults.[181] Thus, starting in 2005 another booster shot was urged for persons 11 through 64 years of age.[182] Vaccine exemptions are available.

Measles

What is measles?

Measles is a contagious disease that produces a pink rash all over the body. It is caused by a virus that affects the respiratory system, skin and eyes. The first symptoms appear about 10 days after becoming infected. A fever, cough, and runny nose develop, and the eyes become red, watery and sensitive to light. The fever may reach 105° F (41°C). Small pink spots with gray-white centers occur inside the mouth. A few days later, pink spots break out on the face. The rash then spreads all over the body. Once the rash reaches the feet—in two or three days—the fever drops and the runny nose and cough disappear. The rash on other parts of the body begins to fade, and the infected person starts to feel better.

Antibiotics and drugs do not work to shorten the duration or alleviate the symptoms of measles once it is contracted. Treatment mainly consists of allowing the disease to run its course. However, cool sponge baths and soothing lotions to relieve the itchy rash may be helpful. Drinking lots of liquids to prevent dehydration is recommended as well. The disease confers permanent immunity; the infected person will not contract it again.

Is measles dangerous?

Prior to the 1960s, most children in the United States and Canada caught measles. Complications from the disease were unlikely. Previously healthy children usually recovered without incident.[1] However, measles can be dangerous in populations newly exposed to the virus,[2] and in malnourished children living in undeveloped countries.[3,4] Ear infections, pneumonia, brain damage (subacute sclerosing panencephalitis), and death are some of the possibilities.[5] In advanced countries, measles can be severe when it infects people living in impoverished communities with poor nutrition, sanitation, and inadequate health care. Complications are also more likely when the disease strikes infants, adults, and anyone with a compromised immune system.[6]

Scare tactics: Doctors and other health authorities often try to frighten parents about measles by exaggerating the risks. For example, vaccine pamphlets published by the CDC claim that 1 out of every 1000 children who contract measles will get encephalitis, an infection of the brain.[7] However, Dr. Robert Mendelsohn, renowned pediatrician and vaccine researcher, had this to say: "The incidence of 1/1000 may be accurate for children who live in conditions of poverty and malnutrition" but for just about everyone else "the incidence of true encephalitis is probably more like 1/10,000 or 1/100,000."[8] Furthermore, about 75 percent of these cases will *not* show evidence of brain damage.[9]

Vitamin A and nutrition: Several studies show that when patients with measles are given vitamin A supplements, their complication rates and chances of dying are significantly reduced. For example, as early as 1932 doctors used cod-liver oil—high in vitamin A—to treat measles and lower mortality by 58 percent.[10]

Studies conducted in 1958 and 1961 confirmed that the wild measles virus has a severe short-term negative effect on immunity and the child's nutritional status, especially vitamin A and nitrogen metabolism.[11,12] Nevertheless, antibiotics—later shown to be ineffective at treating measles—soon replaced vitamin A therapy, and by the 1960s vaccinations gained preference over treatment protocols. During the mid-1980s new studies demonstrated an increased risk of diarrhea, respiratory disease, and death in children with mild vitamin A deficiency.[13,14]

In a 1987 study conducted in Tanzania, Africa, 180 children with measles were randomly divided into two groups and received routine treatment alone or with 200,000 i.u. of orally administered vitamin A. Mortality rates in the vitamin A group were cut in half. In fact, children under two years of age who did not receive vitamin A were nearly eight times more likely to die (Figure 28).[15]

Figure 28:

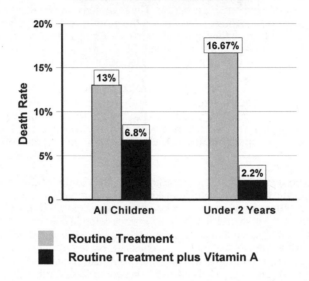

Vitamin A *Reduces* the Measles Death Rate

African children with measles were divided into two groups. The first group received routine treatment. The second group received the same treatment plus 200,000 i.u of vitamin A on hospital admission and again the next day. The death rate in children receiving the vitamin A was half that of those receiving routine treatment alone—just 6.8% compared to 13%. The difference in mortality was even greater in children under 2 years of age—just 2.2% compared to 16.67%. Source: *British Medical Journal* (January 31, 1987):294-96.

In 1990, the *New England Journal of Medicine* confirmed that vitamin A supplements significantly reduce measles complication and death rates.[16] In 1992, researchers measured vitamin A levels in children with measles and determined that deficiencies were associated with lower levels of measles-specific antibodies, higher and longer lasting fevers, and a greater probability of being hospitalized.[17] The authors of the study recommended vitamin A therapy for children under two years of age with severe measles.[18] A 1993 study showed that 72 percent of all measles cases in the U.S. requiring hospitalization are deficient in vitamin A. The greater the deficiency, the worse the complications and higher the probability of dying.[19]

Malnutrition is clearly responsible for higher disease complication and death rates.[20] According to David Morley, infectious disease expert, "Severity of measles is greatest in the developing countries where children have nutritional deficiencies... The child with severe measles and an immune system suppressed by malnutrition secretes the virus three times longer than does a child with normal nutrition."[21] Dr. Viera Scheibner, vaccine researcher, summarizes the data more succinctly: *"Children in Third World countries need improved vitamin A and general nutritional status, not vaccines."*[22]

Fever reducers: Poor nutrition and a vitamin A deficiency are not the only factors known to increase measles complication and mortality rates. Standard treatment protocols may be detrimental as well. For example, when doctors administer antipyretics (fever reducers, such as aspirin) to control the rising temperature in measles patients, greater

Figure 29:

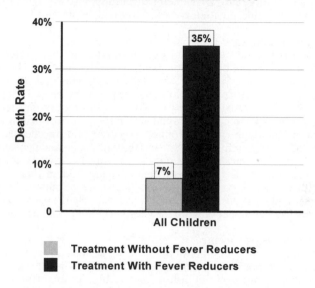

Fever Reducers *Increase* the Measles Death Rate

Treatment Without Fever Reducers

Treatment With Fever Reducers

African children with measles were divided into groups. The first group received routine treatment, including antipyretics (aspirin, salicylates, etc.). The second group did not receive antipyretics. Mortality was five times greater in the group that had their fevers suppressed. Source: Abstract of a 1967-68 measles epidemic study conducted in Ghana.

---

problems are likely. In one study during a measles epidemic in Ghana, Africa, children were divided into two groups. One group received antipyretics—typical treatment at many hospitals. Mortality was five times greater than in the group that did not receive this treatment (Figure 29).[23] Researchers concluded that "children with the most violent, highly febrile form of the disease actually had the best prognosis."[24]

In another study conducted in Afghanistan, 200 children with measles were divided into two groups. Once again, members of one group received aspirin to lower fever. The study revealed that children who received the antipyretics had prolonged illness, more diarrhea, ear infections and respiratory ailments, such as pneumonia, bronchitis and laryngitis, and significantly greater mortality rates.[25] According to Dr. Harold Buttram, who studied the data, "it could be inferred that interference with the natural course of the disease significantly dampened the immune responses of the children."[26] The authors of the study noted that the "adverse effect of antipyretics, which makes the course of the disease longer, facilitates superinfections which give rise to high mortality."[27] This study also suggests that "children suffering from measles should be kept warm enough in order to have fever and pass the disease safely."[28]

Dr. Robert Mendelsohn agrees that fevers should not be suppressed: "Doctors do a great disservice to you and your child when they prescribe drugs to reduce his fever... When your child contracts an infection, the fever that accompanies it is a blessing, not a curse... A rising body temperature simply indicates that the process of healing is speeding up. It is something to rejoice over, not to fear."[29]

Other researchers have noted that "the development of cancer may quite possibly have been given a boost in certain cases through the repression of febrile conditions."[30] In fact, pyrexia (a condition resulting from fever *inducers*) has been used in the prevention and treatment of carcinomas.[31] Despite the evidence implicating antipyretics in prolonging disease and raising mortality rates, Dr. Scheibner ruefully observes that "the relentless suppression of fever in children with measles is still widely practiced."[32]

Does a measles vaccine exist?
In 1758, Francis Home conducted the first experiments to prevent measles by inserting measles-infected blood into deliberate cuts made on healthy people.[33] He claimed that his "variolation" technique caused a milder form of the disease. However, it was not without danger; variolation was known to spread syphilis, tuberculosis, and several other diseases.[34] In 1940, the U.S. military tested an experimental measles vaccine on enlisted personnel. Following severe reactions, the program was ended.[35] In 1954, a team of virologists headed by John F. Enders, an American scientist, found a way to separate the measles virus from other substances and grow it in living cells.[36] In 1960, Enders' vaccine was tested, and in 1963 both a live-virus shot and an inactivated vaccine were licensed. By the mid-1960s, several measles vaccines were being given to millions of young children in the U.S. However, in 1967 the inactivated vaccine was removed from the market because it did not provide long-term immunity and was causing "atypical" measles.[37] By the early 1970s, Canada and other countries had begun nationwide measles vaccination campaigns.[38,39]

How safe is the measles vaccine?
The measles vaccine has a long history of causing serious adverse reactions. The pharmaceutical company responsible for producing the measles vaccine publishes an extensive list of ailments known to have occurred following the shot. Severe afflictions affecting nearly every body system—blood, lymphatic, digestive, cardiovascular, immune, nervous, respiratory, and sensory—have been linked to this "preventive" inoculation. These include: encephalitis, subacute sclerosing panencephalitis (SSPE), Guillain-Barré syndrome, febrile and afebrile convulsions, seizures, ataxia, ocular palsies, anaphylaxis, angioneurotic edema, bronchial spasms, panniculitis, vasculitis, atypical measles, thrombocytopenia, lymph-adenopathy, leukocytosis, pneumonitis, Stevens-Johnson syndrome, erythema multiforme, urticaria, deafness, otitis media, retinitis, optic neuritis, rash, fever, dizziness, headache, and death (Figure 30).[40]

The manufacturer also warns that the measles vaccine "has not been evaluated for carcinogenic or mutagenic potential" and "it is...not known whether [it] can cause fetal harm when administered to a pregnant woman or can affect reproductive capacity." Thus, "it would be prudent to assume that the vaccine strain of virus is...capable of inducing adverse fetal effects... Caution should be exercised when...administered to a nursing woman."[41]

Subacute sclerosing panencephalitis: Scientific documentation confirming adverse reactions to the measles vaccine is well established. For example, subacute sclerosing panencephalitis (SSPE), a slow, progressive disease that begins with mental deterioration and muscle spasms, then progresses over months or years to convulsions, coma, and death, was first recorded following measles vaccine in 1968, shortly after this shot was introduced.[42] The following year, a federal SSPE registry was established to document the growing number of cases being reported.[43] Shortly thereafter, the *Journal of the American Medical Association* published an extensive report on this disturbing new development.[44] By 1997, it was clear that children vaccinated with measles (or MMR) would continue to run the risk of contracting SSPE. For example, researchers documented the case of a 13-year-old girl whose intellectual and physical functioning prior to the development of illness had been very good. After contracting SSPE, "the child verbalized little and was socially inappropriate; her memory and thinking abilities were impaired. She grew progressively worse, and added myoclonic jerks of the upper limbs, with depressed tendon reflexes." The authors concluded that subacute sclerosing panencephalitis was a delayed adverse effect of measles vaccine.[45] In fact, the National Institutes of Health considers SSPE a

Figure 30:

Adverse Reactions: Measles Vaccine

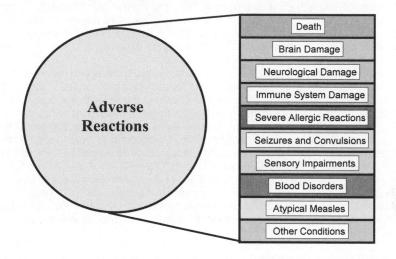

Severe afflictions affecting nearly every body system—blood, lymphatic, digestive, cardiovascular, immune, nervous, respiratory, and sensory—have been linked to the measles vaccine. Source: The vaccine manufacturer's product inserts and the *Physician's Desk Reference* (PDR).

"late" complication of measles, and reports that this slow virus infection occurs "an average of seven years after initial exposure."[46]

Encephalitis and Guillain-Barré syndrome: Other neurological disorders following measles vaccination are well documented in the medical literature. In the United States, shortly after the measles vaccine was introduced, 59 cases of central nervous system damage following vaccination were reported to the CDC.[47] In 1964, the Medical Research Council in Great Britain tested the new measles vaccine and discovered that 1 of every 532 vaccinated children experienced convulsions—more than six times the rate in unvaccinated children.[48] From 1968 to 1974, Great Britain documented 47 cases of encephalitis (brain inflammation) and 122 cases of febrile convulsions following measles vaccination.[49,50] By 1975, Canadian researchers were reporting the same problems. For example, "In a previously well child with no evidence of pre-existing immunologic defect, a fatal encephalitis developed 10 days after administration of measles vaccine."[51] Japanese children were also experiencing encephalitis following their shots.[52] In 1983, *Lancet* published a report identifying 26 additional cases of convulsions after vaccination.[53] In 1984, Germany documented meningoencephalitis in a 15-month-old girl "seven days after measles/mumps vaccination." She died three days later.[54] In 1999, Spanish researchers confirmed that children vaccinated with measles remain at risk for neurological disorders. They present the case of a 16-month-old baby with "self-limiting acute encephalopathy characterized by cerebellar ataxia and alterations in behavior." The child also showed clinical signs of attenuated measles, a classical indication that the condition resulted from the shot. They believe that such reactions may be underreported.[55] Other studies document the occurrence of Guillain-Barré syndrome (GBS)—an autoimmune and nervous system disease resulting in paralysis—following measles vaccination.[56-59] Today, the FDA and CDC continue to receive reports of severe neurological disorders following injections with the measles (or MMR) vaccine.[60]

Blood disorders: Thrombocytopenia, a blood disease resulting in spontaneous bleeding, is a well-known adverse reaction to the measles vaccine. As early as 1966, researchers noted that 86 percent of vaccinated individuals experienced an extreme drop in platelet levels needed for clotting blood.[61] During the 1970s, 1980s, 1990s, and 2000s, wherever measles vaccination campaigns were enforced, including in Sweden,[62] Canada,[63] Germany,[64] Finland,[65] Great Britain,[66] and France,[67] new cases of thrombocytopenia were reported. In 1994, the U.S. Vaccine Safety Committee officially acknowledged thrombocytopenia as an adverse reaction to the measles vaccine.[68] Subsequent data supports this conclusion.[69-71]

Sensory impairments: Optic neuritis (eye damage) and hearing loss following measles (or MMR) vaccination are also well established in the medical literature. In 1978, researchers documented "partial vision loss" 22 days subsequent to the measles vaccine.[72] In 1985, researchers wrote about a 16-month-old baby who began "walking into objects" 14 days after her shot. An ophthalmologic examination revealed minimal light perception, "diffuse chorioretinitis with perivascular retinal edema" and other ocular changes "consistent with measles retinopathy."[73] In another 1985 study, researchers documented "severe bilateral deafness" 10 days subsequent to the measles vaccine.[74] In 1988, the *British Medical Journal* published a report on "total deafness" in one ear 11 days after the measles vaccine.[75] In 1991, the *New England Journal of Medicine* published a report on "permanent bilateral hearing loss" 22 days subsequent to the measles vaccine.[76] And in 1993, several cases of "profound hearing loss" following measles vaccination were documented in the medical literature.[77]

Immune system suppression: In 1981, researchers reported that the measles vaccine depresses the ability of disease-fighting lymphocytes to perform their duties.[78] In 1992, researchers again confirmed that health-enhancing lymphocytes decline in number following measles vaccination.[79] Dr. Richard Moskowitz, vaccine researcher, offers a possible explanation. He believes that the weakened measles virus injected directly into the blood may cause antibodies to inhibit an acute inflammatory response to the virus. Months or years later, during periods of stress, they may begin to attack the body's own cells resulting in an autoimmune crisis.[80] Moskowitz surmised that the unnatural process of vaccination can lead to slow viruses developing in the body. These may bring about the "far less curable chronic diseases of the present."[81] Also, "these illnesses may be more serious than the original disease, involving deeper structures [and] more vital organs."[82]

Inflammatory bowel disease: In 1995, *Lancet* published a landmark study by Dr. Andrew Wakefield and his team of medical researchers showing that babies vaccinated with measles are at greater risk than unvaccinated children to develop inflammatory bowel disease later in life. Scientists believe that the vaccine, which contains attenuated measles virus, provokes the immune system into attacking its own intestinal cells. The study found one case of inflammatory bowel disease for every 142 people vaccinated against measles. In fact, people who received the measles vaccine were 2½ times more likely to develop ulcerative colitis and three times more likely to develop Crohn's disease when compared to unvaccinated controls (Figure 31).[83]

Wakefield's conclusions are supported by other factors: 1) The incidence of inflammatory bowel disease has increased over the past few decades, a period coinciding with the routine use of live measles vaccines.[84,85] 2) At least two studies, one conducted in Sweden, the other by Japanese researchers, seem to confirm a positive association between the measles virus and the development of Crohn's disease.[86,87] (Furthermore, Dr. Viera Scheibner, who analyzed the Swedish data, concluded that "exposure to *natural* [wild-type virus] measles in early infancy *protected* against the bowel diseases.")[88] 3) The measles virus had previously been discovered in the inflamed intestinal walls of bowel disease victims, and "persistent measles virus infection" in Crohn's disease victims had already been confirmed.[89-91] 4) Wakefield's measles-vaccinated cohort had a significantly higher rate of inflammatory bowel disease than his unvaccinated cohort, yet the overall rate in the unvaccinated group was higher than that found in previous studies.[92,93] Therefore, "the

Figure 31:

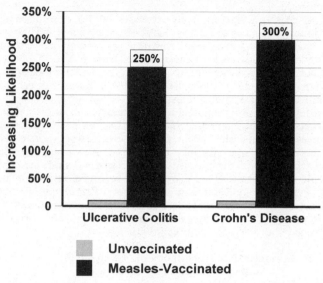

The Measles Vaccine and
Inflammatory Bowel Disease

Unvaccinated

Measles-Vaccinated

People who received the measles vaccine were 2½ times more likely to develop ulcerative colitis and three times more likely to develop Crohn's disease when compared to unvaccinated controls. Source: *Lancet* (April 29, 1995).

---

increased risk of inflammatory bowel disease in the vaccine cohort is not due to an abnormally low prevalence [in the unvaccinated group]" and Wakefield's conclusions may have been understated.[94] 5) In 1998, Dr. Wakefield and his associates published a more sophisticated study in *Lancet*, once again illustrating a probable link between the measles component of the MMR vaccine, intestinal aberrations, and chronic inflammation of the colon.[95]

According to Dr. Albert Knapp, of the Department of Gastroenterology at Lenox Hill Hospital in New York, the link between the measles virus and bowel disease makes sense. It appears that in some people the body is unable to recognize its own intestinal cells, so it develops antibodies that attack them, causing inflammation. Knapp thinks that "vaccination could stimulate the [antibodies] that lead to Crohn's [disease] in certain people who are genetically predisposed to it."[96]

Severe allergic reactions: Some people are hypersensitive to ingredients in the measles vaccine, such as egg proteins (from the chick embryo cell cultures used to propagate the measles virus), neomycin (an antibiotic) and hydrolyzed gelatin.[97] This can lead to anaphylaxis, an extreme allergic reaction that may cause the victim's heart to stop or throat to swell cutting off oxygen, painful abdominal cramps, seizures, shock, collapse, and death.[98] Numerous reports of anaphylaxis following measles (and MMR) vaccination have been documented in England,[99] Norway,[100] Australia,[101] Canada,[102] the USA,[103,104] and Japan.[105]

Atypical measles: From 1963 to 1967, nearly two million doses of the inactivated measles vaccine were given to children before authorities pulled the shot off the market because it was causing a severe form of measles when the youngsters came into contact with the natural virus.[106] The illness is characterized by an atypical rash that progresses in a reverse manner: it starts on the extremities and moves toward the center of the body. Other symptoms include fever, headache, muscle aches, peripheral edema (swelling of the hands and feet), abdominal pain, persistent vomiting, and severe pneumonia.[107] The condition is painful and long-lasting, with some symptoms remaining up to six months after the acute episode.[108]

Often, atypical measles is "incompletely expressed."[109] For example, a rash does not always occur.[110] In such instances, the disease may be misdiagnosed and underreported.[111] Authorities warn practitioners not to confuse it with meningococcemia or rickettsial diseases.[112] Authorities also acknowledge that there is no time limit between vaccination and the onset of atypical measles. It can strike several months or years later, and has proven to be a continuing problem.[113,114] During the 1960s, 1970s and 1980s, it was "a disease of significant morbidity in young adults and some adolescents."[115]

Atypical measles also occurs in children, adolescents and adults who originally received the inactivated vaccine and are later revaccinated with the live measles virus.[116] However, anyone who receives the live measles vaccine may be at risk for a very severe and potentially fatal "vaccine strain measles virus infection," not just those who received the dead vaccine and were later revaccinated with the live virus.[117] For example, a study in *Pediatrics* noted that several people who contracted the disease "had received only attenuated measles virus vaccines."[118] A study published in another issue of *Pediatrics* described cases of "exaggerated natural measles" following live virus measles vaccination.[119] In addition, a report in *Lancet* noted that atypical measles syndrome (AMS) "has also been observed in people immunized with live vaccine preparations."[120]

<u>Congressional Testimony of Wendy Scholl</u>
Mother of a measles vaccine victim

The following excerpt is from a statement made by a distraught mother testifying before Congress. (More adverse reaction reports possibly linked to the measles vaccine may be found in the chapters on MMR and autism.)

My name is Wendy Scholl. I reside in the state of Florida with my husband, Gary, and three daughters, Stacy, Holly, and Jackie. Let me stress that all three of our daughters were born healthy, normal babies. I am here to tell of Stacy's reaction to the measles vaccine...where according to the medical profession, anything within 7 to 10 days after the vaccine to do with neurological sequelae or seizures or brain damage fits a measles reaction....

At 16 months old, Stacy received her measles shot. She was a happy, healthy, normal baby, typical, curious, playful until the 10th day after her shot when I walked into her room to find her laying in her crib, flat on her stomach, her head twisted to one side. Her eyes were glassy and affixed. She was panting, struggling to breathe. Her small body lay in a pool of blood that hung from her mouth. It was a terrifying sight, yet at that point I didn't realize that my happy, bouncing baby was never to be the same.

When we arrived at the emergency room, Stacy's temperature was 107 degrees. The first four days of Stacy's hospital stay she battled for life. She was in a coma and had kidney failure. Her lungs filled with fluid and she had ongoing seizures.

Her diagnosis was 'post-vaccinal encephalitis' and her prognosis was grave. She was paralyzed on her left side, prone to seizures, had visual problems. However, we were told by doctors we were extremely lucky. I didn't feel lucky. We were horrified that this vaccine which was given only to ensure that she would have a safer childhood, almost killed her. I didn't know that the possibility of this type of reaction even existed. But now, it is our reality.[121]

How effective is the measles vaccine?
During the pre-vaccine era, measles was a common childhood illness. Nearly everyone contracted it by the age of 10 and developed permanent immunity as a result.[122] After the vaccine was introduced, measles declined to an average of 3000 cases per year in

Figure 32:

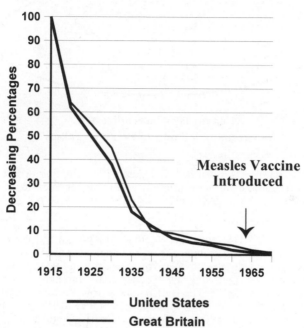

The Measles Death Rate was Decreasing on its Own *Before* the Vaccine was Introduced

Measles Vaccine Introduced

Decreasing Percentages

1915   1925   1935   1945   1955   1965

━━━━━━ **United States**

━━━━━━ **Great Britain**

From 1915 to 1958, *before* the measles vaccine was introduced, the measles death rate in the United States and Great Britain had already declined on its own by 98 percent. Source: *International Mortality Statistics* 1981:182-83.

---

the 1980s, and even fewer cases per year during the 1990s.[123] However, a significant decline in measles began long before the vaccine was introduced. From 1958 to 1962, the number of cases toppled by 38 percent.[124] The measles death rate tumbled on its own even more. In 1900, there were 13.3 measles deaths in the United States per 100,000 population. By 1955, eight years *before* the first measles shot, the death rate had declined on its own by 97.7 percent to .03 deaths per 100,000.[125] Figures published in *International Mortality Statistics* confirm this reduction: from 1915 to 1958, the measles death rate in the U.S. and U.K. declined by 98 percent (Figure 32).[126]

Eradication: In 1933, A.W. Hedrich published a study on epidemiological patterns of measles. He concluded that when 68 percent of children less than 15 years of age are immune to the disease, epidemics do not develop.[127] Today, authorities retain this general idea—that a precise degree of "herd immunity" will prevent epidemics—but are unclear about the level required to achieve it.

In 1991, the CDC concluded that measles outbreaks can be avoided if 70 to 80 percent of two-year-olds in inner cities are vaccinated.[128] A 1992 study published in the *Journal of the American Medical Association* also concluded that "immunization coverage of two-year-olds of 80 percent or less may be sufficient to prevent sustained measles outbreaks

Figure 33:

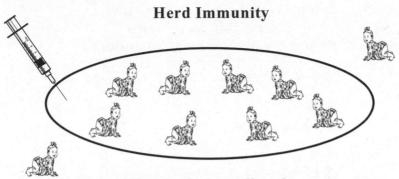

Herd Immunity

**Can measles be eradicated
by vaccinating 8 or 9 of every 10 babies?**

Scientists believe that measles can be eradicated by vaccinating 80% to 100% of the population. Theoretically, such "herd" immunity will interrupt measles transmission and end epidemics. Source: *Infect Med* 1997; 14(4): 297-300, 310.

---

in urban communities."[129] However, the World Health Organization (WHO) estimates that "over 95 percent" of the population must be vaccinated to eliminate the disease.[130] Other authorities acknowledge that "the level of coverage required to prevent transmission of measles is unknown."[131] Outbreaks have occurred in communities where 97 percent of the population was "protected."[132] This has led some researchers to suspect that "indigenous transmission" of measles cannot be stopped unless "close to 100 percent coverage" is achieved with a vaccine that is 90 to 98 percent effective (Figure 33).[133]

When the measles vaccine was introduced in 1963, officials were confident that they could eradicate the disease by 1967.[134] That did not occur. In 1978, the federal government announced that its new goal was to eradicate measles from the country by 1982.[135] That did not occur. In 1990, after examining 320 scientific works from around the world, 180 European medical doctors concluded that "the eradication of measles...would today appear to be an unrealistic goal."[136] Professor D. Levy of Johns Hopkins University also weighed the odds of eradicating measles with mass immunization campaigns and concluded that if current practices [of suppressing natural immunity] continue, by the year 2050 a large part of the population will be at risk and "there could in theory be over 25,000 fatal cases of measles in the USA."[137] Nevertheless, in 1994 authorities once again targeted measles for eradication from the Western Hemisphere, this time by the year 2000.[138] As the year 2000 drew near, the CDC announced its new goal (again) to eradicate measles by 2010.[139]

Immunity: The measles vaccine does not confer permanent immunity—one reason eradication of the disease is so elusive. Epidemics regularly occur in vaccinated populations. Dr. William Atkinson, senior epidemiologist with the CDC, admitted that "measles transmission has been clearly documented among vaccinated persons. In some large outbreaks...over 95 percent of cases have a history of vaccination."[140] In fact, according to WHO, the odds are about 15 times greater that measles will strike those vaccinated against the disease than those who are left alone.[141]

The medical literature is replete with documented vaccine failures. For example, in 1970 and 1971 there was a measles outbreak in St. Louis, Missouri; 50 percent of all cases were in vaccinated people.[142] In 1977, there was an outbreak of measles at the University of California, Los Angeles (UCLA) in a population considered 91 percent immune.[143] In 1978 and 1979, an outbreak of measles occurred in a Rhode Island junior high school.

Only 22 percent of the cases were in unvaccinated students.[144] In 1984, 58 percent of all school-aged children in the U.S. who contracted measles were adequately vaccinated.[145] Authorities claimed that 66 percent of all measles cases that year were "nonpreventable," but 59 percent (992 of 1,669 cases) occurred in people who had been properly vaccinated.[146] Also in 1984, there was a measles outbreak in New Mexico junior high schools; 98 percent of the cases were in recently vaccinated students.[147] During a 1984 outbreak in an Illinois high school, 100 percent of the cases occurred in previously vaccinated students.[148] In 1985, 80 percent of all cases of measles in the U.S. occurred in children who had been properly vaccinated.[149] That same year, there was an outbreak of measles in Corpus Christi, Texas. The student body was fully immunized, with more than 99 percent showing proof of measles vaccination.[150]

In 1985 and 1986, in states with stringent immunization requirements, between 61 and 90 percent of all measles cases occurred in "appropriately" vaccinated individuals.[151] In 1986, during a measles outbreak in Arkansas, it was discovered that 54 percent of all cases were in vaccinated people.[152] That same year, there was an outbreak in Dane County, Wisconsin; 96 percent of the cases had records of prior measles vaccination.[153] In 1987, 72 percent of all measles cases in Minnesota occurred in vaccinated people.[154] In 1988, 69 percent of all school-aged children in the U.S. who contracted measles were vaccinated.[155] In 1989, during a measles outbreak in Quebec, Canada, 58 percent of all school-age cases were previously vaccinated.[156] In the U.S., the number of cases climbed to over 18,000, yet 89 percent of all school-aged measles victims had been vaccinated.[157] In 1990, the CDC recorded more than 27,000 cases of measles, despite high vaccination rates.[158] In 1993, numerous children in the Philippines died from an outbreak of measles "caused by an inferior vaccine."[159] In 1995, 56 percent of all measles cases in the U.S. occurred in people who were previously vaccinated.[160] In 1996, measles outbreaks occurred primarily among children who had prior vaccinations.[161] And in 1999, the CDC continued to document many cases of measles in previously vaccinated individuals (Figure 34).[162]

Vaccination and revaccination: In 1963, the age for measles vaccination was arbitrarily set at nine months. In 1965, the age was raised to 12 months, and raised again in 1976 to 15 months. The vaccine is largely ineffective when given prior to this age.[163] In fact, children vaccinated at 12 to 14 months are three times more likely to contract measles than those vaccinated at a later date.[164]

Despite changes to the measles vaccination schedule, outbreaks continued to occur in fully vaccinated populations. Some answers were provided when researchers studying vaccine efficacy analyzed immune levels of California children who had received a measles shot. Those who were vaccinated for the first time showed an average post-immunization antibody titer level of 73. One year later, the protective antibody levels dropped by 59 percent to 30.[165] Data from this study seemed to confirm the short-lived efficacy of the measles vaccine, and may have contributed to the authorities' answer to an ineffective vaccine: revaccination. However, the California study also examined children who received "booster" doses and found that second shots caused only a modest rise in titer levels. After one year, the level was almost back to where it had been before the second shot. The data indicated that "a booster dose might not have any lasting effect on waning immunity."[166] Nevertheless, the Advisory Committee for Immunization Practices (ACIP) recommended a booster shot to school-aged children (4 to 6 years old)—even though experts acknowledged that the "optimal timing and frequency of boosters" is unknown and controversial.[167] Today, a second shot is administered prior to entering school, although the American Academy of Pediatrics disagreed with this advice and advocated a second shot at 11 to 12 years of age.[168]

Some authorities have other ideas about when and how often to vaccinate. Dr. Ciro A. de Quadros, Immunization Director with the Pan American Health Organization, recommends vaccinating all children nine months to 14 years old followed by an aggressive campaign every four years to vaccinate all children 1 to 4 years old, *regardless of prior disease or vaccination history.*[169]

Figure 34:

Outbreaks of Measles
in Vaccinated Populations

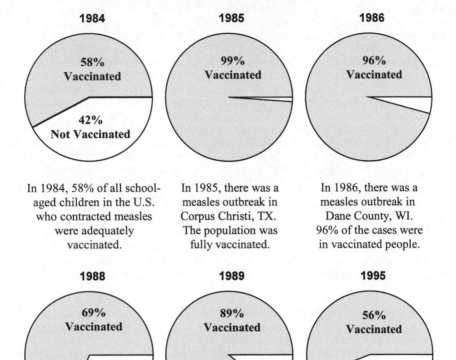

1984

58%
Vaccinated

42%
Not Vaccinated

In 1984, 58% of all school-aged children in the U.S. who contracted measles were adequately vaccinated.

1985

99%
Vaccinated

In 1985, there was a measles outbreak in Corpus Christi, TX. The population was fully vaccinated.

1986

96%
Vaccinated

In 1986, there was a measles outbreak in Dane County, WI. 96% of the cases were in vaccinated people.

1988

69%
Vaccinated

In 1988, 69% of all school-aged children in the U.S. who contracted measles were adequately vaccinated.

1989

89%
Vaccinated

In 1989, 89% of all school-aged children in the U.S. who contracted measles were adequately vaccinated.

1995

56%
Vaccinated

44%
Not Vaccinated

In 1995, 56% of all measles cases in the U.S. occurred in people who were previously vaccinated.

Source: *New England Journal of Medicine* 1987; 316:771-74. *Journal of the American Medical Association* 1990; 263:2467-71. Several CDC *MMWRs*.

Epidemiological changes: The measles vaccine dramatically altered distribution of the disease by shifting incidence rates from age-groups unlikely to experience problems (children 5 to 9 years old) to age-groups most likely to suffer from severe complications (infants, teenagers, and adults). In 1963, *before* the measles vaccine was introduced, it was extremely rare for babies under one year old to develop measles. Their mothers had previously contracted measles naturally and developed protective antibodies that were passed on to their children during birth. These babies were secure from measles for the first 15 months of life (Figure 35).[170]

Figure 35:

Maternal Antibodies Protect Babies

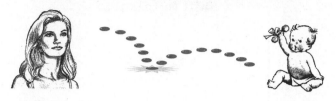

Unvaccinated	**Mama's**
Mother	**Baby**
(Previously contracted	**(Maternal antibodies**
natural measles)	**protect against measles)**

Mothers who contract measles naturally develop protective antibodies that are passed on to their children during birth. These babies are secure from measles for the first 15 months of life. In contrast, babies born to measles-vaccinated mothers are susceptible to the disease during the crucial early months when measles can be especially dangerous. Source: *Pediatrics* 1996; 97:53-58.

After the measles vaccine was introduced, fewer mothers had natural immunity. By 1992, at least 28 percent of all measles cases were now occurring in infants (Figure 36).[171] CDC officials admit this situation is likely to get worse, and attribute it to the growing number of mothers who were vaccinated.[172] In some regions of the country, the problem *is* worse. For example, in Brownsville, Texas, 45 percent of all measles cases were in babies under one year old.[173]

A recent study published in *Pediatrics* confirmed that infants of mothers born after 1963 are 7½ times more likely to contract the disease than infants of mothers born earlier.[174] In 2000, the *Journal of Medical Virology* published a study demonstrating that blood serum taken from women with natural immunity to the measles virus (due to having acquired measles naturally) has the capacity to neutralize many more wild-type measles strains than blood serum taken from vaccinated women. Only two of 20 wild-type viruses were not neutralized by at least 75 percent of the women with natural immunity. In contrast, 10 of the wild-type viruses were unable to be neutralized by at least 75 percent of the vaccinated women.[175] The researchers noted that "with an increasing proportion of mothers being vaccinated, the number of infants susceptible to resistant wild-type viruses may increase dramatically."[176]

Today, a higher percentage of teenagers and adults are suffering from measles than ever before. From 1960 to 1964, *before* the measles vaccine was introduced, only 10 percent of cases were in persons over age 10, and just three percent in persons 15 years and older. By 1977, *after* the vaccine was introduced, 60 percent of all cases occurred in persons over age 10, while 1 of every 4 cases (26 percent) struck persons 15 years and older.[177]

In 1977 and 1978, during a measles outbreak in England, 30 percent of the cases were in persons over 15 years of age.[178] In 1978 and 1979, during an outbreak of measles in Rhode Island, 78 percent of the cases occurred in persons over age 10.[179] In 1995, 37 percent of all cases were occurring in adults 20 years or older.[180] By 1999, the CDC confirmed that at least 50 percent of all measles cases were still occurring in high-risk age groups that were not susceptible to measles during the pre-vaccine era (Figure 37).[181]

The risk of measles-related pneumonia and liver abnormalities is greater in the adolescent and young adult age-groups. According to a study published in the *Journal of Infectious Diseases,* such complications have increased by as much as 20 percent.[182] The risk of death from measles is also much higher for infants and adults than for children.[183]

Figure 36:

The Changing Epidemiology of Measles: A Shift to Infants

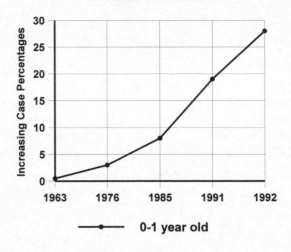

━━●━━ 0-1 year old

In 1963, *before* the measles vaccine was introduced, it was extremely rare for babies under one year old to develop measles. Their mothers had contracted the disease naturally so the babies were protected by maternal antibodies received at birth. By 1992, several years *after* the vaccine was introduced, fewer mothers had natural immunity and 28 percent of all cases were in infants. Source: CDC.

Deadly, Experimental Measles Vaccines: A CDC and WHO Catastrophe

In developing countries where children are malnourished, where health care is inadequate, and measles is common, fatality rates between 5 and 10 percent are possible.[184-186] However, infants up to five months old are usually protected by maternal antibodies that they received during birth.[187-189] Standard measles vaccines do not work in babies under nine months.[190] Thus, authorities reasoned that if an effective vaccine could be developed for this vulnerable period—from 5 to 9 months—the measles death rate could be lowered.

Scientists pinned their hopes for a new vaccine on "high-titer" shots that are 10 to 500 times more potent than standard measles vaccines.[191] In the early 1980s, they tested one of these—the Edmonston-Zagreb (EZ-HT) strain—on Mexican and Gambian babies 4 to 6 months old.[192-195] During the next few years this high-titer measles vaccine was also tested on babies in Guinea-Bissau, Togo, Senegal, Haiti, and impoverished minority communities in Los Angeles, California.[196-202] The general public was informed that EZ-HT "produces a better immunological response than standard vaccines," but studies prove that it was experimental and deadly.[203]

The Senegal study:

From 1987 to 1989, scientists set up a research center near 30 remote villages in central Senegal. Their stated primary objective was to study the clinical efficacy of two high-titer measles vaccines: Edmonston-Zagreb (EZ-HT) and Schwartz (SW-HT).[204] However, researchers had already done several studies demonstrating that high-titer measles vaccines produce a better immunological response than standard vaccines when given to children younger than nine months and as early as four months.[205] Therefore, scientists conducting the Senegal

Figure 37:

The Changing Epidemiology of Measles:
A Shift to Older Age Groups

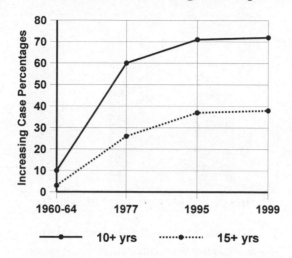

From 1960 to 1964, *before* the measles vaccine was introduced, only 10 percent of cases occurred in persons over age 10, and just 3 percent in persons 15 years or older. By 1977, *after* the measles vaccine was introduced, 60 percent of all cases were in persons over age 10, while 1 of every 4 cases (26 percent) struck persons 15 years and older. This trend continues today. Source: *Hospital Practice,* July 1980. CDC, *MMWR* 2000; 49(25):557-60.

---

study may have had another agenda. In fact, an elaborate "mortality surveillance" was established to check safety, evaluate the vaccination strategy, and perform "independent checks on child deaths."[206]

Researchers may have suspected the vaccine was dangerous when the results of earlier studies began to filter in. But they were probably reluctant to abandon their high-titer shot without testing it at least one more time to be sure. Senegal must have seemed ideal; the region was extremely remote, and less than four percent of the mothers who "consented" to the study were literate.[207]

To begin the study, researchers randomly assigned comparable children to three vaccine groups: a) EZ-HT administered at five months; b) SW-HT given at five months; and c) placebo at five months, followed by a standard low-titer measles vaccine at 10 months. All of the children were followed for up to three years. When the results were tabulated (using eight statistical procedures) it became clear that children who received the high-titer measles vaccines had significantly higher mortality at 41 months than children in the standard low-titer measles vaccine group. But they were not dying from measles. *Most of the deaths were from other common childhood diseases.* Apparently, the high-titer measles vaccines lowered overall immunity making the children fatally susceptible to diarrhea, dysentery, malaria, malnutrition, acute respiratory ailments, and other infectious diseases.[208]

Children who received the Schwartz strain (SW-HT) died of other diseases at a rate *51 percent higher* than children who received a standard vaccine. This translates into 48 excess deaths for every 1000 babies vaccinated. Children who received the Edmonston-Zagreb strain (EZ-HT) died of other diseases at a rate *80 percent higher* than children who received a standard vaccine. There were 75 excess deaths for every 1000 babies vaccinated (Figure 38).[209] Mortality remained consistently high in the second and third year after the EZ-HT

Figure 38:

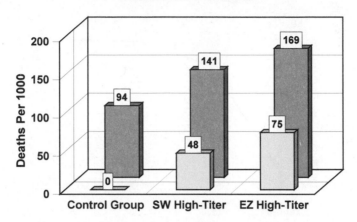

High-Titer Measles Vaccines and Excess Deaths

Total Deaths Per 1000 Babies Vaccinated

Excess Deaths Per 1000 Babies Vaccinated

Senegal babies were vaccinated with either a) a standard measles vaccine (the control group), b) a high-titer Schwartz vaccine (SW-HT), or c) a high-titer Edmonston-Zagreb vaccine (EZ-HT). During the following 36 months, fatality rates were recorded. Children who received the high-titer vaccines died *from other causes* at significantly greater rates. In fact, children who received the SW-HT died of other diseases at a rate *51 percent higher* than children who received a standard vaccine—48 excess deaths for every 1000 babies vaccinated. Children who received EZ-HT died of other diseases at a rate *80 percent higher* than children who received a standard vaccine—75 excess deaths for every 1000 babies vaccinated. Source: *Lancet* (October 12, 1991).

---

vaccine was administered, whereas it declined substantially in the control group. *One of every six babies vaccinated with EZ-HT died within three years* (Figure 39).[210]

When it started to become clear that mortality in the high-titer vaccine groups was excessive, researchers refused to end the study. Instead, they sought out new babies to take part in more tests of their deadly shots.[211] They said "these findings suggest a need to reconsider the use of high-titer measles vaccines early in life *in less developed countries*."[212] [Author's emphasis added.] The implication is that EZ-HT and EZ-SW may be okay for use in *more developed* countries. In fact, the Senegal researchers were willing to develop "other strategies to reduce mortality from early measles," but apparently only *"if these findings are confirmed in other settings."*[213]

The Los Angeles study:
Vaccine researchers were unwilling to abandon their deadly Edmonston-Zagreb high-titer measles vaccine. Instead, they set up a study base in Los Angeles, California. In 1990, three years after the Senegal study was initiated, the first American Black and Hispanic babies were injected with EZ-HT.[214]

The World Health Organization (WHO) and the CDC knew about the high mortality associated with EZ-HT but considered the data "preliminary."[215] Thus, the Los Angeles trials were permitted to occur. However, Dr. Joanne Hatim, an active proponent of vaccine

Figure 39:

Edmonston-Zagreb High-Titer
Measles Vaccine:
1 of Every 6 Vaccinated Babies Died

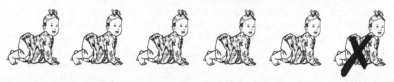

One of every six Senegal babies who received the experimental Edmonston-Zagreb high-titer measles vaccine (EZ-HT) died from other causes within three years. Source: *Lancet* (October 12, 1991).

safety, questioned the experimental study, and was able to muster public outrage.[216] In 1991, the Los Angeles trials were halted, but not before nearly 1500 minority babies were experimented on.[217]

The CDC lied about the Los Angeles study on several points, both before and after it was conducted:

1) The "informed consent" form provided to parents violated U.S. and internationally accepted ethical codes of conduct regulating human experimentation. The mothers and fathers of the babies who were used as research subjects were not informed that EZ-HT was unlicensed in the U.S. It was registered as an investigational new drug to be used for experimental and research purposes only.[218] Nor were they informed of earlier studies in Guinea-Bissau, Senegal, and Haiti where the EZ-HT measles vaccine had shown a significant increase in mortality.[219] The Los Angeles babies were used as sacrificial guinea pigs because it was well established *before* they were injected that this experimental vaccine was a killer.[220]

2) Parents were told that millions of doses of the Edmonston-Zagreb vaccine had already been used in Europe. But the Los Angeles, California babies were not receiving that vaccine; they were being injected with the 10 to 500 times more potent, high-titer shot.[221]

3) The CDC claimed that the communities targeted for the experimental vaccine were hardest hit by a recent outbreak of measles. Babies in Inglewood, East Los Angeles, and West Los Angeles received the shots.[222] However, according to data obtained from the Los Angeles County Department of Health, 14 of 24 regions within Los Angeles County had a greater number of confirmed measles cases than East Los Angeles, and 16 of 24 regions had more measles than West Los Angeles. Inglewood was ranked fourth. In other words, communities targeted for the experimental shots were *not* hardest hit by the recent outbreak of measles.[223]

The three regions chosen to receive the experimental shots were predominantly Black and Hispanic. Eighty-eight percent of the babies were minorities.[224] Several mixed-race and White communities harder hit by the recent outbreak of measles were not chosen to participate in the study.[225]

4) The CDC claimed that no children were adversely affected by the experimental vaccines. However, one baby died from a rare bacterial disease.[226] Furthermore, according to investigative journalist Keidi Obi Awadu, several children "experienced what parents are describing as long-term immune system impairment, seizures and other acute conditions consistent with vaccine-induced injury."[227]

5) Dr. Stephen Hadler, director of the epidemiology and surveillance division of the CDC's national immunization program, claimed that babies died in the earlier studies because they were malnourished and did not have access to adequate health care.[228] However, the Senegal study emphasized that "the three vaccine groups were comparable as regards various social, family, and health characteristics."[229] If the babies vaccinated with high-titer shots

were malnourished, so were the babies in the control group, yet mortality was 80 percent higher in the group receiving EZ-HT.[230] Regarding the claim that babies did not have adequate health care, the Senegal study also noted that "intensive medical care [was] provided during the project."[231] For example, "Free drugs and medical services were provided to all children. As a consequence, overall mortality was substantially lower than during the three preceding years."[232]

6) The Los Angeles study may have had a hidden agenda. In Senegal, researchers established that "there was no significant difference within the study group in mortality by sex,"[233] yet researchers claimed the vaccine had a "mysterious gender bias," with girls more likely to suffer from the vaccine-induced delayed mortality.[234] E. Richard Stiehm, an immunologist at the University of California, Los Angeles, thinks that girls mount a superior immune response to the measles vaccine, then suffer from a hypersensitivity that leaves them immunologically disadvantaged later on. Kenneth Bart, director of the National Vaccine Program Office in Rockville, Maryland, provided a sociological explanation: boys and girls probably get sick equally in the years after vaccination, but girls receive less adequate health care and so die at greater rates. However, Lauri Markowitz, an epidemiologist with the CDC, thinks there may be a biological explanation, and claimed there is no evidence that boys in the earlier studies were treated better than girls. To shed light on this gender enigma, Markowitz planned to measure antibody levels and immune cell counts in Los Angeles children who received the high-titer vaccine.[235] Is it possible that these babies' lives were placed in jeopardy to satisfy scientific curiosity and settle an academic debate?

In 1990, WHO requested 250 million doses of the deadly EZ-HT measles vaccine to be dispensed throughout the world.[236] However, data from Guinea-Bissau, Senegal, and Haiti continued to confirm that EZ-HT doesn't save lives—it increases mortality.[237] By June of 1992, the link was irrefutable; WHO called for a moratorium on use of the disputed vaccine.[238] By some estimates, this may have prevented 18 million baby deaths.[239] Four years later, the CDC issued a tepid letter of regret by declaring, "a mistake was made."[240] Yet, the entire debacle was unnecessary. In the Senegal study conclusion, the authors direct readers to a Togo study that used a *low-titer* measles vaccine and produced a good immunogenic response at six months.[241] Researchers also discussed another Senegal study where standard measles vaccines "were safe, even when given at 4-6 months."[242] Furthermore, "since most complications of measles occur during the 2nd and 3rd weeks after onset, early *treatment* is possible."[243] In fact, "a systematic treatment of complications in [the other Senegal study] reduced the case-fatality rate among children below three years of age by 78 percent."[244] Thus, non-fatal options *were* available.

Mumps

What is mumps?

Mumps is a contagious disease caused by a virus. The illness begins with a fever, headache, muscle aches, and fatigue. Salivary glands beneath the ears along the jaw line become swollen. In some instances, testicles, ovaries, and female breasts may also swell. Treatment mainly consists of allowing the disease to run its course. Medical intervention is seldom required. Symptoms usually disappear within a week. The disease confers permanent immunity; the infected person will not contract it again.[1,2]

Is mumps dangerous?

Mumps is a relatively harmless disease when it is experienced in childhood.[3] Complications are uncommon but can be much more severe when they occur in teenagers and adults.[4-6] For example, orchitis (inflammation of the testes) occurs in about 20 percent of mumps cases in post-pubescent males.[7] This has caused some people to claim mumps will prevent a man from fathering children. However, orchitis usually affects only one testicle; sterility from the ailment is extremely rare.[8,9] Mumps has also been associated with transient meningitis, temporary hearing loss, and inflammation of the ovaries.[10] Full recovery without complications usually follows in 3 to 4 days.[11] Permanent harm from mumps, including death, is rare.[12,13]

Childhood diseases can also have a *favorable* effect on the child's immune system. When children overcome illnesses on their own, they build resistance against other diseases in later life.[14,15] For example, several studies show that women are less likely to develop ovarian cancer if they have had mumps in childhood.[16-19] This may be the best reason several European doctors proclaimed, "there is no plausible medical reason...to immunize girls against mumps."[20]

Does a mumps vaccine exist?

Mumps vaccines were developed in the 1950s. They were tested on orphans and retarded children.[21] Researchers concluded that a "single dose...may be insufficient to produce immunity."[22] In 1967, the first mumps vaccine was licensed; it was put into general use during the 1970s.[23] Today, different mumps vaccines are available using either the Jeryl Lynn, Urabe, Leningrad-Zagreb or Leningrad-3 strains of the live mumps virus.[24]

How is the mumps vaccine made?

In the United States, the Jeryl Lynn strain of the live mumps virus is "propagated in chick embryo cell culture." The growth medium is a buffered salt solution containing amino acids "supplemented with fetal bovine serum." Other ingredients include sucrose, phosphate, glutamate, recombinant human albumin, and neomycin (an antibiotic).[25] Because the mumps vaccine is usually administered by way of the MMR shot, the live measles virus and rubella virus (propagated in "human diploid lung fibroblasts") must be considered elements of the vaccine as well.[26,27]

How safe is the mumps vaccine?

The drug company that produces and distributes the mumps vaccine publishes an extensive list of ailments known to have occurred following the mumps (or MMR) shot. These include aseptic meningitis, encephalitis, diabetes mellitus, orchitis (inflammation of one or both of the testicles), parotitis (the technical name for mumps), atypical mumps, thrombocytopenia (a serious blood disorder), arthritis, otitis media, optic neuritis, anaphylaxis, Guillain-Barré syndrome, pancreatitis, convulsions, seizures, and death.[28]

Meningitis: Several studies have linked the mumps vaccine to meningitis and other complications of the nervous system. For example, as early as 1987 Swedish researchers reported 19 cases of serious neurological sequelae thought to be associated with the Jeryl Lynn strain mumps vaccine.[29] In 1988, Canadian researchers identified a case of mumps meningitis as a potential "post-immunization complication."[30,31] In 1989, German investigators reported 27 cases of neurological disorders related to both the Jeryl Lynn and Urabe strains of the mumps vaccine.[32] *Lancet* reported that meningitis was occurring in some children 21 days following mumps vaccination.[33] A Yugoslavian study documented 115 cases of meningitis within 30 days of mumps vaccination.[34] The *Pediatric Infectious Disease Journal* reported correlations between the mumps vaccine and meningoencephalitis.[35] *Lancet* published data confirming that the mumps virus in the vaccine—not the wild mumps virus—was causing vaccine-related mumps meningitis. This was confirmed when the vaccine-strain virus was isolated from the victims' cerebrospinal fluid.[36-39] The *British Medical Journal* also published data confirming, by way of nucleotide sequencing, that mumps meningoencephalitis is vaccine related.[40] In 1992, *Lancet* published data linking both the Jeryl Lynn and Urabe strains of the mumps vaccine to post-vaccinal meningitis.[41] In 1993, *Lancet* published additional data confirming aseptic meningitis as a well-recognized complication of mumps vaccine, with onset typically occurring 15 to 35 days after receiving the shot.[42] That same year, Japan removed the MMR vaccine from the market because it was reported to be causing encephalitis in 1 of every 1044 people vaccinated.[43] In 1994, the U.S. Institute of Medicine admitted to being able to isolate and identify the mumps vaccine-virus strain from neurologically impaired patients following vaccination. Aseptic meningitis was "officially" recognized as resulting from the mumps vaccine.[44]

Meningitis attack rates: In 1989, European scientists published data showing that mumps meningitis had an attack rate of 1 case per every 1000 children vaccinated.[45] Yet, in 1991 officials *estimated* that mumps meningitis was occurring at a much lower rate of 4.2 cases per one million doses.[46] Japanese researchers reported higher incidence rates: 1 case per 2000 doses in one study,[47] and 6 cases per 2000 doses in another study.[48] In 1992, English researchers documented a similar "virologically confirmed and suspected" mumps vaccine-associated meningitis rate of 1 in 3800 doses.[49] All the cases of "lymphocytic meningitis" and proven mumps meningitis occurred between 17 and 34 days following MMR vaccination.[50]
In 1992, the United Kingdom halted distribution of two brands of MMR vaccine containing the Urabe strain of mumps virus following concern about the risk of meningitis associated with these vaccines.[51] However, in 1993 the company producing these vaccines announced that it will continue to make vaccines that contain the meningitis-causing Urabe mumps strain so that shortages do not cause suspended immunization campaigns.[52]

Diabetes: The mumps vaccine has also been linked to diabetes. In 1975, the *Journal of Pediatrics* published interviews with parents of diabetic children. Several were convinced that onset of the disease followed mumps vaccination.[53] That same year, scientists recorded a case of Type-1 diabetes one month after mumps vaccination.[54] In 1979, researchers revealed that cases of Type-1 diabetes occurred within two years of the mumps vaccine being introduced in Germany.[55] In 1984, German researchers documented more cases of diabetes that occurred 10 days to three weeks following mumps vaccination.[56] In 1986, researchers published data on several children who developed diabetes 2 to 4 weeks after mumps vaccination.[57] By 1990, several new cases of diabetes within 30 days following vaccination were reported.[58] In 1991, scientists reported that diabetes occurred five months following mumps vaccination.[59] Other researchers confirmed diabetes and pancreatitis after mumps vaccination.[60] In 1992, 180 European doctors noted that the mumps vaccine "can trigger diabetes, which only becomes apparent months after vaccination."[61] The *New England Journal of Medicine* showed that viruses can trigger diabetes.[62] (The mumps and MMR shots contain live viruses.) Today, there are continued reports of diabetes following receipt of the MMR vaccine.[63]

Adverse Reaction Report

The following story illustrates the potential damage from the mumps vaccine (or MMR shot): "I had an MMR (measles, mumps and rubella) vaccine at age 36 because I was returning to school and needed it or I couldn't enroll. Within days of the vaccine, I developed mumps-like symptoms that lasted six months: lump in the throat, swelling, difficulty swallowing. Then I developed a rare, recurrent condition called subacute thyroiditis, which

Figure 40:

Outbreaks of Mumps
in Vaccinated Populations

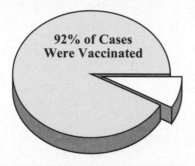

92% of Cases
Were Vaccinated

In 2006, there was a large outbreak of mumps in the United States. Ninety-two percent (92%) of the cases were in people who were previously vaccinated against the disease. Source: CDC, *MMWR* (May 26, 2006); 55(20):559-63.

causes swelling of throat tissue, lungs and thyroid, and disrupts your entire system. The severe, scary symptoms include heart palpitations, swallowing difficulty and shallow breathing. I have landed in the emergency room four times. I am convinced the vaccine had something to do with this rare condition because they have concluded it is viral-based, and they have taken tissue from my thyroid and cultivated mumps from it!"[66]

How effective is the mumps vaccine?
Prior to the mumps vaccine, most children under 10 years of age contracted the disease.[67] During the early 1980s, there were about 4000 cases per year.[68] However, outbreaks of mumps often occur in vaccinated populations. For example, in 1981 during an outbreak of mumps in a Westwood, Massachusetts high school, 94 percent of all cases with known vaccination status occurred in previously vaccinated students. In fact, the vaccinated teenagers were more than twice as likely as the unvaccinated teens to contract the disease.[69]

In 1987, there was an outbreak of mumps in Minnesota schools: 632 of the 769 cases (82 percent) were in previously vaccinated students.[70] That same year, 119 stockbrokers at the Chicago Futures stock exchange caught mumps "following an intensified push for mumps vaccination."[71,72] In 1991, there was an outbreak of mumps in Tennessee schools; 67 of 68 cases (99 percent) were in previously vaccinated students.[73] In 1993, Japan stopped MMR vaccination because it was causing mumps in vaccinated children and other people they associated with.[74] By 1995, there were less than 1000 reported cases in the U.S.[75]

From 2001 to 2003, there were fewer than 300 mumps cases per year in the U.S.[76] However, in 2004 and 2005, there was an epidemic of more than 70,000 cases of mumps in the United Kingdom, despite vaccine coverage of 82 percent.[77] More than 30 percent of the cases were in previously vaccinated persons.[78] During the first four months of 2006, 11 states reported 2,597 cases of mumps—the largest number in a single year since 1991.[79] When the cases with known vaccination status were analyzed, 74 percent had been fully immunized with MMR—they had received the recommended two doses of the mumps vaccine—and 92 percent had received at least one shot of the supposedly "protective" mumps vaccine. Only 8 percent of cases occurred in unvaccinated people (Figure 40).[80]

The CDC believes that several factors contributed to the 2006 multi-state outbreak. For example, the "delayed recognition and diagnosis of mumps" was partially blamed on younger doctors who might not have seen cases of mumps and "might not consider the diagnosis in vaccinated persons."[81] The CDC also blamed several states for not requiring two doses of the MMR vaccine as part of the college admissions process—despite the

Figure 41:
The Changing Epidemiology of Mumps:
A Shift to Older Age Groups

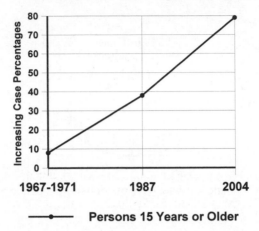

— Persons 15 Years or Older

Before the mumps vaccine was put into general use, just 8 percent of all cases occurred in persons 15 years of age or older. By 1987, several years *after* the vaccine was placed in use, this figure jumped to 38 percent. By 2004, 79 percent of all mumps cases were occurring in this older age group. Source: CDC, *MMWR* (1989); *JAMA* (April 12, 2006).

---

fact that three-quarters of all the mumps cases occurred in people who had been vaccinated twice with MMR, precisely as the CDC recommended.[82] Thus, waning immunity (from ineffective vaccines) was a contributing factor as well.[83]

Epidemiological changes: Years ago, Dr. Robert Mendelsohn noted with great foresight that if immunity from the mumps vaccine proves to be temporary "there is an open question whether, when your child is immunized against mumps at 15 months and escapes this disease in childhood, he may suffer more serious consequences when he contracts it as an adult. If the mumps immunization is given to protect adult males from orchitis—not to prevent children from getting mumps—it would seem reasonable to administer it only to those males who haven't developed natural immunity by the time they reach puberty. They would then be more certain of protection as adults. All girls and countless boys would thus avoid the potential consequences of a hazardous vaccine."[84]

As Dr. Mendelsohn foresaw, the mumps vaccine did indeed shift incidence rates of the disease from young children to teenagers and adults. Mumps in young children is a mild, benign disease. It is a more serious disease when contracted by older age groups.[85] Before the mumps vaccine, most children caught the disease. From 1967 to 1971, before this shot was put into general use, 92 percent of all cases occurred in persons 14 years of age or younger. Just 8 percent of cases occurred in persons 15 years of age or older.[86] By 1987, several years after the vaccine was placed in use, this figure jumped to 38 percent.[87] By 2004, more than 79 percent of all cases were contracted by older persons (Figure 41).[88]

In some areas, an even larger proportion of cases struck older persons. For example, during a 1991 mumps outbreak in Tennessee, 63 of the 68 cases (93 percent) had an average age of 15 years or older.[89] Today, teens and adults continue to contract mumps at greater rates than before the vaccine was introduced. During a large mumps outbreak of more than 2500 cases in early 2006, the median age of persons who caught the disease was 21 years.[90] The rate was highest among persons aged 18-24 years, and was unnaturally high—much greater than during the pre-vaccine era—in adults 25-39 years of age.[91]

Rubella

What is rubella?

Rubella (or German Measles) is a contagious disease caused by a virus. Symptoms include a slight fever, rash, sore throat and runny nose. Lymph nodes on the back of the head, behind the ears, and on the side of the neck may become tender. In some instances, the joints become painful and swollen. Treatment mainly consists of allowing the disease to run its course. Medical intervention is seldom required. Symptoms usually disappear within a few days. Most cases confer permanent immunity; rubella rarely infects the same person twice.[1,2]

Is rubella dangerous?

Rubella is usually a nonthreatening disease when contracted by children. The illness is ordinarily so mild it escapes detection or passes for a cold. However, if a pregnant woman develops rubella during the first trimester, her baby may be born with birth defects.[3]

Does a rubella vaccine exist?

In 1969, the first live-virus rubella vaccine was licensed in the United States. Several European countries, Canada, and Japan also introduced rubella vaccines around this time. In 1979, a more potent live-virus rubella vaccine was sanctioned for use.[4] Today, Merck & Co., Inc. produces Meruvax®II, a live-virus rubella vaccine that is usually provided in combination with measles and mumps vaccines. Merck calls this triple vaccine M-M-R®II.[5] In 2005, the chickenpox vaccine was added to this combination and marketed as ProQuad®.[6]

How is the rubella vaccine made?

Some of the early rubella vaccines (HPV-77/DK12 and /DE5) were produced in dog kidneys and duck embryos (Figure 42).[7-9] However, in 1979 vaccine manufacturers started producing and distributing the Wistar RA27/3 strain of the live rubella virus "adapted to and propagated in WI-38 human diploid lung fibroblasts."[10-12] This vaccine is still in use today. In fact, the current rubella vaccine originated from cell lines obtained from the tissue of aborted human fetuses.[13] (For additional information and a list of similar vaccines, see *Appendix III* on page 309.) According to early rubella vaccine researchers seeking to avoid the problem of "passenger viruses" (vaccine contaminants):

> We decided to isolate a rubella virus directly from naturally infected material.... The opportunity arose...when many rubella-virus infected fetuses became available.... Explant cultures of the dissected organs of this fetus, the 27th in our series of Philadelphia rubella abortuses, were set up. The third explant, which happened to be from kidney, was selected arbitrarily for further study. Fibroblast cells that grew out from this explant could be subcultivated after several weeks. The presence of rubella virus in the supernatant fluids was confirmed. After four subcultivations of the infected kidney fibroblasts, the supernatant fluid was inoculated directly into a WI-38 culture. This then was the genesis of the RA27/3 rubella strain.[14-16]

Other researchers offer a similar account of this vaccine's inception:

> Two groups of human fetuses, 8 to 20 weeks of age, were used for the initiation of diploid cell strains. The first group consisted of normal embryos obtained by hysterotomy and flown from Scandinavia... The second group represented spontaneous abortions obtained from the gynecologic service of the Philadelphia General Hospital. Intact fetuses of both groups were kept at 0° to 4° C from the time of abortion until used.... The human diploid cell strains were initiated from surgically and spontaneously aborted fetuses.... The WI-38 strain...originally derived from fetal lung.[17,18]

Figure 42:

History of the Rubella Vaccine

1969-1973: HPV-77/DK12
Propagated in dog kidneys (DK)

1970-1976: Cendehill strain
Least effective of the rubella vaccines

1969-1978: HPV-77/DE5
Propagated in duck embryos (DE)

1979-2002+: RA27/3
Propagated in lung tissue
of aborted human fetuses

The growth medium for the current rubella vaccine is a buffered salt solution "supplemented with fetal bovine serum." This vaccine also contains human serum albumin, neomycin (an antibiotic), sorbitol, and hydrolyzed gelatin stabilizer (an animal protein substance made from boiled cows or pigs).[19-21] The measles and mumps vaccines (often administered in combination with the rubella vaccine) are "propagated in chick embryo cell culture."[22] The chickenpox vaccine (often administered in combination with the measles, mumps and rubella vaccines)[23] is derived from a live varicella virus "introduced into human embryonic lung cell cultures, adapted to and propagated in embryonic guinea pig cell cultures and finally propagated in human diploid (fetal tissue) cell cultures."[24] This vaccine also contains monosodium L-glutamate (MSG).[25]

How safe is the rubella vaccine?

The drug company that produces the rubella vaccine publishes an extensive list of ailments known to have occurred following the rubella (or MMR) shot. These include arthritis, arthralgia, myalgia, encephalitis, Guillain-Barré syndrome, thrombocytopenia, leukocytosis, polyneuritis, polyneuropathy, optic neuritis, anaphylaxis, and death.[26] Numerous studies and frequent reports filed with the FDA's Vaccine Adverse Event Reporting System (VAERS) confirm these and other afflictions following rubella (or MMR) vaccination.[27]

Arthritis: As early as 1969—the same year that the rubella vaccine was initially licensed—scientists knew that the rubella vaccine was causing serious problems. The *New England Journal of Medicine* published a study documenting "arthritis after rubella vaccination."[28] The *American Journal of Diseases of Children* also noted cases of "transient arthritis" after rubella vaccination.[29] In 1971, the *American Journal of Diseases of Children* published another study showing that 10 percent of children developed joint problems following their rubella shots.[30] That same year, the *American Journal of Epidemiology* showed that 25 percent of women in their 20s, and 50 percent of women aged 25 to 33, had adverse joint symptoms following rubella vaccination.[31]

In 1972, the *Journal of the American Medical Association* published data showing that 46 percent of women above 25 years of age developed acute arthritis following rubella vaccination.[32] That same year, the *American Journal of Epidemiology* published a study documenting "joint reactions in children vaccinated against rubella."[33] The *Journal of Pediatrics* also reported on several cases of "recurrent joint symptoms" in babies starting 2 to 7 weeks following their rubella vaccinations.[34] In addition, the *American Journal of Public Health* published a report on "joint symptoms following an area-wide rubella immunization campaign."[35]

Figure 43:

The Rubella Vaccine and Arthritis

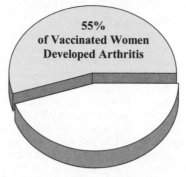

55%
of Vaccinated Women
Developed Arthritis

In a study of adult women who were vaccinated against rubella, 55 percent developed arthritis or joint pain within four weeks. Source: *Annals of the Rheumatic Diseases* 1986; 45:110-114. Additional studies confirm "chronic arthritis" after rubella vaccination.

In 1973, another study published by the *American Journal of Diseases of Children* documented several youngsters with recurrent arthritis following their rubella vaccinations.[36] In 1977, the *Journal of Arthritis and Rheumatism* published a study documenting "chronic arthropathy associated with rubella vaccination."[37] In 1980, two additional studies and secret data from Merck Research Laboratories confirmed that incidence rates for arthritis and arthralgia following rubella vaccination are generally much higher in women than in children. Up to 1 out of every 4 women vaccinated was injured by the shot. Moreover, adverse reactions in women tended to be more severe and of longer duration, sometimes lasting for years.[38-41]

In 1982, data published in both the *American Journal of Epidemiology* and *Lancet* once again confirmed that "joint reactions" and "rubella-associated arthritis" were occurring after rubella shots.[42,43] In 1984, *Lancet* again reported that chronic arthritis persisted for up to seven years in several women following their rubella shots.[44] In 1985, the *Journal of Infectious Diseases* recorded cases of chronic arthritis in women vaccinated against rubella. The author of the study also documented a case of rheumatoid arthritis with "joint destruction" that began after rubella vaccination and lasted for over 20 years.[45] In 1986, a study published in *Annals of the Rheumatic Diseases,* showed that 55 percent of women vaccinated against rubella developed arthritis or joint pain within four weeks (Figure 43).[46]

In 1991, the U.S. Vaccine Safety Committee acknowledged that the rubella vaccine causes both acute and long-term arthritis.[47] In 1992, *Clinical Infectious Diseases* published a study documenting cases of "chronic arthritis" after rubella vaccination.[48] That same year, the *British Medical Journal* reasserted that the rubella component of the MMR vaccine "is associated with an increased risk of episodes of joint and limb symptoms."[49] In 1996, researchers once again published data on "chronic arthropathy and musculoskeletal symptoms associated with rubella vaccines."[50] In 1997, the *Journal of the American Medical Association* published additional data on the risk of chronic arthropathy among rubella-vaccinated women.[51] In 1998, the *Journal of Infectious Diseases* published yet another paper on "rubella vaccine-induced joint manifestations.[52]

In 2002, *Clinical and Experimental Rheumatology* published an analysis of the Vaccine Adverse Event Reporting System (VAERS) database. The study examined "the incidence rate of chronic arthritis adverse reactions reported following adult rubella (and hepatitis B) vaccinations." (Chronic arthritis is defined as persisting for at least one year.) The report concluded that the incidence rates "were statistically significant." Furthermore, the chronic arthritis adverse reactions following rubella vaccination primarily affected females at a mean onset of 10-11 days following vaccination. An autoimmune etiology was presumed.[53] Today, these debilitating adverse reactions still occur; many people continue to experience severe joint problems and arthritis-like symptoms following their rubella or MMR vaccinations.[54]

Nervous system and blood disorders: As early as 1970, the *Journal of the American Medical Association* published reports of paralysis following rubella vaccination.[55] In 1972, the *Journal of Pediatrics* confirmed a loss of physical sensation and difficulty walking following rubella shots.[56] That same year, the *New York State Journal of Medicine* published data on thrombocytopenia (a serious blood disorder) associated with rubella vaccination.[57] In 1974, a study published in the *American Journal of Diseases of Children* once again documented neurological disorders following rubella shots. With one strain of the vaccine virus, researchers found "polyneuropathies" occurring at a rate of 2.2 cases per 1000 doses. Symptoms persisted for more than 2½ years in several children.[58] In 1977, the *British Medical Journal* published a paper on "diffuse myelitis associated with rubella vaccination."[59] In 1982, *Archives of Neurology* published data on optic neuritis and myelitis following rubella vaccination.[60] In 1991, the *New England Journal of Medicine* acknowledged the occurrence of "bilateral hearing loss" after measles and rubella vaccination.[61] That same year, the U.S. Institute of Medicine reported several cases of nerve pain, numbness, Guillain-Barré syndrome, and transverse myelitis following rubella vaccination.[62] In 1994, the *European Journal of Pediatrics* published data by German researchers tracing a case of Guillain-Barré syndrome in a young teenager to the rubella portion of the MMR vaccine.[63] Today, the FDA continues to receive reports of neurological disorders following receipt of the rubella or MMR vaccine.[64]

Diabetes: In 1947, prior to national immunization campaigns, there were an estimated 600,000 cases of diabetes in the United States.[65] By 1976, less than 10 years after mass inoculations with the mumps and rubella vaccines (licensed in 1967 and 1969, respectively), more than 10 million people in the U.S. were afflicted with diabetes—despite a population increase of just 50 percent.[66] By 2005, nearly 21 million people—7 percent of the population—harbored this disease.[67] In fact, about 1 of every 500 children and teenagers now have diabetes.[68] Even more astonishing, nearly 10 percent of all U.S. citizens aged 20 years and older have this disease.[69] What could be causing such drastic increases in diabetes cases?

Since 1968, "there has been increasing interest in the possibility that viral infection may play a part in the etiology of diabetes mellitus."[70] According to *Lancet,* "One virus consistently produces diabetes in man—the congenitally acquired rubella virus."[71] In fact, up to 20 percent of all persons affected by congenital rubella syndrome (CRS) develop Type-1 diabetes *up to 20 years later.*[72] This is particularly significant for a couple of reasons. First, it indicates that the rubella virus can remain dormant for many years. Studies have confirmed this.[73-75] Secondly, if the wild rubella virus can cause illness, so can the manufactured rubella virus in the vaccine. Dr. Harris Coulter, testifying before Congress on the relationship between vaccinations and juvenile-onset diabetes (type-1), spoke to this issue: "Of the three vaccines making up the MMR shot, the rubella component is the major suspect because rubella itself, like mumps, is known to be a cause of diabetes, and the action of the vaccine resembles that of the disease. If the disease can cause diabetes, so can the vaccine."[76]

In 1982, researchers documented "rubella-specific immune complexes" consisting of rubella viruses and the antibodies to them. These immune complexes attack the insulin-producing pancreas, and were found in persons vaccinated against rubella. According to the study authors, "Rubella-specific immune complex formation is frequent after vaccination and could be demonstrated in two-thirds of an unselected group of vaccinates." These immune complexes were not found in persons who contracted rubella naturally nor in those who were not infected by rubella.[77]

In 1986, researchers published data showing that diabetes could be induced in laboratory animals by infecting them with the rubella virus. They considered the most probable cause an immunological reaction—the formation of an autoimmune state in which the body becomes allergic to itself.[78] In 1989, scientists infected human pancreatic islet cells with rubella virus and noted "significant reductions in levels of secreted insulin."[79] In 1997, Dr. Coulter, who analyzed these studies, concluded that "Diabetes after rubella vaccination probably represents a combined effect: the virus attacks the islet cells of the pancreas in an organism which has already been weakened by an autoimmune reaction to the same virus."[80] Today, diabetes continues to afflict an ever increasing number of people.

Chronic fatigue syndrome: Scientific studies have linked the new rubella vaccine introduced in 1979 to chronic fatigue syndrome, a debilitating immune system disorder. The first reports of this disease began surfacing in the medical literature in 1982 when *Lancet* published data on patients with persistent unexplained symptoms, including chronic fatigue. Affected individuals had elevated viral antibodies, and the ailment was initially labeled post-viral syndrome or Epstein-Barr virus infection.[81] In 1986, the *Journal of Immuno-Pharmacology* published new data on mechanisms of autoimmunity, causing researchers to suspect that "rubella reinfection...could account for the viral antibodies found in patients with chronic fatigue."[82,83] In 1988, *Medical Hypotheses* published additional research showing that although patients with chronic fatigue syndromes have elevated IgG serum antibodies to multiple common viruses, "only IgG rubella antibodies are positively correlated with the intensity of symptoms."[84] According to the author of the study, "In countries that routinely immunize children with the new [rubella] vaccine, adults might be persistently reexposed to the more provocative antigens of the new vaccine due to respiratory secretions..."[85] In other words, the rubella virus lingers in recently vaccinated children and can be spread to hypersensitive adults. Reinfection produces multiple viral antibodies resulting in "the characteristic symptoms in adult women who are over-represented in the patient population."[86] Thus, "the possible role of rubella immunization in the etiology of chronic fatigue syndromes deserves further study."[87] In 1991, *Clinical Ecology* published a new study confirming that the vaccine strain of the rubella virus was a causative agent in the development of chronic fatigue syndrome.[88]

Adverse Reaction Reports

This section contains a few adverse reaction reports that appear to be linked to the rubella portion of the MMR shot.[89] (Additional adverse reaction reports possibly linked to the rubella vaccine may be found in the chapters on MMR and autism.)
- "My child caught rubella two weeks after her MMR."
- "My granddaughter received MMR and reacted with a low grade fever and a rash that our local emergency room nurse said is 'looking a lot like rubella.' She said this before she was informed that the child received MMR 10 days prior."
- "My baby daughter has been extremely ill for three weeks following her 12-month well-visit, which included the MMR shot. She experienced fever up to 102 degrees, vomiting, diarrhea, complete loss of appetite, and pain in her joints (knees, ankles, elbows and wrists). She has been learning American Sign Language, and began signing 'hurt' and pointing to her joints. It has been heartbreaking to see her lose the ability to stand and walk. The physicians originally agreed that her fever and symptoms were a result of the MMR live viruses. After a couple of weeks, they said that her illnesses were unrelated—even though her symptoms remained the same. I took a perfectly healthy, happy little girl to the doctor and our lives have been a nightmare. I will definitely trust my instincts and not take another chance, even though our pediatric office has a policy of denying treatment if children are not up-to-date on their shots."
- "My daughter is four years old. She had a reaction to her vaccine when she was 12 months old. Between 5 and 7 days after, she had high-pitched screaming that would last for 2 to 3 hours at a time. After taking her to the hospital, they found nothing wrong. She has had ankle pains for three years. She gets her 'ankle medicine' nearly every night."
- "My daughter died after receiving the MMR shot. Within hours, it put her into sudden onset diabetes. When I brought her to the doctor, he said her panting and lethargy were

not serious. (The shot put her into diabetes and she was going into acidosis.) We brought her into emergency the next day but she died from complications (brain swelling and convulsions from the diabetes). I said all along that it was the MMR that kicked it off. The doctors insisted I was wrong and that it was some unknown virus from 'somewhere' that kicked it off. I kept saying, 'Come on! You just shot her full of a live-virus vaccine and you are telling me that it was an unknown virus that killed her? Do I look that stupid?'"

▸ "I am a nursing student. Within three weeks of taking the MMR vaccine I became weak, tired, and sluggish. This led to numbness in both hands and feet. I developed Guillain-Barré syndrome and was hospitalized for two months. I was unable to walk, had difficulty moving my upper limbs, suffered urinary and abdominal problems, partial facial paralysis, and I lost a substantial amount of weight. Previously, I was an active, healthy woman."

▸ "I am a new mom. When I was discharged from the hospital after giving birth, the nurse said I needed to get the rubella shot. Shortly after coming home, I started having headaches that wouldn't go away. I finally called my doctor after being home almost a week with continuous headaches. She told me it was probably tension headaches from the stress of being a new mom, and to try some caffeine. Today, almost two weeks since I had my baby, I am still experiencing these headaches, so I decided to look up some of the side effects of the rubella vaccine. Sure enough, mild to severe headaches is listed, along with joint pain. I am so glad I have chosen not to vaccinate my daughter."

▸ "After the birth of my daughter, my obstetrician recommended the MMR vaccine since I didn't have antibodies. A week after the shot, a rash appeared all over my body. Two weeks later, I had severe joint pain which alternated from my knee to ankle to wrist. The joint pain lasted seven days and then severe fatigue set in. My doctor immediately said this was not related to the vaccine."

▸ "I am a 57-year-old registered nurse who was, as a condition of employment, required to take MMR. About 14 days later I developed a rash with lesions in my right eye, fever, and joint pain. My joint pain has not gone away but has become chronic, and sometimes unbearable. I have been put on a variety of drugs which I had terrible reactions to and was even hospitalized for. I have been unable to work. I filed a worker's compensation claim, which they are trying to deny."

How effective is the rubella vaccine?

Prior to the introduction of the rubella vaccine in 1969, thousands of cases of rubella circulated throughout society. Most children contracted the disease and developed permanent protection. As a result, about 85 percent of the adult population was naturally immune; just 15 percent were susceptible to the disease.[90,91] After the vaccine was introduced, researchers began to notice that cases of rubella were occurring in vaccinated populations. For example, in 1971 during an outbreak of rubella in Casper, Wyoming, 73 percent of the cases occurred in previously vaccinated children.[92,93] In 1973, the *Australian Journal of Medical Technology* published a study showing that 80 percent of all army recruits who had been vaccinated against rubella just four months earlier still contracted the disease.[94] In 1980, more than 10 years after a national immunization campaign with the rubella vaccine was instituted, *Pediatrics* published data indicating that about 15 percent of children in a well-vaccinated community remained susceptible to rubella.[95] In 1980, 1985, and again in 1987, serological analyses confirmed that about 15 percent of the adult population, including women of childbearing age, were still not protected from the disease—the same percentage as before vaccinations.[96-98] Scientists are doubtful that higher vaccination rates—even 80 to 95 percent—will solve this dilemma.[99]

The *Journal of the America Medical Association* published data showing that antibody levels after rubella vaccinations fell to half their high point within four years.[100] The Minnesota Department of Health reported that 50 percent of all rubella cases were in vaccinated persons.[101] Additional data confirmed that many people vaccinated against rubella had no evidence of immunity within a few years. For example, Dr. Stanley Plotkin, Professor of Pediatrics at the University of Pennsylvania School of Medicine, showed that 36 percent of adolescent females who had been vaccinated against rubella lacked serological proof of immunity.[102]

When people are vaccinated against rubella, high levels of rubella antibodies are detected in their blood. However, *Current Problems in Pediatrics* published data showing that these people may still catch the disease.[103] The *Journal of Infectious Diseases* also published data showing that several people vaccinated against rubella and who later caught the disease (vaccine failures) had abundant antibodies to the rubella virus.[104] Thus, antibody levels are not good indicators of immunity.

Vaccine strategies: Mass rubella vaccination campaigns were never intended to protect vaccine recipients; the disease is usually harmless in children. Instead, the goal has always been to protect the unborn fetuses of rubella-susceptible pregnant women. As Dr. James Cherry, Professor of Pediatrics at UCLA, noted, "The point of rubella immunization is not prevention of rubella but prevention of the congenital rubella syndrome."[105] Therefore, the vaccine's capacity to reduce the number of rubella cases is not nearly as significant as it's ability (or lack thereof) to protect fetuses from rubella virus-related birth defects.

When the rubella vaccine was introduced, authorities had to decide on one of two strategies: a) the U.S. preference to vaccinate one-year-olds and children 5 to 9 years old, or b) the U.K. preference to vaccinate susceptible females of childbearing age, mainly 11 to 14 year old girls.[106] Scientists continue to debate the merits of each plan. Swiss researchers assert that "there is no plausible medical reason...to immunize...boys against rubella."[107] However, if all youngsters, male and female, are vaccinated, the wild virus should theoretically have fewer hosts to infect, and pregnant women would be less likely to contract the disease.[108,109] But if the vaccine only offers temporary immunity, as studies indicate, and wears off in a few years, females vaccinated as children may actually have greater likelihoods of contracting rubella during their childbearing years.[110,111] Furthermore, research has shown that "most persons who contract rubella as adults do so through contact with other adults."[112] Therefore, some authorities argue that since children are not the primary "herd" infecting pregnant women, they should not be targeted for vaccination.[113] Is it ethical for one herd—children—to be force-inoculated, denied natural immunity, and subjected to all of the potential side effects of the vaccine, so that another herd—the unborn fetuses of rubella-susceptible pregnant women—may be theoretically protected?[114]

On the other hand, if all children are given the opportunity to achieve natural immunity, by the time girls reach childbearing age about 85 percent will be naturally protected.[115] Then, susceptible females—the one true, small group at risk—can be targeted for vaccination. However, there is a potentially serious problem with this strategy as well. When 11 to 14 year-old girls are targeted for vaccination, pregnant or soon-to-be-pregnant women (and their fetuses) are subjected to a greater risk of accidental exposure to the rubella virus. In fact, the medical literature is replete with examples of pregnant women who were inadvertently injected with the rubella vaccine.[116] There are also many cases of rubella-vaccinated women who gave birth to babies with congenital rubella syndrome (CRS).[117-120]

These many valid concerns have caused some researchers to argue against mandating this vaccine.[121] One outspoken scientist cautioned members of U.S. and Canadian national immunization advisory boards that *"even the most desirable goal never justifies means that violate essential rights, particularly when complications of vaccination can occur."*[122] Regardless, vaccine policymakers in the U.S. today recommend a combination of *both* strategies: one dose of the rubella vaccine (via MMR) at 12 to 15 months of age plus a booster shot at 4 to 6 years. However, "those who have not previously received the second dose should complete the schedule by age 11 to 12 years."[123]

Epidemiological changes: Vaccine strategies have drastically altered the disease landscape. In 1980, Dr. James Cherry noted that rubella vaccinations shifted age groups susceptible to the ailment: "Essentially, we have controlled the disease in persons 14 years of age or younger but have given it a free hand in those 15 or older."[124] From 1966 to 1968, *before* the rubella vaccine was licensed, 77 percent of all cases occurred in persons 14 years of age or younger. Just 23 percent occurred in persons 15 years of age or older.[125] By 1975, however, 62 percent of all rubella cases were in the 15-or-older group. In 1976 and 1977, this figure increased to more than 70 percent.[126] By 1990, 81 percent of all

Figure 44:

The Changing Epidemiology of Rubella:
A Shift to Older Age Groups

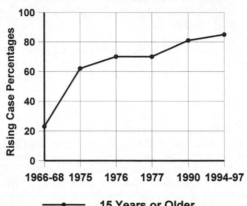

Copyright © NZM

From 1966 to 1968, *before* the rubella vaccine was licensed, just 23 percent of all rubella cases occurred in persons 15 years of age or older. By 1975, just a few years *after* the rubella vaccine was introduced, 62 percent of all rubella cases were in the 15-or-older group. In 1976 and 1977, this figure rose to more than 70 percent. By 1997, 85 percent of all rubella cases were in persons 15 years of age or older. Source: CDC *MMWRs*.

rubella cases occurred in this older age group, with the greatest increases in persons 15 to 29 years old—the prime childbearing years.[127] From 1994 to 1997 this trend continued, with 85 percent of all rubella cases occurring in persons 15 years or older (Figure 44).[128]

Congenital rubella syndrome (CRS):
In 1941, Sir Norman Gregg, an Australian ophthalmologist, noticed that some women who caught rubella early in pregnancy gave birth to babies with disabilities, such as eye defects, hearing loss, heart disease, and learning problems.[129] Although some defects are permanent, others are short-lived or correctable.[130] However, not all pregnant women exposed to the virus give birth to injured babies.[131,132] Congenital rubella syndrome (CRS) occurs in less than 25 percent of infants born to women who contract rubella during the first trimester of pregnancy.[133] The risk of a single congenital defect declines to about 15 percent by the 16th week of pregnancy.[134] Defects are rare when the maternal infection occurs after the 20th week of gestation.[135]

Since 1969, when the rubella vaccine was introduced, the number of rubella cases has steadily declined. For example, in 1970 more than 56,000 cases were recorded in the U.S.; 3,904 in 1980; 1,125 in 1990; just 152 in 2000.[136,137] Authorities use this as evidence of the vaccine's efficacy and benefit to society. However, as noted earlier, the vaccine's capacity to reduce the number of rubella cases is inconsequential if it is unable to protect the unborn child from birth defects.[138] In fact, when the official data is analyzed, it becomes clear that CRS cases actually *increased* after the vaccine was introduced.[139,140]

In 1966, the year the government began keeping statistics on congenital rubella syndrome, there were 11 cases reported in the United States. In 1967, there were just 10 cases, with 14 more reported the following year. However, in 1969 the rubella vaccine was introduced and the CDC recorded 31 cases of CRS. In 1970, CRS cases skyrocketed to 77—a greater than 600 percent increase over pre-vaccine numbers. In 1971, there were another 68 cases. These figures remained high in later years (Figure 45).[141] Adjustments for annual population variances do not alter the results (Figure 46).[142]

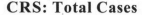

Figure 45:

CRS: Total Cases

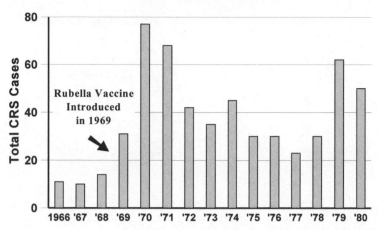

Government figures show that cases of congenital rubella syndrome (CRS) *increased* after the rubella vaccine was introduced. Source: CDC, *MMWR* (October 25, 1996).

Figure 46:

CRS Cases: Population-adjusted

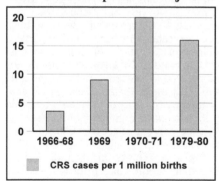

Cases of congenital rubella syndrome (CRS), adjusted for annual population variances, *increased* after the rubella vaccine was introduced. Source: CDC. Cited in a Public Health Information Sheet by the *March of Dimes Birth Defects Foundation* (October 1984).   © NZM

In 1966, before the vaccine was introduced, the CDC recorded 46,925 cases of rubella and 11 cases of congenital rubella syndrome. During the 1980s, rubella cases declined. The average number of CRS cases per year declined as well, but still remained higher than before rubella vaccination campaigns were initiated (11.7 cases per year in the 1960s versus 13.1 cases per year in the 1980s).[143] By 1991, there were just 1,401 cases of rubella, but the CDC recorded 47 cases of CRS. In 1992, there were just 160 cases of rubella and 11 cases of CRS—the exact number of CRS cases recorded by the CDC more than 25 years earlier in 1966 *before* the vaccine was introduced.[144]

Abortions: Some doctors recommend abortions to non-immune pregnant women when they are exposed to the rubella virus.[145] By terminating pregnancies suspected of harboring rubella-infected babies, CRS statistics are artificially reduced. Dr. James Cherry addressed this issue when he noticed that cases of CRS were declining even though the number of rubella infections in women of childbearing age remained stable.[146] Another researcher, Dr. Jean Joncas, also addressed this issue by noting that "the number of therapeutic abortions performed" when rubella is confirmed in pregnant women is rarely considered in evaluating decreases in the incidence of CRS.[147] In one study in which therapeutic abortions were counted, the result was "a 10 percent increase in the incidence of CRS cases, and the real rate was probably much higher."[148]

Figure 47:
Doctors Refuse the Rubella Vaccine

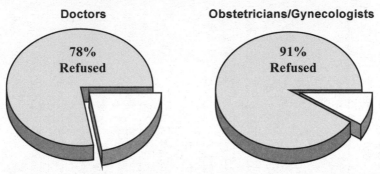

Doctors   Obstetricians/Gynecologists

78%
Refused

91%
Refused

Copyright © NZM

In one study, 78 percent of the doctors and 91 percent of the obstetricians and gynecologists (who work daily with pregnant women) refused to take a rubella shot. Source: *Journal of the American Medical Association* 1981; 245(7):711-13.

What do doctors think about the rubella vaccine?

Medical policymakers understand that "hospital employees are as likely to be susceptible [to rubella] as the general public."[149-151] In fact, they believe that outbreaks in healthcare facilities are of particular concern because "pregnant women are often dependent on hospital-based services, and it is quite possible that a single infected hospital employee could transmit rubella to several susceptible pregnant patients."[152] Thus, many hospitals require all employees to be vaccinated against rubella. In Evanston, Illinois, a 46-year-old social worker was fired from her hospital job when she refused the shot. Yet, doctors who work at these hospitals exempt themselves from the rubella vaccine by claiming they are not employees of the hospital.[153] They are the *least* likely to participate in rubella vaccination campaigns.

The *New England Journal of Medicine* reported that one-third of all hospital employees rejected rubella shots; 81 percent of the doctors refused the vaccine, with senior staff physicians having an even lower participation rate.[154] The *Journal of the American Medical Association* reported that 47 percent of all employees at the University of Southern California Medical Center would not comply with a rubella vaccination campaign; 78 percent of the doctors would not consent to the shot, while 91 percent of the obstetricians and gynecologists (who work daily with pregnant women) refused to participate (Figure 47).[155,156]

When the doctors were questioned about their refusals, they confessed to being concerned about adverse reactions and did not think rubella vaccination was a priority. (A study published in the *Journal of the American Medical Association* showed that 50 percent of all people vaccinated against rubella complained of adverse reactions.)[157] Even when these doctors were confronted with information that the potential for an outbreak existed, that the vaccine was safe, and that a history of previous rubella infection was an unreliable predictor of immunity, they still could not be persuaded to be vaccinated nor to endorse a rubella vaccination program. According to proponents of the vaccine, "Such reluctance on the part of physicians—especially influential, senior physicians—presents a formidable obstacle to convincing nonphysicians that such a program is safe, useful, and necessary."[158] This prompted Dr. Robert Mendelsohn to pose an ethical question: "If doctors themselves are afraid of the vaccine, why on earth should the law require that you and other parents allow them to administer it to your kids?"[159]

MMR
(Measles, Mumps, Rubella)

What is MMR?
MMR is an abbreviation for measles, mumps, and rubella—three common childhood illnesses up until the mid-1970s. Vaccines are available for each of these diseases. However, in the 1980s they were combined into a single "three-in-one" MMR shot. (For important information about these three diseases and their respective vaccines, read the separate chapters on measles, mumps and rubella.)

How is the MMR vaccine made?
According to the U.S. manufacturer, Merck & Company, Inc., the current MMR vaccine—MMR® II—contains attenuated live measles and mumps viruses propagated in chick embryo cell culture, plus "the Wistar RA 27/3 strain of live attenuated rubella virus propagated in WI-38 human diploid lung fibroblasts."[1] Studies published in *American Journal of Diseases of Children* and *American Journal of Epidemiology,* reveal that the rubella strain was cultured from an aborted human fetus.[2,3] (See *Appendix III* on page 313.) In addition, the growth medium for the three live viruses that are needed to produce the MMR vaccine is a buffered salt solution "supplemented with fetal bovine serum."[4] Other ingredients include sucrose, phosphate, glutamate, recombinant human albumin, sorbitol, hydrolyzed gelatin stabilizer, and approximately 25mcg of neomycin (an antibiotic).[5] The MMR vaccine does not contain a preservative. In fact, according to the FDA, MMR-II *never* contained thimerosal, a potentially dangerous chemical used in some vaccines.[6] However, trace amounts of mercury were detected in an earlier MMR formulation.[7]

How safe is the MMR vaccine?
The drug company that makes the MMR vaccine publishes an extensive list of warnings, contraindications, and adverse reactions associated with this triple shot. These may be found in the vaccine package insert[8] (available from any doctor giving MMR) and in the *Physician's Desk Reference* (PDR) at the library.[9] The following afflictions affecting nearly every body system—blood, lymphatic, digestive, cardiovascular, immune, nervous, respiratory, and sensory—have been reported following receipt of the MMR shot: encephalitis, encephalopathy, neurological disorders, seizure disorders, convulsions, learning disabilities, subacute sclerosing panencephalitis (SSPE), demyelination of the nerve sheaths, Guillain-Barré syndrome (paralysis), muscle incoordination, deafness, panniculitis, vasculitis, optic neuritis (including partial or total blindness), retinitis, otitis media, bronchial spasms, fever, headache, joint pain, arthritis (acute and chronic), transverse myelitis, thrombocytopenia (blood clotting disorders and spontaneous bleeding), anaphylaxis (severe allergic reactions), lymphadenopathy, leukocytosis, pneumonitis, Stevens-Johnson syndrome, erythema multiforme, urticaria, pancreatitis, parotitis, inflammatory bowel disease, Crohn's disease, ulcerative colitis, meningitis, diabetes, autism, immune disorders, and death (Figure 48).[10,11]

Adverse Reaction Reports

This section contains unsolicited adverse reaction reports associated with the MMR vaccine. They are typical of the daily emails received by the *Thinktwice Global Vaccine Institute* (www.thinktwice.com).[12]

▸ "My 12-month-old received his MMR shot on a Friday. The following Friday he had a 104 degree temperature and became violently ill. The doctor said it was a stomach virus. But on Monday morning he woke up with a rash all over. I took him to the doctor and was very upset to learn that this is very common."

▸ "When my daughter was just over one year old, she received her MMR vaccination. Later that day she had a high fever and I put her to bed. I was busy doing housework downstairs and got this 'mother's intuition' that something was wrong. I rushed upstairs

Figure 48:

Adverse Reactions: MMR Vaccine

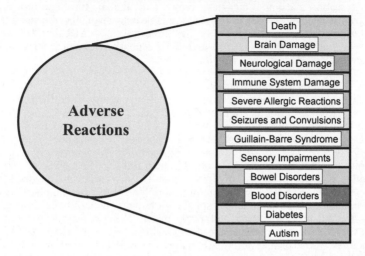

Severe afflictions affecting nearly every body system—blood, lymphatic, digestive, cardiovascular, immune, nervous, respiratory, and sensory—have been linked to the MMR vaccine. Source: Merck & Co., Inc. "M-M-R® II (Measles, Mumps, and Rubella Virus Vaccine Live)." Product insert from the vaccine manufacturer (December 2007); *Physician's Desk Reference* (PDR), 61st edition (2006); Vaccine Adverse Event Reporting System (VAERS); Multiple studies.

---

to find her blue and not breathing. I called a nurse. My daughter was convulsing, so I was instructed to reach down her throat to open her air passage. She was rushed to the hospital and they immediately put her into a cool bath. She was in the hospital for almost a week. Had it not been for my gut feeling that something was wrong, my baby would not be with me today."

▶ "Recently, my 13-month-old had his MMR. He now has constant high fevers and seizures, which he never had. He is a totally different boy. This is devastating."

▶ "Our son developed seizures after his MMR vaccine at 14 months. Today, after two years of anti-epilepsy medications, he has totally regressed. We decided to stop all medications five weeks ago and his grand mal fits have stopped. We are now left with a child experiencing severe constipation and bowel problems."

▶ "My son is 14 months old. Seven days ago he had his MMR. As soon as the nurse gave it, his glands started swelling about one hour after. He has had a high temperature and is not sleeping that well at night, and also not wanting his food. Today, his left arm is very, very red. It looks like he has been scalded by a red-hot kettle. We made an appointment at the doctors and they said that it's a reaction to the MMR. She also said that it looks like his arm has been stung, but I said to her, 'No way my son has been stung.' We came home, but now the red inflamed arm seems to be going further up to his shoulder. I am so scared."

▶ "My granddaughter had an MMR. When she first got it she soon had a stiff neck and knots in the glands in her groin. At first they said it was the shot and that it was quite common. Now, four weeks later she still has the problem. She is not back to walking like she was. Maybe she's afraid that it will hurt. The doctor now says that she has had a virus and that is the problem. I'm really worried."

▸ "I am writing from Canada. All the arguments about vaccines saving lives and preventing diseases mean nothing when your child becomes one of those that someone has decided is expendable for the sake of maintaining the program. Until two years ago, I was not against vaccinations—my ten year old had been fully vaccinated. His only reaction was a high fever and fussiness for a few days after each DPT. Then, two years ago, my then 14-month-old son received the MMR vaccine. Nine days later, he developed a fever and a severe measles-like rash. I had been warned that many children have a mild reaction between 1 and 6 weeks. Because my son's case was severe, I took him to be examined as instructed. I was told he was allergic to food or something in his environment but that it could not possibly be a reaction to the MMR. As a mother, my instincts told me otherwise but I proceeded as advised. The following morning, my son's appearance had completely changed. He looked as though he had been scalded from the top of his head to the tip of his toes. I was extremely worried. A nurse-friend advised me to call the Nursing Hotline. The adverse reaction for the MMR vaccine was read to me over the phone from the *Centers for Disease Control Handbook*. There were three major symptoms: 1) fever, 2) transient rash, and 3) thrombocytopenia, or internal bleeding, that I was told would present itself as bruising. Later that day, I noticed that his legs were turning blue and purple. I rushed him to emergency. By the time we arrived, the bruising had spread up his body to his chest. He was immediately administered adrenaline, steroids and prescription-strength antihistamines. Like the night before, the attending physician could not tell me what was wrong with my son but refused to even entertain the idea that he might be reacting to the MMR. I was dumbfounded! He had all three symptoms of an adverse reaction to MMR—and within the specified time frame. It took almost a month, but thankfully my son recovered with no obvious long-term damage. Deeply alarmed by the refusal of the medical community to explore the possibility that MMR was the culprit, I called our public health office and provided a detailed account of what had transpired. I had taken photos of my son which I offered to submit to Public Health, but was told that the Chief Medical Officer would contact me as part of the investigation and I could provide the photos at that time. No follow-up ever occurred. A few weeks later, I received a letter from the Chief Medical Officer dismissing the case without explanation and simply stating that my son should continue to follow the vaccination schedule. Upon receipt of the letter, I was in shock. I called back to Public Health and spoke with the intake nurse who had handled the case earlier. She was as stunned as I was. I know that I do not have 'scientific proof' that MMR was the culprit, but neither did the medical community have proof that it was not. When you look at the timing and the adverse symptoms, it is almost certain that MMR was the problem. That is even more true now, two years later, when he has failed to react to anything else in his food or environment. At the very least, the Chief Medical Officer should have maintained an open file on my son with a big question mark, but that never happened. I withheld his next MMR vaccine. Even more than the terrifying ordeal, the reaction of the medical community has made me totally distrust the vaccine program. If we could be confident that the medical community was properly recording and investigating adverse reactions when they do occur, then we might be able to have some trust in the system. But they are not. How many other cases like that of my son have been swept under the carpet rather than reported and investigated so they could help to sound the alarm that a problem exists? We have no idea what is really happening out there because the medical community and pharmaceutical companies are terrified of having their programs put at risk. If they had our children's best interests at heart, and knew that a sizable number of children are having serious adverse reactions, some vaccines would be pulled for further investigation. MMR could be administered as three separate vaccines, and they could try to develop new non-threatening tests to determine which children are at risk for a reaction. By engaging in denials and cover-ups, the medical community itself is undermining public confidence. I was stunned when I did my own research and learned that doctors in Britain and Switzerland had written letters arguing that the MMR vaccine was not adequately tested before it was approved. My son, like all the others who have been tragically damaged or who have lost their lives, is one too many."

▸ "Three days ago my friend's 15-month-old daughter was hospitalized after experiencing a high fever and her first seizure. The hospital put the baby through a series of tests, including a CAT scan and CBC. My friend told me he thought it was a reaction to the MMR vaccine she recently received. However, the doctors were puzzled and disallowed this explanation."

▸ "My friend's 15-month-old daughter received an MMR vaccine. Within eight days she was hospitalized. My friend called to see what I could find out about Stevens-Johnson syndrome. They told her that her daughter may die as a result of this."

▸ "A dear friend lost her 15-month-old daughter two weeks after her MMR. She was healthy and showed no signs of illness yet died suddenly in her sleep one afternoon. The post mortem revealed a viral infection and traces of pneumonia, but her mother and I find it very hard to believe that the vaccine wasn't to blame."

▸ "One week after the MMR shot for my 16-month-old daughter, she had diarrhea. The next day she had three seizures. What steps should be taken once a reaction has occurred? I want to be sure it is documented and the government made aware."

▸ "Ten days after MMR vaccine was injected into our daughter, she was dead. Two days ago I carried my daughter to her grave. We were told to possibly expect a mild reaction after 10 days; she was only seventeen months old. We believe our daughter died to save others, and that she holds the key. We will seek justice and bring all the lies to a stop and have the perpetrators locked up for crimes against humanity. All those little children, and for what? We are dealing with nothing short of a holocaust—government sanctioned corporate profiteering and killing at taxpayers' expense."

▸ "My daughter had a serious reaction to MMR at 22 months. She developed brain damage after a fever of 106 degrees. She also has seizures which are unresponsive to medication, damage to the nerves of her eyes, and learning disabilities that she battles every day. We took her case to court and lost. The doctor who testified on their behalf stated that the government only called him in when they wanted a finding in their favor. What a setup! Of course *they* don't have to live with the frustrations and expense of raising these vaccine-damaged children."

▸ "Are there more people like me who have lost children to diabetes from the MMR shot? Can you send me studies, data, or personal stories that you have concerning other babies, such as mine, who went into sudden onset diabetes after getting the MMR shot?"

▸ "My once healthy son reacted eight days after his MMR when he developed urticaria which was treated with antihistamine. He soon started to have epileptic seizures, and one by one tried many of the anti-convulsant drugs with little or no effect. Years later, and for no obvious reason, the seizures really took hold and, to cut this long and tragic story short, he underwent emergency brain surgery at the age of 9 years. After that he was a changed youngster, his personality was lost and he behaved in a basic, instinctive way. The part of the brain which was removed from the frontal region was tested in an independent lab. The measles virus was found. A second test was carried out to ascertain whether this was a 'wild' measles virus or if it was from the MMR vaccine. Yes, you've guessed already—it was a vaccine virus. As if things weren't bad enough, no medic or politician will listen to real-life stories such as this. How on earth are we to make progress if those in authority keep their ears closed? Our son is now 16 years old and has spent most of his life battling against the odds. All this because we wanted to do our best and protect him by taking him along for his vaccinations. The very best of luck to everyone."

▸ "Three days after my daughter received her MMR, she started blinking her eyes and sniffling a lot. She's been doing this for 2½ months now. Is there a link between the MMR and facial tics?"

▸ "Five days after my healthy 19-month-old son had his MMR shot, he developed croup with a temperature of 104. Of course, his doctor says they are not related."

▸ "When my daughter was 2 years old, she received her MMR shot. Five days later, she had a high fever and seizures. Now she has a hearing loss."

▸ "My daughter received her 2nd MMR when she was three years old. Shortly after, she started having a problem with her hearing. Can MMR damage hearing?"

▸ "I became aware of the truth almost too late after my youngest had been 'poisoned' by vaccination as a baby. When she started school, she had a terrible response to the MMR serum at the tender age of five and almost died. (Her doctor at that time even blamed the nasty stuff! He was a rarity.)"

▸ "My son recently contracted SSPE, a measles-virus illness [which is invariably fatal]. It all started 3 years ago when his health deteriorated to where he could not function—no walking, talking or head movement whatsoever. My son never had measles but he had the MMR vaccination when he was 9 years old. The gestation period for SSPE is from 2 to 12 years. It doesn't take a brain surgeon to figure out what caused my son's ailment but trying to prove it is a different matter."

▸ "My 12-year-old had a seizure within 10 minutes of his second MMR. His head rolled side to side and his arms jerked a couple of times. He was unaware of this, so he must have blanked out. Afterwards, he felt woozy, very tired, and had a headache at the bridge of his nose. Also, his arm that got the shot was numb. The feeling in it gradually returned over the course of an hour."

▸ "At the age of 14, the doctor said my MMR from previous years was obsolete, so they gave me another shot. I walked out of the office, passed out immediately, awoke, vomited profusely, and passed out again. My mother screamed for help. Can you believe they actually tried to charge my mother for another visit!?"

▸ "I have a 15-year-old daughter. We recently moved to the U.S. from the U.K. without her medical records. Upon arrival we were required to give her complete immunizations. I strongly objected but felt pushed into re-immunization because of state laws to get her into school. After her second MMR she has been complaining of dizzy spells and continuous headaches. Is there a link between over-immunization of MMR and this sickness?"

▸ "When I was a child, I was given MMR. Almost seven days to the hour I became ill: fever, sweats, throwing up even the slightest amount of fluid or food. This went on for a month or so. The doctors would not even consider that the shots caused the illness. Later, they wanted me to have the second MMR; my parents refused. The doctors went through the usual tantrums and said I wouldn't be able to attend school. When my parents said 'Fine, he won't go,' the doctors gave in. At about the age of 18, I had a blood screening and was told I didn't have all of the MMR vaccine. Forgetting the episode as a child, I let them give me the shot. Seven days later I was sick again, but not as severe."

▸ "When I was fifteen, there was a supposed outbreak of measles. Parents were told that in order for their children to continue attending public school, they were required to get MMR. So, my parents dutifully obeyed. Two days later, I was feeling kind of sick, but not quite enough to stay home from school. Over the course of that day, I began to feel weaker and weaker, and my fever grew. By the time I got home and was able to take my temperature, it was up to 104. I remember laying on the couch, and although I was covered by about six blankets, I was shivering so badly that the entire couch was shaking. The next minute I was so hot that I would throw off the blankets. I had no interest in food or drink and was unable to even hold water down. I went to bed that night, and after about four hours finally fell into an exhausted sleep. When I woke up the next morning, I had a headache so severe that I was seeing double. I am not sure how high my fever got. A week later, my oldest brother's girlfriend died at the age of sixteen. The cause of death was ruled the MMR booster shot. She had been perfectly healthy before this. I was given the shot at the same location on the same day as the girl who died. I vowed never to get a shot again, and haven't since then."

▸ "I was told that I wouldn't be allowed to register for my college classes if I didn't have the MMR. I was very distressed because I knew of the side effects, but I also wanted to continue my education. So, feeling I had no other option, I got the shot. The nurse administered the vaccine. I told her I felt ill, but she assured me I'd be just fine. Upon standing, I vomited on the floor. She said it was my 'nerves' and that I would get over it. I paid for the shot, feeling very dizzy and faint. I told the front desk lady that I was feeling faint and having tunnel vision. She seemed unconcerned. Thinking fresh air would help me, I somehow stumbled to the door and made it to my car. I am still unsure how I made it that far safely. I had to lie in my car in the parking lot for half an hour before I could drive home. Once home, I felt feverish and went directly to bed. I stayed there for three days battling what felt like the flu, complete with a lack of energy, muscle aches, and a fever. I called the doctor's office and was told it was 'normal' for patients to experience those symptoms post vaccination. I didn't return for my second dose. It confirmed that I won't put any children I may have through that. I can only imagine what a baby would feel, being unable to vocalize her discomfort aside from crying. It breaks my heart."

▸ "I was told by the nursing school where I am enrolled, "No vaccine, no school." Even though I had all the normal vaccines as a child, I was unable to show this. Five days after I received the MMR vaccine, I was so ill that I ended up in the emergency room. The doctor told me that the MMR did not cause my sickness, and my nursing school supervisor said it was a virus. Why does the medical establishment deny vaccine reactions? Why can't they tell us this important information and let us make educated responsible decisions. The irony is that I got the vaccine and now I'm so sick that I can't go to school."

▸ "My daughter received a double dose of the MMR vaccine because her pediatrician told me that she got the first one too early. Now she has a major mood disorder and has been diagnosed as clinically depressed and learning disabled. She can be sweet and bright, but when her bad mood overtakes her, she can be abusive, hostile, cruel and out of control."

▸ "My college refused to admit me without an MMR vaccine. I had a terrible reaction and was rushed to the hospital with piercing screams, a high temperature and delirium. Now I have trouble focusing, and can be scattered and forgetful. I can't stand change and don't have the energy and drive that I once had. My family thinks I developed obsessive-compulsive disorder. I am very bright, but nearly blew my scholarship after the shot."

▸ "I'm a chiropractor. The other day, one of my patients informed me that she tried to get an acquaintance of hers to at least study up on vaccines to make an informed choice. This lady looked at her as if 'how dare she believe that vaccines are not the best thing to do.' She said this lady called her in tears the other day saying that she wished she had taken the time to listen to my patient and do the research because her child started having seizures the same day that she got MMR."

▸ "My daughter had MMR when she was traveling abroad at the age of 28, one year ago. Shortly after the shot she noticed that her ear was bothering her, that her glands seemed swollen. Since then, she has not felt well. Her head feels dizzy, her ears are plugged, and she has a buzzing in her head that hurts when loud sounds are around her. She has had a general feeling of malaise and other symptoms such as pain in her sigmoid area, a numbness running down her leg, and other very strange things. Have you ever heard of this type of reaction?"

▸ "Today, shortly after I was inoculated with the MMR vaccine, I began feeling faint and short of breath. After ten minutes of holding my head between my knees in a dirty gas station bathroom, I decided I could drive the 20 miles home."

▸ "Five years ago, I was given an MMR shot and within days was suffering from ulcerative colitis. I now spend my days rushing to the bathroom (10-20 times daily), suffering severely from the disease. Doctors say that UC is incurable and they suggest removing my colon. What can I do? I want my life back."

How effective is the MMR vaccine?
Prior to the introduction of the measles, mumps and rubella vaccines, thousands of cases of measles, mumps and rubella occurred every year. Today, these numbers are greatly reduced. However, unlike the natural diseases, the MMR vaccine does not confer permanent immunity. For example, measles epidemics regularly occur in vaccinated populations. According to the CDC, "measles transmission has been clearly documented among vaccinated persons. In some large outbreaks...over 95 percent of cases have a history of vaccination."[13] Outbreaks of mumps and rubella often occur in vaccinated people as well.[14] Evidently, immunity is short-lived. The *Journal of the America Medical Association* published data showing that antibody levels after rubella vaccinations fell to half their high point within four years.[15] The medical literature contains many examples of MMR vaccine failures. Thus, people who receive MMR may still be susceptible to the three diseases.

In a study conducted by scientists from the Direct Health 2000 clinic in Eltham, South London, England, half of all children vaccinated with MMR were found to have "zero or very low immunity" against measles and mumps. According to Dr. Sarah Dean, who

Figure 49:

MMR Booster Doses:
Do Doctors and Nurses Recommend Them?

Doctors & Nurses

Doctors

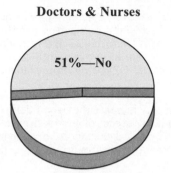

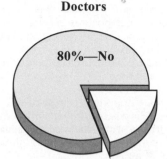

51 percent of all surveyed U.K. doctors and nurses had reservations about or disagreed with the policy of giving booster doses.

80 percent of all surveyed U.K. doctors would not "unequivocally recommend" a second dose of MMR to a wavering parent.

Source: *British Medical Journal* (January 13, 2001); 322:82-85.

oversaw the study, "This means there could be a lot of children who think they have got the umbrella protection" yet remain at risk. Dean believes that young children's immune systems cannot cope with more than one virus at a time.[16] Yet, a second dose of MMR was added to immunization schedules.

The *British Medical Journal* published a survey of doctor's and nurse's attitudes toward booster doses of MMR. Fifty-one percent of all U.K. doctors and nurses had reservations about or disagreed with the policy of giving an MMR booster shot, and 80 percent of all U.K. doctors would not "unequivocally recommend" the second dose to a wavering parent (Figure 49).[17]

MMR and Autism

Many parents report that their perfectly healthy children became autistic after receiving the MMR vaccine. (Autism is a complex autoimmune and developmental disability. Common symptoms include inadequate verbal and social skills, repetitive behavior patterns, little or no interest in human contact, self-destructive behavior, and gastrointestinal anomalies.)[18-20] The affected children were developing normally, then regressed after receiving the triple shot, losing their previously acquired skills. The medical community vociferously denies any connection between the MMR vaccine and autism. However, in 1998 *Lancet* published a landmark study by Dr. Andrew Wakefield linking the onset of autistic symptoms to the MMR vaccine.[21] Wakefield and his world-class team of medical experts investigated previously normal children who subsequently suffered from intestinal abnormalities and regressive developmental disorder, including a loss of acquired skills. In most cases, "onset of symptoms was after measles, mumps, and rubella immunisation."[22] Further research uncovered a possible explanation:

> Atypical patterns of exposure to common childhood infections —measles, mumps, rubella and chickenpox—have been associated with autism and autistic regression.... A close temporal relationship in the exposure to two of these

infections during periods of susceptibility may compound both the risk and severity of autism.... Although historically, these rare patterns of exposure may have accounted for only a small proportion of autism, the widespread use of a combination of the candidate agents in a single vaccine [MMR] may have changed this.[23]

An earlier study published in the *American Journal of Epidemiology* identified in utero and infant exposures as periods of apparent susceptibility, when both the brain and immune system are undergoing rapid development.[24] Thus, fetuses and young children are especially prone to adverse consequences if they contract two or more viral infections concurrently. Wakefield elaborated on the increased perils of being exposed to more than one virus at a time:

> One important pattern of infection that may increase the risk of delayed disease is where different viruses interact, either with each other or both interact with the host immune system simultaneously. Virologic data support the possibility of a compound effect of multiple concurrent viral exposures influencing...the risk of autism.[25]

Is it safer to receive MMR as three separate shots?
Dr. Wakefield theorized that if a child who is exposed to two or more *wild* viral infections around the same time is at increased risk for autism, then a child who is injected with three live viruses via the MMR vaccine is equally susceptible to the ailment, if not more so. Thus, Wakefield proposed separating the measles, mumps and rubella vaccines from the three-in-one MMR shot—the way they were in the 1970s prior to being combined—and administering them individually over the course of several weeks or months. His solution would satisfy immunization recommendations designed to protect against the three diseases while safeguarding against the risk of autism:

> If, following thorough independent scientific investigation, it emerges that autistic...disorders are causally related to a compound influence of the component viruses of MMR, whether these viruses have been encountered naturally or in the vaccine, then through judicious use of the vaccines, one may have a means for preventing the disease [autism]. Spacing the single vaccines, thereby dissociating the exposures that, together, may constitute the risk, provides a way of not only preventing the acute measles, mumps and rubella infections, but also, potentially, the risk of one of the most devastating diseases that it has been our misfortune to encounter.[26]

For families that elect to vaccinate their children, Wakefield's proposal to separate the shots seems like a prudent approach, especially since recipients of MMR are being injected with three different live viruses—contained within a chemical mixture of three diverse and potent drugs—all at once. Furthermore, the medical and scientific literature contains evidence linking the MMR vaccine to a multitude of serious adverse reactions. The MMR vaccine manufacturer, plus numerous unsolicited personal stories, confirm the tragic possibilities.[27] Thus, when Wakefield's research was first publicized, concerned parents quickly rejected MMR and demanded instead the individual shots. Several doctors initially supported Wakefield's recommendation and complied with their clients' requests. However, *the individual measles, mumps and rubella vaccines are capable of causing severe adverse reactions* as well. These are also listed by the manufacturer and documented in numerous studies.[28] (Note: In 2010, Dr. Wakefield was found guilty of professional misconduct and struck off the medical register. Read more in the Autism chapter.)

MMR was initially administered as three separate shots, rarely at the same time. Thus, early reports of adverse consequences could be attributed to a particular vaccine. Later, when the three-in-one MMR vaccine replaced the individual vaccines it became much more difficult to link a bad reaction to either the measles, mumps, or rubella portions of the shot. Today, MMR is often given with other vaccines as well, making it even more difficult to determine whether one vaccine in particular caused an adverse reaction, or if all of the vaccines given at once overwhelmed the recipient's immune system. (For more information about this, read the chapter on multiple vaccines given simultaneously.)

Why are the three vaccines combined?

The three vaccines—measles, mumps and rubella—are combined into a single shot for *convenience,* not safety or efficacy. In fact, when 180 Swiss physicians analyzed 320 scientific works from around the world they concluded that *there is no medical foundation for combining measles, mumps and rubella into a single shot.*[29] Speaking as a group, these doctors formally rejected a compulsory MMR immunization campaign, but not before making several observations:

> One thing is...unmistakably clear from the example of the USA: the MMR immunization campaign...has elements of compulsion that work right into the sphere of individual rights. Since the USA has enforced a 95 percent immunization level by means of obligatory vaccination, unexpected epidemics now make rigorous, police-enforced measures necessary, with quarantines, exclusions from school, and house-to-house vaccinations. An obligatory MMR *booster* vaccination has already been implemented...
>
> Similar experiences have been recorded in other countries with high levels of immunization. Moreover, recent investigations...have convincingly shown that eradication of the three diseases of measles, rubella, and mumps is in practice impossible. The rational basis of every immunization strategy that rests upon the mass vaccination of infants is thereby invalidated...
>
> These three childhood diseases necessitate the fulfillment of three completely different objectives to which it is impossible to do justice with a single combined injection... After a careful analysis of the relevant material [we, the 180 unified physicians] reject the state MMR immunization campaign... [and] advocate a very restrained, individually adjusted immunization practice which takes account of the different nature of the problems relating to the three childhood diseases, does not fundamentally alter the epidemiology of the three diseases, and respects parents' freedom of choice.[30]

Can the three vaccines be administered separately?

Yes. The three vaccines—for measles, mumps and rubella—can be administered separately because they are manufactured individually. Details can be found in the *Physician's Desk Reference* at the library.[31] However, doctors and health authorities in the United States, England and other countries are unlikely to offer this option to their clients.[32] In fact, most doctors refuse to honor parental requests for the individual vaccines. They claim that if these vaccines are administered separately, children will remain vulnerable to disease.

Here are typical comments made by parents seeking the individual vaccines:[33]

▶ "I read that ultra-sensitive kids do better with individual components of MMR rather than the three-in-one shot. Our son has had sensory issues so we would like to have him vaccinated separately, but I can't find the individual vaccines and our doctor won't help."

▶ "How can we get the MMR vaccine administered to our son in three separate doses instead of one MMR shot? Our health department says that it's impossible."

In England, the British Medical Association formally banned making single vaccines for measles, mumps, and rubella available. Doctors who oppose this ban risk losing their licenses to practice. For example, Peter Mansfield, a U.K. doctor who believes that families should have the right to choose single vaccinations instead of the controversial MMR, and who has been offering them as an alternative, was accused by the General Medical Council of putting children at risk; he faced a disciplinary hearing that nearly forced him to end his medical career.[34]

Figure 50:

MMR, Crohn's Disease, and Autism:
What Do Nurses Think?

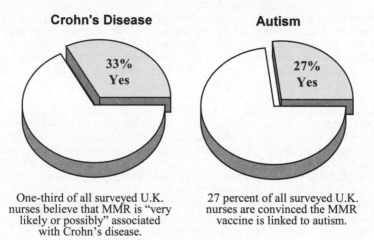

Crohn's Disease

33%
Yes

Autism

27%
Yes

One-third of all surveyed U.K. nurses believe that MMR is "very likely or possibly" associated with Crohn's disease.

27 percent of all surveyed U.K. nurses are convinced the MMR vaccine is linked to autism.

Source: *British Medical Journal* (January 13, 2001); 322:82-85.

What do nurses think?

British researchers questioned nurses about MMR's possible link to new diseases. One-third believe that MMR is "very likely or possibly" associated with Crohn's disease, and 27 percent are convinced the MMR vaccine is linked to autism (Figure 50).[35]

Adverse Reaction Reports: MMR and Autism

This section contains unsolicited adverse reaction reports linking the MMR vaccine to autism or autistic-like behaviors. They are typical of the daily emails received by the *Thinktwice Global Vaccine Institute* (www.thinktwice.com).[36]

▶ "After my son's MMR at 12 months, his development and personality changed. He would stare off and not notice anything, not even the waving of my hand in front of his face. His personality became nothing—he lost all words and still has none. It is so hard to see my only son lose his personality and life to a shot."

▶ "My son received the MMR shot shortly after his first birthday. I complained to his doctor when he did not walk, talk or respond as a normal one-year-old. I was told that the shots would not have that reaction. He was diagnosed as mentally retarded, autistic, and Tourette's syndrome. I am convinced that he has these problems due to the shots. He suffered severe diarrhea, etc.—all of the symptoms. I pray that something will be done to stop the government from mandating these shots so that another child (and parent) will not have to suffer this. It has truly been an emotional roller coaster raising him. Although he has been in a special school since kindergarten, the calls to pick him up because he had a bathroom accident, is hitting, tics are out of control, etc., has been very overwhelming."

▶ "At 12 months, my daughter received her first MMR vaccine. Within the hour she began vomiting and developed a fever of 103. We went to emergency and when she got in to see a doctor (an hour later) she had developed a rash. The doctor confirmed that it was indeed a measles rash in reaction to the vaccine (he also quoted something like less than 2 percent of cases end up with the rash) but stated that the vomiting was likely because she may have been sick prior to the vaccination. Public Health required the reaction to be reported, which I did, and I got a letter back advising that her next MMR immunization be done in a 'hospital setting.' My daughter did not eat all weekend. When she was 3 years old, we noticed some speech issues. As parents, we could not understand more than 75 percent of her sentences. Others could never understand her. She went for speech therapy. In the process, screenings were done and she also had sensory integration dysfunction (SID). I went into her journal and was able to determine that only since her first birthday did she start displaying the symptoms that became the basis of the SID diagnosis. (Nobody could touch or tickle her. She would smell everything—paper, pencils, cloth, plastic, toys, string—before using it, like a compulsion.) She went from being a contented child to an anxious, inconsolable child. I was a diehard immunization advocate, but after that experience I think vaccines are not all they are hyped up to be by the medical profession!"

▸ "My sister's son is six years old and has received all of his vaccines. When he was a year old he could say ten words. He was a happy baby. At 15 months he got his MMR vaccine. Shortly after, his sister was born. Since around that time he started to change little by little. He stopped talking and began to act differently. He would point at things rather than say what he wanted. He did not always turn his head when people called him. He would go in his own world and some of his behavior seemed autistic. He would cover his ears when he heard noise. His behavior became more difficult to deal with. He was paranoid and screamed when they took him in public and also when visitors came by. He always had to have something in his hand that he would bang up against things. Today, he still feels the need to twirl something in his hand or bang something. He also needs to release energy and nervousness from his body by running back and forth."

▸ "My son is vaccine-injured. After his 15-month vaccines, he could no longer stand, quit talking, quit turning his head when his name was called, and had terrible diarrhea that still isn't resolved six years later. He is autistic, and his spinal fluid contains vaccine-strain measles virus."

▸ "When our beautiful, healthy, only son was 15 months old, he was given his routine MMR. In four days he was at death's door with meningitis. He could no longer speak, walk, eat, or see. His behavior could best be described as autistic."

▸ "I watched my normal son regress into autism two weeks following his MMR shot at 15 months. His pediatrician failed us. The government failed us. The Institute for Health, the FDA and the CDC failed us. They all lie and deceive and are motivated by money. Autism doesn't run in my family. My daughter, age 5, is completely normal and healthy. My son stopped talking since that vaccine. It's no coincidence that he became very sick and visited the doctor seven times following the MMR. Nobody helped us. Nobody helped our son. Two years later, his school district is failing us, lying to us, doctoring his educational records. Since autism has entered my life, I have given up support for this country and our school system. I don't wave the flag and it's very sad that the U.S. doesn't have any choice but to focus on terrorism rather than our forgotten learning-disabled children."

▸ "My 10-year-old son was healthy until nine days after his MMR vaccine at age 16 months. He had two febrile seizures and a measles rash, then lost his few words of speech over the next week."

▸ "My granddaughter was vaccinated for MMR. Ten days later, she stopped talking, standing, and has developed a shakiness that affects her whole upper body. EEG, MRI, Rett syndrome testing, blood tests, have all come back negative. Doctors say they have never seen this before. They want to do a spinal tap. I am so afraid of the risks to the baby. She is 17 months old and her immune system has been shot down by the MMR."

▸ "I am a new mother of a beautiful 5-month-old girl whose 8-year-old half-brother was stricken with severe epilepsy and mild autism following his MMR shots when he was 18 months old. He has suffered more than 50 seizures, some requiring hospitalization."

▸ "We are concerned parents of a 23-month-old toddler. At 12 months he seemed quite normal. He spoke a few words, waved bye-bye and threw a ball when asked. Now he shows signs of autistic-like behavior. He does not talk, he walks on his toes, and flaps his arms constantly. At times he seems to be in his own world, running back and forth aimlessly. He does not give eye contact and does not indicate his needs. When his name is called, he does not acknowledge the caller. I strongly feel...that my son is a victim of some adverse effect caused by the MMR vaccine."

▶ "My friend works for a lady who has three autistic children, two boys and one girl. The girl was two years old when she got her MMR, and within 48 hours she could no longer speak or function like a 2-year-old. She was later diagnosed with autism, the same for the boys. I starting reading everything and now have knowledge to make my own decision. I understand my legal rights and how to get my kids exempt from these harmful vaccines."

▶ "My first child received MMR when I was pregnant and exposed my unborn child to the rubella virus. He was born profoundly deaf with ADHD and autistic traits."

▶ "When my son was a baby, I got him all of the required shots. He reacted badly to MMR and has since been diagnosed with pervasive developmental disorder."

▶ "My friend had a normal child react to the MMR vaccine and to this day is autistic."

▶ "My stepson was adversely affected by his MMR. He has seizures and is autistic."

▶ "Exactly 14 days after my son's MMR, he had measles-type and mumps-type reactions. He is now autistic. He also has leaky gut syndrome and asthma. My son was in PERFECT health up until the day of his reaction. He lost all powers of speech on that day and has never regained them."

▶ "Prior to my son's MMR vaccine he said loads of words. Now he has very little speech and is autistic. If I could turn back the clock, I would, but now I have to live with the knowledge that we did not protect him; we let them damage him beyond repair."

▶ "My grandson had his MMR vaccine and immediately showed signs that were puzzling to us. He stopped talking, only screamed, and started to walk on his toes. Doctors were no help. We were finally told he has 'autistic traits.' There are four more babies in our family and the parents are all worried that this might also happen to their children. My question: Is it the mercury in vaccines that does this, or is it the three shots together?"

▶ "I feel that my country is letting me down. My daughter developed early with her speech at under six months old. She was such a happy baby who loved nothing more than physical contact. And then came the imminent choice of the MMR. After much deliberation, I decided to vaccinate her. I wish I could turn back time. Her speech disappeared, her early skills had also gone, and suddenly it seemed as if she had forgotten everything she once knew. It was as if someone had stolen my daughter away from me. Of course, physically she looked the same, but the baby I knew was locked inside her own mind. We are awaiting diagnosis of autistic spectrum disorder, and while the doctors are fine talking about her condition, the room falls silent at the mention of MMR. We know what that shot has done to our child. Isn't it blatantly obvious to the rest of the world? I've come to the conclusion that the world has gone mad, but amongst the madness I'm focused on staying sane and being the voice of my daughter. One day our silent children will speak for themselves."

▶ "My son became autistic due to a single dose of MMR. People who do not believe that there is a connection haven't had to live the nightmare. Thankfully, after his reaction to the vaccine we did research and he never received another dose. I must constantly fight with his schools because most doctors refuse to acknowledge a connection between MMR and autism. I will do anything to help reform and/or ban the vaccine that changed my son's life and future. With or without anyone's help, no matter what roadblocks are put in my way, I will make sure the word gets out to both the parents of the victimized children as well as to the rest of the unknowing public. This is a cause I am dedicated to no matter where it leads me. They will never find a cure until they freely admit the cause. Not one more lost child! May God bless all the victims of this preventable disease."

Is the MMR vaccine mandatory?
Although the CDC recommends that most children receive two doses of MMR, each state offers legal exemptions to the shots.

Where can I get more information about MMR?
For more information about MMR, please read the individual chapters on measles, mumps and rubella. The chapter on autism also has a lot of important data pertaining to the MMR vaccine.

Autism

In 1943, the well-known child psychiatrist, Dr. Leo Kanner, announced his discovery of 11 cases of a new mental disorder. He noted that "the condition differs markedly and uniquely from anything reported so far..."[1] This condition soon became known as autism.

What is autism?
Autism (often referred to as autistic spectrum disorder, Asperger's syndrome, or pervasive developmental disorder) is a complex developmental disability—a neurological derangement that affects the functioning of the brain. This condition usually appears during the first three years of life and often strikes following an early childhood of apparently normal development. Mental and social regression are not uncommon. Although the severity of the affliction varies from child to child, the following symptoms are typical: inadequate verbal and social skills, impaired speech, repetition of words, bizarre or repetitive behavior patterns, uncontrollable head-banging, screaming fits, arm flapping, little or no interest in human contact, unresponsiveness to parents and other people, extreme resistance to minor changes in the home environment, self-destructive behavior, hypersensitivity to sensory stimuli, and an inability to care for oneself.[2,3]

How common is autism?
According to several researchers who investigated Kanner's claims, autism was extremely rare prior to 1943.[4] Using Kanner's own case definition of autism, Dr. Darold Treffert calculated a rate in Wisconsin (from 1949-1969) of less than 1 in 10,000 (.00007).[5] In 1966, Dr. Victor Lotter published the first epidemiological study of autism in England and found the rate to be 4.1 per 10,000 children.[6] However, by the 1980s over 4500 new cases were being reported every year in the United States alone.[7] In 1997, the CDC reported that 1 of every 500 children is autistic (20 per 10,000).[8] In 2007, the CDC showed that autism affects 1 of every 150 U.S. children (67 per 10,000).[9] In 2009, new research by the CDC raised the autism rate to 1 in 110, and much worse for boys.[10] That same year, a study in *Pediatrics* showed that autism affects 1 of every 91 children (110 per 10,000).[11] In 2011, a new study published in the *American Journal of Psychiatry* found that 1 of every 38 children (263 per 10,000) has an autism spectrum disorder.[12] "We have an epidemic on our hands," exclaimed Congressional representative Christopher Smith.[13] Congressman Chip Pickering described the epidemic in more sobering terms: *"More children will be diagnosed with autism this year than AIDS, diabetes and cancer combined."*[14]

What causes autism?
When the first cases of autism began to appear in the 1940s, researchers were puzzled by the high incidence of autistic children being born into well-educated families. Over 90 percent of the parents were high school graduates. Nearly three-fourths of the fathers and one-half of the mothers had graduated from college. Many had professional careers. As a result, scientists unsuccessfully tried to link autism to genetic factors in upper class populations.[15] Meanwhile, psychiatrists, unaware of the neurological basis of the illness, sought psychological explanations. The mother was accused of not providing an emotionally secure home environment, and presumed to be the cause of her afflicted child's ailment.[16,17]

Today, researchers have discounted these earlier notions but still do not have a complete understanding of this condition. Although autism has been linked to biological and neurological differences in the brain, and genetic factors appear to play a role in the etiology of this disease, no single cause has been identified.[18] However, recent dramatic increases in the number of children stricken with this debilitating ailment—coincident with the introduction of new vaccines—may shed some light on this medical mystery.

Autism and compulsory vaccination programs:
The first cases of autism in the United States occurred at a time shortly after the pertussis vaccine became available. When the pertussis vaccine was initially introduced (during

the late 1930s), only the rich and educated parents who sought the very best for their children, and who could afford a private doctor, were in a position to request the newest medical advancements. (Remember how researchers were puzzled by the high incidence of autistic children being born into well-educated and "upper class" families.) However, by the 1960s and 1970s parents all over the country, within every income and educational level, were seeking help for their autistic children. Socioeconomic disparities began to disappear during this period. Today, autism is evenly distributed among all social classes and ethnic groups.[19] Once again this puzzled the researchers. Many simply concluded that earlier studies were flawed, but there is an explanation. Free vaccinations at public health clinics didn't yet exist in the 1940s and 1950s. Compulsory vaccination programs were still on the horizon. However, as vaccine programs grew, parents from across the socioeconomic spectrum gained equal access to them. The growing number of children suffering from this new illness directly coincided with the increasing popularity of the mandated vaccination programs during these same years. Autistic children were now being discovered within every kind of family in dreadfully greater numbers than ever before imagined.[20]

The same correlations between autism and childhood vaccination programs may be found in other countries as well. When the United States ended World War II and occupied Japan, a mandatory vaccine program was established. The first autistic Japanese child was diagnosed in 1945.[21] Hundreds of new cases of autism were being diagnosed annually in Japanese children shortly thereafter.[22]

Europe began promoting the pertussis vaccine in the 1950s; the first cases of autism began to appear there in the same decade. In England, the pertussis vaccine wasn't promoted on a large scale until the late 1950s. Shortly thereafter, in 1962, the National Society for Autistic Children in Britain was established.[23]

In the 1980s and 1990s, cases of autism soared once again. For example, the California Department of Health examined the number of people with autism requiring developmental resources. There were increases each year from 1987 to 1998, with an overall increase of 273 percent during this period. Services for all other developmental disabilities increased by no more than 50 percent during this same period.[24] The U.S. Department of Education (DOE) showed even greater increases: from 1991 to 1997, the number of children with autism requiring special education services increased 556 percent.[25] In fact, DOE figures show higher rates of autism in every state.[26] Other countries have experienced similar increases.[27] Impartial autism researchers do not attribute these increases to better diagnostic skills nor to expanded diagnostic categories. Several analysts implicate vaccines—especially the three-in-one live-virus MMR shot introduced and vigorously marketed during this period (see pages 143-154). Analysts also blame the busier vaccine schedule and greater number of mercury-containing vaccines mandated for children (see pages 164-175.) In fact, each year as the number of required vaccines rise, autism cases soar (Figure 51).[28,29] Aluminum-containing vaccines may also be a factor (see pages 175-177).

MMR: A Link to Autism

In 1995, Dr. James Oleske, a pediatric immunologist, tested an autistic child thought to have been damaged by an MMR vaccine and found that his measles titers (antibody levels) were three times higher than normal. Dr. Oleske continued his research and discovered this same pattern in other autistic patients. His findings were presented at a National Institutes of Health (NIH) meeting.[30]

In 1996, Dr. Hugh Fudenberg, director of the NeuroImmuno Therapeutics Research Foundation in Spartanburg, South Carolina, published a pilot study on infantile onset autism and noted that 75 percent of his subjects exhibited their initial symptoms within one week of vaccination.[31] That same year, Dr. Sudhir Gupta, world-renowned immunologist, also noted an apparent association between the onset of autistic symptoms and vaccination, especially MMR. He presented his findings at the National Autism Association in Chicago.[32] Dr. Bernard Rimland, director of the internationally recognized Autism Research Institute, spoke at the 1996 Chicago conference on autism as well. He believes that overzealous childhood vaccine programs are a leading cause of current epidemics of autism.[33]

Figure 51:

Vaccines and Autism

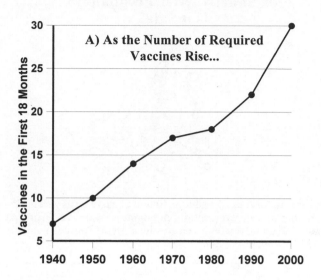

A) As the Number of Required Vaccines Rise...

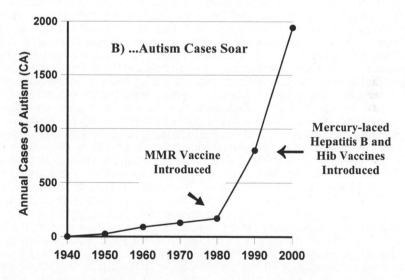

B) ...Autism Cases Soar

MMR Vaccine Introduced

Mercury-laced Hepatitis B and Hib Vaccines Introduced

In the 1940s and 1950s, children received DPT and smallpox vaccines. By 2000, babies under 1½ years of age were required to receive *30 doses* of various vaccine and chemical compounds, including inoculations for hepatitis B, DTaP, Hib, polio, MMR, chickenpox, and pneumococcal disease. Cases of autism skyrocketed during this period. Source: Children's Hospital of Philadelphia; Centers for Disease Control and Prevention; California Department of Health and Human Services.

Figure 52:

The MMR Vaccine Before, During, or Shortly After Pregnancy: Is it Safe?

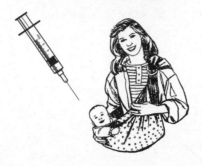

According to Dr. Edward Yazbak, the administration of a live virus vaccine booster (MMR or rubella) to a mother around conception, pregnancy, or delivery (postpartum) "may not be safe or wise" and could result in a child with autism. Source: Yazbak, E. "Autism: Is There a Vaccine Connection," 2000.

In 1998, *Lancet* published a landmark study by Dr. Andrew Wakefield linking the onset of autistic symptoms to the MMR vaccine.[34] Wakefield and his world-class team of medical experts investigated previously normal children who subsequently suffered from intestinal abnormalities and regressive developmental disorder, including a loss of acquired skills. In most cases, "onset of symptoms was after measles, mumps, and rubella immunisation." Furthermore, "the uniformity of the intestinal pathological changes and the fact that previous studies have found intestinal dysfunction in children with autistic-spectrum disorders, suggests that the connection is real and reflects a unique disease process."[35]

In 1999, Dr. Edward Yazbak published two separate studies showing significant correlations between MMR and autism. In the first study, mothers who received an MMR vaccine prior to conception and again in the postpartum period (shortly after giving birth) increased their child's risk of autism when they breastfed their child *and* later permitted the child to receive an MMR vaccine.[36] In Yazbak's second study, six of seven children (86%) born to mothers who received an MMR vaccine prior to conception and again during pregnancy were diagnosed with autism. The seventh child had developmental problems.[37]

In 2000, Dr. Yazbak published a third study demonstrating that "the administration of a live virus vaccine booster (MMR) to a mother around conception, pregnancy, or delivery" may result in a child with autism or pervasive developmental disorder (PDD). In this study, 22 of 22 mothers (100%) who had received a live virus vaccine [during this crucial period] "had at least one child develop autism in connection with or following such a vaccination.... In many instances, the children's autistic manifestations reportedly started or worsened after they received their first MMR vaccine." Dr. Yazbak concluded that giving live virus vaccines (MMR or rubella) to a mother just before or during early pregnancy, or in the postpartum period, "may not be safe or wise.... The role of vaccines in precipitating autism should therefore become the focus of extensive and unbiased research."[38] (Figure 52)

The following story describes one woman's experience after receiving MMR just prior to conceiving: "My son was conceived shortly after I had received MMR (and Rhogam) after a miscarriage. He was hurt in utero from the vaccines I received. From birth, he did not make eye contact. He was further hurt by DPT (screaming episode) and MMR (digestive disorders) that he received from the pediatrician. My son did not speak until 3 ½ years old, and could not read until after being treated by a naturopathic doctor at age 13. All his life he suffered from digestive problems, malnutrition, low IQ, and sensory disorders. Not only is my son vaccine-injured, but the many MMR vaccines and Rhogam that I received postpartum after each of my pregnancies have caused my health to break down, and I quite literally was plucked off my deathbed by naturopathic interventions. I have been trying to recover my health for several years. I will continue to fight to bring out the truth and help my son receive the care he needs to be well."[39]

On April 6, 2000, Congress gathered several parents of MMR-damaged children, and experts, to study the apparent connection between MMR and autism. Extensive excerpts from this hearing—and other congressional hearings on autism—are posted on the *Thinktwice Global Vaccine Institute* website.[40]

Studies "Disproving" an MMR-Autism Link

Shortly after Dr. Wakefield's research showing correlations between MMR and autism was published in the February 1998 issue of *Lancet,* this important public health issue gained international recognition. Headline stories in major newspapers throughout the world spread the news that a scientific link had finally been discovered providing some answers to the horrendous epidemics of autism. However, incredulous authorities sought to discredit Wakefield's data and any link between vaccines and developmental disorders. Thus, two studies purporting to disprove correlations between MMR and autism were rushed into publication. During Wakefield's congressional testimony, he reviewed these extemporaneous studies and laid to rest any doubts regarding their biased study designs.

The Finnish study: In the first study, the "Finnish" paper—funded by Merck,[41] the manufacturer of the MMR vaccine—researchers identified adverse events following an MMR vaccination campaign in Finland during the three weeks post-vaccination. They located 31 individuals who experienced severe gastrointestinal symptoms (diarrhea and vomiting) after MMR and noted that none had a diagnosis of inflammatory bowel disease or autism. On this basis, they concluded that there was no evidence for MMR-associated inflammatory bowel disease or autism.[42]

Wakefield's response: "No one has ever suggested that acute gastrointestinal symptoms within three weeks of MMR is a risk for autism or inflammatory bowel disease. Parents reported *behavioral changes* as the initial presenting feature in their children. Thirty-one children is far too small a number, and the children are still too young to assess risk of inflammatory bowel disease. Peltola, et al. tested the *wrong* hypothesis."[43]

The Taylor study: In the second study, the "Taylor" paper, researchers again sought to dismiss any relationship between MMR and autism. They reasoned that if a causal link exists, there should have been an escalation in the number of children with autism in the first groups of children eligible for the triple shot. In England, MMR was introduced in 1988. The authors of this study claimed that MMR was administered during each child's second year of life. Thus, children born in 1987 should have been the first group to show an increase in cases of autism. However, since a rise in autism began in children born a few years before 1987, they concluded that MMR could not have been responsible for the higher rate.[44]

Wakefield's response: "There was a crucial omission from the paper by Taylor, et al. In 1988—with the introduction of the MMR in the U.K.—a 'catch-up' campaign was instituted which targeted pre-school children *of one to four years of age* who had not previously received monovalent measles, mumps, or rubella vaccines.... Corroboration of this comes in the form of a contemporaneous paper from Dr. Christine Miller, previously of the PHLS, who stated: 'Although the program will be aimed mainly at the one to four year age groups, where it will have the maximum effect, MMR vaccine can be given at any age.'[45] Taylor et al's omission of the crucial information on the catch-up campaign led the reader to believe that those, and only those, born in 1987 were the first children eligible for MMR. They were challenged on this omission in a subsequent letter to the *Lancet.*[46] In their reply they acknowledged that they were aware of the catch-up campaign and admitted that no fewer than 36 autistic children in their data-set were born before 1987 and had, therefore, received their MMR over the age of two years.... Since they were aware that their cohort contained children who received the MMR after the age of two years *it was not scientifically legitimate to test the hypothesis that a step-up should be seen in those born in 1987*. The fact that the step-up occurs in those born in 1986 is alarming, and would be consistent with an association with MMR. Such were the anxieties about the quality of this study that it was recently the subject of a special, and highly critical debate at the *Royal Statistical Society* in London. The conclusion reached was that Taylor et al's study design was wrong."[47]

The Ongoing MMR-Autism Controversy

Shortly after the April 2000 congressional hearings on autism, Japanese researchers duplicated Dr. Andrew Wakefield's study. They isolated vaccine strains of the measles virus from patients with ulcerative colitis and autism and noted that these "results are concordant with the exposure history of patients." In other words, they confirmed that some cases of autistic enterocolitis, a new syndrome of gastrointestinal complications and developmental regression in children, are apparently linked to the MMR vaccine.[48,49]

On May 16, 2000, and again on August 9, 2000, Congressman Dan Burton wrote to Donna Shalala, Secretary of Health and Human Services (HHS), requesting that she assemble a panel of experts "who are free of financial conflicts of interest" to review the existing scientific research into a possible link between the MMR vaccine and autism.[50] Burton's requests were denied.

In September of 2000, the *American Journal of Gastroenterology* published another study by Dr. Andrew Wakefield that followed up on his earlier work linking developmental disorders and behavioral regression with bowel symptoms. Of 60 children with autism and/or other disintegrative disorders, chronic colitis was identified in 53 (88 percent) compared with just one of 22 (4.5 percent) in pediatric controls. Wakefield concluded that "a new variant of inflammatory bowel disease is present in this group of children with developmental disorders."[51]

Three months later, another study by Dr. Andrew Wakefield, published in *Adverse Drug Reaction and Toxicologica Reviews,* documented 170 cases of children who developed autism shortly after the MMR vaccine. Apparently, in children who are genetically susceptible to autism, the MMR vaccine may damage the intestines, allowing food byproducts called peptides to pass through the intestinal walls, damaging the brain. Wakefield also reviewed earlier studies that were used to validate licensing the MMR vaccine. As early as 1968, researchers knew that measles could cause gut illnesses. Therefore, the gastrointestinal tract was a likely site for *delayed* pathology. Researchers were also aware that measles vaccines had been linked to *delayed* encephalopathic events. Yet, the original safety studies on the MMR vaccine did not observe adverse events beyond 28 days, and rarely for this period of time. Wakefield concluded that the MMR vaccine trials were too short to observe long-term problems like autism, and that "a significant index of suspicion exists without evidence of safety."[52-54]

On April 23, 2001, just two days before another scheduled hearing on autism,[55] the newly created Institute of Medicine (IOM) Immunization Review Committee, issued a report concluding that "the evidence favors rejection of the causal relationship at the population level between MMR vaccine and autistic spectrum disorders." However, "the proposed biological models linking MMR vaccination to autism spectrum disorders, although far from established, are nevertheless not disproved."[56]

The MMR-Autism Controversy in the United Kingdom

On September 2, 2001, a survey conducted in the United Kingdom indicated that a majority of parents wanted a public inquiry into MMR safety and its possible link to autism.[57] The U.K. government refused to publicly air scientific arguments. According to one outraged citizen, "Of course there should be a public inquiry since no parent should be forced to give chemicals to their children. A verdict of 'there is nothing to suggest MMR is unsafe' is not the same as 'MMR *is* safe.'"[58] Another concerned parent stated that "the refusal to hold an inquiry indicates something to hide. I love my son more than anything in the world. They're going to have to come up with a bit more in the way of factual reassurance [than] sneering references to the 'chattering classes.'"[59] Others claimed "the government long ago lost all credibility on safety issues," and that authorities should "stop treating very able adults with real concerns as idiots."[60] An Irish parent, whose son became autistic after his MMR injections, ruefully noted that the British government appears to be involved in a coverup. Yet, to another U.K. citizen, the solution is simple: "Let the people who understand matters give us arguments to help us decide."[61]

In December 2001, public concern regarding MMR drew Prime Minister Tony Blair into the vaccine debate. Several doctors, lawmakers and the media demanded to know whether Blair's 19-month-old son, Leo, received the MMR vaccine. Blair refused to answer the question despite his government's assurances that MMR is safe, and advice to parents to have the shot administered to their children. Parents were outraged at Blair's silence regarding his son's vaccination records, but the Prime Minister claimed it invaded his son's privacy.[62-64] (Dr. Wakefield's wife, Carmel, was more forthright: "As Andy's work was unfolding, we had to reappraise our policy on vaccinating our own children, so our second two children have not had MMR vaccination.")[65]

Tony Blair and the U.K. government also criticized parents who were abandoning the combined MMR shot for the individual measles, mumps, and rubella vaccines. Blair claimed this would place children at risk of contracting the diseases, and he cited Japan as an example of the dangers. Japan stopped using MMR in 1993 when they switched to using three separate injections because the triple vaccine was causing outbreaks of meningitis and other dangerous side effects. But Japan's Health Ministry refuted Blair's claim. Withdrawing the MMR vaccine did *not* cause an increase in deaths from measles. A spokesman said that more people had died from measles during the period when MMR was being used.[66]

In the midst of this mounting controversy over an apparent link between MMR and autism, Dr. Andrew Wakefield was fired from his post at the Royal Free Hospital Medical School in London. "I have been asked to go because my research results are unpopular," he stated. "I did not wish to leave but I have agreed to stand down in the hope that my going will take the political pressure off my colleagues and allow them to get on with the job of looking after the many sick children we have seen." Many parents, especially those involved in his research, were angry at the hospital's decision. But Wakefield added that "I have not done anything wrong. I have no intention of stopping my investigations."[67] In fact, Wakefield was hired as the Director of Autism Research for the International Child Development Resource Center in Florida. His new post completed a world-class team of autism specialists.[68]

The Denmark MMR-autism study:

According to the Institute of Medicine, Committee on Immunization Safety Review, "it is important to recognize the inherent methodological limitations of epidemiological [population-based] studies in establishing [an MMR-autism] causality."[69,70] Nevertheless, on November 7, 2002, CDC researchers published an epidemiological (population-based) study of MMR-autism rates in Denmark. More than 500,000 MMR-vaccinated versus MMR-unvaccinated children born from 1991 through 1998 were included in the analysis. Although a link between MMR and autism was seemingly disproved, and the CDC was quick to tout the results as conclusive, there were many significant defects in the study design:[71,72]

- The study did not differentiate between classical (early onset) autism and regressive autism, the type associated with MMR.
- Data regarding *when* the first autistic symptoms were noted (how soon before or after MMR vaccination) was omitted from the analysis.
- Data on the number of children with *autistic spectrum disorders* (in contrast to a strict diagnosis of *autism*) was underreported and incomplete.

- Only psychiatric records were used, not medical records, so there was no data on the presence or absence of measles virus in the gastrointestinal tract. Biological—not epidemiological—research will provide the best evidence either supporting or disputing an MMR-autism link.
- The study covered eight birth cohorts, but two of these included babies only one or two years old, too young in most cases to have received MMR. This could skew the data in favor of "no MMR causality."
- Vaccinated children were listed as unvaccinated if they were diagnosed with autism before they received MMR. Later reclassifications confound data and diminish study credibility.

Other important considerations:
- Denmark removed mercury-based vaccines from the market prior to the birth dates of the children studied. In contrast, children in the United States and England were repeatedly exposed to neurotoxic levels of mercury (mainly from maternal and infant vaccines) before receiving MMR. Thus, U.S. and U.K. children may have had more debilitated immune systems with less ability to effectively respond to the measles or rubella viruses in the MMR vaccine.[73]
- According to Dr. Greg Poland, a measles vaccine expert at the Mayo Clinic in Rochester, Minnesota, a study in one country might not always relate to people in another. Barbara Loe Fisher, co-founder and president of the National Vaccine Information Center, agrees that this study might not apply to American children. She notes that the Danish "are a genetically homogeneous people, and we are not."[74]
- Prior to this study, health officials vigorously defended earlier, flawed studies that rejected a link between MMR and autism. In this study, the authors confess that earlier studies designed to evaluate the suggested link between MMR vaccination and autism did not have "sufficient statistical power to detect an association."[75] In other word, earlier studies *were* flawed, but now we are expected to have confidence in this one. (A recent study published in the *Journal of the American Medical Association* found that one of every three medical studies are eventually contradicted.)[76]

Government-suppressed data:
On November 21, 2002, Congressman Dan Burton wrote to President Bush urging him to host a White House conference "to galvanize a national effort to determine why autism has reached epidemic proportions."[77] Four days later, attorney's for the U.S. government responded by asking a federal court to conceal important documents linking vaccines to autism. They argued that only the government has the right to decide what vaccine evidence can be released to the public. According to Jeff Kim, a lawyer representing hundreds of families whose children became autistic after receiving MMR, sealing important documents and creating "a shroud of secrecy" over them solely benefits vaccine manufacturers.[78] A few days later, the *New York Times* published a commentary by Stephen Gillers, a legal ethicist, providing clarity on this issue: "When a court is asked to suppress information that might help vindicate legal claims, or that reveals a continuing public danger or unethical behavior by powerful people or institutions, secrecy is intolerable. The harm is made worse when a judge, a public official, is asked to use public power to inflict it."[79]

The Wakefield witch hunt:
In 2004, *Lancet* "retracted" its publication of Dr. Andrew Wakefield's 1998 landmark study linking the onset of autistic symptoms (and Crohn's disease) to the MMR vaccine.[80] The U.K.'s General Medical Council (GMC) used this as an opportunity to levy four misconduct charges against the doctor at the heart of the MMR controversy: 1) he failed to obtain GMC permission before his work appeared in print; 2) he published inadequately founded research; 3) he obtained funding improperly; and 4) he subjected children to "unnecessary and invasive investigations."[81] If found guilty, Wakefield could lose his medical license. However, by July 2006, after nearly two years of investigations, the GMC had indicated that it may drop the charges.[82] The news that Dr. Wakefield might not face

charges was welcomed by his many supporters. According to Rosemary Kessick, the mother of an autistic boy whose treatment is part of the investigation, the GMC purposely smeared Dr. Wakefield to boost public confidence in MMR. In addition, "Hundreds of autistic children with the serious bowel disease first identified by Dr. Wakefield have been unable to get any treatment in the U.K., and the drawn-out investigation has played a major role in this disgraceful state of affairs."[83] Jackie Fletcher, director of JABS, a U.K. support group for vaccine-damaged children, declared: "It has been an absolute witch hunt. All he was guilty of was listening to what parents said, clinically investigating the children and then reporting his findings. All he did was hold up a red flag and say, 'There's something going on that needs to be investigated further.'"[84] (Note: The GMC did not drop its case against Dr. Wakefield. It dragged on for several years and by May 2010 he was found guilty of professional misconduct and struck off the medical register.)[85]

Where are the autistic Amish?

In April 2005, Dan Olmsted, a reporter for United Press International, began searching the Amish community for cases of autism. He began his quest in Lancaster County, the heart of Pennsylvania Dutch country, where statistically there should have been at least 130 people with autism.[86] However, the Amish, who still ride horse-and-buggies, also shun modern medicine and do not vaccinate their children. This may have been the reason Olmsted had a difficult time finding autistic Amish. When he finally located an Amish family with an autistic child, the mother gave the following explanation: "Unfortunately our autistic daughter, who's doing very well—she's been diagnosed with very, very severe autism—is adopted from China, and so she would have had all her vaccines in China before we got her, and then she had most of her vaccines given to her in the United States before we got her. So, we're probably not the pure case you're looking for."[87] (Photographs of the child taken in China before she was vaccinated show a smiling, alert child looking directly into the camera.)[88]

Olmsted eventually located another autistic child in the Amish community, and she was vaccinated prior to her disability as well. According to Stacey-Jean, a member of the Amish community, "Almost every Amish family I know has had somebody from the health department knock on our door and try to convince us to get vaccines for our children. The younger Amish more and more are getting vaccines. It's a minority of children who vaccinate, but that is changing now. There's one family that we know; their daughter had a vaccine reaction [around 15 months of age] and is now autistic. She was walking and functioning and a happy, bright child, and 24 hours after she had her vaccine, her legs went limp and she had a typical high-pitched scream. They called the doctor and he said it was fine, that a lot of high-pitched screaming goes along with it. She completely quit speaking, quit making eye contact with people. She went into her own world."[89]

Where are the autistic children at Homefirst® Health Services?

In metropolitan Chicago, thousands of children are cared for by Homefirst Health Services, an alternative medical facility where babies are often delivered at home and are rarely vaccinated. According to Dr. Mayer Eisenstein, Homefirst's medical director who founded the practice in 1973, "We have a fairly large practice. We have about 30,000 or 35,000 children that we've taken care of over the years, and I don't think we have a single case of autism in children delivered by us who never received vaccines." Dr. Paul Schattauer, who has been with Homefirst for 20 years, confirmed Eisenstein's observations: "In my practice I don't see autism. Sometimes...you feel like you've got a pretty big secret."[90] (Homefirst's patients also have significantly less asthma and diabetes compared to national rates. Eisenstein noted that, "In the alternative medicine network which Homefirst is part of, there are virtually no cases of childhood asthma, in contrast to the overall Blue Cross rate of childhood asthma which is about 10 percent.")[91]

"Some supposed experts will tell you that the increase in autism reflects only greater awareness. That is nonsense."—Dr. Bernard Rimland, autism expert[92]

A warning cry:

In February 2006, Dr. Peter Fletcher, former Chief Scientific Officer at the U.K. Department of Health, and former Medical Assessor to the Committee on Safety of Medicines (responsible for deciding if vaccines are safe), publicly acknowledged that he has seen a "steady accumulation of evidence" from scientists worldwide that the MMR vaccine is causing brain damage in some children. Also, "the refusal by governments to evaluate the risks properly will make this one of the greatest scandals in medical history."[93] Dr. Fletcher had more to say:

> There are very powerful people in positions of great authority in Britain and elsewhere who have staked their reputations and careers on the safety of MMR, and they are willing to do almost anything to protect themselves.
>
> Clinical and scientific data is steadily accumulating that the live measles virus in MMR can cause brain, gut and immune system damage in a subset of vulnerable children. There's no one conclusive piece of scientific evidence, no 'smoking gun,' because there very rarely is when adverse drug reactions are first suspected. When vaccine damage in very young children is involved, it is harder to prove the links. But it is the steady accumulation of evidence, from a number of respected universities, teaching hospitals and laboratories around the world, that matters here. There's far too much to ignore. Yet government health authorities are, it seems, more than happy to do so. Why isn't the government taking this massive public health problem more seriously? This official complacency is utterly inexplicable.
>
> When scientists first raised fears of a possible link between mad cow disease and an apparently new, variant form of Creutzfeldt-Jakob disease (CJD) they had detected in just 20 or 30 patients, everybody panicked and millions of cows were slaughtered. Yet, there has been a tenfold increase in autism and related forms of brain damage over the past 15 years, roughly coinciding with MMR's introduction, and an extremely worrying increase in childhood inflammatory bowel diseases and immune disorders such as diabetes, and no one in authority will even admit it's happening, let alone try to investigate the causes.
>
> It's entirely possible that the immune systems of a small minority simply cannot cope with the challenge of the three live viruses in the MMR jab and the ever-increasing vaccine load in general.[94]

Mercury in Vaccines: A Link to Autism

In 1929, Eli Lilly, a vaccine manufacturer, developed and registered thimerosal under the trade name Merthiolate.[95] Thimerosal is nearly 50 percent mercury by weight.[96] Mercury is the most toxic element on earth, after plutonium.[97] Even very low concentrations—whether inhaled, eaten, or placed on the skin—can cause nervous system and brain damage.[98] In the 1930s, thimerosal was added to vaccines as an anti-bacterial preservative.[99] Some of the children who received these vaccines showed telltale signs of neurological damage and mercury poisoning. Many of these children were later diagnosed with autism.[100,101]

For most of the past 80 years, medical authorities have ignored the evidence and denied that mercury in vaccines is a serious problem. As a result, thousands of new babies who could have been saved were permanently damaged or killed. The pertussis vaccine, which became available in the 1930s and 1940s (and later, DPT), was among the first to contain mercury (see Table 4, page 174). In the 1990s, additional mercury-laced vaccines were added to the mandatory schedule of childhood shots. For example, starting in 1991, infants were compelled to receive several doses of the mercury-laced hepatitis B vaccine, the first shot just hours after birth. Multiple doses of the mercury-laced haemophilus influenzae type B (Hib) vaccine were given to babies as well.

Throughout the infamous era of mercury-tainted vaccines (sadly, still occurring), outraged parents of vaccine-damaged children pleaded with anyone who would listen: Why is mercury being injected into our precious babies? No one had an answer. In fact, the medical community refused to even acknowledge their pleas —despite a secret memo from 1991. Apparently, Merck had calculated that 6-month-old babies who received their recommended shots could receive a mercury dose up to 87 times higher than federal guidelines for the maximum daily consumption of mercury from fish![102] Eventually, even callous pharmaceutical executives and their industry collaborators (i.e., the AAP, FDA and CDC) had to capitulate. Thus, in July 1999, the American Academy of Pediatrics (AAP) and the United States Public Health Service issued a joint statement recommending the removal of thimerosal from vaccines. This was welcome news, but was it sincere?

In July 1999, health officials recommended that vaccine manufacturers eliminate thimerosal as a preservative "as soon as possible."[103] However, newly released documents show that the CDC was simultaneously working behind the scenes to discourage thimerosal's removal. For example, when a major vaccine manufacturer—SmithKline Beecham—contacted the CDC shortly after its announcement, and offered to immediately begin supplying mercury-free DTaP vaccines for children, the CDC rejected the offer.[104,105] Perhaps a sharp plunge in autism rates would seem too obvious. One federal official declared, "If CDC were basing its decision on safety alone, it would have taken SmithKline up on its offer. That's a no-brainer, so there were other considerations. Immediate withdrawal would send a strong message: 'We messed up!' I don't think they wanted to send that message to parents, the public, or those considering legal action."[106]

The CDC was also concerned that "an immediate withdrawal might discredit international vaccine programs."[107] The World Health Organization (WHO) has urged the CDC against banning thimerosal in U.S. vaccines because it might elicit objections to WHO's immunization programs overseas. WHO is now injecting children in developing countries with the same quantities of mercury that U.S. doctors were giving American children at their highest exposures, but in less time.[108] According to John Clements, WHO vaccine advisor, "My mandate...is to make sure...that 100 million are immunized...this year, next year and for many years to come, and that will have to be with thimerosal-containing vaccines."[109]

The Simpsonwood Gathering

In June 2000, a top-secret meeting of health officials and government scientists occurred at the secluded Simpsonwood conference center in Norcross, Georgia. Although the Centers for Disease Control and Prevention (CDC) convened the meeting, no public announcement was made of the gathering. Just 52 private invitations were issued. Participants included high-level officials from the CDC, FDA, top vaccine specialists from the World Health Organization, and representatives from every major vaccine manufacturer, including Merck, GlaxoSmithKline, Wyeth and Aventis Pasteur. All of the participants were repeatedly warned that the scientific data under discussion was "embargoed." Note-taking and photocopies of documents were strictly prohibited. No papers could leave the room.[110-112]

The federal health officials and industry representatives had assembled to discuss an alarming new study that confirmed a link between thimerosal (mercury) in childhood vaccines and neurological damage, including recent dramatic increases in autistic spectrum disorders. Tom Verstraeten, a CDC epidemiologist, had analyzed the agency's massive Vaccine Safety Datalink (VSD) database (distinct from VAERS) containing thousands of medical records of vaccinated children and was "stunned" by what he saw: "We have found statistically significant relationships between exposure [to mercury in vaccines] and outcomes. At two months of age, developmental delay; exposure at three months, tics; at six months, attention deficit disorder. Exposure at one, three and six months, language and speech delays—the entire category of neurodevelopmental delays."[113] Verstraeten also discussed previous studies showing a link between mercury and neurodevelopmental disorders.[114] Since 1991, when the CDC and FDA started requiring newborn infants to receive multiple doses of thimerosal-laced hepatitis B vaccines, thimerosal-laced haemophilus influenzae type B (Hib) vaccines, and the already mandated thimerosal-laced diphtheria, tetanus and pertussis shots (via DPT and DTaP), cases of autism skyrocketed.

Dr. Bill Weil, with the American Academy of Pediatrics (AAP), told the group, "You can play with this all you want," but the results "are statistically significant."[115] Dr. Richard

Johnston, an immunologist and pediatrician, exclaimed, "I do not want my grandson to get a thimerosal-containing vaccine until we know better what is going on."[116] Yet, instead of taking quick action to warn parents and recall the unsafe shots, this shameless group of 52 vaccine proponents spent the next two days calculating how to cover up the truth.[117]

"We are in a bad position from the standpoint of defending any lawsuits," said Dr. Robert Brent, a pediatrician.[118] However, Dr. Robert Chen, head of vaccine safety for the CDC, congratulated his group for their apparent success thus far at concealing the facts, and expressed relief that "given the sensitivity of the information, we have been able to keep it out of the hands of, let's say, less responsible hands."[119] Dr. John Clements, WHO vaccine advisor, was more blunt, declaring that perhaps the CDC study "should not have been done at all because the outcome could have, to some extent, been predicted." He stated that "the research results have to be handled," and warned that the study "will be taken by others and used in ways beyond the control of this group."[120]

How to "handle" undesirable scientific data:

At the Simpsonwood gathering, a plot was hatched. To begin, the CDC relinquished control of its vast database on childhood vaccines—the very same database Tom Verstraeten used to confirm a link between thimerosal-laced vaccines and autism. Although the VSD database was public property—developed at taxpayer expense—it was turned over to a private health insurance agency, ensuring that it could not be accessed by non-collaborators for additional research.[121] Three years later, Verstraeten had reworked the data and published a new version of his original study in the November 2003 issue of *Pediatrics*. However, this time "no consistent significant associations were found between thimerosal-containing vaccines and neurodevelopmental outcomes."[122] [Dr. Mark Geier, an independent scientist, eventually gained access to the VSD data. His findings, published in a recent issue of the *Journal of the Neurological Sciences,* are summarized on pages 170-171.]

After the Simpsonwood gathering, the CDC also instructed the Institute of Medicine (IOM), i.e., the National Academy of Sciences, to produce a new study with contrived results: no correlation between thimerosal and brain disorders. According to Dr. Marie McCormick, who chaired the IOM's Immunization Safety Review Committee in January 2001, the CDC "wants us to declare, well, that these things are pretty safe." In fact, "we are not ever going to come down that [autism] is a true side effect" of thimerosal.[123] In transcripts of the meeting, the committee's chief staffer, Kathleen Stratton, predicted that the IOM would conclude that the evidence was "inadequate to accept or reject a causal relation" between thimerosal and autism. Apparently, that was what "Walt wants"—a reference to Dr. Walter Orenstein, director of the CDC's National Immunization Program.[124]

To complete the deception, the CDC would need additional "proof" that thimerosal-laced vaccines are safe. They never intended to conduct honest science; rather, their goal was to establish a plausible defense, insulate manufacturers against liability, while producing justification for continuing mandatory vaccine campaigns. For example, in May 2001, Dr. Gordon Douglas, then-director of strategic planning for vaccine research at the National Institutes of Health, assured a Princeton University gathering that "four current studies are taking place *to rule out the proposed link between autism and thimerosal.*" Furthermore, "in order to undo the harmful effects of research claiming to link the [measles] vaccine to an elevated risk of autism, we need to conduct and publicize additional studies to assure parents of safety."[125] Douglas formerly served as president of vaccinations for Merck.

The Simpsonwood gathering places all CDC-sponsored research into question. Although this civic institution was originally entrusted with a lofty mandate to protect our children, it has degenerated into a private arm of the pharmaceutical industry. The CDC has lost its ethical bearings and cannot be trusted to objectively oversee scientific studies whose outcomes affect the health and welfare of our youngest, most innocent members of society. Who is looking after our children—the brain-trust of our future—if policy trumps science, and profits trump safety? "The CDC is guilty of incompetence and gross negligence" says Mark Blaxill, vice president of Safe Minds, a nonprofit organization concerned about mercury in medicines. "The damage caused by vaccine exposure is massive. It's bigger than asbestos, bigger than tobacco, bigger than anything you've ever seen."[126]

Children versus profits:

On July 18, 2000, Congress held additional hearings to find out why mercury is put into vaccines.[127] On October 25, 2000, Chairman Dan Burton wrote another letter to the U.S. Health and Human Services Secretary, Donna Shalala, requesting an immediate recall of all vaccines containing thimerosal, but the FDA refused to recall any of the numerous thimerosal-containing vaccines.[128] Instead, they suggested a phase-out over several years, permitting drug companies to continue selling their dangerous mercury-laden products to innocent children and unsuspecting parents.[129,130] Doctors were encouraged to participate in this debacle. To make matters worse, Merck continued to sell hepatitis B vaccines containing mercury for two years after issuing a press release declaring "Now, Merck's infant vaccine line is free of all preservatives." Parents expecting mercury-free vaccines were deceived.[131]

How safe are children in developing countries?

In May 2001, WHO committed to "develop a strong advocacy campaign to *support* the ongoing use of thimerosal."[132] In fact, the U.S. government continues to ship mercury-laced vaccines to developing countries—some of which are now experiencing dramatic increases in rates of autism. In China, where the disease was virtually unknown prior to 1999 when U.S. manufacturers introduced mercury-laced vaccines, by June 2005 there were more than 1.8 million Chinese autistics. Autistic disorders are also rising quickly in India, Nicaragua and other developing countries that are now using thimerosal-laced vaccines.[133]

Thimerosal safety test:

On June 19 and 20, 2002, Congress initiated another hearing to investigate *"The Status of Research into Vaccine Safety and Autism."* In the second day of proceedings, Congressman Dan Burton produced a memo indicating that the FDA was aware that thimerosal in vaccines was dangerous. In fact, in the only study of thimerosal ever conducted prior to permitting it to be used in children's vaccines, the poisonous substance killed all of the test subjects:[134,135]

How much mercury do vaccines contain?

According to the FDA, thimerosal, which is almost 50 percent mercury by weight, has been one of the most widely used preservatives in vaccines. A vaccine containing 0.01% thimerosal as a preservative contains 50 micrograms (mcg) of thimerosal per 1 ml dose, or approximately 25mcg of mercury per 0.5 ml dose.[136] In the mid-1980s, babies received four 25mcg doses of mercury-laced DPT vaccines (100mcg by 18 months). In the early 1990s, four 25mcg doses of the mercury-laced Hib vaccine and three 12.5mcg doses of the mercury-laced hepatitis B vaccine were added to the vaccine schedule (237.5 mcg by 18 months). In the late 1990s, three 12.5mcg doses of the mercury-laced influenza vaccine were recommended, bringing the total possible mercury exposure by 18 months of age to 275mcg (Figure 53).[137]

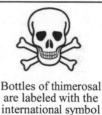

Bottles of thimerosal are labeled with the international symbol for poison: a skull and crossbones.

In 2009, several vaccines (i.e., for some brands of influenza, meningococcal and tetanus) still contained high concentrations of mercury (see *Appendix I* on page 307).[138]

The term 'preservative-free' indicates that no preservative (thimerosal or otherwise) is used in the vaccine; however, "traces used during the manufacturing process may be present in the final formulation. In other words, *some vaccines that are 'preservative-free' may contain traces of thimerosal.* Similarly, the term 'thimerosal-reduced' usually indicates that thimerosal is not added as a vaccine preservative, but trace amounts may remain from use in the manufacturing process."[139]

A different kind of immunity:

On November 13, 2002, lawmakers introduced a Homeland Security bill that included an "Eli Lilly rider"—a provision protecting drug companies from thimerosal lawsuits. "It looks like payback," a lawyer noted, considering "the industry spent millions bankrolling [political] campaigns." Media sleuths could not discover who sponsored the provision.[140]

Figure 53:

Cumulative Mercury Exposure
by 18 Months of Age

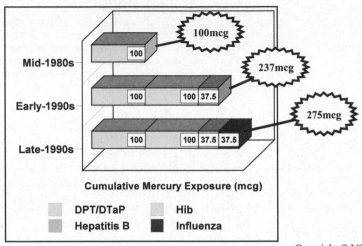

Cumulative Mercury Exposure (mcg)

DPT/DTaP   Hib

Hepatitis B   Influenza

In the mid-1980s, babies received four 25mcg doses of mercury-laced DPT vaccines (100mcg by 18 months). In the early 1990s, four 25mcg doses of the mercury-laced Hib vaccine and three 12.5mcg doses of the mercury-laced hepatitis B vaccine were added to the immunization schedule (237.5mcg by 18 months). In the late 1990s, three 12.5mcg doses of the thimerosal-laced influenza vaccine were recommended, bringing the total possible mercury exposure by 18 months to 275mcg. Source: CDC childhood immunization schedules.

The Pichichero thimerosal study:

On November 30, 2002, a new study concluded that mercury in vaccines is not harmful —*despite warning against the use of thimerosal-laced shots in low weight, premature infants.* Additional incongruities also cast doubt on the study results. For example:

- The study was too small to make definitive conclusions (40 subjects; 21 controls).
- Researchers waited several days to analyze blood, urine and stool samples. Thus, *peak* mercury levels in recently vaccinated babies were not assessed.
- Certain predisposed babies have more trouble processing mercury. Yet, mercury levels in *damaged* children were not evaluated.
- The lead author of this study, Dr. Michael Pichichero, had a clear conflict of interest. He was paid to do other studies for Eli Lilly, the pharmaceutical company that was being sued for producing thimerosal used in vaccines.[141,142]

The Danish thimerosal study:

In October 2003, Danish researchers published a large population study comparing children who received a thimerosal-containing vaccine versus children who received a thimerosal-free vaccine. The authors of the study concluded that "the results do not support a causal relationship between childhood vaccination with thimerosal-containing vaccines and development of autistic spectrum disorders."[143] However, the researchers were affiliated with Statens Serum Institut, a Danish business enterprise receiving more than 80 percent of its profits from vaccines. In fact, Statens Serum Institut manufactured the now discontinued thimerosal-laced pertussis vaccine that was investigated in their own study, and not surprisingly, found to be safe. They also provided the diphtheria and tetanus components of a major thimerosal-laced DTaP vaccine sold in the United States.[144]

Ethylmercury (in vaccines) versus methylmercury:

Health officials often claim that ethylmercury—the type of mercury found in vaccines containing thimerosal—should not be compared to methylmercury, a well-established neurotoxin. However, in 1977 a Russian study found that adults exposed to much lower concentrations of ethylmercury than those given to American children still suffered brain damage years later.[145] Russia banned thimerosal from children's vaccines more than 20 years ago. Austria, Great Britain, Japan, and all of the Scandinavian countries also removed thimerosal from childhood vaccines.[146] In 1985, the *Archives of Toxicology* published a comparative study that administered similar doses of ethylmercury and methylmercury to rats. The ethylmercury-treated rats had higher concentrations of inorganic mercury in their kidneys and brains.[147] More recently, in August 2005, a study funded by the National Institutes of Health also found that ethylmercury is *more* toxic to the brain than methylmercury. It crosses the blood-brain barrier at a quicker rate and converts to inorganic mercury (which is more difficult to excrete and stays in the brain longer) at much higher concentrations: ethylmercury at 34 percent, versus methylmercury at 7 percent.[148]

Immunity for drug companies:

Although public outrage forced legislators to yank the Eli Lilly rider from the 2002 Homeland Security bill, three years later, in December 2005, it was once again surreptitiously slipped into unrelated, must-pass legislation—granting immunity to drug companies from liability for injuries caused by their products. According to Laura Bono, board chair of the National Autism Association, "Families of vaccine-injured children have witnessed the emotional, physical, and financial devastation caused by the pharmaceutical industry's reckless disregard for safety standards. Now, the misplaced priorities of Senate leadership have sacrificed public health and basic civil rights to the greed of an industry willing to overlook safety concerns for the sake of profit.... I am afraid for American citizens who could be one shot away from a lifelong disability far worse than the disease it was meant to prevent and be left with no legal recourse for pursuing compensation for their injuries. We should all be very concerned about the future of public health and civil rights now that the rules have changed so drastically."[149]

The Geier thimerosal studies:

Dr. Mark Geier is a medical doctor and geneticist, a former research scientist at the National Institutes of Health, and a former professor at Johns Hopkins University. From 2003 through 2008, he and his son, David, published several studies showing a link between autistic spectrum disorders and thimerosal-containing vaccines. For example, an analysis of the federal government's Vaccine Adverse Event Reporting System (VAERS) database "showed statistical increases in the incidence rate of autism, mental retardation, and speech disorders" after children received thimerosal-containing vaccines when compared with children who received thimerosal-free vaccines. In fact, "there was a 2-fold to 6-fold increased incidence of neurodevelopmental disorders" following additional doses of mercury-containing shots (Figure 54).[150] A follow-up study published in the *Journal of American Physicians and Surgeons,* confirmed that children vaccinated with thimerosal-containing vaccines "have higher rates of speech disorders, autism, and heart arrest" and that "the relative risk of each of these disorders correlated with increasing doses of mercury" contained in the shots.[151] Another study by the Geiers found that children with autism excrete significantly higher concentrations of mercury from their bodies during chelation therapy—a treatment for heavy metal poisoning—than non-autistic children.[152] In a 2006 study, the Geiers analyzed trends in the child immunization schedule and compared the number of autism cases and speech ailments before and after thimerosal-free vaccines were introduced. The results show that "the trends in newly diagnosed neurodevelopmental disorders correspond directly to the expansion and subsequent contraction of the cumulative mercury dose to which children were exposed from thimerosal-containing vaccines through the U.S. immunization schedule."[153] Two 2007 Geier studies, published in the *Journal of Toxicology and Environmental Health,* confirmed statistical correlations between the total mercury content that children received from their vaccines and the severity of autistic symptoms.[154,155]

Figure 54:

Statistical Increases in Neurodevelopmental Disorders After Children Received Thimerosal-Containing Vaccines

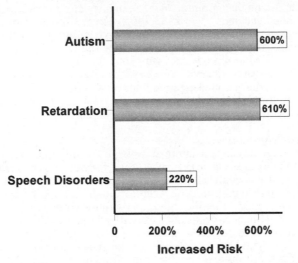

An analysis of the federal Vaccine Adverse Event Reporting System (VAERS) database "showed statistical increases in the incidence rate of autism, mental retardation, and speech disorders" after children received thimerosal-containing vaccines when compared with children who received thimerosal-free vaccines. Source: *Exp Biol Med* 2003;228:660-664.

In August 2008, the *Journal of the Neurological Sciences* published a new study by Drs. Heather Young and Mark Geier that analyzed the vaccination records of more than 278,000 children during a 7-year period (1990-1996). The amount of mercury that these children received from their thimerosal-containing vaccines was compared to how often they were diagnosed with medical disorders. The study protocol was approved by the CDC. The results showed that disorders without a biologically plausible link to mercury exposure—pneumonia, congenital anomalies, and failure to thrive—did not occur at greater rates in children with greater exposure to mercury from their thimerosal-containing vaccines. In contrast, there was "a significant association between mercury exposure from thimerosal-containing vaccines and neurodevelopmental disorders"—a correlation that is biologically plausible. Infants (birth cohorts) with the most mercury from their vaccines had significantly higher rates of autism, autistic spectrum disorders, tics, attention deficit disorder, and emotional disturbances—2 to 4 times higher—when compared to infants who received less mercury from their shots.[156] [This study utilized the CDC's Vaccine Safety Datalink database and confirms the original findings that led to the secret Simpsonwood gathering.]

The Montreal thimerosal studies:
In July 2006, *Pediatrics* published an epidemiological study that assessed rates of pervasive developmental disorder (PDD) in Montreal children. The authors of the study concluded that thimerosal-laced shots did not cause autistic spectrum disorders. In fact, "the prevalence of pervasive developmental disorder in thimerosal-free birth cohorts was significantly higher than in thimerosal-exposed cohorts."[157] In other words, the dangerous preservative actually appeared to protect against neurological damage! According to the

authors of the study, factors accounting for the increased prevalence of PDD include: a broadening of diagnostic concepts and criteria, increased awareness, better identification of children with PDD, and improved access to services.[158]

In March of 2007, new findings by Dr. David Ayoub were presented at a National Autism Association (NAA) meeting *confirming* a link between mercury-containing vaccines and rates of pervasive developmental disorder in Montreal. The peak rate of 1 in 87 children diagnosed with PDD occurred after they were injected with the highest concentrations of thimerosal-containing vaccines. In addition, the new data revealed flaws in the 2006 Montreal study. For example:

- The original study monitored a single Montreal school district. The new study broadened the data to include all five Montreal school districts.
- The original study claimed that children were not exposed to thimerosal-containing vaccines post-1996 although several mercury-containing vaccines were administered well beyond 1996.
- The study reported PDD rates in children from Montreal but vaccination rates were taken from Quebec City—a totally different population cohort.[159]

Karen McDonough, NAA-Chicago president, responded to the new data: "It's irresponsible that such flawed data [the original Montreal *Pediatrics* study] was published in a medical journal. This new information confirms a relationship between vaccines and autism that can't be explained by better diagnosing or changing diagnostic criteria."[160] Dr. David Ayoub and Dr. Yazbak, co-authors of the new Montreal study (along with Monica Ruscitti) detailed the study flaws in letters to *Pediatrics,* which the journal refused to publish. The editor, Dr. Jerold F. Lucey stated in a reply, "I believe the evidence of no link between [vaccines] and autism is sufficient. It's not worth publishing more on this subject."[161]

The Generation Rescue study:
On June 26, 2007, Generation Rescue, a nonprofit institution, published the results of a study that it commissioned comparing rates of autism (and other neurological disorders) in vaccinated versus completely unvaccinated children. The $200,000 survey, conducted by SurveyUSA, an independent research firm, collected data on 17,674 children. Here is a summary of the most notable findings:

- Vaccinated boys (ages 11-17) were *112 percent* more likely to have autism, *158 percent* more likely to have a neurological disorder, and *317 percent* more likely to suffer from ADHD, than unvaccinated boys (Figure 55).
- Vaccinated children (ages 4-17) were *120 percent* more likely to have asthma.[162,163]

The 'better diagnosis' theory of autism:
Although medical authorities would like to convince parents that the rise in autism is caused by better diagnosis—not vaccines—Dr. Boyd Haley, one of the world's foremost authorities on mercury toxicity, and head of the chemistry department at the University of Kentucky, dismisses this ruse with a logical question: "If the epidemic is truly an artifact of poor diagnosis, then where are all of the 20-year-old autistics?" Furthermore, "you couldn't even construct a study that shows thimerosal is safe. It's just too darn toxic. If you inject thimerosal into an animal, its brain will sicken. If you apply it to living tissue, the cells die. If you put it in a petri dish, the culture dies. Knowing these things, it would be shocking if one could inject it into an infant *without* causing damage."[164]

Where does the AAP stand on thimerosal in vaccines?
The American Academy of Pediatrics' (AAP) policy on mercury exposure states, "Mercury in all its forms is toxic to the fetus and children, and efforts should be made to reduce exposure to the extent possible to pregnant women and children as well as the general population."[165] Yet, the AAP supports giving pregnant women and infants flu vaccines that contain high concentrations of mercury.[166] For example, when New York state legislators considered banning thimerosal from medical products, the AAP officially opposed such legislation because it "sends the wrong message to New York parents and

Figure 55:

Vaccinated (vs. Unvaccinated) Boys
are More Likely to Suffer from
Autism and Other Neurological Disorders

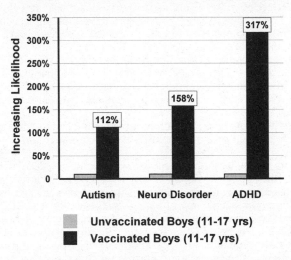

Unvaccinated Boys (11-17 yrs)

Vaccinated Boys (11-17 yrs)

A recent survey conducted by an independent research firm collected data on 17,674 children and found that vaccinated boys (ages 11-17) were *112 percent* more likely to have autism, *158 percent* more likely to have a neurological disorder, and *317 percent* more likely to suffer from ADHD, than unvaccinated boys. *Science Daily* (June 26, 2007).

---

pregnant women, and in fact all New Yorkers."[167] The AAP's stance on this issue has some parents suspecting that a full removal of mercury from vaccines would create a significant drop in autism rates, making the connection between vaccines and autistic spectrum disorders painfully clear. According to one distraught parent, "It's heartbreaking that the AAP is not dedicating more time to the medical needs of our children...and equally saddening that they support the use of a poisonous substance. This also sends the wrong message. It says, 'We don't want to see if the autism rates go down.'"[168] Another distraught parent wondered, "How can pediatricians tell us not to let our kids eat too much fish, but then aggressively oppose legislation to halt direct injection of mercury? Whose side are they on—our kids' or the pharmaceutical industry's?"[169]

Pregnant women, infants, and mercury-laced vaccines:
In February 2006, the CDC's Advisory Committee for Immunization Practices (ACIP) repeated its recommendation that infants up to 24 months old receive multiple doses of flu vaccines—despite containing high quantities of mercury—and even expanded its recommendation to 59 months of age! The ACIP also recommends flu vaccines for pregnant women.[170,171] In May 2007, the ACIP repeated its improbable assertion that mercury-laced flu vaccines for pregnant women are safe.[172] The Institute of Medicine previously recommended that mercury *not* be injected into these sensitive populations.[173] Many flu shots still contain 25mcg of mercury, an amount that is considered grossly unsafe under Environmental Protection Agency (EPA) guidelines. Concerned father, Christian McIlwain, responds: "Children and fetuses are still being exposed unnecessarily to this neurotoxin. With the recently added recommendations that influenza vaccines be given to women during any stage of pregnancy, and children from age 6 months and up, the amount of early-age thimerosal through recommended vaccines has increased drastically in the last two years."[174] Clair

Bothell, board chair of the National Autism Association is more direct: "When it comes to discussing thimerosal, it's hard to tell where the pharmaceutical industry leaves off and where the CDC begins. The blurring of these lines is not in the best interests of public health."[175]

The CDC "early thimerosal exposure" study:

On September 27, 2007, the *New England Journal of Medicine* published a study funded by the CDC that concluded that a causal association between early exposure to mercury from thimerosal-containing vaccines and deficits in neuro-psychological functioning at 7 to 10 years of age is not supported.[176] In fact, the authors of this study claimed that babies with higher levels of mercury actually performed *better* on several tests. If this study is to be believed, mercury appears to be a well-documented neurotoxin except when it accumulates in babies by way of vaccines. Higher concentrations of mercury from vaccines apparently *improve* motor skills and cognitive dexterity.

Although the authors of this study concluded that a link between mercury in vaccines and deficits in neuropsychological functioning is not supported, this conclusion is deceptive because the study was unable to *disprove* a causal relationship. In fact, this study actually confirmed associations detected in other studies, such as poorer language ability and increased rates of motor and verbal tics. In addition, this study had several design flaws and potential conflicts of interest that appear to have biased its results away from even stronger correlations between mercury in vaccines and neuropsychological deficits:[177]

- The study had a small sample size, with few children in the highest and lowest exposure groups, limiting the ability to detect statistical associations.
- Researchers did not factor in rehabilitative interventions, such as speech therapy, that may have lessened the negative effects of thimerosal exposure.
- The lead author of the study, Dr. William Thompson, was a former employee of Merck, a major manufacturer of thimerosal-containing vaccines. Other authors of the study received consulting fees, lecture fees, and/or grant support from Merck, Sanofi Pasteur, GlaxoSmithKline, MedImmune, Wyeth, Abbott, and/or Novartis —vaccine manufacturers with vested interests in disproving correlations between their products and debilities.
- Children were excluded from the study if they had certain conditions recorded in their medical records, such as encephalitis or meningitis.
- Newborns weighing 5 pounds, 8 ounces or less (9 percent of births) were excluded from the study even though low weight infants may be more susceptible to ingestion.
- Children with attention deficit hyperactivity disorder (ADHD) were allowed to take their medication until the day before testing.
- More than 1 of every 20 children tested was excluded from the final analysis.

Despite this study's many limitations, several statistical correlations were found between early exposure to mercury in vaccines and neuropsychological deficits at a later age:[178]

- Higher prenatal exposure to mercury was associated with significantly poorer performance on backward recall IQ development.
- Higher mercury exposure from birth to 7 months was associated with significantly poorer performance on behavioral regulation, and a higher likelihood of motor and speech tics.
- Higher mercury exposure during the first 28 days of life was associated with significantly poorer performance on speech articulation.
- Among girls, increased neonatal mercury exposure was associated with significantly lower verbal IQ scores.

> *"If you inject thimerosal into an animal, its brain will sicken. If you apply it to living tissue, the cells die. If you put it in a petri dish, the culture dies. Knowing these things, it would be shocking if one could inject it into an infant without causing damage."*
> —Dr. Boyd Haley, mercury-toxicity expert

Table 4:
History of Mercury in Vaccines

1929: Eli Lilly develops and registers thimerosal—which is approximately 50 percent mercury by weight—under the trade name Merthiolate. It is used in over-the-counter ointments and added to vaccines as an anti-bacterial preservative.

1974: Eli Lilly stops manufacturing vaccines, but several other companies continue using thimerosal in vaccines.

1982: The FDA recommends banning thimerosal from over-the-counter products —but not from vaccines—because of its toxicity and ineffectiveness.

1991: Three doses of the thimerosal-laced hepatitis B shot are added to the vaccine schedule, starting at birth; four doses of the thimerosal-laced Hib shot are added to the schedule, starting at 2 months; babies also receive four doses of DPT or DTaP, starting at 2 months (most brands contain thimerosal).

1997: The CDC reported that 1 of every 500 children in the U.S. is autistic.

July 1999: The FDA, CDC and American Academy of Pediatrics (AAP) announce that thimerosal will be phased out of vaccines. Manufacturers may keep producing mercury-containing shots, and doctors are encouraged to keep vaccinating children with the tainted vaccines for several more years, until old stock is used up.

August 1999: Congressman Dan Burton begins a 3-year probe into the link between vaccines and autism. Several hearings are held, including one in July 2000 on Mercury in Medicine.

June 2000: A top secret "Simpsonwood" gathering among health officials and vaccine producers is held to discuss a new CDC study showing a statistical link between thimerosal-containing vaccines and autism. An official asserts that the study results "have to be handled."

October 2001: The Institute of Medicine admits that a causal relationship between thimerosal-containing vaccines and neurological disorders is "biologically plausible."

November 2002: Lawmakers surreptitiously try to pass a law preventing parents from suing vaccine manufacturers. Also, the "Pichichero" study is published, claiming thimerosal in safe.

2003-2012: Several studies either confirm or deny a link between thimerosal-laced vaccines and autism. For example:
- In October 2003, a Danish study claimed no link between vaccines and autism. In November 2003, the reworked "CDC-Simpsonwood-Verstraeten" study claimed no link between vaccines and neurodevelopmental disorders. Dr. Mark Geier published a series of studies confirming a link between thimerosal-laced vaccines and autism. Researchers discredited a Montreal study that claimed thimerosal-laced vaccines are not harmful. In June 2007, Generation Rescue confirmed the vaccine-autism link. In September 2007, the CDC funded a study that found several correlations between thimerosal-laced vaccines and neuropsychological outcomes, yet concluded that such a link was not supported.
- The CDC repeated its recommendation that pregnant women, infants and children continue receiving the mercury-laced flu shot.
- New studies confirm that autism is more prevalent than ever before estimated, affecting 1 of every 91 children or 1 of every 38 children.

© NZM

This study also acknowledged several earlier studies that found important links between thimerosal-containing vaccines and neuropsychological deficits:
- In a previous vaccine safety analysis published in *Pediatrics,* post-neonatal exposure to thimerosal in vaccines was associated with an increased risk of language delays.[179]
- A 2004 *Pediatrics* study found that mercury from vaccines in the first year of life correlated with an increased risk of tics, a finding similar to that found in this study[180]
- A study of 12,000 British children found an association between mercury in vaccines and poorer prosocial behavior (actions meant to benefit others or society as a whole).[181]
- Studies of prenatal exposure to methylmercury from fish intake have shown negative associations with language and spatial abilities, attention span, and dexterity.[182,183]
- Previous studies have reported negative effects of thimerosal exposure on neuronal cells, biochemical pathways, and animal behavior.[184]

Did autism rates improve after mercury-laced vaccines were discontinued?
From 1999 through 2002, several mercury-laced vaccines were phased out of the recommended immunization schedule. They were replaced with low-mercury, or "thimerosal-free," vaccines. Today, authorities claim that autism rates have not declined after the mercury phaseout, and use this to support their contention that vaccines are safe.[185,186] (If mercury in vaccines contributed to autism, then rates should have dropped after mercury was removed.) However, during this so-called "phaseout" period, authorities actually *added* mercury-laced flu shots to the list of vaccines urged for all babies 6 to 23 months of age.[187,188] Soon thereafter, the CDC also added *pregnant women in their first trimester* to the list of people officially recommended—and actively encouraged—to receive mercury-laced flu vaccines.[189,190]

In addition to these dubious actions during this greatly publicized "phaseout" of mercury, four doses of a new vaccine with high *aluminum* content were added to the immunization schedule (for pneumococcal disease).[191] Two doses of another aluminum-containing vaccine (for hepatitis A) were added in 2005[192]—a 20% increase in aluminum content since the mercury phaseout (Figure 56).[193] Thus, millions of infants in utero and babies continued to receive unnaturally high doses of neurotoxic chemicals—mercury and aluminum—long after unsuspecting parents were led to believe that vaccines were purified and made safe.

Aluminum in Vaccines: A Link to Autism

Several vaccines contain high amounts of aluminum (see *Appendix II* on page 308). Babies receive multiple doses of these aluminum-containing shots. For example, the hepatitis B vaccine (Engerix-B) is given at birth, 2 and 6 months of age. Each dose has 250 micrograms (mcg) of aluminum. The DTaP shot (Infanrix) is given at 2, 4, 6 and 15 months. Each dose has 625mcg of aluminum. The Hib vaccine (Pedvax) is given at 2, 4 and 12 months. Each dose has 225mcg of aluminum. The pneumococcal vaccine (PCV/Prevnar) is given at 2, 4, 6 and 12 months. Each dose contains 125mcg of aluminum. The hepatitis A vaccine (Havrix) is given at 12 and 18 months. Each dose has 250mcg of aluminum. Thus, babies who follow the CDC immunization schedule are injected with nearly 5000mcg (5mg!) of aluminum by 18 months of age (Figure 57).[194,195] (Since some shot dates are variable, *babies may receive up to 1,475mcg of aluminum at their 12-month or 15-month checkups!*)

Aluminum is neurotoxic, even in minute quantities, and has a long history of well-documented hazards.[196,197] In 1927, Dr. Victor Vaughn, a toxicologist with the University of Michigan, testified before the Federal Trade Commission that "all salts of aluminum are poisonous when injected subcutaneously or intravenously."[198] According to the American Academy of Pediatrics, "Aluminum is now being implicated as interfering with a variety of cellular and metabolic processes in the nervous system and in other tissues."[199] This has led some researchers to speculate that aluminum may be linked to autism.[200,201] Some evidence appears to support this possibility. For example, in 1997 the *New England Journal of Medicine* published data showing that premature babies injected with aluminum build up toxic levels in the blood, bones and brain, and that aluminum toxicity can lead to neurological damage, including mental handicaps at 18 months of age.[202]

The FDA is aware that aluminum is dangerous. In a critical document on drug evaluation, the following statement is made: "Research indicates that patients with impaired kidney function, including premature neonates, who receive [injections] of aluminum at greater than 4 to 5mcg per kilogram of body weight per day, accumulate aluminum at levels associated with central nervous system and bone toxicity. Tissue loading may occur at even lower rates."[203] This means that for a 6 pound baby, 11-14mcg would be toxic. The hepatitis B vaccine given at birth contains 250mcg of aluminum—*20 times higher than safety levels!* Babies weigh about 12 pounds (5.5kg) at two months of age when they receive 1,225mcg of aluminum from their vaccines—*50 times higher than safety levels!*[204]

Of course, healthy babies without impaired kidney function may be able to handle more aluminum. However, no one knows how much more because such studies were never conducted. In addition, babies are not screened for kidney strength prior to vaccination. Therefore, it's impossible to know ahead of time which babies will succumb to aluminum poisoning. Instead, parents are expected to play Russian Roulette with their children.

Figure 56:

Vaccines Containing Aluminum
Were *Added* to the Immunization Schedule
When Mercury-Laced Vaccines Were Removed

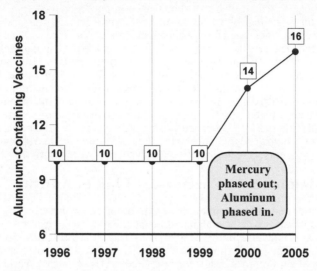

Copyright © NZM

From 1999 through 2002, several mercury-laced vaccines were phased out of the recommended immunization schedule. They were replaced with low-mercury, or "thimerosal-free," vaccines. However, during this so-called "phaseout" period, four doses of a new vaccine containing high *aluminum* content were added to the childhood immunization schedule (for pneumococcal disease). Two doses of another aluminum-containing vaccine (for Hib) were added in 2005—a 20% increase in aluminum content since the mercury phaseout.

The CDC, like the FDA, is also aware that aluminum is dangerous. For example, in June 2000, Dr. Tom Verstraeten, CDC epidemiologist, made the following comment to a group of concerned scientists: "The results [for aluminum] were almost identical to ethylmercury because the amount of aluminum [in vaccines] goes along almost exactly with the mercury." He was referring to a landmark study that found "statistically significant relationships" between both aluminum and mercury in vaccines and neurodevelopmental delays.[205] Dr. John Clements, WHO vaccine advisor, provided another telling statement: "Aluminum is not perceived, I believe, by the public as a dangerous metal. Therefore, we are in a much more comfortable wicket in terms of defending its presence in vaccines."[206]

Autism cases compensated in federal court:

In May 2011, a new study was published in the *Pace Environmental Law Review* revealing that for more than 20 years the federal Vaccine Injury Compensation Program (VICP) has been quietly awarding monetary compensation for vaccine injuries to children with brain damage and autism while the federal government was publicly denying that vaccines can cause autism. Authors of the study investigated children who were awarded compensation by the government for vaccine injuries resulting in brain damage. They found that 83 of these children were diagnosed with autism. They also found that autism is at least three times more prevalent among vaccine injured children than among children in the general U.S. population today.[207] Several vaccine safety advocacy groups, including Safe Minds and the National Autism Association, issued press releases calling for an immediate Congressional investigation.[208]

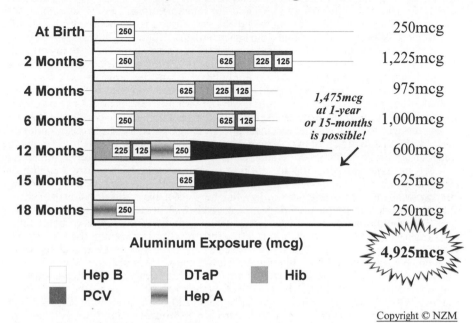

Cumulative Aluminum Exposure by 18 Months of Age

		Aluminum Exposure (mcg)	
At Birth	250		250mcg
2 Months	250 / 625 / 225 / 125		1,225mcg
4 Months	625 / 225 / 125		975mcg
6 Months	250 / 625 / 125	*1,475mcg at 1-year or 15-months is possible!*	1,000mcg
12 Months	225 / 125 / 250		600mcg
15 Months	625		625mcg
18 Months	250		250mcg

Aluminum Exposure (mcg)

☆ **4,925mcg** ☆

☐ Hep B ☐ DTaP ▨ Hib
■ PCV ▨ Hep A

The hepatitis B vaccine (Engerix-B) is given at birth, 2 and 6 months. Each dose contains 250mcg of aluminum. The DTaP shot (Infanrix) is given at 2, 4, 6 and 15 months. Each dose contains 625mcg of aluminum. The Hib vaccine (Pedvax) is given at 2, 4 and 12 months. Each dose contains 225mcg of aluminum. The pneumococcal vaccine (PCV/Prevnar) is given at 2, 4, 6 and 12 months. Each dose contains 125mcg of aluminum. The hepatitis A vaccine (Havrix) is given at 12 and 18 months. Each dose contains 250mcg of aluminum. Thus, babies who follow the recommended immunization schedule are injected with nearly 5000mcg (5mg!) of aluminum by 18 months of age. (Since some shot dates are variable, *babies may receive up to 1,475mcg of aluminum at their 12-month or 15-month checkups!*) Source: Vaccine product inserts and the CDC's immunization schedule, 2011.

Vaccines and Autism: Adverse Reaction Reports[209]

▸ "I am a new grandmother of a beautiful granddaughter. She was a perfectly healthy baby that was alert, happy and made wonderful eye contact. My daughter took her for her first set of shots at two months. The next day she was very lethargic and unresponsive. She also cried a lot and could not hold her head up. Within five days she was rushed to the hospital with seizures. The doctors would not even discuss the possibility of the shots being the cause. They ran every test and could not find a thing wrong with her. After three days, they sent her home. One week later, we were back in the ER with seizures for four hours. She makes little eye contact and is very easily upset. Three more days in the hospital with a diagnosis of acid reflux! When did that ever cause seizures? Finally, the neurologist admitted that sometimes vaccines will cause seizures and push a child into autism."

▸ "My son had his first shot at four months old, then went on a catch-up schedule to get him up to date. About 6 to 7 days after his shots, his breathing became labored, he had a high fever and he came out in bruises. He was already in the hospital due to his prematurity so all the tests were done to find out what was wrong. The day before he had his shots we were told he could come home the following week. Imagine our surprise when 3 months later he was still in the hospital. They could not find anything wrong with him and let us bring him home. They told us that the problems were from his prematurity, which we believed. After his 2nd, 3rd and 4th immunizations, I knew something was wrong. He went from a fun-loving, beautiful, smart boy to an autistic child with a lot of problems. When he was 18 months old I gave birth to a daughter. They gave her hepatitis B and vitamin K shots. I had specifically asked for this not to happen. With my preemie, they will not accept that the immunizations caused the autism. If you saw him one year ago and then saw him now you would not believe he was the same child."

▸ "Several years ago our only child, who was two years old, was diagnosed autistic. I checked her shot records but was told it was not vaccines. She is now 14 years old and still severely autistic. The problem is, now I have four more autistic children. I believed the doctors who told us it was not vaccines. Now we are the parents of five autistic children."

▸ "I have an autistic child in my second grade classroom. His parents told me that he was perfectly healthy until he had his shots at the age of two. Now he can barely communicate or keep up with our schedule of learning. I am concerned about my 4-month-old granddaughter. She is to have her second immunization this week. I have expressed my concerns with my son and daughter-in-law, but they need to make this decision themselves. When you work with an autistic child, you desperately want to save others from this disease."

▸ "I am the mother of a 4 ½ year old boy who is now in the process of being tested for autism. My son was a happy and carefree little boy until he went in for his four-year well-check to receive his booster shots. My son changed—his smile, his speech regressed, he seemed withdrawn and not like the little boy I knew. I was scared and confused, so I called his doctor. We told her how our son changed suddenly and drastically after his shots. Of course, I was told that there is no link between his behavior and the vaccinations, that this is the age when children are usually diagnosed—it is just a coincidence that the vaccines that are given at his well-check is usually the time when a child is diagnosed."

▸ "One day after receiving her immunizations, my four-year-old niece went into seizures. She slept for two days. After waking up, she had infantile behavior and strongly resembled a mentally challenged child, with automatic movements and actions. She spent eight more days in the hospital, then was sent to a children's hospital for physical, speech, music, and other therapies. There have been slight changes; at first she was running into walls when walking, biting, staring blankly, and no verbalization. She is still on oral steroids, and now mimicking some words, holding things, not as much biting, but now licking things. My sister was told that her 4-year-old is on a 1-year-old verbal level, but a 1-month-old level as far as focusing and recognizing. An infectious disease specialist said that it was probably a combination of an infection and the shots, but not the shots alone. She is now being told that it was just a coincidence that she had the shots the previous day."

▸ "My beautiful, four-year-old grandson is not talking, and showing signs of autism. He was a vibrant, healthy baby, and was growing well until his baby shots at the age of 14 months. Within a two-week period after receiving his shots, he stopped giving eye contact, seemed to turn inward, and has never been the same. He is developing well physically, but mentally and emotionally he is very delayed. My daughter suffers daily from his emotional and mental disability. It breaks my heart to see this. I don't know if he will ever be able to live a normal life. Someone has committed a horrible crime against these young children."

Where can I get more information about autism?

The MMR chapter has more information about autism, including personal stories linking this triple shot to pervasive developmental disorders. The *Thinktwice Global Vaccine Institute* (www.thinktwice.com) lists important autism organizations and other resources.

"Aluminum is not perceived, I believe, by the public as a dangerous metal. Therefore, we are in a much more comfortable wicket in terms of defending its presence in vaccines."
—Dr. John Clements, World Health Organization (WHO) vaccine advisor

Hepatitis A

What is hepatitis A?

Hepatitis A is a contagious liver disease usually transmitted through contaminated food or water, or by coming into close contact with someone who is already infected. Symptoms may be similar to the flu, with low-grade fever, loss of appetite, fatigue and abdominal pain. Jaundice is possible.[1,2] The disease is rarely as serious as other types of viral hepatitis.[3] For example, the case-fatality rate among all age groups is less than one-third of one percent—about 3 deaths per 1000 cases—mainly in adults greater than 50 years of age.[4-6] Most people who are infected recover completely.[7] In children younger than 6 years of age, 70 percent of hepatitis A infections are asymptomatic—there is no fever, fatigue or jaundice; the child is simply a carrier of the disease.[8] In older children and adults, symptoms are more likely.[9] There is no risk of long-term or chronic hepatitis A infection. Once you contract the disease and recover—typically in less than 2 months—you will not get it again.[10]

How prevalent is hepatitis A and who is most at risk?

In 2005, there were 4,488 cases of hepatitis A reported in the United States; just 208 of these were in children under 5 years of age. Just 14 cases were in children under 1 year of age.[11] The groups at greatest risk of contracting hepatitis A are persons traveling to regions of the world with high rates of this disease, men who have sex with other men, illicit drug users, and persons with blood clotting disorders.[12] Young children are *not* among the groups at greatest risk.[13-15]

Does a hepatitis A vaccine exist?

Today, two monovalent hepatitis A vaccines are available in the United States: Vaqta® by Merck, and Havrix® by GlaxoSmithKline. They are recommended for persons 12 months of age and older.[16] Combination vaccines containing hepatitis A are available as well. For example, Twinrix® contains both the hepatitis A and hepatitis B vaccines for persons 18 years of age or older.[17] In 2007, the FDA approved an "accelerated dosing schedule" for this combination shot: three doses administered within three weeks, with another booster dose one year later.[18]

How safe is the hepatitis A vaccine?

The hepatitis A vaccine is "derived from hepatitis A virus grown in human MRC-5 diploid fibroblasts" (originated from aborted fetal tissue). Each dose also contains aluminum, sodium borate, sodium chloride, bovine albumin and formaldehyde.[19] (See *Appendices II, III* and *IV* on pages 308-310 for more information.) Several serious 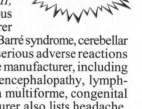 adverse reactions have been reported by the vaccine manufacturer following receipt of the hepatitis A vaccine. These include Guillain-Barré syndrome, cerebellar ataxia, encephalitis and thrombocytopenia.[20] In addition, other serious adverse reactions following administration of this vaccine have been reported to the manufacturer, including anaphylaxis, brachial plexus neuropathy, transverse myelitis, encephalopathy, lymphadenopathy, syncope, meningitis, hepatitis, diabetes, erythema multiforme, congenital abnormality, and multiple sclerosis.[21,22] The vaccine manufacturer also lists headache, upper respiratory infection, ear infection, menstruation disorder, myalgia, asthma, wheezing, allergic reactions, dermatitis, and diarrhea as commonly reported side effects of this vaccine.[23] The Vaccine Adverse Event Reporting System (VAERS), jointly operated by the CDC and FDA, also receives numerous independent reports confirming "neurologic, hematologic, and autoimmune syndromes" linked to this vaccine.[24,25]

The following adverse reaction associated with the hepatitis A vaccine is typical of the daily emails received by the *Thinktwice Global Vaccine Institute* (www.thinktwice.com): "Are there any doctor recommendations against administering the hepatitis A vaccine to a 2-year-old with a fever? A co-worker's son had a seizure last night for the first time.

The circumstances seem to point towards an allergic reaction to the vaccination. The 2-year-old was admitted to the emergency room last night after the parents heard muffled gasping from the crib. I'm afraid to think of what would have happened had they not awoken."[26]

How effective is the hepatitis A vaccine?

According to the CDC, "the overall incidence of hepatitis A has declined in the United States over the past several decades primarily as a result of better hygienic and sanitary conditions."[27] For example, in the early 1970s, about 55,000 cases of hepatitis A were reported each year in the United States. By the early 1990s, before a hepatitis A vaccine was introduced, less than 25,000 cases were reported each year—a greater than 50 percent reduction.[28]

According to the hepatitis A vaccine manufacturer, the duration of protection "is unknown at present."[29] For example, in a 6-year follow-up study of children and adolescents who received 2 doses of the hepatitis A vaccine, researchers were only able to note "detectable" levels of anti-hepatitis A antibodies in test subjects—a measure far short of the "protective" levels sought.[30] In other words, immunity is most likely brief; additional booster shots may be recommended in the future. Also, the incubation period of hepatitis A (the time between being exposed to the disease and showing symptoms) can be 50 days.[31] Therefore, when a child receives the vaccine and contracts the disease shortly thereafter, the vaccine will not be implicated as defective or causative. Instead, the child may be blamed for harboring a pre-existing condition.[32]

Is the hepatitis A vaccine mandatory?

Although children are not among the groups at greatest risk from this disease, authorities believe that "routine vaccination of children is the most effective way to reduce hepatitis A incidence nationwide."[33] Yet in 2004, *after* children under 5 years of age began receiving the CDC's recommended hepatitis A vaccine, there was a 26 percent *increase* in the number of children under 5 years of age who contracted the disease: 231 cases in 2003 versus 291 cases in 2004.[34,35] In other words, children are being subjected to all of the potential hazards of this vaccine, with limited or questionable personal benefits, as part of an overall immunization strategy to protect high risk groups whose members are either difficult to reach or have rejected the shot. Parents may legally exempt their children from this vaccine—and from other "mandatory" shots as well.

Hepatitis B

What is hepatitis B?
Hepatitis B is a viral infection. Symptoms may be similar to the flu, including weakness, loss of appetite, nausea, vomiting, a low-grade fever, diarrhea, sore muscles and joint pain.[1] A swollen liver and jaundice (yellowing of the skin and eyes) are possible as well. In some instances, individuals who contract this disease are carriers of the virus yet exhibit few or none of these symptoms. Acute hepatitis B usually runs its course within a few months. Most patients do not require hospital care and 95 percent recover completely; they will not contract the disease again.[2,3] Long-term or chronic hepatitis B infections can be serious. Authorities estimate that about 20 percent of chronic cases eventually progress to liver damage, causing about 4,500 deaths annually.[4]

How is hepatitis B contracted?
In the United States, about half of all new cases among adults occur through sexual transmission. The virus is spread through contact with the body fluids—blood, saliva and semen—of an infected person. (The virus remains communicable outside of the body for at least one week.) The incubation period—how long it takes to show signs of the disease after being exposed—ranges from 6 weeks to 6 months. People who inject illegal drugs account for another 15 percent of new cases, mainly by sharing needles with infected persons. It is also possible to contract hepatitis B by being stuck with a used needle, through improperly screened blood transfusions, or during birth when the virus passes from an infected mother to her baby.[5]

How prevalent is hepatitis B?
In 2004, there were 6,212 cases of hepatitis B reported in the United States.[6] In 2005, there were 5,119 documented cases in the U.S.[7] Nevertheless, authorities estimate that more than 1 million Americans have chronic hepatitis B infection—approximately one-third of one percent of the population.[8] Some experts dispute this figure and assert that in North America, Europe and Australia, true carriers of the virus represent less than one-tenth of one percent of the population.[9]

Who is most at risk?
The groups at greatest risk of contracting hepatitis B are heterosexuals engaging in unprotected sex with multiple sex partners, prostitutes, sexually active homosexual men, intravenous drug users, healthcare and public safety workers exposed to infected body fluids, and household contacts of persons with chronic hepatitis B infection.[10] Infants born to infected mothers have a greater chance of acquiring this disease than babies born to non-infected mothers. (Concerned pregnant women can be tested.)[11] However, children rarely develop this disease. In the U.S., less than one percent of all cases occur in persons less than 15 years of age.[12,13] The disease is even more uncommon in babies and toddlers. For example, in 2004 there were just 10 cases of hepatitis B in children under 5 years of age.[14] In 2005, there were only 5 cases of hepatitis B in this age group (Figure 58).[15]

Black Americans contract hepatitis B at higher rates than Asians and at rates 2 to 3 times greater than Whites. For example, in 2003 there were 2,724 reported cases of hepatitis B among Whites (who comprise about 75 percent of the U.S. population) and 1,235 cases among Blacks (12 percent of the U.S. population). This translates into a rate of 1.2 cases per 100,000 population for Whites and 3.3 cases per 100,000 for Blacks (Figure 59).[16,17]

Persistent exposure to hepatitis B may provide benefits. For example, the *American Journal of Epidemiology* published a study showing that healthcare workers increase their risk of contracting hepatitis B through frequency of contact with blood, but not through frequency of contact with patients. The authors of the study concluded that healthcare workers may become passively immunized, rather than infected, through continuous exposure to low levels of hepatitis B.[18]

Figure 58:

Hepatitis B Cases by Age Group: United States, 2005

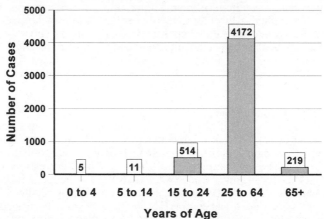

In the United States, less than 1 percent of all reported hepatitis B cases occur in persons less than 15 years of age. The disease is even more uncommon in babies and toddlers. For example, in 2005 there were just 5 cases of hepatitis B in children under 5 years of age. Source: CDC, *MMWR* (March 30, 2007); Vol. 54, No. 53: Table 3.

Does a hepatitis B vaccine exist?

In 1981, the Food and Drug Administration (FDA) licensed a plasma-derived hepatitis B vaccine. It contained hepatitis B antigens (disease matter) extracted from individuals infected with hepatitis B. This vaccine was later withdrawn from the market because vaccines derived from human blood are capable of transmitting unforeseen and potentially dangerous viruses. In 1986, the first of several genetically engineered (synthetic recombinant) vaccines was licensed for use on the general population. Today, two hepatitis B vaccines are available in the U.S. and elsewhere: Merck's Recombivax HB®—a viral vaccine containing 5mcg of hepatitis B surface antigen, treated in phosphate buffer with formaldehyde, plus 250-500mcg of aluminum;[19] and GlaxoSmithKline's Engerix-B®—containing aluminum, sodium chloride, and "trace amounts of thimerosal."[20] (See *Appendix II* on aluminum.) Combination vaccines containing hepatitis B are available as well.

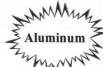

How safe is the hepatitis B vaccine?

Several studies, including one by the *New England Journal of Medicine* and another by the *Institute of Medicine,* have investigated the probability that recipients of the plasma-derived hepatitis B vaccine may have received shots contaminated with undetected viruses, especially HIV, a precursor to AIDS.[21,22] The clinical studies used to assess the safety of the current hepatitis B vaccine were comprised of just 147 healthy infants and children who were monitored for just 5 days after each shot.[23] This is not a large enough sample nor long enough time period to determine true rates of adverse events. In fact, the manufacturer admits that "broad use of the vaccine could reveal adverse reactions not observed in clinical trials."[24] Adult test subjects were monitored for only 5 days after each shot as well. Still, systemic complaints were reported following 15 percent of the injections. These included arthralgia, myalgia, paresthesia, back pain, neck pain, lymphadenopathy, headache, fever, malaise, chills, vomiting, diarrhea, abdominal pains, upper respiratory infection, earache, and hypotension.[25]

Figure 59:

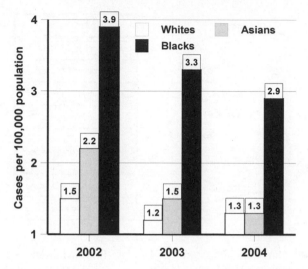

Hepatitis B Cases by Race

Black Americans contract hepatitis B at higher rates than Asians and at rates 2 to 3 times greater than Whites. Source: CDC, *MMWRs:* (June 16, 2006), Vol. 53, No. 53.; (April 22, 2005), Vol. 52, No. 54.; (April 30, 2004), Vol. 51, No. 53.

The manufacturer also lists several serious adverse reactions that have been reported after the hepatitis B vaccine was licensed and mass marketed. These include arthritis, Guillain-Barré syndrome, multiple sclerosis, myelitis, transverse myelitis, lupus, thrombocytopenia, vasculitis, seizures, peripheral neuropathy, Bell's palsy, radiculopathy, encephalitis, Stevens-Johnson syndrome, eczema, alopecia (loss of hair), anaphylaxis, bronchial spasms, herpes zoster, tachycardia, optic neuritis, visual disturbances, and hearing disorders.[26] Although official fact sheets[27] and other public endorsements[28] of the hepatitis B vaccine minimize or deny serious reactions, numerous studies published in medical and scientific journals throughout the world,[29] plus frequent reports filed with the FDA's Vaccine Adverse Event Reporting System (VAERS),[30] confirm these and other afflictions following hepatitis B vaccination (Figure 60). Some of these studies are summarized in the sections below.

Arthritis: In 1990, shortly after the hepatitis B vaccine was introduced, the *British Medical Journal* documented a link between this vaccine and polyarthritis (painful inflammation of five or more joints).[31] That same year, the *Journal of Rheumatology* published a paper on "reactive" arthritis after hepatitis B vaccination.[32] In 1994, the *British Journal of Rheumatology* published data documenting rheumatoid arthritis after hepatitis B vaccination.[33] That same year, the *British Medical Journal* published three additional papers confirming a correlation between the hepatitis B vaccine and reactive arthritis.[34-36] In 1995, the *Scandinavian Journal of Rheumatology* published two papers documenting cases of arthritis following hepatitis B vaccination.[37,38] That same year, the *Irish Medical Journal* published data showing links between this vaccine and arthropathy.[39] In 1997, the *British Journal of Rheumatology* published two additional studies documenting several case histories of "inflammatory polyarthritis" after hepatitis B vaccination.[40,41] In 1998, rheumatoid arthritis after recombinant hepatitis B vaccination was documented once again in the *Journal of Rheumatology*.[42] That same year, the French journal, *Revue de Medecine Interne,* published a study on adult-onset Still's disease—a rare and painful type of arthritis—after hepatitis A and B vaccination.[43]

Figure 60:
Adverse Reactions: Hepatitis B Vaccine

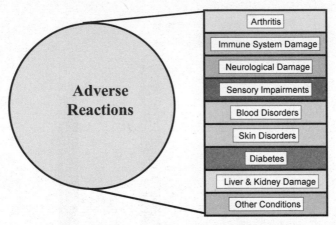

Severe adverse reactions—including arthritis, Guillain-Barré syndrome, multiple sclerosis, myelitis, lupus, thrombocytopenia, encephalitis, allergic skin reactions, visual disturbances, and hearing disorders—have been linked to the hepatitis B vaccine. Source: The vaccine manufacturer; reports filed with the Vaccine Adverse Event Reporting System (VAERS); numerous case studies published in medical and scientific journals throughout the world.

In 1999, *Rheumatology* documented rheumatic disorders after hepatitis B vaccination.[44] In 2000, the American College of Rheumatology published a paper in their peer-reviewed journal, *Arthritis & Rheumatism,* showing Sjogren's syndrome—a rare form of chronic arthritis—after hepatitis B vaccination.[45]

Autoimmune and neurological disorders (including multiple sclerosis): As early as 1983, the *New England Journal of Medicine* published a study showing polyneuropathy —the simultaneous malfunction of several nerves—after hepatitis B vaccination.[46] In 1988, the *American Journal of Epidemiology* showed multiple "neurologic adverse events" after hepatitis B vaccination, including several cases of Bell's palsy, Guillain-Barré syndrome, lumbar radiculopathy, brachial plexus neuropathy, optic neuritis and transverse myelitis.[47] That same year, *Archives of Internal Medicine* wrote about myasthenia gravis—a severe, chronic autoimmune neuromuscular disease—after hepatitis B vaccination.[48] In 1991, *Lancet* published a paper documenting central nervous system demyelination after recombinant hepatitis B vaccination.[49] In 1992, *Nephron* published data linking systemic lupus erythematosus (SLE)—a chronic autoimmune disease affecting multiple organs—to hepatitis B vaccination.[50] Also in 1992, *Clinical Infectious Diseases* published a paper linking Evan's disease—a rare autoimmune and blood disorder with a high fatality rate—to hepatitis B vaccination.[51] That same year, the French journal, *Therapie,* published a study on "peripheral facial paralysis" after hepatitis B vaccination.[52] In addition, *Infectious Disease News* published a paper noting several cases of neurological damage resembling multiple sclerosis after hepatitis B vaccination.[53] In 1993, the *Journal of Hepatology* published a paper on transverse myelitis—inflammation of the spinal cord—following hepatitis B vaccination.[54] That same year, the French journal, *La Nouvelle Presse Médicale,* published data confirming "acute myelitis" after hepatitis B vaccination.[55] Also in 1993, *Clinical Infectious Diseases* documented "classic multiple sclerosis" after hepatitis B vaccination.[56] In 1994, *Archives of Pediatric and Adolescent Medicine* published data linking lupus to hepatitis B vaccination.[57] That same year, the Scandinavian journal, *Acta Neurologica Scandinavica,* published a paper on acute cerebellar ataxia—severe loss of balance and motor coordination—after recombinant hepatitis B vaccination.[58] In 1995, the Journal of *Neurology, Neurosurgery, and Psychiatry* published a study on central nervous system demyelination after vaccination with hepatitis B.[59] That same year, the *American Journal of Neuroradiology* also documented myelitis after hepatitis B vaccination. The authors of this study suggested that adverse reactions of this nature may be underreported because symptoms can be delayed.[60] In 1996, both *Nephron* and the French journal, *Anne Dermatol Venereol,* published studies linking lupus erythematosus to the hepatitis B vaccine.[61,62] That same year, the *Journal of Hepatology* published a paper linking leukoencephalitis—inflammation of the white substance of the brain—to hepatitis B vaccination.[63] Also in 1996, the *New England Journal of Medicine* documented cryoglobulinemia—a rare autoimmune disease causing impaired circulation, bleeding and other serious problems—after hepatitis B vaccination.[64] The *Journal of Autoimmunity* also documented hepatitis B vaccine-induced autoimmunity.[65] In 1997, the *Indian Journal of Pediatrics* published a study linking Guillain-Barré syndrome —an autoimmune disease causing nerve damage, muscle weakness and paralysis—to the hepatitis B vaccine.[66] That same year, the *Journal of Korean Medical Science* documented acute myelitis after hepatitis B vaccination.[67] Also in 1997, "mental nerve neuropathy" following hepatitis B vaccination was documented.[68] In addition, the *Journal of the American Medical Association* published data on 46 people—mostly women—who lost their hair after hepatitis B vaccination.[69] In 1998, both systemic lupus erythematosus and thrombocytopenia were documented in recipients of the hepatitis B vaccine.[70] In 1999, the *American Journal of Gastroenterology* published additional data on hair loss after hepatitis B vaccination.[71] That same year, *Autoimmunity* documented demyelinating polyneuropathy after hepatitis B vaccination, while *Neurology* published data correlating multiple sclerosis and encephalitis with hepatitis B vaccination.[72,73] That same year, *La Nouvelle Presse Médicale* documented cervical myelitis after hepatitis B vaccination.[74] In 2000, *Neurology* published data linking multiple sclerosis to the hepatitis B vaccine.[75] That same year, the *Journal of the Medical Association of Thailand* wrote about Guillain-Barré syndrome following recombinant hepatitis B vaccination.[76] In 2001, *Clinical Infectious Diseases* published a paper on leukoencephalitis after hepatitis B vaccination.[77] In 2004, *Neurology* published a study showing that hepatitis B vaccination is associated with a statistically significant elevated risk of multiple sclerosis.[78] In 2006, *Chinese Medical Journal* documented multiple sclerosis after hepatitis B vaccination.[79] In 2008, *Neurology* published two new studies showing a statistically significant correlation between hepatitis B vaccination in children and the development of pediatric multiple sclerosis (central nervous system demyelination) more than three years later.[80,81]

Sensory impairments: Several medical and scientific publications have documented vision and hearing disorders following hepatitis B vaccination. For example, in 1987 *Lancet* published a paper on uveitis—inflammation of the inner layer of the eye often leading to blindness—after hepatitis B vaccination.[82] In 1993, *Lancet* published additional data documenting vision loss and eosinophilia—an allergic blood disorder—following hepatitis B vaccination.[83] In 1994, *Optometry and Vision Science* wrote about optic neuritis after hepatitis B vaccination.[84] In 1995, the *Archives of Ophthalmology* documented epitheliopathy—a rare eye disorder causing vision impairment—after hepatitis B vaccination.[85] In 1996, *Lancet* published a paper documenting an "occlusion of the central retinal vein" following hepatitis B vaccination.[86] That same year, the *American Journal of Ophthalmology* wrote about bilateral white dot syndrome—causing a loss of visual acuity in both eyes—after hepatitis B vaccination.[87] Also in 1996, *La Nouvelle Presse Médicale* documented neuropapillitis—inflammation and deterioration of the optic nerve—after hepatitis B vaccination,[88] and another French journal, *Annales D Oto-Laryngologie Et De Chirurgie Cervico-Faciale,* documented hearing loss after hepatitis B vaccination.[89] In 1997, *La Nouvelle Presse Médicale* published two separate papers documenting several cases of occlusion of the central retinal vein following hepatitis B vaccination.[90,91] That same year, *Nephrology Dialysis Transplantation* confirmed the occurrence of optic neuritis after hepatitis B vaccination.[92] In addition, *International Ophthalmology* documented "ophthalmic complications" in recipients of this vaccine.[93] Also in 1997, *Annals of the New York Academy of Sciences*, and the international journal, *Auris, Nasus, Larynx,* both documented hearing loss subsequent to hepatitis B vaccination.[94,95] In 1998, the *Journal of French Ophthalmology* published data on epitheliopathy after hepatitis B vaccination.[96] In 1999, the *British Journal of Ophthalmology* confirmed optic neuritis after hepatitis B vaccination.[97] That same year, the Scandinavian journal, *Acta Ophthalmologica Scandinavica*, published data on papilledema —swelling of the optic disk—after hepatitis B vaccination.[98] In 2001, the German publication, *Klin Monatsbl Augenheilkd,* also documented optic neuritis after hepatitis B shots.[99]

Blood disorders: In 1990, shortly after the hepatitis B vaccine was mass marketed, the *British Medical Journal* documented vasculitis—inflammation of the blood vessels —following hepatitis B vaccination.[100] In 1993, another British medical journal, *Thorax,* confirmed the occurrence of this disorder following hepatitis B vaccination.[101] That same year, *Lancet* published a study on Eosinophilia, an allergic blood disorder, after hepatitis B vaccination.[102] In 1994, and again in 1995, *Lancet* documented thrombocytopenia—a serious disease causing excessive bleeding, bruising and clotting problems—after hepatitis B vaccination.[103,104] In 1998, the *Scandinavian Journal of Infectious Diseases* also confirmed the occurrence of thrombocytopenia in several patients who were recently vaccinated against hepatitis B.[105] In 1998, *Archives of Disease in Children* published data showing that thrombocytopenia occurs as an adverse reaction to hepatitis B vaccination.[106] In 1999, the *European Journal of Pediatrics* confirmed once again that thrombocytopenia can occur following vaccination with hepatitis B and MMR.[107] That same year, the *Journal of Rheumatology* published two important papers, the first showing a link between vasculitis and hepatitis B vaccination.[108] The second paper documented erythermalgia—vascular spasms in the hands and feet causing burning pain—after hepatitis B vaccination.[109] In 2000, *Clinical and Experimental Rheumatology* studied cases of polyarteritis nodosa—a rare, systemic, necrotizing (cell-damaging) type of vasculitis—after hepatitis B vaccination.[110] That same year, the *British Journal of Haematology* documented severe pancytopenia—a dangerous reduction of blood cells—after hepatitis B vaccination.[111] In 2001, the *Journal of Rheumatology* published additional data confirming the possibility of vasculitis after recombinant hepatitis B vaccination.[112] That same year, the Italian journal, *Haematologica,* confirmed thrombocytopenia as an adverse possibility following hepatitis B vaccination.[113]

Skin disorders: In 1989, the *New England Journal of Medicine* documented erythema nodosum—a painful inflammation of the skin with tender lumps—following hepatitis B vaccination.[114] In 1993, the *Journal of Rheumatology* documented cases of both erythema nodosum and Takayasu's arteritis—a rare form of vasculitis—after hepatitis B vaccination.[115] That same year, the Swedish journal, *Acta Dermato-Venereologica,* wrote about lichen ruber planus—an itchy skin eruption characterized by hard, thick lesions grouped together and resembling algae or fungus growing on rocks—after hepatitis B vaccination.[116] In 1994, *Archives of Dermatology* also documented lichen planus after hepatitis B vaccination.[117] That same year, *Pediatric Dermatology* showed a link between erythema multiforme—an inflammatory skin disease—and hepatitis B vaccination.[118] In 1997, the *Australasian Journal of Dermatology* confirmed "lichenoid reactions" (lichen planus) due to hepatitis B vaccination.[119] That same year, the *Journal of the American Academy of Dermatology* wrote about anetoderma—localized wrinkles, loss of elasticity, and atrophy of the skin—following hepatitis B vaccination.[120] In 1998, the *British Journal of Dermatology* published two papers documenting skin disorders after hepatitis B vaccination: one on lichen planus,[121] the other on urticaria and angioedema—allergic skin disorders characterized by burning, itching, and painful wheals.[122] In 1999, the *International Journal of Dermatology* also documented lichen planus after hepatitis B vaccination.[123] In 2000, *Clinical and Experimental Dermatology* published data linking erythema multiforme to the hepatitis B vaccine.[124] That same year, the *Nepal Journal of Dermatology* documented lichen planus after hepatitis B vaccination.[125] In 2001, the *Journal of the American Academy of Dermatology* published a paper on lichen planus after hepatitis B vaccination[126] and *Pediatric Dermatology* documented the occurrence of "lichenoid eruption" following this shot.[127]

Diabetes, liver and kidney disorders: In 1994, *Lancet* documented liver dysfunction after hepatitis B vaccination.[128] In 1995, *Clinical Nephrology* published a paper on nephrotic syndrome—kidney damage—after hepatitis B vaccination.[129] In 1996, the *New Zealand Medical Journal* published two papers linking the hepatitis B vaccine to epidemics of insulin-dependent diabetes mellitus (IDDM). The author of the studies found that in the three years following a well organized, newly instituted national hepatitis B immunization campaign, there was a 60 percent increase in cases of IDDM.[130,131] In 1997, *Intensive Care Medicine* wrote about liver inflammation and acute respiratory distress following hepatitis B vaccination.[132] In 2000, *Pediatric Nephrology* confirmed the possibility of being stricken with nephrotic syndrome after hepatitis B vaccination.[133] Other publications have also documented adverse reactions to this vaccine.[134-144]

Adverse Reaction Reports

This section contains unsolicited adverse reaction reports associated with the hepatitis B vaccine, typical of the daily emails received by the *Thinktwice Global Vaccine Institute*.[145]

▸ "After our son was born, they injected him with hepatitis B vaccine, even though he was not breathing and had an apgar of two. He immediately suffered a seven minute seizure. They gave us no reason for this other than to say it was probably caused by metabolic acidosis. Now our son has Sensory Integration Dysfunction. We are desperate for answers."

▸ "My grandson had his first hepatitis B vaccine when he was only hours old, and the second one about a month later. He has had several seizures since and his skin breaks out in a red itchy rash."

▸ "My son was profoundly damaged by the hepatitis B vaccine he was given at birth. (He was featured on ABC's '20/20' program which questioned the vaccine's safety.) We have had a grueling journey, made all the more staggering by virtue of my own conventional public health training. Needless to say, I made a complete about-face on the vaccine issue while flying by the seat of my pants to save my son. When we refused additional vaccines, one pediatrician reported us to social services, and we were dropped from a federal developmental assistance program. No one helped us for almost two years, even though we went to many specialists. I want to inform and assist other parents."

▸ "Can you please tell me if the hepatitis B shot is given at birth. My pediatrician says he has no record of any shot being given to our daughter at birth, but I remember the band-aid. My daughter was diagnosed at two days old with 'moderate' hearing loss. However, when she was born, she was very alert and immediately turned to the sound of my husband's voice. Everyone in the room noticed. I feel something is not right."

▸ "Our daughter was born healthy but we allowed her to get the hepatitis B vaccine, and at three days old she started having seizures. After a week in the local children's hospital surrounded by the best doctors and nurses it was discovered that she had suffered a stroke. We had to keep her on phenobarbital for about eight weeks until they felt it safe that the seizures had stopped. They have never been able to determine what caused it."

▸ "My daughter received the hepatitis B shot at 16 hours old and suffered from insomnia, irritability, agitation, abdominal pains, cramps, and crying-screaming for 12 hours straight."

▸ "My grandson had a hepatitis B vaccine at two days old. He was sent home from the hospital and returned later in the afternoon to the emergency room because he wasn't breathing properly. A few days later he was having seizures. One month later he again had the vaccination and ended up at the ER again with the same problem. Doctors keep telling us that it is not because of the vaccination, however we went through the same thing twice right after the vaccine. My grandson is now on an apnea monitor and I feel he will have problems forever, and that we have lost our freedom with him by the poor little thing being attached to this machine. The doctors are denying that this could be from the vaccination, but I am very concerned about letting him have the third shot."

▸ "My little boy was injured by a hepatitis B vaccine given to him when he was only three days old. The adverse reaction was so severe that he had an aneurysm rupture in his brain, died three times and was resuscitated each time. He has many complications and is severely brain damaged. His life was taken from him. He is now two-and-a-half years old and is just learning how to hold up his head. He has seizure disorder, epilepsy, cortical blindness, a feeding tube, and is immobile."

▸ "My son was healthy until five days after he received his hepatitis B vaccination. He has since been chronically ill for two years."

▸ "I took my daughter to the doctor at one month old. I let the pediatric office give her a hepatitis B immunization. That evening she woke up from her nap with terror-like screaming and her body trembling."

▸ "My husband and I have been accused of 'shaken baby syndrome' and our child is in foster care. We believe that he has been damaged by the hepatitis B vaccine. He received all three of his hepatitis B shots by the time he was two months old. Now they are saying that he had them too soon and he has to have another, that it will take a court order to stop this. I am terrified of what will happen if he gets another shot. He was born six weeks premature and reacted badly to his shots. After the first, he cried and had a head circumference growth of 4.25cm in four days. After the second shot he stopped breathing. He had brain swelling, bleeding in the brain and behind the eyes. He has multiple problems from this, and because of his symptoms we have been arrested for child abuse. My husband is still in jail. I am out on bail. I did not know about vaccine damage before it happened to us."

▸ "I know of parents who were charged with shaken baby syndrome after a bad reaction to the hepatitis B vaccine. The child was taken away, given a second shot, had another bad reaction, and was hospitalized with brain and eye damage. This is a typical VAERS reaction to the hepatitis B vaccine. Doctors are in denial. Is there anything you can do?"

▸ "Our daughter received a hepatitis B vaccine. She was then hospitalized with a fever and thrombocytopenia (a serious blood disorder)."

▸ "Do you have a number I can reach to report a reverse reaction to hepatitis B vaccination causing my son to get type 1 diabetes?"

▸ "Our friend had a four month old son in good health until three weeks ago when he received the hepatitis B shot. He immediately started vomiting, had diarrhea and a fever. These symptoms left after a few days. Yesterday, he was laid down for his nap. When his parents tried to wake him, he was not breathing. They rushed him to a clinic. He was then transferred to Children's Hospital in New Orleans. A CAT scan and MRI revealed 'blood behind the eyes with two areas of past bleeding and one area of recent bleeding in the brain.' The first conclusion the doctors arrived at was 'shaken baby syndrome.' The parents were devastated and are still in a state of shock, both from the implied accusation and their concern for their child. You have never met more loving, caring, gentle people than these two. Their baby's life signs are now stable, but he is completely unresponsive."

▸ "I am a mother of three boys—six years, four years, and almost seven months. But the problem with my family is, we no longer have our seven month old baby. We lost our dear baby when he was almost two months old. He passed away after receiving just one shot of the hepatitis B vaccine! He was born healthy, ate well, went for his checkup like my other children. The doctor commented on how well he was doing, and how healthy he was. Then he asked me if I would like to give him the one shot now and the others in two weeks. IF I WOULD HAVE ONLY KNOWN! I thought I was doing the right thing for my child, and even better than having him get all at once. From the day he passed away I knew it was the shot. I could not see anything else wrong with him. My mind will never be at peace. If I had only known what vaccines can do, and have done, I may have reconsidered, so I thank you for putting out so much information on this. I didn't know at the time what may have happened, but I will do what I have to do to save another life."

▸ "My 5-year-old daughter slumped to the floor after receiving her second dose of the hepatitis B vaccine. That is when the nurse gave us a side-effects sheet and was telling me when to bring her back for another shot."

▸ "Our 6-year-old son became ill after his first dose of hepatitis B vaccine. He had a fever of 103 degrees for five days. After his second dose he had a fever that did not go away. Three months later he was diagnosed with rheumatic fever. One month later his blood counts dropped and he was rediagnosed with A.L.L. leukemia."

▸ "My 7-year-old had a hepatitis B and varicella shot. One month later I took her back to the doctor because she said her ears were ringing, and she was acting strange. The doctor assured me nothing was wrong and gave her a second hepatitis B shot. Two weeks later she began having seizures. She twitches, falls, and has a hard time breathing. She is now on 625mg of Depakote daily. Can you shed some light on this?"

▸ "My son was required to get the hepatitis B vaccine in order to stay in school. I decided to give it to both my children since my daughter would be required to have it. My son, seven, now wakes up with arthritis in his legs to a point where he can't walk. My daughter, nine, has times when she can't even move her neck, and she has debilitating dizzy spells. The doctors tell me that the neck pain is caused by a strep infection, which she no longer has, but still has the pain, and the dizzy spells are caused by hypotension, which she has never had problems with before. Are there any doctors that you know of who are not bought by big government and will tell me how to effectively treat my children? Also, is there somewhere I can go to get involved in the eradication of this vaccine and help save other children and parents from the pain that our family has gone through?"

▸ "I'm writing to ask what might have happened to my 11-year-old daughter when she received her second hepatitis B shot. After the nurse injected the shot into her arm she got up and almost tripped into the next examination room across the hall and fell flat to the ground. I went to pick her up not knowing what had happened, and when I lifted her up she was lifeless, and then her body started to shake. It was very frightening."

▸ "My son received the hepatitis B vaccine. Within days he displayed cold and flu-like symptoms. It quickly escalated into a high fever with itchy, red hives all over his body, with severe joint pain and swelling. He was hospitalized within 10 days of the shot. He is now diagnosed with juvenile rheumatoid arthritis and is on several medications. Prior to the shot he was a very healthy, active boy who played sports."

▸ "My 14-year-old daughter contracted mononucleosis and suffered an abnormal amount of illness since her first hepatitis B shot. Prior to the shot, she competed in the National Junior Olympics and has always been an 'A' student. This has changed. She currently is suffering from chronic fatigue, dizziness, memory loss and sore joints. We have put her through a series of medical tests. She has evidence of an autoimmune disease. They want to treat her with immuno-suppressive drugs or intravenous gamma globulin. This is her life. This just breaks my heart. I write this with tears in my eyes. Please help."

▸ "I am from Russia, where they do not have the hepatitis B vaccine. When I came to America, I was required to have the vaccine in order to attend school or summer camps. I received it at the age of 14 and I developed optic neuritis by my 15th birthday. I had become blind. Not only was this a complete shock, but it was very painful, since my optic nerve had swollen so much. To make matters worse, I was diagnosed with multiple sclerosis."

▸ "I am concerned about my 18-year-old sister who has been getting grand mal seizures for three years now, ever since she was vaccinated against hepatitis B. She got her first seizure the day of the shot and is now taking medication. She has recently been complaining of even more annoying symptoms, such as constantly seeing flashing lights and dark spots, which make it difficult for her to read and concentrate on things. The doctor said that the seizures could be atrophying her occipital lobe, and that seizure activity could even be spreading to the temporal lobe, which could start to affect her intelligence."

▸ "My daughter, at 23, got a hepatitis B shot and has been sick ever since. She seems to have chronic fatigue syndrome."

▸ "I am a 33-year-old white female. I became very ill about three weeks after receiving the 2nd dose of the hepatitis B vaccine, which was required by my university. I have been experiencing joint pain, vasculitis, and fever for the past two months. My doctors brush off the possibility that my problems are a reaction to the vaccine. When I contacted the county health department and CDC, they denied the vaccine causing these kind of problems."

▸ "I was given the hepatitis B vaccine by my employers. They said it was safe and could not cause side effects. This was obviously untrue because I had a reaction. After ten years of constant ill health I was diagnosed with chronic fatigue syndrome."

▸ "I was given a vaccine against hepatitis B by my employers. The day after vaccination I was very ill—pains in all parts of my body. This illness never fully went away. I have been attending doctors ever since, with constant infection, severe headaches, fatigue, insomnia, loss of libido. There is no doubt that these symptoms began with the vaccination.

I have been hospitalized on three different occasions for tests. Doctors do not want to look at the possibility that the vaccine was related to my illness. My quality of life is destroyed and there does not seem to be any way of getting better."

▸ "Ever since I received the hepatitis B vaccine I have had weakness and heaviness in my legs, among other symptoms. I've seen several doctors and had many tests to determine what is wrong with me. I am in the category of multiple sclerosis-like symptoms, but no doctor has been able to rule-out or rule-in any specific diagnosis."

▸ "I was forced to receive the hepatitis B vaccine because my job placed me at 'high' risk. At first I experienced weird symptoms, then developed multiple sclerosis."

▸ "My son was healthy until he got a hepatitis B vaccine while in the service. Shortly after that he came down with the 'flu' and then he was diagnosed with multiple sclerosis."

▸ "My husband had to get the hepatitis B vaccine for work. He became ill after the first shot but was never told of any adverse reactions, so he continued. After all three shots he became so weak he couldn't work or even function in a normal capacity."

▸ "I was a registered nurse until I had an autoimmune reaction to hepatitis B vaccine. I am now disabled."

▸ "I talked to a doctor who is a professor of molecular biology at Baylor College of Medicine. Her brother, who is also a PhD, had an adverse reaction to the hepatitis B vaccine and is now bedridden. I am a registered nurse who had a reaction to the same vaccine. My life has been totally altered by this. Mine was an autoimmune reaction. I was 44 years old when it happened. I know several other nurses across the country and a doctor in Hawaii that have lupus or multiple sclerosis after taking the same type of recombinant vaccine."

▸ "My 62-year-old mother was told that she was exposed to hepatitis and needed the vaccine. Within two months she began having major problems with joint pain and arthritis. She has seen many doctors who tell her this is part of growing old. However, after seeing a special on '20/20' I began to piece together the truth."

▸ "Shortly after receiving hepatitis B shots, I was diagnosed with a rare autoimmune disease called ocular myasthenia gravis. My neurologist is aware that immunizations trigger these diseases, yet the public is kept in the dark. I'll never have another vaccine."

▸ "Ten years ago I did not believe the medical and governmental communities could be so wrong about vaccinations. I am convinced they are wrong and are too arrogant to look at all the facts. I feel justified in my understanding and beliefs because I was once a medical doctor. My children and I enjoyed excellent health until we received our hepatitis B vaccine series. Within a short period, my daughter developed type 1 diabetes, and my son and I developed Behcet's disease. My Behcet's has since attacked my central nervous system and I am in poor shape. [Behcet's disease causes canker sores in the mouth, on the genitals, arthritis, and inflammation of the eyes, digestive tract, brain and spinal cord.] I am disabled due to the brain injury and have been forced to retire. Isn't it all very curious—all three of us developing autoimmune diseases after receiving hepatitis B vaccinations."

Hepatitis B Vaccine Reaction Reports
Outnumber Reported Disease Cases in Children

The National Vaccine Information Center (NVIC) released figures which show that the number of hepatitis B vaccine-associated serious adverse event and death reports in American children under the age of 14 outnumber the reported cases of hepatitis B disease in that age group. Analysis of raw computer data in the government-operated Vaccine Adverse Event Reporting System (VAERS) confirms that in 1996 there were 872 serious adverse events reported to VAERS in children under 14 years of age who had been injected with hepatitis B vaccine. The children were either taken to a hospital emergency room, had life threatening health problems, were hospitalized or were left disabled following vaccination. Forty-eight children died after they were injected with hepatitis B vaccine in 1996. By contrast, during that same year only 279 cases of hepatitis B disease were reported in children under age 14 (Figure 61).[146] From 1992 through 2005, there were 36,788 hepatitis B vaccine-related adverse events reported to VAERS in all age groups, including 14,800 serious adverse events and 781 deaths (Figure 62).[147]

Figure 61:
Hepatitis B Vaccine Adverse Reactions
Versus Cases of the Disease
(in Children Under 14 Years of Age)

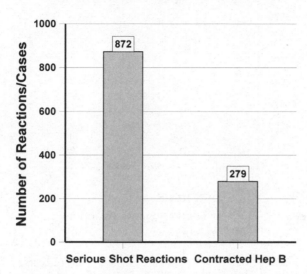

In 1996, there were 872 *U.S. government-documented* serious adverse reactions to the hepatitis B vaccine in children under 14 years of age. They were either hospitalized, had life-threatening health problems, or were left disabled following vaccination; 48 of these children died. By contrast, in 1996 only 279 cases of hepatitis B disease were reported in children under age 14. Source: VAERS; NVIC Press Release (January 27, 1999).

The U.S. had one of the lowest rates of hepatitis B in the world even before a vaccine was in use. In 1990, a year before the CDC ordered all children to get the shot, there were 21,102 cases of hepatitis B reported in the U.S. (population 248 million). In 1996, 10,637 cases were reported. According to CDC, "Hepatitis B continues to decline in most states, primarily because of a decrease in the number of cases among injecting drug users and, to a lesser extent, among both homosexuals and heterosexuals of both sexes."[148]

"As more states mandate hepatitis B vaccination, NVIC is getting more reports of children dying or suffering rashes, fevers, seizures, arthritis, diabetes, chronic fatigue and other autoimmune and brain dysfunction following their hepatitis B shots," said NVIC co-founder and president Barbara Loe Fisher. "Newborn babies are dying shortly after their shots and their deaths are being written off as sudden infant death syndrome. Parents should have the right to give their informed consent to vaccination, and Congress should give emergency priority funding to independent scientists who can take an unbiased look at this vaccine, instead of leaving the search for truth in the hands of government officials who have already decided to force every child to the vaccine," she said.[149]

Drug companies marketing the genetically engineered recombinant DNA hepatitis B vaccine in the U.S. used studies to demonstrate safety which only monitored children for 4 or 5 days after vaccination. Professor Bonnie Dunbar, Ph.D., a Texas cell biologist and pioneering vaccine researcher, said "It takes weeks and sometimes months for autoimmune disorders, such as rheumatoid arthritis, to develop following vaccination. No basic science research or controlled, long term studies into the side effects of this vaccine have been conducted in American babies, children or adults."[150]

Figure 62:
Hepatitis B Vaccine Adverse Reactions
(All Ages)

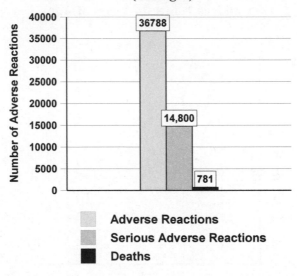

Adverse Reactions

Serious Adverse Reactions

Deaths

From 1992 through 2005, there were 36,788 *officially reported* adverse reactions to the hepatitis B vaccine in all age groups. 14,800 of these were "serious," leading to hospitalization, life-threatening health problems, or disabilities; 781 people died. Source: VAERS.

France Ends Hepatitis B Vaccination Program for Children:
In July, 1998, 15,000 French citizens belonging to 15 associations filed a lawsuit against the French government for misleading the public about the risks and benefits associated with the hepatitis B vaccine. Hundreds—perhaps thousands—of innocent French citizens have suffered from autoimmune and neurological disorders, including multiple sclerosis, following hepatitis B vaccination.[151] As a result, in October 1998, France became the first country to halt hepatitis B vaccine requirements for entry into school.[152]

★ Congressional Hearing: May 18, 1999 ★
Hepatitis B Vaccine: Helping or Hurting Public Health
Chairman John L. Mica

Recent news reports have questioned the safety of hepatitis B vaccines and have suggested an association between the vaccine and multiple sclerosis and other autoimmune disorders. Our job here today is not to "prove" whether or not this vaccine "causes" illnesses or deaths. Instead, we have created a forum for asking questions about what scientific evidence does exist and whether further studies should be completed. Specifically, I would like this hearing to examine the following issues: First, what is being done to study the adverse reactions reported in the Vaccine Adverse Event Reporting System (VAERS)? Second, do the benefits of administering the vaccine to infants outweigh the risks? Third, what process does the CDC employ to make a recommendation for a vaccine? What role do pharmaceutical companies play in that process? Do conflicts of interest exist? Fourth, what disclosure is required before the vaccine is given? Is it adequate? [For example], when a parent takes their child in for a vaccine, they are supposed to be given an information sheet outlining the risks and benefits of the vaccine. While most states mandating vaccinations allow exemptions, the information sheet does not tell parents that these exemptions exist.[153]

Testimony of Michael Belkin
Father of a vaccine victim

My daughter Lyla Rose Belkin died on September 16, 1998 at the age of five weeks, about 15 hours after receiving her second hepatitis B vaccine booster shot. Lyla was a lively, alert 5-week-old baby when I last held her in my arms. Little did I imagine as she gazed intently into my eyes with all the innocence and wonder of a newborn child that she would die that night. She was never ill before receiving the hepatitis B shot that afternoon. At her final feeding that night, she was extremely agitated, noisy and feisty—and then she fell asleep suddenly and stopped breathing. The autopsy ruled out choking. The NY Medical Examiner ruled her death sudden infant death syndrome (SIDS).

But the NY Medical Examiner (Dr. Persechino) neglected to mention Lyla's swollen brain or the hepatitis B vaccine in the autopsy report. The coroner spoke to my wife and I and our pediatrician (Dr. Zullo) the day of the autopsy and clearly stated that her brain was swollen. The pediatrician, Dr. Zullo's notes of that conversation, are: *"brain swollen...not sure cause yet...could not see how recombinant vaccine could cause problem."*

SIDS is a diagnosis of exclusion—it wasn't this, it wasn't that, everything has been ruled out and we don't know what it was. *A swollen brain is not SIDS.* Through conversations with other experienced pathologists, I subsequently discovered that brain inflammation is a classic adverse reaction to vaccination (with any vaccine) in the medical literature. I set out to do an investigation of the hepatitis B vaccine.... These are my conclusions, supported by the following pages of text and analysis that are too lengthy to present in entirety in the time allotted for this appearance. Please read the results of my investigation, as it will help you understand the magnitude of the hepatitis B vaccine issue:

- Newborn babies are not at risk of contracting hepatitis B disease unless their mother is infected.
- Hepatitis B is primarily a disease of junkies, gays, and promiscuous heterosexuals.
- The vaccine is given to babies because health authorities couldn't get those risk groups to take the vaccine.
- Adverse reactions outnumber cases of the disease in government statistics.
- Nothing is being done to investigate those adverse reactions.
- Those adverse reactions include numerous deaths, convulsions and arthritic conditions that occur within days after hepatitis B vaccination.
- The CDC is misrepresenting hypothetical, estimated disease statistics as real cases of the disease.
- The Advisory Committee on Immunization Practices (ACIP) is recommending new vaccines for premature infants without having scientific studies proving it is safe.
- The U.S. vaccine recommendation process is hopelessly compromised by conflicts of interest with vaccine manufacturers, the American Academy of Pediatrics, and the CDC.

Question: Why did the ACIP establish a policy mandating that newborn babies not at risk of the disease be automatically administered the 3-shot hepatitis B vaccine as their first involuntary indoctrination into the pediatric care of America?

Answer: In the CDC and ACIP's own words, almost every newborn U.S. baby is now greeted on its entry into the world by a vaccine injection against a sexually transmitted disease for which the baby is not at risk—because they couldn't get the junkies, prostitutes, homosexuals and promiscuous heterosexuals to take the shot. *That is the essence of the hepatitis B universal vaccination program.*

Question: Why not just screen the mother to see if she is infected with hep B (since that's about the only way for a baby to get the disease), instead of vaccinating all infants?

Answer: Selling vaccines is extremely profitable and the process of mandating vaccines is fraught with conflicts of interest between vaccine manufacturers, the ACIP and the American Academy of Pediatrics. The business model of having the government mandate that everyone must buy your product is a monopolist's delight.

Question: What studies are being done on the data from the FDA's Vaccine Adverse Event Reporting System (VAERS).

Answer: Absolutely nothing. The 25,000 reports are going into a drawer and being forgotten. [See the **United States Vaccination Policy Flowchart** on the following page.]

Question: Why do the CDC, ACIP and Merck say that there are 140,000-320,000 new infections/yr (70,000-160,000 symptomatic infections/yr) when their own CDC data shows only 10,000 reported cases per year?

Answer: They are passing off estimated, hypothetical numbers as actual cases. **This is statistical fraud.** In the financial world such misrepresentation would lead to criminal charges. If a company inflated its earnings or revenues by 300% (as the CDC does with hepatitis B disease statistics) and foisted those figures off as official data (and not some back-of-the-envelope guesstimate)—that company would be investigated by the SEC and sued by shareholders. Go try to audit those 320,000 supposed new infections/year. You will not find them. The whole exercise is designed to increase public hysteria about the risk of a low-risk disease so the CDC can extend it's pervasive influence and Merck can increase it's $900 million/year vaccine revenues.

Question: What process does the Center for Disease Control employ to make a vaccine recommendation?

Answer: I attended the February ACIP meeting in Atlanta and was absolutely appalled. Every vote by the Committee on new vaccine mandates was unanimous (except for one dissenting vote on rotavirus vaccine for premature infants). There was hardly any discussion of adverse reactions; the ACIP simply rubber-stamped every proposal on the agenda. I call it "Vaccination Without Representation." In one instance, the ACIP passed a recommendation for rotavirus vaccine for premature infants *even though no scientific studies had been done showing it was medically safe.*

What Should Be Done? This Committee should investigate the 1991 ACIP recommendation establishing universal hepatitis B vaccination of newborn babies, and if (as with the rotavirus vaccine example) no studies were done to prove this was safe in a broad sample of racially and genetically diverse babies less than 48 hours old before they established that recommendation, then the CDC has been experimenting on babies like guinea pigs and this Committee should suspend that universal immunization policy. In addition, VAERS data strongly suggests *combining multiple vaccines may be convenient and profitable for pediatricians—but fatal or debilitating for infants.* This is another matter for independent scientists to audit.[154]

Testimony of J. Barthelow Classen, MD
Physician and vaccine researcher

Thank you for the opportunity to discuss my findings on the association between hepatitis B vaccine and insulin-dependent diabetes.... We found that the incidence of diabetes rose 60 percent in New Zealand following a massive hepatitis B immunization program. The CDC initiated a study to verify our findings. Their preliminary data has been published and shows hepatitis B immunization, when given starting after 8 weeks of age, is associated with a 90 percent increase in the risk of diabetes, supporting our findings.... Our data on diabetes shows that vaccine-induced diabetes may occur three or more years following immunization. If we immunized every child after 8 weeks of life with the hepatitis B vaccine there may be an extra 4,000 to 5,000 cases of diabetes per year. We estimate there are 10,000 cases of vaccine-induced diabetes in the U.S. each year. On average, each case may cost $1 million in lost productivity and medical expenses. The estimated liability cost of the vaccine-induced diabetes is over $10 billion per year. The current cumulative liabilities to the U.S. government and to manufacturers could exceed $250 billion....[155]

"We estimate there are 10,000 cases of vaccine-induced diabetes in the U.S. each year. On average, each case may cost $1 million in lost productivity and medical expenses." —J. Barthelow Classen, MD

United States Vaccination Policy Flowchart*

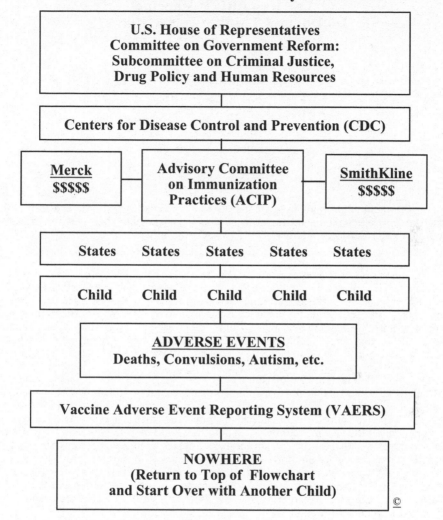

U.S. House of Representatives
Committee on Government Reform:
Subcommittee on Criminal Justice,
Drug Policy and Human Resources

Centers for Disease Control and Prevention (CDC)

Merck
$$$$$

Advisory Committee
on Immunization
Practices (ACIP)

SmithKline
$$$$$

States   States   States   States   States

Child   Child   Child   Child   Child

ADVERSE EVENTS
Deaths, Convulsions, Autism, etc.

Vaccine Adverse Event Reporting System (VAERS)

NOWHERE
(Return to Top of Flowchart
and Start Over with Another Child)

©

*Flowchart developed by Michael Belkin, father of a vaccine victim.

The hepatitis B vaccine and AIDS:

In 1978, the New York Blood Center in Manhattan, New York injected 1083 gay men with an experimental hepatitis B vaccine that was developed in chimpanzees and produced by Merck. Shortly thereafter, homosexual men in San Francisco, Los Angeles, Denver, Chicago and St. Louis also received three shots of this experimental vaccine over a period of three months. In 1980, 20 percent of the gay men who volunteered for the hepatitis B vaccine experiment in Manhattan were found to be HIV-positive—the highest incidence of HIV anywhere in the world, including Africa. In 1981, the AIDS epidemic became official. Although there is no proof that the infamous hepatitis B vaccine experiments on gay men caused AIDS, there is no question that AIDS erupted in the U.S. shortly thereafter.[156]

The Hepatitis B Vaccine:
Do Doctors Think it is Necessary?

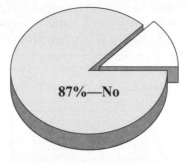

87%—No

Surveys in medical journals indicate that up to 87 percent of pediatricians and family practitioners do not believe the hepatitis B vaccine is needed by their newborn patients. Source: *Pediatrics* 1993; 91:699-702. *Journal of Family Practice* 1993; 36:153-57.

How effective is the current hepatitis B vaccine?

Hepatitis B vaccine efficacy is defined by injecting subjects with the shot then measuring the number of anti-hepatitis B antibodies that are produced in the blood. These antibodies must meet or exceed a predetermined level established by researchers, a basis presumed to provide protective benefits. Scientists call this "seroprotection." According to this definition, the vaccine is considered "highly immunogenic" when antibody levels are measured shortly after the last dose of the 3-dose vaccine regimen is administered.[157] However, according to the vaccine manufacturer, "the duration of the protective effect in healthy vaccinees is unknown."[158] In fact, follow-up studies just 5 to 9 years later show that approximately half of all vaccinated people fail to maintain protective antibody levels.[159,160] For example, a study published in the *New England Journal of Medicine* showed that after five years antibody levels (presumed to correlate with immunity) declined sharply or no longer existed in 42 percent of the vaccine recipients. In addition, 34 of the 773 subjects (4.4 percent!) became infected with the virus.[161,162] In another study, fewer than 40 percent of the vaccine recipients had protective antibody levels after 5 years.[163] A similar study showed that 48 percent of the vaccine recipients had inadequate antibody levels after just four years.[164] In fact, according to the World Health Organization, up to "60 percent of adults will lose all detectable antibody to hepatitis B vaccine within 6 to 10 years."[165] The medical literature is replete with corroborating data documenting vaccine failures.[166,167]

Is the hepatitis B vaccine mandatory?

In 1991, the CDC recommended that all infants receive the hepatitis B vaccine. Today, states mandate this shot. Yet, surveys in medical journals indicate that up to 87 percent of pediatricians and family practitioners do not believe this vaccine is needed by their newborn patients (Figure 63).[168,169] However, "because a vaccination strategy limited to high-risk individuals has failed," and since children are "accessible," they are now compelled to receive the three-shot series beginning at birth.[170] In other words, because high-risk groups are difficult to reach or have rejected this vaccine, authorities are targeting babies —even though babies are not likely to contract this disease. They are being subjected to all of the risks of this vaccine without the expected benefit. Due to waning efficacy or partial immunity, older children are compelled to receive booster doses as well. In addition, some companies are demanding hepatitis B shots for adults as a condition of employment. Grown-ups must carefully weigh the risks and benefits. Parents should know that each state permits them to legally exempt their children from "mandatory" shots.

Meningitis

- Haemophilus Influenzae type B (Hib disease)
- Streptococcus pneumoniae (Pneumococcal disease)
- Neisseria meningitidis (Meningococcal disease)

What is meningitis?

Meningitis is an infection of the fluid surrounding a person's spinal cord and brain. Common symptoms include a high fever, headache, and a stiff neck. Nausea, vomiting, and sleepiness are also possible. In infants, usual symptoms may be difficult to notice. The baby may simply appear inactive, irritable, or refuse to eat. As the disease progresses, seizures sometimes occur.[1]

What causes meningitis?

Meningitis can be caused by a virus or bacterium. Viral meningitis (also called aseptic meningitis) is fairly common, usually less severe, and dissipates without treatment.[2] In fact, no specific treatment is available for viral meningitis. Antibiotics do not work against viruses.[3] In contrast, bacterial meningitis can be serious, and may cause hearing loss, learning disabilities, and other neurological damage, including death in a small percentage of cases when treatment is delayed.[4,5] The disease is diagnosed by performing a spinal tap—by inserting a needle into the lower back to obtain fluid from the spinal canal. Once proper identification of the responsible pathogen has been determined, antibiotics can be administered.[6]

Bacterial meningitis:

Bacterial meningitis is caused by at least three different classifications of bacteria: 1) *Haemophilus influenzae;* 2) *Streptococcus pneumoniae;* and 3) *Neisseria meningitidis* (Figure 64).[7] Each class of bacteria contains several different strains (sometimes called serogroups or serotypes) that can cause meningitis. For example, at least three meningitis-causing strains of haemophilus influenzae have been identified: strains B, E, and F.[8] Haemophilus influenzae type B (Hib) is the most well-known strain. Approximately 90 strains of streptococcus pneumoniae (pneumococcal disease) have been identified.[9] Scientists know of at least 13 strains of neisseria meningitidis (meningococcal disease), such as B, C, and Y.[10]

Bacterial pathogens are contagious, spread through coughing and kissing. However, they are not easily spread via casual contact or by simply breathing the air where an infected person has been. None of the bacteria that cause meningitis are as contagious as ailments like the common cold or flu.[11]

Are vaccines available for bacterial meningitis?

Several vaccines have been developed to combat bacterial meningitis. However, each vaccine is only designed to protect against one or more strains of just one class of bacteria. For example, the haemophilus influenzae vaccine (type B, the Hib shot) will not protect against meningitis caused by haemophilus influenzae type E or type F. Nor will it protect against meningitis caused by the many different strains of streptococcus pneumoniae or neisseria meningitidis. The streptococcus pneumoniae and neisseria meningitidis vaccines were developed with the same inherent limitations. They are only designed to protect against a few of the many different meningitis-causing strains that have been identified.[12-14] For more specific information about vaccines that were developed to combat bacterial meningitis, read the chapters on haemophilus influenzae type B (Hib), pneumococcal disease, and meningococcal disease.

Figure 64:

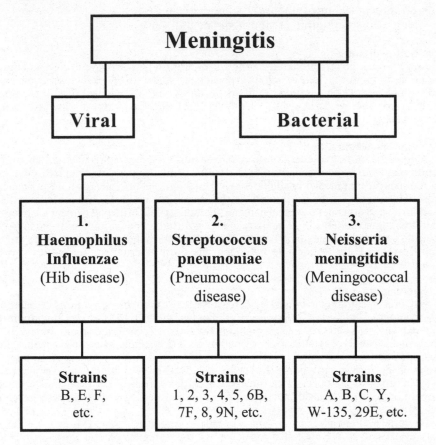

Meningitis can be caused by a virus or bacterium. Viral meningitis is usually less severe. Bacterial meningitis can be serious. Each class of bacteria contains multiple strains.

Haemophilus Influenzae
Type B (Hib)

What is Haemophilus influenzae type b?

Haemophilus influenzae type b, or Hib (no relation to the flu), is a serious bacterial infection. Meningitis (inflammation of the membranes surrounding the brain and spinal cord) occurs in about half of the cases.[1] Around 25 percent of all Hib infections cause hearing loss, neurological problems, or pneumonia.[2-4] Nearly 15 percent of cases result in epiglottitis (inflammation of the throat).[5] The case-fatality rate is about four percent.[6,7]

Hib is spread through sneezing, coughing, and secretions from an infected person. Treatment mainly consists of intravenously administered antibiotics. Oxygen therapy and other medical interventions may also be required.

How prevalent is Hib?

During the 1970s and 1980s, there were an estimated 16,000 to 20,000 Hib infections per year in the United States.[8,9] (Official statistics were not kept, so these figures may have been inflated when the vaccine was developed.) Rates tumbled starting in the 1990s, with just 329 cases of Hib in American children under five years of age in 1994, 259 cases in 1995, and an average of 272 cases per year from 1996 through 2000.[10-13] However, Hib infections occurred at a much lower rate during the 1940s and 1950s than during the 1970s and 1980s. In fact, *Hib rates jumped by 400 percent between 1946 and 1986.*[14-16]

What caused Hib rates to dramatically increase?

Several factors indicate that mass immunization campaigns with pertussis and other non-Hib vaccines may have been responsible for the unprecedented epidemics of invasive bacterial infections, such as Hib, during the 1970s and 1980s. Let's look at some of these possible factors:

1) Introduction of the pertussis vaccine. The pertussis vaccine became available in 1936 and was put into general use during the 1940s—a period coinciding with the start of Hib's dramatic rise. Mass immunization campaigns and mandatory state vaccine laws for entry into school were established in the 1960s.

2) The peak age of invasive Hib disease. Hib-induced meningitis peaks in children 6-7 months of age.[17] The DPT vaccine is administered at 2, 4, and 6 months. A probable link between the DPT vaccine and invasive bacterial infections is further strengthened by data showing that the number of cases in babies less than three months old has remained stable since 1942.[18]

3) "Provocative" disease. Several studies confirm that vaccinations can "provoke" or cause new diseases. For example, the *Journal of Infectious Diseases* published a study confirming "disease accentuation after immunization."[19] More recently, the CDC conducted a study of polio victims and discovered that "a significantly higher proportion of cases [when compared to matched control children] received a DPT injection within 30 days before paralysis onset." Authors of the study concluded that DPT injections are an important cause of provocative disease.[20]

4) The Swedish experiment. In 1979, Sweden stopped vaccinating with pertussis due to an unacceptably high incidence of adverse reactions and insufficient protective benefits.[21] In 1986, Sweden decided to revisit the DPT controversy because a new and supposedly safer "acellular" pertussis vaccine became available. Sweden tested this new vaccine (two separate versions) on 2,840 children, and quickly ended further testing when it was discovered that the vaccine was a) insufficiently effective at preventing whooping cough, and b) responsible for causing several deaths *and a statistically significant number of invasive bacterial infections.*[22,23]

5) Japanese data. In 1975, Japan stopped vaccinating infants with pertussis. Instead, the vaccination age was raised to two years. In 1981, Japan switched to the acellular pertussis vaccine and continued its policy of not vaccinating children under two years of age.[24]

A few years later, researchers studied meningitis mortality rates in Japan between the years of 1971 and 1985.[25] According to research scientist Dr. Viera Scheibner, who analyzed the data, there was "a clear decline in the incidence of meningitis [in children up to two years of age] after 1975, while meningitis cases skyrocketed in two and three year olds, clearly reflecting the consequences of the shift in vaccination age to two years."[26] In other words, the national mortality rate for Hib-induced meningitis declined in babies that were not vaccinated with DPT, and increased in DPT-vaccinated toddlers (Figure 65).

Who is most susceptible to Hib?

Sixty percent of all Hib cases occur in children less than 12 months of age, and 90 percent occur in children less than five years of age.[27] Native American Indians, Eskimo children, African-Americans, and children from lower socioeconomic families are all at increased risk of contracting Hib.[28-30] For example, in the U.S., African-American children are four times as likely to contract Hib as white children.[31] Some researchers attribute this to genetic predispositions.[32,33] Other researchers claim that "minority children are much more likely to live in crowded conditions that increase the likelihood of Hib transmission."[34] Several studies confirm that living in crowded conditions place children at greater risk.[35-38] Studies also show that children placed in day care,[39-42] parental smoking,[43,44] a history of ear infections, an already weakened immune system, and previous hospitalizations are high risk factors for contracting Hib as well.[45-49] However, breastfeeding was found to have a "protective effect" against Hib infections.[50-52]

Hib may not be as communicable as authorities originally believed. In fact, "the contagious potential of invasive Hib disease is considered to be limited." Two studies found that Hib does not spread easily. Out of 772 children who came into contact with an infected child, none of the 185 children in the first study, and only one of the 587 children in the second study, caught the disease.[53,54]

Thirty percent of all healthy people are carriers of the microorganism responsible for "causing" Hib, yet they never show symptoms of the disease.[55] Apparently, some people are naturally immune without having been vaccinated. Perhaps other factors besides being exposed to the Hib germ (such as good nutrition and a healthy immune system) help determine whether illness will occur.

Does a Hib vaccine exist?

If, as the evidence suggests, Hib epidemics resulted from mass immunization campaigns with non-Hib vaccines, there is a great irony in seeing new vaccines developed to combat diseases created by old vaccines. Nevertheless, in 1985 the first of several Hib vaccines was licensed for use in the United States. This vaccine was ineffective in children under age two, so it was quickly recommended for all children two years old or older—even though 75 percent of all Hib cases occur *before* the age of two years.[56-59]

From 1987 to 1990 several new "conjugated" Hib vaccines were licensed for use in the U.S. By 1991, Hib vaccines were recommended for use in infants as young as 2 months.[60,61] Today, three conjugate Hib vaccines are licensed for use in infants as young as six weeks: HibTITER®, produced by Wyeth; ActHIB®, by Sanofi Pasteur; and PedvaxHIB®, manufactured by Merck. In addition, two combination vaccines containing Hib are also available: TriHIBit®, combined with DTaP; and Comvax®, combined with hepatitis B.[62-65]

How is the Hib vaccine made?

According to Merck, "haemophilus influenzae type b and Neisseria meningitidis serogroup B are grown in complex fermentation media."[66] The final product is formulated to contain 225mcg of aluminum.[67] (For more information on aluminum, see *Appendix II*.) Other Hib vaccines are coupled with diphtheria or 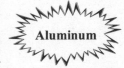 tetanus toxoids. Depending on which Hib vaccine (or combination shot) is under consideration, common ingredients may include: sodium chloride, ammonium sulfate, formalin (a solution of formaldehyde and methanol), sucrose, pertussis antigens, and "a trace amount of thimerosal"—a mercury derivative.[68,69]

Figure 65:

Hib-Meningitis Mortality Rates *Declined* when DPT Vaccinations were Stopped

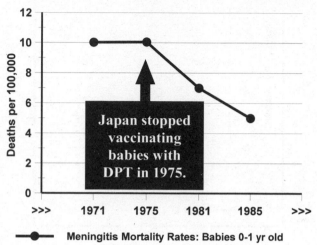

— ● — Meningitis Mortality Rates: Babies 0-1 yr old

In 1975, Japan stopped vaccinating babies with DPT. During the next several years, Hib-meningitis mortality rates dramatically declined. Source: Mortality statistics, Japanese Ministry of Health.

How safe is the Hib vaccine?

Hib vaccines are often administered simultaneously with other vaccines. Thus, when a child experiences an adverse reaction to the shot, it is often difficult to ascertain which component of the vaccine (or of the several simultaneously administered vaccines) is responsible. Nevertheless, the medical literature contains copious documentation confirming possible correlations between the Hib vaccine and serious ailments, including: Guillain-Barré syndrome, early onset Hib disease, transverse myelitis (paralysis of the spinal cord), aseptic meningitis, invasive pneumococcal disease, upper respiratory infection, otitis media (ear infection), thrombocytopenia (a decrease in blood platelets leading to internal bleeding), erythema multiforme (allergic skin disease), fever, rash, hives, vomiting, diarrhea, high-pitched crying, seizures, convulsions, and sudden infant death syndrome.[70-79]

The Hib Vaccine and Type 1 Diabetes

Important research indicates that the Hib vaccine may also be causally linked to rising epidemics of type 1 diabetes. Sharp increases of insulin-dependent diabetes mellitus have been recorded in the United States, England, and other European countries following mass immunization campaigns with the Hib vaccine.[80,81] In a landmark study published in both the *British Medical Journal* and *Autoimmunity,* more than 200,000 Finnish children were split into three groups.[82,83] The first group received NO doses of the Hib vaccine. The second group received one dose of the Hib vaccine (at 24 months of age). The third group received four doses of the Hib vaccine (at 3, 4, 6, and 18 months of age). At ages 7 and 10, the total number of cases of type 1 diabetes in all three groups was tallied.

Results: At age 7, there were 54 more cases per 100,000 children in the group that received four doses of the Hib vaccine when compared to the group that received no doses—a 26 percent increase![84,85] At age 10, there were 58 more cases per 100,000 children in the

Figure 66:

The Hib Vaccine and Rising Diabetes Rates

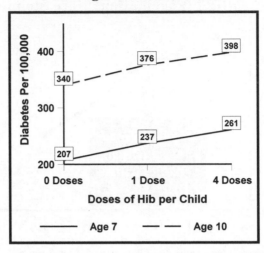

More than 200,000 Hib-vaccinated and non-vaccinated children were compared. One group received no doses; another group received 1 dose; the third group received 4 doses of the Hib vaccine. At ages 7 and 10, the number of cases of type 1 diabetes in all three groups was tallied. At age 7, there were 54 more cases per 100,000 children in the group that received 4 doses of the Hib vaccine vs. the group that received no doses—a 26% increase. At age 10, there were 58 more cases per 100,000 children in the group that received 4 doses vs. the group that received no doses. According to experts, "the potential risk of the vaccine exceeds the potential benefit." Source: *BMJ* (Oct. 23, 1999); *Autoimmunity* 2002;35(4):247-53.

---

group that received four doses of the Hib vaccine when compared to the group that received no doses.[86] Based on an annual birth rate of about 4 million children, in the United States alone this translates into 2,300 additional (and avoidable) cases of diabetes every year.[87] (Each case of insulin-dependent diabetes is estimated to cost more than $1 million in medical costs and lost productivity.)[88] By contrast, the Hib vaccine is expected to prevent a much smaller number of severe disabilities.[89] These figures depict significant differences. According to some experts who analyzed the data, a causal relationship between the Hib vaccine and type 1 diabetes is supported (Figure 66).[90] Furthermore, "the increased risk of diabetes in the vaccinated group exceeds the expected decreased risk of complications of Hib meningitis."[91] Thus, these experts issued a warning to the public that, in their estimation, "the potential risk of the vaccine exceeds the potential benefit."[92]

Adverse Reaction Reports

This section contains unsolicited adverse reaction reports associated with the Hib vaccine.[93,94]

▸ "I am writing for help. My daughter was born a healthy baby girl and was progressing great. Then I got a reminder in the mail that said it was time for her shots. I made an appointment, got her shots, and one week later my daughter was dead. The autopsy report came back as 'Haemophilus influenzae.' She was not ill in any way, but now my baby is dead. They keep saying it can't happen, but what more proof do they need? I have a dead baby who died of the disease that she was supposed to be immune to."

▸ "I have a son who was diagnosed with diabetes six months after his first Hib shot. Two of his friends were also diagnosed six months after their first Hib shot. There is no history of diabetes in any of these families."

▸ "My daughter received a Hib vaccine a few months before she was diagnosed with type 1 diabetes."

▸ "My child has attention deficit hyperactivity disorder (ADHD) and we think it may be connected to his Hib vaccine."

▸ "My daughter received the Hib shot and within eight hours became sick. She was unwell for three days."

▸ "My daughter's sleeping problems started at 3 months old when she received her Hib vaccine. From 8pm to 5am I could not make her sleep for four weeks."

▸ "I had my 3½ month-old baby vaccinated with Hib, DPT and polio. She went from being a content baby that woke on average twice a night to waking every hour to 90 minutes. We are now three months down the line and she still wakes in pain (throwing her head back with her back arching) every two hours."

▸ "Six days after my 7-month-old baby received his 3rd Hib and hepatitis B vaccine, he started throwing up baby foods. I don't mean spitting up; I mean forcefully throwing up that lasted for 4-5 hours until his stomach was empty. We got pushed off by the pediatrician for the past two months, but finally I convinced him that something is indeed wrong as my baby isn't growing properly. We are now seeing specialists. The pediatric allergist only showed an egg allergy. Now we're seeing another specialist. My parents feel the vaccines are to blame. Have you ever heard of vaccines causing problems like this?"

▸ "A child I once cared for recently died at 15 months of age from a reaction to the Hib vaccine. It seemed like SIDS because he died in his sleep."

▸ "Our 10-year-old daughter was diagnosed with diabetes [a few months after she received her Hib vaccine]."

How effective is the Hib vaccine?

Children are at risk of contracting Hib disease following their Hib vaccinations. For example, doctors have been warned by the CDC that cases of Hib may occur after vaccination, "prior to the onset of the protective effects of the vaccine."[95] This same warning is published by all three of the Hib vaccine manufacturers in their product inserts.[96] Other research warns of "increased susceptibility" to the disease during the first seven days after vaccination.[97] The American Academy of Pediatrics has warned doctors to warn parents to look for signs of the disease in their children following vaccination.[98] In fact, several studies found that Hib-vaccinated children are 2 to 6 times more likely than non-Hib-vaccinated children to contract Hib disease during the first week following vaccination.[99-103] Additional research has confirmed that antibody levels *decline* rather than increase immediately following Hib vaccinations[104,105] —even with the newer conjugated Hib vaccines[106] —placing the child at *greater* risk for invasive disease.

From 1998 to 2000, 32 percent of all children aged 6 months to 5 years with confirmed Hib disease had received three or more doses of Hib vaccine, including many who had received a booster dose 14 or more days before onset of their illness.[107] In one study of children who contracted Hib at least three weeks after their shot, more than 70 percent developed meningitis.[108]

Although the evidence suggests that minority children are at greater risk of contracting Hib,[109] at least one study found the conjugated Hib vaccine to be ineffective at preventing Hib disease among a group of minority children.[110]

Efficacy of the Hib vaccine in combination with other vaccines:

Vaccine manufacturers often combine vaccines—a practice that pediatricians favor—even when studies indicate that overall efficacy may be suppressed. For example, the Hib vaccine is often given along with the DTaP shot. However, scientists recently discovered that "when Hib conjugates were combined with DPT vaccines containing acellular pertussis, Hib antibody response was lowered." In fact, antibody levels were "five to ten times lower" in groups receiving the combined vaccines compared with groups receiving vaccines separately.

Even so, because convenience is evidently more important than efficacy, vaccine authorities "encourage introduction of DTPa-Hib [diphtheria, tetanus, and acellular pertussis with Hib] combinations to facilitate the inclusion of Hib into the already crowded childhood immunization schedule."[111] In another study where children 12 to 15 months of age were given a booster dose of the Hib vaccine concurrently with DTaP and Prevnar, "some suppression of the Hib antibody response was observed."[112,113]

Did Haemophilus influenzae type B (Hib) vaccines cause increases in Haemophilus influenzae type E (Hie) and type F (Hif) bacterial infections?

There are several different types of haemophilus influenzae, including types a, b, c, d, e, and f. The "b" type is just one strain—the only one for which a vaccine was created. Prior to the introduction of the Hib vaccine, haemophilus influenzae type b was the most common cause of bacterial meningitis in the United States.[114] The other strains rarely caused invasive disease. However, new cases of meningitis caused by non-type b strains of haemophilus influenzae are on the rise. Scientists believe the Hib vaccine may be responsible. For example, in 1989, *prior* to the introduction of the new conjugated Hib vaccine, the rate of invasive haemophilus influenzae type f disease (Hif) was 0.5 cases per 1 million population. By 1994, a few years *after* the Hib vaccine was mandated, the rate nearly quadrupled to 1.9 cases per 1 million population.[115] Even more alarming is the case-fatality rate of this virulent strain: 21 percent among children and 30 percent among adults.[116]

Several studies confirm that Hib vaccines may actually be causing *increases* in the number and severity of invasive haemophilus influenzae infections.[117-119] For example, a study presented at the National Academy of Sciences noted that "vaccination against particular (targeted) serotypes may cause an increase in carriage of (and diseases attributed to) nontargeted serotypes."[120] Research published in a 2000 issue of *Epidemiology and Infection* noted that "After the introduction of Hib immunization in children, invasive Hib infections in unimmunized adults also declined, *but the overall rate of invasive haemophilus influenzae disease in adults increased."*[121] The study authors issued a warning: "Physicians and microbiologists should be aware of the changing epidemiology, the high associated mortality and high risk of underlying disease."[122]

In 2007, *Clinical Infectious Diseases* published new data confirming that the incidence of invasive haemophilus influenzae disease is *increasing* among adults. For example, between 1996 and 2004 (after the Hib vaccine was introduced) Illinois recorded a 169 percent escalation. Compared with 1996, cases of invasive haemophilus influenzae disease in 2004 were 2.9 times more likely among persons aged 18-64 years and 3.6 times more likely among persons 65 years and older. The vaccine appears to have decreased cases of haemophilus influenzae type b in children at the expense of "replacement" types of the disease in adults. Isolates taken from infected adults indicate that only 15 percent were type b while 85 percent were non-type b. Ironically, researchers do not consider this a failing of the Hib vaccine; instead, "it raises the question whether a [new] vaccine will need to be developed."[123,124]

Did Hib vaccines cause increases in non-Hib bacterial infections?

During the same period when bacterial infections associated with Hib disease *decreased* (beginning around 1991 when U.S. authorities mandated the new conjugated Hib vaccine), bacterial infections associated with pneumococcal and meningococcal disease dramatically *increased.* Before the 1990s, Haemophilus influenzae type b was the leading cause of bacterial meningitis among children less than five years of age.[125] Today, Streptococcus pneumoniae and Neisseria meningitidis are the leading causes of bacterial meningitis.[126] This is due to *real* increases in case numbers, not just because the Hib vaccine reduced Hib disease knocking it from the leader's platform. (This is the official explanation/fabrication promoted by the CDC.)[127] For example, the U.K. experienced a nearly 400 percent increase in annual meningococcal cases after the Hib vaccine was introduced.[128] Thus, the Hib vaccine may have artificially suppressed one type of bacterial infections (Hib-related), while simultaneously provoking into prominence two other types of bacterial infections: pneumococcus and meningococcus. Of course, new vaccines were quickly developed to combat the increased incidence of these diseases.

Pneumococcal Disease
Prevnar 13® (for children)

What is pneumococcal disease?
Pneumococcal disease, or *streptococcus pneumoniae,* is a serious bacterial illness that can cause meningitis, pneumonia, ear infections, sinusitis, and bacteremia (an infection of the blood). The pneumococcal pathogen consists of approximately 90 different strains, including serogroups 1, 2, 3, 4, 5, 6B, 7F, 8, 9N, 9V, 10A, 18C, 26, 54, 68, and so on.[1,2]

How prevalent is pneumococcal disease?
During the 1980s and 1990s, the annual incidence of pneumococcal disease in the United States was an estimated "10 to 30 cases per 100,000 persons."[3] In children under 5 years old, about 15 percent of cases are meningitis while the rest are usually blood infections.[4] According to the Centers for Disease Control and Prevention (CDC), this translated into about 700 cases of meningitis, 13,000 blood infections, and approximately 200 deaths annually.[5]

Bacterial infections associated with pneumococcal (and meningococcal) disease appear to have dramatically *increased* in the U.S. following mandated Hib vaccinations. Streptococcus pneumoniae has overtaken Hib as the leading cause of bacterial meningitis.[6] Other countries are experiencing similar increases in bacterial infections following mass vaccination campaigns with the Hib vaccine. In Finland, where pneumococcal disease has increased since 1993, a team of researchers speculated that "the increase in invasive pneumococcal infections is causally related to the disappearance of Hib disease."[7,8] Following an outbreak of bacterial infections in Iceland, researchers considered this "another possible example of upsurge in pneumococcal disease after Hib control."[9]

Who is most susceptible to pneumococcal disease?
Persons 65 years and older, children under two years of age, immuno-compromised adults, and the chronically ill are at greatest risk of contracting pneumococcal disease. Most healthy children are not at risk. In fact, according to the Red Book Report of the Committee on Infectious Diseases published by the American Academy of Pediatrics, "[Pneumococcal infections in children] are more likely to occur when predisposing conditions exist, including immunoglobulin deficiency, Hodgkin's disease, congenital or acquired immunodeficiency (including HIV), nephrotic syndrome, some viral upper respiratory tract infections, splenic dysfunction, splenectomy and organ transplantation."[10]

Does a pneumococcal vaccine exist?
Two "polysaccharide" pneumococcal vaccines, Pneumovax® by Merck and Pnu-Imune® by Wyeth, have been available since the 1970s. They are mainly recommended for seniors and high risk children over 2 years of age.[11,12] Many people refer to them as "pneumonia" vaccines for adults. They are not recommended for younger children. (For more information about these two vaccines, see the chapter on Pneumonia.)

In February 2010, the FDA approved a new diphtheria-conjugated pneumococcal vaccine—Prevnar 13®—for children under six years of age.[13] Prevnar 13, produced by Wyeth, is designed to protect against 13 of the approximately 90 different pneumococcal strains capable of causing bacterial disease (Figure 67).[14] This vaccine was developed to replace the original Prevnar—PCV7—introduced ten years earlier. Prevnar 13 is administered as a four dose series starting at two months of age.[15]

How safe is Prevnar 13?
The number and severity of adverse reactions to Prevnar 13 are similar to those reported after PCV7.[16] According to the American Academy of Pediatrics (AAP), "Available data suggest that [the pneumococcal vaccine] may prove to be among the most reactogenic vaccine of those currently used."[17] In fact, studies documenting the most commonly reported

Figure 67:

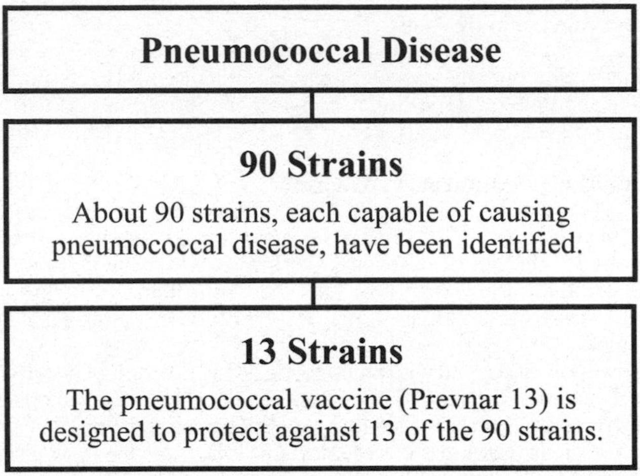

Pneumococcal Disease

90 Strains
About 90 strains, each capable of causing pneumococcal disease, have been identified.

13 Strains
The pneumococcal vaccine (Prevnar 13) is designed to protect against 13 of the 90 strains.

The conjugate pneumococcal vaccine (Prevnar 13) is designed to protect against 13 of the approximately 90 different pneumococcal strains capable of causing bacterial disease. Source: The vaccine manufacturer's package inserts.

adverse reactions confirm that many children who receive this vaccine experience diarrhea, irritability, a rash or hives, and tenderness at the injection site "interfering with limb movement."[18-20] Nearly 20 percent of babies refuse to eat, and about 13 percent will vomit, following their pneumococcal shots.[21]

Serious adverse events were reported in 8.2 percent of infants and toddlers who received Prevnar 13.[22] The package insert by the vaccine manufacturer lists several serious adverse reactions that occurred during trials of the vaccine. Although the manufacturer does not admit a causative relationship between the vaccine and many of these reactions, parents who are considering this vaccine may wish to weigh the implications. Such reactions included 162 visits to the emergency room and 24 hospitalizations within 3 days of a dose for various ailments, such as congestive heart failure, aplastic anemia, autoimmune disease, diabetes mellitus, neutropenia, thrombocytopenia, pneumonia, bronchiolitis, colitis, otitis media, asthma, wheezing, croup, seizures, hypotonic-hyporesponsive episode, and several deaths, many attributed to SIDS.[23] In fact, the vaccine manufacturer admits that "there have been spontaneous reports of apnea (temporary cessation of breathing) in temporal association with the administration of Prevnar."[24] Additional adverse reactions identified from postmarketing experience include blood and lymphatic system disorders, such as lymphadenopathy, and immune system disorders, such as anaphylactic/anaphylactoid reaction and shock.[25]

Vaccine ingredients: 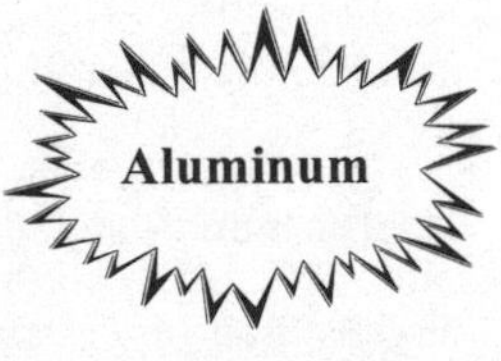
Each dose of the pneumococcal vaccine contains 13 modified strains of streptococcus pneumoniae, CRM$_{197}$ (a "variant of diphtheria toxin isolated from cultures of *corynebacterium diphtheriae*"), polysorbate 80, and 125mcg of aluminum.[26] Aluminum is neurotoxic, even in very small amounts, and has a long history of known and documented hazards.[27] In fact, according to the American Academy of Pediatrics, "Aluminum is now being implicated as interfering with a variety of cellular and metabolic processes in the nervous system and in other tissues."[28]

More recent, unpublished research led by Canadian neuroscientist Chris Shaw shows a link between the aluminum hydroxide used in vaccines, and symptoms associated with Parkinson's, ALS (Lou Gehrig's Disease), and Alzheimer's. Mice injected with this common vaccine ingredient developed statistically significant increases in memory loss, anxiety, allergic skin reactions, and nerve cell damage. According to Shaw, "This is suspicious. Either this link is known by industry and it has never been made public, or industry was never made to do these studies. I'm not sure which is scarier."[29] Nevertheless, pediatricians continue to inject millions of babies every year with the aluminum-containing Prevnar vaccine and other aluminum-containing shots. (For more information about aluminum, read *Aluminum in Vaccines* on page 175, and see *Appendix II* on page 308.)

The Pneumococcal Vaccine and Type 1 Diabetes

Dr. Barthelow Classen, an immunologist at Classen Immunotherapies, testified before the Food and Drug Administration (FDA) that the conjugated pneumococcal vaccine for children "could cause a major epidemic of diabetes."[30] Classen's landmark study published in the *British Medical Journal* and *Autoimmunity* showed a causal relationship between the conjugated Hib vaccine and insulin-dependent diabetes.[31,32] The conjugated pneumococcal vaccine is technologically similar to the Hib vaccine with one notable difference: the pneumococcal vaccine contains seven different bacterial strains "so its toxicity may be seven times as great as the currently marketed Hib vaccines."[33] Classen calculates that this vaccine will cause 28,000 cases of insulin dependent diabetes every year in the United States alone.[34] "These cases of diabetes may not occur until 3½ to 10 years following immunization."[35] Classen believes the risks greatly exceed the benefits, and told the FDA that it should abandon plans to approve this vaccine until methods are developed to give the vaccine without inducing diabetes.[36]

Adverse Reaction Reports

Parents have observed serious health problems in their children after they were vaccinated with Prevnar. A few of their unsolicited personal experiences are reprinted below.[37-39]

▸ "I had a baby that was perfectly healthy, happy, okay until she got her Prevnar vaccine. Thirty hours later, she's in the hospital having seizures that they can't stop. You're not going to tell me it's not related to the vaccine." [This child slipped in an out of a coma for 45 days, until she died. Tremors shook her little body during most of this time.]

▸ "My 6-month-old received the Prevnar vaccine two days ago. Her temperature went to 102.6° and she vomited that evening. The injection site is very inflamed—it looks like a burn and has a large knot under it that...extends from the site like a finger."

▸ "My daughter was given a Prevnar and Hib vaccination together at 9 months. Three days later she threw her head back, her eyes rolled back in her head, and she was unresponsive. I rushed her to the doctor and was told that she had an ear infection, and sometimes children do that to drain the infection out of their ears. She was not unresponsive very long. So I thought, well maybe the doctor was right. But she was having a seizure in front of the doctor, and was never really observed for anything else. She continued to do this for the next two years. It took us the whole two years to finally get an EEG done, which showed nothing. After the results, I was actually told that she was just doing this for attention. Yeah, right. We were finally referred to a children's hospital. She had four more EEG's and two MRI's, which of course showed nothing. We tried eight different medicines which only made her lose her hair and weight. We were also told she had cerebral palsy, although she had no symptoms of any health problems until she received the shots. Of course, all of the doctors say that the shots did not cause any of her problems. But she was normal until this happened. She was even rolling over at two months and crawling at six months. She was starting to talk at seven months. She quit talking, and quit walking altogether. Thank you for listening. My daughter will not receive any more vaccinations ever!"

▸ "My 10-month-old son received Prevnar four days ago. Since then he has been vomiting and developed a rash on his body. I will not let him receive the vaccine again."

▸ "My 12-month-old daughter just received [Prevnar, DTaP, chickenpox and Hib vaccines]. She vomited for 3 hours and had diarrhea." [This baby was admitted to the hospital and diagnosed with pneumonia.]

▸ "I am a mother of 18-month-old twins. Both received the Prevnar shot on June 18, 2007 and both have been experiencing daily reactions since the injection from soreness, wheezing, fever, rash, and diarrhea. The onsets of fevers were noted with both children within the first 6 hours of injection. My son was taken to the emergency room by ambulance within 12 hours of injection for a febrile seizure. He was taken a second time the following morning (within 24 hours of injection). Neither child could walk the first 48 hours after the shot. They reverted to crawling. Both broke out in a rash on the 5th day after injection, and both children continue to have diarrhea and a noticeable difference in gassiness since the shot. This weekend, the 12th day after their shots, both babies woke with a 101 degree fever. The fevers do not respond to Motrin. At 11pm I went in to check on the babies as they were both feverish all day. My son was in the midst of his 3rd seizure, this one lasting much longer and more severe than the first ones. We rushed him to the ER where he underwent a CAT Scan and Spinal Tap to rule out any viral or brain issues. None were reported. He was transported to another hospital where he could be evaluated by a specialist and underwent EEG. Again, he was given a clean bill of health and released. According to the doctors, there are no hidden ailments causing these seizures; the suspected culprit is the Prevnar injection. The doctors have advised that the good news is our son should grow out of these seizures by 5 or 6 years of age. However, now that his fever threshold has been broken, he will likely continue having these seizures every time he becomes feverish until it is outgrown. Although they have advised the seizures are not damaging, we are to notify our doctor every time my son's fevers rises above 101, and have been told to take him to the ER if a seizure lasts more than 5 minutes. All three seizures were 7-10 minutes or longer so far. We have found numerous reports on the federal VAERS site that show the same reactions, and our doctor has made a reporting as well. We have noted that there appears to be a larger number of seizures reported by male children, though both male and female reports exist in the 2007 database. We have found that hospitalization/ER visits were common within the first 3 days, 14 days, and 30 days after the injection. My husband and I are most upset that we were not told that U.S. law does not require this vaccine. This statement is not listed on the 'Notice to Parents' nor is there any indication of seizures as a possible side effect. The seizures are not noted on the manufacturer's website. This vaccine was not given with the benefit of proper warnings. Our fear is that our son and daughter will continue to suffer these adverse reactions in some form or another for days to come. As concerned and affected parents, we want to let everyone know what has happened to our children."

▸ "Is it possible to rule out a vaccine, Prevnar, as having an association with an 'atypical' seizure? My 29-month-old healthy son received a third dose of Prevnar during his recent 'well check' visit. I questioned this at the time as I had not expected a vaccine on this day. In fact, from literature I have since read, it indicated that the four recommended doses should be given on a regular schedule up until 15 months of age. I still have not received an answer as to why my son was a candidate for this third dose at almost 2½ years of age. Less than 72 hours later, I awoke to find my son limp and barely breathing. He was completely unresponsive, eyes wide open and his lips began to turn blue, followed by bubbly drool coming from his mouth. We arrived at the ER by ambulance approximately 45 minutes later. Only then did he begin to 'come to.' This frightening experience repeated itself 10 days later— a similar state of unresponsiveness, eyes open, drooling, etc. for about 45 minutes. It was the second episode that caused the doctors to speculate that my son might be having seizures. This came as a complete shock to my husband and myself as he does not possess any precluding characteristics: no family history, no trauma or injuries. He was a healthy full-term baby with no prior illnesses. Further, I have a 5½ year old daughter who likewise is very healthy with no neurological problems. (She, on the contrary, received NO Prevnar, as it was not available evidently when she was an infant, thank goodness!) That same day, my son received an EEG. The results came back 'normal.' However, my pediatrician suggested we see a neurologist because of the severity and length of time of my son's seizures. The neurologist concurred that this was an emergency. Two days later we arrived at Denver children's hospital where my son was monitored on a more advanced EEG for 18 hours. We were prescribed Depakote and sent home. All my concerns/suspicions about Prevnar have been dismissed by the doctors."

How effective is the pneumococcal vaccine?

The efficacy of Prevnar 13 against pneumococcal disease was *inferred* from comparative studies seeking "non-inferiority" to the original Prevnar (PCV7). However, the original Prevnar was similarly based upon a comparison to babies injected with another vaccine.[40] A true controlled study comparing babies vaccinated with pneumococcus—either Prevnar or Prevnar 13—to non-vaccinated babies was never conducted. According to the manufacturer, three of the 13 strains in the vaccine did not meet the pre-specified non-inferiority criterion, and "the duration of protection from immunization is not known."[41]

In practical terms, it may be nearly impossible to tell how well the pneumococcal shot really works because its efficacy is only determined by its protection against bacterial disease caused by the 13 strains included in the vaccine. According to the manufacturer, "Prevnar 13 will not protect against *streptococcus pneumoniae* serotypes that are not in the vaccine."[42] In fact, scientists have known for some time that *streptococcus pneumoniae* are subject to "changes in capsular type by recombination."[43] This has caused researchers to issue warnings that pneumococcal vaccines only targeting some strains of the disease "may increase carriage of and disease from serotypes not included in the vaccine."[44,45] Scientists writing for the *Journal of Molecular Microbiology* concur, and conclude that "this has implications for the long-term efficacy of conjugate pneumococcal vaccines that will protect against only a limited number of serotypes."[46]

In 2007, the *Pediatric Infectious Disease Journal* published data confirming "serotype replacement," where less prevalent (but more severe) pneumococcal strains replace strains targeted by the vaccine.[47] During 2000, the year in which Prevnar was licensed, 65 percent of all pneumoccocal cases were caused by strains in the vaccine. By 2004, just 27 percent of all pneumococcal cases were caused by vaccine strains; 73 percent of all cases were due to non-vaccine strains![48] Furthermore, the non-vaccine strains isolated from patients' respiratory tracts are more resistant to antibiotics and multidrug treatments.[49] Vaccine strains of pneumococcal disease have also become more resistant to antibiotics.[50]

In 2007, the *Journal of the American Medical Association* also published data showing that non-vaccine strains of pneumococcal disease are replacing the strains targeted by Prevnar. For example, ever since the vaccine was introduced, "the incidence of non-PCV7 serotype disease more than doubled among Alaska Native children."[51] In addition, the new strains are more dangerous. Compared with illness prior to Prevnar vaccination, "current cases are more likely to be hospitalized and to be diagnosed with pneumonia and empyema"[52] (a life-threatening infection causing pus and fluid to accumulate in the lung cavity).

It is also important to note that Prevnar 13 will not protect against bacterial infections caused by haemophilus influenzae type b or meningococcus.[53] Thus, when a child is vaccinated and still contracts bacterial disease, including meningitis, blood infections or pneumonia, unless the diagnosis is confirmed using very specific serological methods, antigen testing, or culture data, no one will know which strain of which bacterial pathogen—Hib, pneumococcus, or meningococcus—was responsible.[54] As a result, doctors and other authorities will find it difficult to confirm (and thus easier to deny) the existence of "vaccine failures."

The pneumococcal vaccine and otitis media:

The vaccine industry promotes this shot as a prophylactic against ear infections (otitis media). However, this is a deceptive tactic because the manufacturer admits that "children who received Prevnar appear to be at *increased* risk of otitis media due to pneumococcal serotypes not represented in the vaccine."[55] Apparently, Prevnar is "indicated for active immunization of infants and toddlers against otitis media *caused by serotypes included in the vaccine.*"[56] However, "because otitis media is caused by many organisms other than serotypes of streptococcus pneumoniae represented in the vaccine, *protection against all causes of otitis media is expected to be low.*"[57] [Italics added for emphasis.]

Simultaneous administration with other vaccines:
When the pneumococcal vaccine is administered along with other vaccines, it may interfere with the presumed efficacy of those vaccines. A few examples, taken from the vaccine manufacturer, are listed below:[58,59]
Hib: When the Hib vaccine was administered with Prevnar, Hib antibodies "were lower" after the 4th dose.
Pertussis: "Although some inconsistent differences in response to pertussis antigens were observed, the clinical relevance is unknown."
Polio: The polio vaccine contains three types of polio virus. "The [antibody] response to two doses of IPV [inactivated polio virus] given concomitantly with Prevnar...was lower for [polio virus] type 1."

Conflicts of interest?
Unbiased vaccine safety and efficacy standards are essential. Prevnar clinical trials and industry practices seem to be riddled with conflicts of interest. For example:
- Wyeth-Lederle Laboratories, the company that developed Prevnar and stands to gain the most from its universal use among children, provided a grant to pay for the studies that "proved" the safety and efficacy of the shot.[60-62]
- Drs. Steven Black and Henry Shinefield of Kaiser Permanente, the scientists who oversaw the major clinical trials used to "prove" the safety and efficacy of the vaccine, are closely associated with American Home Products, the parent company of Wyeth-Lederle Laboratories.[63]
- Dr. Kathryn Edwards, an outspoken advocate of Prevnar, was paid by Wyeth-Lederle Laboratories $255,000 per year from 1996 to 1998 to study Prevnar (and other pneumococcal vaccines).[64-66] Yet, she sat on the FDA's Vaccine Advisory Committee as a full-time member helping to recommend which vaccines to license.[67]
- Dr. Jerome Klein has been paid by vaccine manufacturers to testify against vaccine-injured children.[68] He often convinced the court that any relationship between vaccinations and death is "merely coincidental."[69] He was also the chief editor of a vaccine website promoting Prevnar—a forum that was paid for by an "unrestricted" grant from Wyeth-Lederle Laboratories.[70,71] Yet, Dr. Klein was a member of the National Vaccine Advisory Committee (NVAC) that recommends vaccines to the U.S. government.[72]
- Dr. Margaret Rennels "participated in virtually all phases" of the testing of the RotaShield rotavirus vaccine.[73] When suspicions grew that the vaccine was unsafe, Dr. Rennels allayed concerns by writing an article entitled "Lack of an apparent association between intussusception and wild or vaccine rotavirus infection."[74] Shortly after being licensed and marketed, the now infamous RotaShield vaccine was withdrawn from the market due to the large number of intussusception injuries that it caused.[75] Dr. Rennels was also an outspoken advocate of pneumococcal vaccines.[76] Several vaccine manufacturers (including Wyeth) donated more than $2.5 million to the university where she worked.[77,78] Rennels conducted a study that "proved" the safety of Prevnar[79] —not unlike her paper on the rotavirus vaccine that "proved" the safety of Rotashield. She also became a member of the Committee on Infectious Diseases that makes vaccine recommendations for the American Academy of Pediatrics.[80]

Is the pneumococcal vaccine mandatory?
Prevnar 13 is included in the CDC's recommended childhood immunization schedule. This vaccine is expensive—about $450 for the 4-dose series.[81] With mandatory laws in place, this vaccine is expected to provide over $5 billion in sales over the next few years for its manufacturer.[82] Of course, each state offers legal exemptions to the shots.

Meningococcal Disease
(Neisseria Meningitidis)

What is meningococcal disease?

Meningococcal disease, or *neisseria meningitidis,* is a serious bacterial illness that can cause meningitis and meningococcemia, or septicaemia (blood poisoning). High fever, headache and stiff neck are common symptoms of meningitis in anyone over the age of two years.[1] In babies, the classic symptoms may be more difficult to notice.[2] The meningococcal pathogen consists of at least 13 different strains, including serogroups A, B, C, Y, W-135, 29E, and Z.[3]

How prevalent and serious is meningococcal disease?

Meningococcal disease is relatively rare.[4] According to the CDC, 1400 to 2800 cases occur each year in the United States, a rate of approximately 1 or 2 cases for every 200,000 people.[5] Of 14 million students in colleges nationwide, about 100 contract this disease each year.[6] About 10 percent of the population carries the bacteria in its nonpathogenic form.[7] None of the bacteria that cause meningitis—including neisseria meningitidis—are as contagious as ailments like the common cold or flu.[8] Bacterial meningitis can be treated with antibiotics.[9] The case fatality rate is approximately 10 percent.[10] About 15 percent of cases result in hearing loss or other sequelae.[11]

Other countries also report few cases of meningococcus. For example, in 1998, Australia reported 421 cases of the disease, Canada had just 126 cases, and Japan made only six notifications.[12] The British Department of Health admits that "Meningococcal infection is relatively rare, affecting approximately 5 in 100,000 people a year in the U.K."[13] However, according to the British Office of National Statistics, meningococcal infection is now the leading cause of death in British children aged 1-5 years.[14] In the U.S., neisseria meningitidis has become the leading cause of bacterial meningitis in children and young adults.[15]

How did meningococcus become the leading cause of bacterial meningitis?

Current evidence suggests that bacterial infections associated with pneumococcal and meningococcal disease increased shortly after the Hib vaccine was introduced. For example, in New South Wales, Australia, the number of cases of meningococcal disease jumped by more than 700 percent between 1988 (*before* the Hib vaccine was introduced) and 1993 (*after* a nationwide Hib vaccination campaign was launched).[16,17] The rise in Australia was so significant that doctors were being advised on new methods to combat the alarming increases.[18]

In Britain, during much of the 1980s, *before* the Hib vaccine was put into general use, about 600 cases of meningococcal disease occurred annually.[19] Large-scale use of the conjugated Hib vaccine began in the early 1990s. During the 1994/1995 notification period, *after* the Hib vaccine was introduced, 1,555 cases of meningococcal disease were laboratory confirmed—a 150 percent increase![20] Four years later, during the 1998/1999 notification period, 2,962 cases were laboratory confirmed.[21] This represents an additional 90 percent rise. The British Department of Health acknowledged that although some of this increase may be due to improvements in reporting, "it is likely that this represents a real increase."[22] In other words, it seems as though the Hib vaccine may not have reduced the overall number of bacterial infections, such as meningitis and blood toxicity, but rather simply caused different bacterial agents—pneumococcus and meningococcus—to assume prominence.

Studies confirm the ability of an essentially dormant microorganism (or of a previously nonexistent microorganism) to emerge into prominence as a serious health threat—often with catastrophic virulence.[23,24] These new and sometimes deadly strains can mutate from preexisting pathogens, from overuse of antibiotics, *or from vaccines that provoke into existence "atypical" diseases.* Atypical strains of measles are well documented in the medical literature.[25] Now, atypical meningitis has been identified.[26] A cluster of 17 "atypically variant strains of C. meningo-septicum" were recently isolated from newborns and immunocompromised patients. Studies indicate that this new species is composed of many subgroups and is resistant to antimicrobial agents, including multiple antibiotics. This atypical pathogen causes meningitis, pneumonia, endocarditis, and blood infections. In addition, it is extremely virulent: a death rate as high as 55 percent has been reported in one nursery outbreak. Officials fear that epidemics may occur.[27]

Who is most susceptible to meningococcal disease?

Persons most susceptible to the infection are often immunocompromised, suffering from various medical conditions, such as a chronic underlying illness.[28] Infants and children have disproportionately higher rates of this disease, but nearly two-thirds of all cases occur in persons aged 15 years and older.[29] Anyone having direct contact with an infected person's oral secretions (such as a boyfriend or girlfriend) may be at increased risk of acquiring the infection.[30] College students living on-campus, especially freshmen, appear to be at higher risk than those residing off campus. However, incidence among college students "usually is similar to or somewhat lower than that observed among persons in the general population of similar age."[31] Active or passive smoking, household crowding, and persons of low socioeconomic status have also been associated with increased risk.[32]

Does a meningococcal vaccine exist?

A vaccine designed to protect against just four of the 13 different strains of meningococcus (A, C, Y, and W-135) has been available in the U.S. since 1981. Menomune® is approved for use in persons 2 years of age and older.[33] In the U.K., three meningococcal vaccines are in use. In Canada, five meningococcal vaccines are available.

In January of 2005, a new meningococcal vaccine—Menactra® (MCV4)—was licensed by the FDA. One month later, the CDC added it to their list of recommended shots, mainly for preadolescents at ages 11 or 12, and for first-year college students living in dormitories. Like its predecessor, MCV4 is designed to protect against just four of the 13 distinct strains of meningococcus.[34] In July of 2007, the CDC recommended that *all* adolescents 11 to 18 years of age receive MCV4.[35] By April of 2011, this vaccine was approved for persons 9 months through 55 years of age.[36] In January of 2011, a third meningococcal vaccine —Menveo®—was licensed by the FDA for use in persons 2 to 55 years of age.[37]

Vaccine ingredients:

Menomune is a "freeze-dried preparation" of group-specific antigens from *neisseria meningitidis,* A, C, Y and W-135, cultivated with "Mueller Hinton agar and Watson Scherp media." Although "no preservative is added during manufacture," the 6 ml vial of diluent for the vaccine contains "sterile, pyrogen-free distilled water to which thimerosal (mercury derivative)" is added as a preservative. Each dose is also formulated to contain lactose added as a stabilizer.[38]

The Menactra vaccine "contains *neisseria meningitidis* serogroup A, C, Y and W-135 capsular polysaccharide antigens individually conjugated to diphtheria toxoid protein." They are then "purified by centrifugation, detergent precipitation, alcohol precipitation, solvent extraction and diafiltration." *Corynebacterium diphtheriae* cultures "are grown in a modified Mueller and Miller medium and detoxified with formaldehyde." Each dose is "formulated in sodium phosphate buffered isotonic sodium chloride solution."[39]

How safe is the meningococcal vaccine?

In the United Kingdom, a nationwide meningococcal vaccine campaign was initiated in November 1999. Less than one year later, by September 2000, the British Committee on Safety of Medicines (CSM) had already received 7,742 Yellow Card reports—suspected adverse reactions—following administration of the "meningitis" shot, including at least 12 deaths.[40] The British government tried convincing the public that most of the deaths were caused by sudden infant death syndrome (SIDS).[41]

In the United States, the Vaccine Adverse Event Reporting System (VAERS) receives reports of adverse events following the administration of childhood shots, including the Menomune vaccine.[42] Anaphylaxis (a severe allergic reaction) and neurologic disorders, including seizures and loss of physical sensations, have been documented among vaccine recipients.[43] In addition, the manufacturer acknowledges that although a cause and effect relationship has not been established, IgA nephropathy—a serious kidney disorder—has occurred following vaccinations with Menomune.[44]

Studies that were used to demonstrate the safety of the new Sanofi Pasteur meningococcal vaccine compared adverse reaction rates between recipients of Menactra (MCV4) and recipients of Menomune. They did not compare adverse reactions between recipients of Menactra and recipients of a true placebo. (There was no comparison to a non-vaccinated population.)[45] This skews the data making the vaccine appear less reactive. Apparently, there were "no important differences in rates of malaise, diarrhea, anorexia, vomiting, or rash" between the two vaccine groups.[46] However, in one study among persons aged 11-18 years, approximately half of the participants experienced at least one systemic adverse reaction, and nearly 5 percent (about one of every 20 people vaccinated) experienced at least one *severe* systemic reaction.[47] Non-systemic reactions were common as well. For example, 13 percent of those who received this vaccine reported pain that limited movement in the arm of injection.[48] Among persons aged 18-55 years, 62 percent experienced at least one systemic adverse reaction, and nearly 4 percent had at least one *severe* systemic reaction.[49]

Adverse Reaction Reports

Shortly after this new vaccine (Menactra, or MCV4) was officially certified as safe by the FDA and placed on the market for mass consumption, several people were stricken with Guillain-Barré syndrome (GBS) following their shots.[50] GBS is a serious neurologic disorder involving inflammatory demyelination of nerves. The ailment is characterized by "the subacute onset of progressive, symmetrical weakness in the legs and arms, with loss of reflexes. Sensory abnormalities, involvement of cranial nerves, and paralysis of respiratory muscles can also occur. A small proportion of patients die, and 20 percent of hospitalized patients can have prolonged disability."[51] Here are a few excerpts from pertinent case reports:

▸ Case 1: "A male aged 18 years was vaccinated with MCV4; 15 days later, he experienced tingling in his feet and hands.... Sixteen days after vaccination, he was hospitalized.... He was observed for 3 days, discharged, and then readmitted 2 days later with bilateral facial weakness and increasing lower extremity weakness. Patellar, triceps, and biceps deep tendon reflexes were absent. Nerve conduction studies...revealed worsening motor nerve conduction velocities consistent with Guillain-Barré syndrome."

▸ Case 2: "A male aged 17 years was vaccinated with MCV4; approximately 25 days later, he had difficulty walking, followed by difficulty moving from a standing to a seated position.... Thirty-two days after vaccination, he was hospitalized with bilateral muscle weakness of upper and lower extremities with absent deep tendon reflexes."

▸ Case 3: "A female aged 17 years.... Fourteen days after vaccination with MCV4, she reported numbness of toes and tongue, and had a lump in her throat. These symptoms were followed by numbness of thighs and fingertips, arm weakness, inability to run, difficulty walking, and falling. Sixteen days after vaccination, she was hospitalized, and neurologic examination revealed decreased tone, weakness of both arms and legs, and reflexes reduced or absent in ankles, knees and arms."

▸ Case 4: "A female aged 18 years was vaccinated with MCV4.... Thirty-one days after vaccination, the patient reported numbness of legs and had trouble standing on her toes. The next morning she could not stand. The patient was admitted to the hospital and physical examination revealed decreased muscle strength in ankles and wrists bilaterally, and reduced biceps, knee, and ankle deep tendon reflexes."

▸ Case 5: "A female aged 18 years was vaccinated with MCV4; 14 days later, she experienced heaviness in her legs when walking upstairs. During the next 8 days, her difficulty walking around continued, and she had bilateral leg pain. Subsequently, she reported headache, back and neck pain, vomiting, and tingling in both hands. She became unable to walk and...was hospitalized for progressive weakness and inability to walk...."

Weakness progressed to include paralysis of arms, difficulty swallowing, and respiratory compromise."

These five cases of GBS occurred in the Eastern United States within a six-week period. All of the victims were 17 or 18 years old; symptom onset was 14 to 31 days after Menactra vaccination.[52] On October 20, 2006, the FDA and CDC alerted consumers and healthcare providers about 17 confirmed cases of GBS following routine administration of the Menactra vaccine. These cases were in older teens and people aged 20 or greater. GBS occurred within six weeks following injection with Menactra.[53] At least two law firms started representing victims of the shot.[54,55] Nevertheless, this vaccine was not removed from the market. Instead, Sanofi Pasteur, the vaccine manufacturer, updated the package insert "to reflect that GBS has been reported in association with the vaccine."[56] The FDA and CDC "are continuing to monitor the situation."[57] However, just two weeks later, on November 3, 2006, the CDC's Advisory Committee on Immunization Practices (ACIP) recommended "resumption of immunization for all groups previously recommended to receive routine Menactra immunization."[58]

How effective is the meningococcal vaccine?

Menomune efficacy rates are unreliable.[59] Antibody levels decline markedly within the first three years following vaccination.[60] The vaccine is ineffective in children under two years of age. Therefore, even though meningococcal disease rates are highest among children under 24 months old, the vaccine is not indicated for this age group.[61] In children 24 to 36 months old, the vaccine is only 52 percent effective.[62] In a three-year study of children who were less than 4 years old at the time of vaccination, efficacy of the "A" strain in the vaccine declined to less than 10 percent.[63] Menactra efficacy "was inferred from the demonstration of immunologic equivalence" to Menomune.[64] According to the manufacturer, Menactra vaccine was "non-inferior" to Menomune.[65]

Authorities often promote the meningococcal vaccine by publicizing the annual number of cases and deaths caused by the disease. However, this is deceitful because the vaccine will not prevent many of these unfortunate tragedies. This is because the meningococcal vaccine is only indicated for the prevention of meningococcal disease caused by 4 of the 13 known strains (Figure 68).[66] The meningococcal vaccine does not contain—and will not protect against—the B strain of meningococcus, the most prevalent cause of meningococcal disease in developed countries.[67] For example, the King County, Washington Health Department reported that from January 2000 through 2006, 64 percent of all strain-identified cases of meningococcal disease among teenagers could not have been prevented with a meningococcal vaccine because they were caused by a serotype not included in the shot.[68]

The B strain is also the most virulent of all the strains, the most common serotype causing meningococcal meningitis and a disproportionate number of fatalities.[69,70] For example, during the 2002/2003 epidemiological year, 82 percent of all laboratory confirmed cases of meningococcal disease—and 73 percent of all meningococcal deaths—in the United Kingdom, Wales and Northern Ireland, were caused by serogroup B.[71] In France, 58 percent of all meningococcal cases between 1999 and 2002 were from serotype B.[72] In the United States, approximately one-third of all meningococcal cases, and more than 50 percent of all cases in infants, are caused by the B strain.[73,74]

The meningococcal vaccine may be causing more virulent strains of the disease. For example, in a recent issue of the *Journal of Clinical Microbiology,* vaccine researchers investigating a fierce, new strain of meningococcus "examine whether mass vaccination against a single serogroup of meningococci would contribute to the emergence of a non-vaccine-preventable serogroup of meningococci, such as the potentially hypervirulent [newly discovered B strain]."[75] Again, they believe that a cluster of new B strain meningococcal cases "is possibly related to the mass immunization campaign" conducted earlier in the region to control the spread of serogroup C meningococci.[76]

Scientists have suspected for some time that meningococcal bacteria have the ability to perform switches of their capsule type. For example, serogroup B incidence rates in Oregon more than doubled from the 1987-1992 period to the 1995-1996 period.[77] Even more astounding, during this same period "the age-specific incidence rate of serogroup

Figure 68:

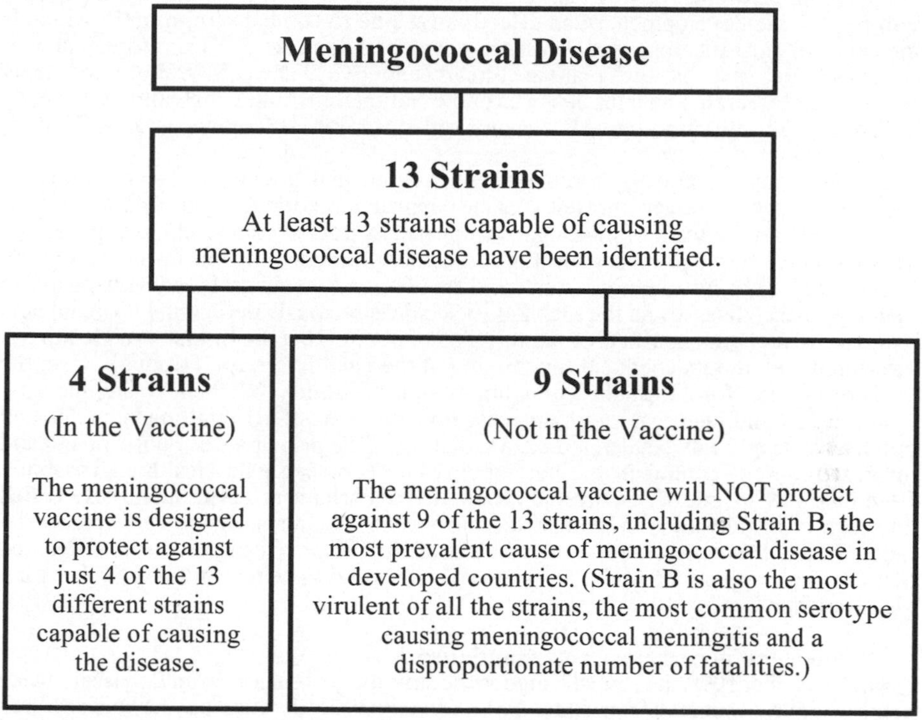

Meningococcal Disease

13 Strains

At least 13 strains capable of causing meningococcal disease have been identified.

4 Strains

(In the Vaccine)

The meningococcal vaccine is designed to protect against just 4 of the 13 different strains capable of causing the disease.

9 Strains

(Not in the Vaccine)

The meningococcal vaccine will NOT protect against 9 of the 13 strains, including Strain B, the most prevalent cause of meningococcal disease in developed countries. (Strain B is also the most virulent of all the strains, the most common serotype causing meningococcal meningitis and a disproportionate number of fatalities.)

The meningococcal vaccine is designed to protect against just 4 of the 13 different strains capable of causing meningococcal disease. Source: Vaccine manufacturer's package inserts.

© NZM

B disease among 15 through 19 year-olds increased 13-fold (from 0.5 to 6.4 cases per 100,000)."[78] Recent research published in the *Indian Journal of Medical Microbiology* affirmed that "meningococci have the capacity to exchange the genetic material responsible for capsule production and thereby switch from serogroup B to C or vice versa."[79] In fact, the study authors conclude that "capsule switching may become an important mechanism of virulence with the widespread use of vaccines that provide serogroup-specific protection."[80] This may be the reason why "the prevalence of meningococci with reduced susceptibility to penicillin is increasing."[81]

Prospective recipients of the meningococcal vaccine should also realize that it will not protect against bacterial meningitis caused by pneumococcus, haemophilus influenzae type b, or newly emerging atypical strains.[82] Thus, when a person is vaccinated and still contracts bacterial disease, it will be difficult to determine whether the vaccine failed, whether the disease was caused by the vaccine, by a strain not included in the shot, or by a completely different bacterial pathogen. The following story typifies the possibilities:

"When I was in high school, my parents had me vaccinated for meningitis. Following my meningitis vaccination, I ended up in the hospital with a major infection that attacked every area of my system. My parents told me that for the first two days that I was hospitalized I did not even recognize them. The doctors performed a lumbar puncture on me. This procedure involved freezing my mid-section so the doctors could insert a large needle into the pit of my spinal cord to withdraw fluid for testing. Their diagnosis was meningitis. I remained hospitalized for three weeks. They did not want to even consider that my meningitis vaccination could have caused my nearly fatal disease."[83]

Future developments:
Vaccine researchers believe that "ultimately, the prevention of meningococcal disease will require the development of an effective vaccine to combat serogroup B, which is the cause of most meningococcal cases in developed countries."[84] Therefore, it should come as no surprise that such plans are already underway. The U.S. Walter Reed Army Institute of Research, under the auspices of the National Institutes of Health, has already begun testing a new "Meningitis B" vaccine called "Group B Meningococcal 44/76 MOS NOMV 5D."[85]

New Zealand has also begun testing a new, experimental "Meningitis B" vaccine called MeNZB™. Large segments of the New Zealand population were used as guinea pigs. However, shortly thereafter a team of investigative journalists published a scathing exposé, *The Meningococcal Gold Rush,* documenting numerous problems with this ill-fated program. In summary: "The information parents and the public are being provided with regarding meningococcal disease and the MeNZB™ vaccine is seriously deficient. [There is] new evidence of apparent conflicts of interest, and our belief that the Ministry of Health has interfered with the independent functioning of the Health Research Council, form the basis of our call for a formal Royal Commission of Inquiry. We believe the integrity, ethics, safety and justification for the mass immunisation of 1.15 million New Zealand children is deeply flawed, dangerous, a violation of the principles of public health and informed consent, contrary to the Nuremberg Code, in breach of the Health and Disability Commissioner's Code of Practice and various acts of Parliament.... The public has a vested interest in being fully informed on all issues surrounding the administration of an experimental medicine to all New Zealanders under the age of 20."[86] The investigative team also noted that "it would appear the MeNZB™ vaccine is intended to be redeveloped further for a global market."[87]

Is the meningococcal vaccine mandatory?
In November 1999, the United Kingdom became the first country to initiate a nationwide meningococcal vaccination campaign.[88] By January 2001, the vaccine was being offered to everyone under 18 years of age.[89] However, England does *not* have mandatory vaccination laws. Parents who wish to receive the vaccine must sign a form providing their consent.[90]

In the United States, the position of the American Academy of Pediatrics (AAP) is that "universal vaccination [with meningococcal vaccine] is not necessary."[91,92] The Advisory Committee on Immunization Practices (ACIP) conducted a financial analysis of vaccination for all college students and determined that it is not likely to be cost-effective. For example, vaccination of college freshmen who live in dormitories might prevent "16 to 30 cases of meningococcal disease" each year at an estimated cost of more than $600,000 per case![93] Still, the AAP and ACIP recommend that college students and their parents "be informed by healthcare providers of the risks of meningococcal disease."[94] As a result, many colleges now have written policies on meningococcal vaccination.[95]

Despite the many safety and efficacy concerns surrounding this vaccine, and a concession by the CDC that "decisions about who to target for vaccination require understanding of the groups at risk, the burden of disease, and the potential benefits of vaccination,"[96] a national campaign is being aimed at middle school students. In fact, "by 2008, the goal will be routine vaccination with MCV4 (Menactra) of all adolescents beginning at age 11 years."[97] According to Dr. Carol Baker, professor of pediatrics at Baylor College of Medicine in Houston, Texas, "This was the first adolescent vaccine, and we knew there were others coming. We really wanted to build a platform for routinely vaccinating the 11- to 12-year-olds with the recommended vaccines."[98] Of course, if this vaccine is mandatory in your state for school entry, or is required for enrollment in a particular college, exemptions are possible.

Chickenpox

What is chickenpox?

Chickenpox, or varicella, is a contagious disease caused by a virus. The technical name for this virus is herpes varicella zoster, a member of the herpes virus family. Chickenpox is considered by many experts to be a relatively harmless childhood ailment: "It is generally a benign, self-limiting disease."[1] Symptoms include a fever, runny nose, sore throat, and an itchy skin rash which can appear anywhere on the body. The rash and disease usually disappear after one or two weeks. The disease usually confers permanent immunity; it is rarely contracted again.

Is chickenpox dangerous?

Chickenpox can be itchy and uncomfortable for a few days. Serious problems are rare. In fact, before a chickenpox vaccine was introduced, doctors recommended exposing children to the virus, and parents organized "chickenpox parties" because complication rates increase when the disease is contracted by teenagers or adults.[2] Prior to the chickenpox vaccine, every year, of the millions of people in the U.S. who contracted this disease, about 100 died from related complications.[3] Many of these were in adults who did not have chickenpox as a child, or in previously unhealthy children—youngsters with already weakened immune systems from other diseases, such as AIDS, leukemia, or cancer.[4-6]

Does a chickenpox vaccine exist?

A chickenpox vaccine has been available since the 1970s but authorities were reluctant to license and promote it because the disease is rarely dangerous and confers lifelong immunity. The vaccine, however, contains a weakened form of the virus; once injected, it remains in the body indefinitely.[7] Authorities were concerned that it could reawaken years after the vaccination and cause serious problems. Also, long-term studies were not conducted. If the vaccine were to be mass-produced and foisted on the public, our society would be subjected to a very large uncontrolled experiment. Researchers would not have a complete picture until after a generation of children were vaccinated. According to Dr. Arthur Lavin, of the Department of Pediatrics at St. Luke's Medical Center in Cleveland, Ohio, we don't know the risks involved in "injecting mutated DNA" (the chickenpox vaccine) into a "host genome" (children).[8] Also, if immunity from the vaccine were to prove temporary, like other vaccines, children who are prevented from contracting the disease naturally, due to widespread use of the shot, might become more susceptible to chickenpox during adulthood when the disease can be serious.[9]

The chickenpox vaccine was originally developed for children with leukemia or weak immune systems, a small population at greater risk for complications from the disease.[10] But vaccine manufacturers sought a wider market for their lucrative product. Merck invested millions of dollars in this vaccine, and according to Samuel Katz, Chairman of Pediatrics at Duke University, and head of a vaccine committee at the National Academy of Sciences, "Merck isn't going to make back its investment in that vaccine by just distributing it to kids with cancer. They're going to be interested in pushing for use in the normal population."[11] However, a study conducted in 1985 by the Centers for Disease Control and Prevention (CDC) determined that the medical costs of treating chickenpox did not warrant spending the money on a national vaccination campaign.[12] Thus, chickenpox manufacturers would have to bide their time since authorities could not rationalize promoting this vaccine.

Despite these concerns, in 1995 the chickenpox vaccine—Varivax®—was licensed for use in the U.S. Shortly thereafter, it was "mandated" in several states because it was "predicted to save $5.40 for every $1 spent on a vaccination program" when the indirect costs of missed work were factored in.[13,14] In other words, the vaccine was not being promoted as essential, but rather as cost-effective, because moms and dads would no longer have to stay home (an average of one day)[15,16] to care for their sick children. (More recent studies question the true cost-effectiveness of this vaccine when two doses, rather than one, are given and when adverse reactions to the vaccine are factored into the analyses.)[17,18]

How is the chickenpox vaccine made?

Official prescribing information issued June 2009 by Merck & Co., Inc., the manufacturer of Varivax®, states: "The virus was initially obtained from a child with natural varicella, then introduced into human embryonic lung cell cultures, adapted to and propagated in embryonic guinea pig cell cultures, and finally propagated in human diploid cell cultures" (fetal tissue).[19] It also contains a cluster of chemical additives. These include: sucrose, hydrolyzed gelatin, sodium chloride, monosodium L-glutamate (MSG), sodium phosphate, potassium phosphate, potassium chloride, and "residual components of MRC-5 cells including DNA and protein...EDTA, neomycin (an antibiotic), and fetal bovine serum."[20]

How safe is the chickenpox vaccine?

The Vaccine Adverse Event Reporting System (VAERS), the federal databank established by Congress in 1986 to document adverse reactions to vaccines, received nearly 10,000 reports involving the chickenpox vaccine between the months of March 1995 and December 1999, a period of less than five years.[21] The Food and Drug Administration (FDA) and CDC studied 6,574 of these reports—those filed between March 17, 1995 and July 25, 1998—then published their findings in the September 13, 2000 edition of the *Journal of the American Medical Association.*[22] Here is a summary of their findings:

Adverse Reactions to the Chickenpox Vaccine: A Summary of FDA and CDC Data

Adverse reactions in recipients of the chickenpox vaccine occurred at a rate of 67.5 per 100,000 doses sold. Approximately 4 percent of reports described "serious" adverse reactions. By FDA definition, "serious" reactions refer to deaths, life-threatening events, hospitalizations, persistent or significant disabilities, and other incidents of medical importance. For example, the data analyzed in this study included numerous cases of neurological disorders, immune system damage, blood disorders, brain inflammation, seizures, and death (Figure 69).[23]

These figures do not take into account the FDA's own admission that "potentially substantial underreporting" made the figures "highly variable fractions of actual event numbers."[24] Nor do these figures take into account that "doses sold" (about 9.7 million through July 1998) is a CDC "projection" for which no reliable documentation can be found. Authors of the study based their figures on oral and private "unpublished data" from the CDC.[25,26] In some parts of the country vaccination rates were below 10 percent.[27,28] If the CDC inflated their estimate of the actual number of doses sold, or if the doctors who bought the vaccine for resale to their patients didn't use up all of their stock, the true rate of adverse reactions associated with the chickenpox vaccine is much higher.

If we take the FDA analysis of VAERS data at face value, serious reactions to the chickenpox vaccine occurred at a rate of 4 percent. This included victims in *all* age groups. However, children under 4 years of age had serious reactions at a rate of 6.3 percent; children under 2 years old had serious reactions at a rate of 9.2 percent; and children vaccinated (by mistake) between birth and their first birthday had serious reactions at an astonishing rate of 14 percent! (Figure 70)[29]

The FDA and CDC findings included a few case histories. For example:[30]

▸ One healthy 18-month-old boy who "had no history of allergy or any prior post-vaccinal adverse event" prior to receiving the chickenpox vaccine (along with others), was admitted to the intensive care unit four days later with a low platelet count. "He began to bleed from the mouth...and died two days later from cerebral hemorrhage."

▸ Another child "without previous convulsions" had an absence seizure three days after varicella vaccine. Following his second dose one month later, he reacted with two generalized tonic-clonic seizures. The researchers noted, "This patient's positive rechallenge for seizure activity *increases suspicion that varicella vaccine may be more than a coincidental factor in observations of postvaccinal convulsions*" [author's emphasis added].

▸ A four-year-old girl developed hemiparesis (partial paralysis on one side of the body) two weeks after receiving the chickenpox vaccine. Medical investigators concluded

Figure 69:

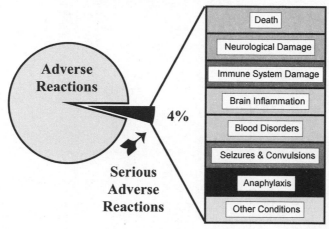

Adverse Reactions:
Chickenpox Vaccine

About four percent of all adverse reactions associated with the chickenpox vaccine are considered "serious." Source: The FDA's Vaccine Adverse Event Reporting System (VAERS), as documented in the *J of the American Medical Assoc.* (September 13, 2000).

---

that "her apparent cerebro-vascular accident assumes particular importance after a recent description of a significant statistical association between natural chickenpox and subsequent ischemic strokes in children." [Interpretation: researchers believe that the vaccine caused her serious disorder.]

Herpes Zoster (Shingles): The FDA and CDC findings also include numerous reports of vaccine recipients developing herpes zoster, or shingles, a painful skin eruption that can last for several weeks. This affliction can occur again and again, months or years following the shot. Once the varicella virus is injected into the body, it remains there indefinitely and can reactivate when immunity declines. According to Dr. Dennis Klinman of the FDA's Center for Biologics Evaluation and Research, and the author of a recently published study in *Nature Medicine,* reactivation of the latent infection can occur following inoculation with the live virus chickenpox vaccine: "As immunity declines, the latent virus wakes up."[31,32] Earlier studies published in both the *New England Journal of Medicine* and the *Pediatric Infectious Disease Journal* already showed this link between the chickenpox vaccine and herpes zoster.[33,34]

According to Dr. James Cherry, a professor of pediatrics at Mattel Children's Hospital at the University of California, Los Angeles, "Our immunity is stimulated by being exposed to the chickenpox. When that stimulation goes away, our protection is going to decrease, so we'll see more cases of shingles. My guess is that we're going to be giving doses of the [chickenpox] vaccine to 30- and 40-year-olds to prevent shingles. The better we do in [eradicating chickenpox], the more we're going to see shingles."[35] Dr. Gary Goldman, an expert varicella research analyst hired by the CDC in 1995 to collect data and monitor trends associated with the newly introduced chickenpox vaccine, is even more candid:

"Chickenpox is generally a benign, self-limiting disease."—Merck, vaccine manufacturer

Figure 70:

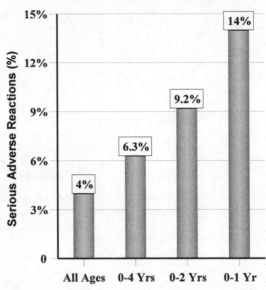

Serious Adverse Reactions: Chickenpox Vaccine

Serious adverse reaction rates dramatically increase in younger age groups receiving the chickenpox vaccine. Source: *J. of the American Medical Association* (Sept. 13, 2000).

"The universal varicella vaccination program in the United States...will leave our population vulnerable to shingles epidemics."[36,37] In fact, "there appears to be no way to avoid a mass epidemic of shingles lasting as long as several generations among adults."[38]

The FDA, CDC and vaccine manufacturer may have traded a relatively mild childhood disease—chickenpox—for a much more serious ailment.[39-41] In fact, shingles causes five times as many hospitalizations and three times as many deaths as chickenpox.[42,43] (The FDA recently licensed a new shingles vaccine—Zostavax—manufactured by Merck,[44] the same company that developed Varivax, the chickenpox vaccine that may be *causing* epidemics of shingles. In other words, a new vaccine was produced to treat a problem wrought by an earlier vaccine.)

Adverse Reactions: Shingles

The *Thinktwice Global Vaccine Institute* receives unsolicited reports of shingles outbreaks following chickenpox vaccination:[45]
 ▸ "My twins were immunized with the chickenpox vaccine. Ever since they received the shot, they have had a recurring rash that looks like chickenpox. It first showed up three days after vaccinations. Nothing works to treat the bumps. The bumps are concentrated in one area, typical of shingles. Our doctors deny it, so basically we just have to deal with this. I wish I had never vaccinated them against chickenpox. My other children caught chickenpox naturally and it never hurt any of them. Please pass this letter on to others who are considering this vaccine so they can make a better decision."
 ▸ "My mother-in-law caught shingles. The doctor said he is seeing a lot more of these lately. Do you think it has anything to do with the chickenpox vaccine?"

More evidence that shingles outbreaks may be induced by the chickenpox vaccine can be found in the following case report:

▸ A 2-year-old boy received the chickenpox vaccine. Twenty-eight months later, he developed "breakthrough chickenpox" with intensely itchy lesions. At the age of 5 years, he had a painful shingles eruption on the back of his neck that lasted for 45 days. Nine months later, he had another outbreak of shingles on his left nipple and the left side of his back. The pain was severe and the rash left scars. Two months later, he had yet another shingles outbreak.[46]

Secondary transmission of the disease: When the chickenpox vaccine was first licensed, product inserts from the chickenpox vaccine manufacturer contained a warning that vaccinated individuals "may" be capable of transmitting the vaccine virus to close contacts, and that vaccine recipients "should avoid close association with susceptible high risk individuals" such as newborns, pregnant women, and immunocompromised people.[47] The *Journal of Pediatrics* published a study confirming that vaccinated children can spread the disease, often with disastrous consequences. For example, a pregnant woman who caught chickenpox from her vaccinated son chose to abort the fetus rather than risk giving birth to a prenatally-injured baby.[48] Chickenpox vaccine data reported to VAERS includes numerous cases of these "unintentional exposures." As a result, the CDC and FDA had to admit that "secondary transmission of the virus can occur."[49] Product labels for the chickenpox vaccine listed "secondary transmission" of the vaccine virus as a known adverse event possibility.[50] Today, the vaccine manufacturer acknowledges that the transmission of vaccine virus may occur between "healthy vaccinees" and "healthy susceptible contacts." Thus, "vaccine recipients should attempt to avoid, whenever possible, close association with susceptible high-risk individuals for up to six weeks."[51] In other words, children vaccinated with the chickenpox shot are mobile carriers of the virus, and can spread this highly contagious disease to every susceptible person they come into contact with.

Shifting age distributions: Prior to licensing the chickenpox vaccine, an important theoretical study was conducted to determine the effects of a national chickenpox vaccination campaign. This study, later published in the *American J of Epidemiology*, concluded that immunization would shift the age distribution of chickenpox cases from children, who are not likely to experience problems with this disease, to teenagers and adults, who have higher complication rates.[52,53] In fact, adults are 10 times more likely to require hospitalization and 25 times more likely to die from chickenpox than children.[54] Yet, this did not stop authorities from licensing and mandating this vaccine. In response, Dr. William Osheroff, medical director of a popular Health Management Organization (HMO), chose not to recommend Varivax. He correctly summarized the pertinent issues: "This is a very benign disease in children but the vaccine may create a false sense of security as these children get older and find themselves non-immune. Chickenpox as an adult is a serious disease."[55]

Before the vaccine became available, more than 90 percent of people entering their 20s were immune to varicella, mainly due to natural chickenpox infection.[56] Thus, very few adults contracted this disease. Infants were usually protected as well because their mothers, who contracted chickenpox as children, had protective antibodies that they passed on to their babies in utero (during pregnancy). However, as more children receive the vaccine and lose the opportunity to acquire natural immunity, moms will no longer be able to protect their babies and the disease is likely to shift to infants, another age group at greater risk for complications. Anyone who doubts this possibility merely has to look at what officials did with measles. Before the vaccine was introduced, less than one-half of one percent of all babies contracted measles. Today, following years of mass immunizations, about 30 percent of all measles cases now occur in babies under one year of age.[57]

Additional confirmation of adverse reactions:
Since 1995, when this vaccine was first licensed for use in the United States, the vaccine manufacturer added at least 17 adverse events to product warning labels.[58,59] Subsequent studies have linked previously unknown adverse reactions to the chickenpox vaccine.[60-62] Common reactions that have been reported following chickenpox vaccination include upper and lower respiratory illness, gastrointestinal disorders, ear infection, eye complaints,

swollen lymph nodes, headache, muscle pain, joint pain, fatigue, malaise, disturbed sleep, loss of appetite, diarrhea, vomiting, and a chickenpox-like rash on the body (often occurring within a few days to three or four weeks following the shot).[63,64]

Serious reactions that have been reported following chickenpox vaccination include anaphylaxis (a sudden, severe, and potentially fatal allergic reaction), thrombocytopenia (a dangerous blood disorder characterized by a low platelet count), Henoch-Schönlein purpura (inflammation of the blood vessels), encephalitis (inflammation of the brain), transverse myelitis (a neurological disorder characterized by inflammation of the spinal cord), Guillain-Barré syndrome (a disorder in which the body's immune system attacks the nervous system resulting in muscle weakness and paralysis), Bell's palsy (facial nerve damage characterized by twitching, drooling, drooping eyelids and corners of the mouth, loss of taste, and facial paralysis), seizures, aseptic meningitis (inflammation of the tissues that cover the brain), Stevens-Johnson syndrome (a potentially deadly skin disease), pneumonia, pharyngitis, secondary bacterial infections, and herpes zoster (shingles).[65]

Numerous adverse reaction reports filed with the government substantiate the extensive list of reactions that have been documented following administration of the chickenpox vaccine. Here are some other "side effects" reported to VAERS: hemolytic streptococcal infection, erythema multiforme, arthritis, arthralgia, petechiae, cellulitis, vasculitis, Kawasaki syndrome, aplastic anemia, encephalopathy, ataxia, optic neuritis, demyelinating syndromes, multiple sclerosis, hypokinesia, paresthesia, hypotonia, convulsions, hemiparesis, and death.[66] Many of the serious ailments are commonly recognized complications of natural chickenpox thoroughly documented in the medical literature.[67-83] Therefore, as the FDA's Varicella Vaccine Safety Surveillance report noted, they "bolster suspicions of relationships with" and are "plausible as potential effects of" the chickenpox vaccine.[84]

Adverse Reaction Reports

The *Thinktwice Global Vaccine Institute* receives unsolicited reports of adverse reactions following chickenpox vaccination. A few of them are reproduced below:[85]

▸ "My five-year-old son received the chickenpox vaccine. Two weeks later I took him to the doctor because I noticed a lot of bruising. Four days later I took him back to the doctor for blood work. That evening I was instructed to rush him to the children's hospital. He was diagnosed with ITP and had to have intravenous immunoglobulin transfusions. Two months later his platelets skyrocketed then dropped. This is related to the chickenpox vaccine because he showed no other virus or illness prior to his diagnosis."

▸ "I did not want to immunize my daughter with chickenpox, but relented. She had a fever of 105 degrees for five days. The doctor said she had a stomach virus, yet she never vomited or had diarrhea. I knew it was not a stomach virus. They just brushed my concerns aside when I asked if it could be from the shot. Now, every time she is exposed to chickenpox, she gets sick. She runs a high fever and is lethargic for three or four days."

▸ "My nephew had a very serious reaction to the chickenpox vaccine. He looked like a child with cancer. All of his hair fell out including eyebrows. He was very pale and weak. It took him several months to get back to normal."

▸ "My husband became paralyzed after immigration required him to have a chickenpox vaccine (at age 50)! I read in the newspaper that it can cause an autoimmune attack on the spine leading to paralysis."

FDA adverse reaction reports: The following case reports were taken directly from the FDA's Vaccine Adverse Event Reporting System (VAERS).[86]

▸ 107121: A 1-year-old child developed a rash, vomited, let out a shrill scream, went into cardiac arrest and died, four days after receiving the chickenpox vaccine.

▸ 158878: A 14-month-old baby girl acquired chickenpox one day after receiving the chickenpox vaccine. Two days later she developed cellulitis that required hospitalization and surgery on her labia.

▸ 279453: A 15-month-old baby developed life-threatening respiratory distress after receiving the chickenpox vaccine. Hospitalization was required.

▸ 131631: A 2-year-old baby became dazed and passed out approximately five minutes after receiving the chickenpox vaccine.

▸ 87553: A 2-year-old baby developed pericarditis, vasculitis, liver damage, and swollen lips two weeks after her chickenpox shot. Hospitalization was required.

▸ 79983: A 2-year-old baby developed acute autoimmune hemolytic anemia 12 days after receiving the chickenpox vaccine. Hospitalization was required.

▸ 121661: A 3-year-old child received the chickenpox vaccine. Nine days later he was paralyzed, unable to walk or urinate. He was hospitalized for 7 days.

▸ 106164: A 4-year-old child developed a "varicella-like rash" six days after his chickenpox vaccine, and was hospitalized with staphylococcal bacteremia.

▸ 122210: A 4-year-old child developed kidney damage two days after receiving the chickenpox vaccine. Two weeks later, she contracted chickenpox and a super-infection. Hospitalization was required.

▸ 80082: A 4-year-old child developed lymphocytic leukemia, headaches, leg pain, bruises, and decreased hemoglobin and platelet counts starting the day after his chickenpox vaccine. He was hospitalized for 28 days.

▸ 88834: A 5-year-old child developed vasculitis and Stevens-Johnson syndrome five weeks after her chickenpox vaccine. She required 10 days in the hospital.

▸ 175928: An 8-year-old child became dizzy and confused three days after receiving the chickenpox vaccine. The child developed seizures and was life-flighted to the hospital.

▸ 275714: An 8-year-old boy vomited and lost consciousness 10 minutes after receiving the chickenpox vaccine. He was unresponsive, diagnosed with acute respiratory distress, and rushed to the emergency room.

▸ 218460: A 9-year-old girl developed Guillain-Barré syndrome after receiving the chickenpox vaccine. She spent five weeks in the hospital.

▸ 114146: A 9-year-old child developed a serious blood disorder 13 days after receiving the chickenpox vaccine. Hospitalization was required.

▸ 219497: Four days after receiving the chickenpox vaccine, this child became unresponsive, developed a focal seizure and started foaming at the mouth. Hospitalization was required.

▸ 90120: A 12-year-old child developed Guillain-Barré syndrome 12 days after receiving the chickenpox vaccine.

Chickenpox vaccine administered with other vaccines:
Among all adverse reaction reports in the recently analyzed VAERS data, 82 percent of the victims received only the chickenpox vaccine. The remaining 18 percent were simultaneously injected with the chickenpox vaccine and MMR, or the chickenpox vaccine and other vaccine combinations.[87] Sometimes the delicate immune systems of young children react poorly to multiple vaccines administered all at once. These children may have serious adverse reactions. The following real-life experience recounted by a concerned mother illuminates the possibilities:

▸ "Last week my 5-year-old daughter received DTaP, MMR, IPV and chickenpox vaccines. Two days later she had at least two complex partial seizures (staring, pupils not contracting when a flashlight was shone into her eyes, unresponsive; during the second one, she was asleep but fingers of both hands were twitching rhythmically). She was hospitalized and recovered the same day, although she had to stay there for two days for observation. The pediatrician, as well as the hospital doctors, dismissed our concerns that the vaccines could have been the cause. A day after returning from the hospital my daughter had a high fever, vomiting and diarrhea. We were told she had picked up a stomach bug at the hospital."[88]

VAERS data and the vaccine manufacturer's warning labels are only two sources of information about adverse reactions to vaccines. The National Vaccine Information Center (NVIC) also monitors damage from the shots. Barbara Loe Fisher, president of NVIC, commented on the FDA study: "We have been waiting for the FDA to follow up on VAERS reports and then disclose and utilize the VAERS data to increase our knowledge about vaccine reactions and possible high risk factors. This is how parents and Congress

Figure 71:

The Chickenpox Vaccine & Doctor Mistakes

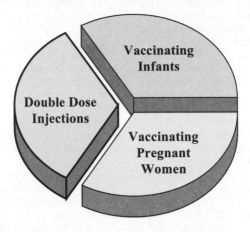

Doctor mistakes account for many of the avoidable adverse reactions associated with the chickenpox vaccine. (This chart does not reflect actual percentages.) Source: *Journal of the American Medical Association* (September 13, 2000).

---

expected the Vaccine Adverse Event Reporting System to be utilized when it was centralized under the National Childhood Vaccine Injury Act of 1986."[89] Fisher applauded public release of the VAERS data but challenged the authors' conclusions minimizing adverse reactions: "We have been getting reports from parents that their children are suffering high fevers, chickenpox lesions, shingles, brain damage, and dying after chickenpox vaccination, *especially when the vaccine is given at the same time [in combination with other vaccines]*. This FDA report confirms our concern that the chickenpox vaccine may be more reactive than anticipated in individuals with both known and unknown biological high risk factors."[90]

Doctor mistakes:
Doctor mistakes account for many of the avoidable adverse reactions to the chickenpox vaccine. These result from a) shots given to infants younger than 12 months, b) double dose injections, and c) vaccinations of pregnant women (Figure 71).[91] Several of the VAERS reports describe women who gave birth to babies with malformations, such as Down syndrome, following "gestational varicella vaccine exposure."[92] Pregnant women should not receive the chickenpox vaccine. Instead, doctors may recommend varicella zoster immune globulin (VZIG)—made from the blood of varicella-infected donors—to "persons at high risk for complications" after they have been exposed to chickenpox.[93] A blood test is also available for persons who are uncertain whether they have natural immunity to chickenpox. Many of these people will find that they are immune.[94]

How effective is the chickenpox vaccine?
In all pre-licensure trials, some vaccinated children contracted chickenpox.[95,96] According to the vaccine manufacturer, "The duration of protection...is unknown."[97] Furthermore, "in a highly vaccinated population, immunity for some individuals may wane due to lack of exposure to natural varicella as a result of shifting epidemiology."[98] Thus, "post-marketing surveillance studies are ongoing to evaluate the need and timing for booster vaccination."[99]

The chickenpox vaccine is not effective in babies under 12 months.[100] In addition, the chickenpox vaccine may be less effective in children when administered in combination with other vaccines. For example, in clinical studies comparing chickenpox vaccine efficacy rates, anti-varicella virus antibody levels were decreased when an investigational chickenpox vaccine was administered concomitantly with DTaP, MMR, Hib, and other shots.[101]

"Vaccine failures" and/or the development of a rash virtually identical to chickenpox, account for many of the documented (and undocumented) complaints associated with this shot.[102] According to an FDA report, about 1 in 10 vaccinated children develop "breakthrough disease" following exposure to chickenpox.[103] Actual statistics are worse because some people do not report their reactions, and because vaccinated children who contract shingles or some other disease as a result of the shot are not listed as recipients of an ineffective or failed vaccine.

In March 2007, the *New England Journal of Medicine* published a study that examined ten years of chickenpox vaccine data in 350,000 subjects to assess the "loss of vaccine-induced immunity to varicella over time."[104] Several important points were made:

- The annual rate of "breakthrough" varicella (cases that occurred in previously vaccinated people) significantly increased with time since vaccination. Nearly 10 percent of all chickenpox cases were breakthrough disease.
- Children who had been vaccinated at least five years previously, were twice as likely to have moderate-to-severe disease (when compared with more recently vaccinated children). Severe disease was linked with complications, such as pneumonia and skin superinfections.
- The vaccine shifted demographics over time. Before the vaccine was introduced, most cases of chickenpox occurred in children between 3 and 6 years of age. By 2004, only 30 percent of cases were in children under the age of 6 years. Older people have become more jeopardized.
- Waning of immunity may result in increased susceptibility later in life, when the risk of severe complications is greater than that in childhood.[105]

Mild chickenpox: Authorities often claim that children who contract chickenpox after having been vaccinated have milder cases—a lower fever and fewer lesions.[106,107] This is the same claim authorities have made, and continue to make, with regard to the measles vaccine. However, some experts believe that a "milder" case of the disease may be detrimental, a sign that the vaccine is suppressing the illness which could lead to more serious chronic ailments. Dr. Harold Buttram, pediatrician and vaccine researcher, comments on a little-known study where antipyretics (fever reducers) were used to lower body temperature and inhibit the typical skin rash associated with measles. "Those children who were treated with [fever reducers] had significantly prolonged duration of illness and increased incidence of respiratory complications.... Children with the most violent, highly febrile form of the disease and marked skin rash actually had the best prognosis for recovery.... It could be inferred that interference with the natural course of the disease significantly dampened the immune responses of the children. If this is true, it may be assumed that [vaccines] may have a comparable effect."[108,109]

Vaccine storage requirements: The chickenpox vaccine is highly susceptible to improper maintenance. Even authorities are unsure about the best way to preserve its potency. Initially, they required physicians to store the vaccine frozen at a temperature of 5°F or colder, and it had to be used within 30 minutes of reconstitution.[110,111] Later, they claimed it could be refrigerated between 36°F and 46°F "as long as the vaccine is not kept at those temperatures for more than 72 hours before administration."[112] One doctor, voicing the concerns of other pediatricians, had this to say: "I can tell you that the handling, storage, and temperature requirements for this vaccine in the clinic are terrible. Maintaining it in an assuredly effective state is a very delicate proposition."[113]

> *"Children with the most violent, highly febrile form of [chickenpox] and marked skin rash actually had the best prognosis for recovery."*
> —*Dr. Harold Buttram,* commenting on the undesirability of "mild" chickenpox

Is the chickenpox vaccine mandatory?

This vaccine has been added to the growing list of mandatory shots. However, according to Barbara Loe Fisher, president of the National Vaccine Information Center, the chickenpox vaccine should not have been mandated. "There are too many questions about the true adverse event and efficacy profile of this...live virus vaccine."[114] Dr. John Close, a California-based medical practitioner, echoed Fisher's concerns: "The list of those who would constitute high-risk individuals is fairly extensive.... I have seen reports of serious adverse reactions up to four percent.... I have not found any reliable reports assessing the completeness of immunity conferred.... Of all the vaccines available at this point, this is the one I would be reluctant to make mandatory."[115]

In June of 2007, the CDC's Advisory Committee on Immunization Practices (ACIP) updated (once again) its previous recommendations "for the prevention of varicella in children, adolescents and adults."[116] Official guidelines were initially established in 1995, then revised in 1999, 2005 and 2006. Concerns about the vaccine's waning efficacy over time, and the increasing number of older people who are becoming more susceptible to the disease, have impelled authorities to constantly fiddle with chickenpox vaccine recommendations. Two doses are now advocated for most people. In addition, healthcare providers have been commanded to use "standing orders" to ensure that women (without evidence of immunity to chickenpox) who have recently given birth, or have otherwise terminated a pregnancy, are vaccinated before discharge from the facility.[117] Also, "women should be counseled to avoid conception for one month after each dose of varicella vaccine" (to avoid the risk of birth defects).[118] Complete varicella vaccine guidelines are published by the CDC. Of course, legal exemptions are permitted. Read your state vaccine laws for more information.

Rotavirus

What is rotavirus?

Rotavirus is a common cause of diarrhea and vomiting in children. It occurs most often in the winter months. Symptoms typically last from 3 to 8 days and may include a fever and abdominal pain. Although babies 6 months to 2 years are most vulnerable to rotavirus infection, nearly all children are exposed to this contagious microbe at least once by the time they are 5 years old. The illness causes partial immunity because repeat infections are less severe. In most cases, rotavirus is mild enough that parents can care for their children at home. However, in severe cases dehydration and death are possible. Over 80 percent of all rotavirus deaths occur in poor countries where babies are malnourished and there is limited access to advanced healthcare. In the United States, about 20 deaths per year are attributed to this disease.[1-8]

Treatment mainly consists of preventing dehydration by giving fluids until the disease runs its course. In serious cases, frequent vomiting makes oral hydration ineffective. Babies unable to keep down liquids risk dying from dehydration and require intravenous fluids.[9]

The first rotavirus vaccine:

In August 1998, the FDA's Vaccines and Related Biological Products Advisory Committee (VRBPAC) licensed the first rotavirus vaccine—RotaShield—for all infants. In March 1999, the CDC's Advisory Committee on Immunization Practices (ACIP) added this drug to its list of universally recommended childhood vaccines. Consequently, parents assumed that this vaccine was safe and had their precious babies vaccinated. They trusted the FDA, CDC and vaccine manufacturer to make their recommendations based on the best science available and the healthcare interests of our nation. After all, when vaccines are licensed and mandated, millions of babies nationwide are affected. Nevertheless, this vaccine was brought to market without adequate safety oversight. In October 1999, sales of this vaccine were terminated because it was linked to numerous cases of intussusception—a serious intestinal blockage—and infant deaths.[10,11]

★ Congressional Hearing: June 15, 2000 ★
Conflicts of Interest and Vaccine Development

On June 15, 2000, a congressional hearing before the Committee on Government Reform was held to determine if "the entire process [of licensing and recommending vaccines] has been polluted and the public trust has been violated."[12] Members of the FDA and CDC advisory committees apparently knew about the potential dangers of the rotavirus vaccine *prior* to it having been licensed and recommended for every child in the country. They even questioned whether the benefits of the vaccine justified the costs, but this didn't stop them from unanimously approving it. Perhaps their financial ties to the vaccine industry caused a serious lapse of judgment. For example, Dr. Kathryn Edwards, a physician on the FDA's advisory committee who voted to recommend the rotavirus vaccine, received $255,000 per year in research funds from Wyeth-Lederle, the drug company that made the rotavirus vaccine.[13,14] As another example, Dr. Paul Offit, a member of the CDC's advisory committee who voted to recommend the rotavirus vaccine, held a lucrative patent on another rotavirus vaccine under development. In addition, he was paid by the drug industry to travel around the country and teach doctors that vaccines are safe.[15] In fact, Congress discovered that 60 percent of the FDA advisory committee members who voted to license this defective rotavirus vaccine, and 50 percent of the CDC advisory committee members who voted to add it to the recommended childhood vaccine schedule, had financial ties to the drug company that produced the vaccine or to two other companies developing their own potentially lucrative rotavirus vaccines—Merck and SmithKline Beecham.[16]

According to Congressman Dan Burton, who chaired the congressional hearing, "Families need to have confidence that the vaccines that their children take are safe, effective and very necessary. Doctors need to feel confident that when the FDA licenses a drug, that it's really safe and that the pharmaceutical industry has not influenced the decision-making process. Maintaining the highest level of integrity over the entire spectrum of vaccine development and implementation is essential. The Department of Health and Human Services has a responsibility to the American public to ensure the integrity of this process by working diligently to appoint individuals that are totally without financial ties to the vaccine industry to serve on these and all vaccine-related panels. No individual who stands to gain financially from the decisions regarding vaccines that may be mandated for use should be participating in the discussion or policymaking for vaccines."[17]

Despite this important congressional exposé, no one at the FDA, CDC or Department of Health and Human Services (HHS) was willing to acknowledge a problem with current "conflict of interest" rules. Instead, they thumbed their noses at the congressional hearing. For example, the FDA's senior associate commissioner Linda Suydam confirmed that the FDA was *not* planning to reform its policies. Her explanation was unequivocal: "Both the law and policies allow us to use people who have financial ties."[18] Nor was the CDC or HHS planning to make recommended changes.[19]

To date, the vaccine approval and recommendation process remains largely unchanged. For example, in January 2006, the *New England Journal of Medicine* published a crucial study of a new rotavirus vaccine—RotaTeq®—that would be used by the FDA and CDC as a basis for licensing and universally recommending this vaccine.[20] Yet, authors of the study included Paul Offit and H. Fred Clark, co-owners of the patent on this vaccine (along with Dr. Stanley Plotkin).[21,22] In addition, several other members of the study team who were supposed to be objectively evaluating the safety and efficacy of this vaccine, were paid consulting fees, lecture fees, and/or provided grant support by Merck, the vaccine manufacturer, or by GlaxoSmithKline, the maker of another rotavirus vaccine soon to be approved as well. Some study team members even owned stock in Merck, whose equity value would increase by positive evaluations of this vaccine.[23] Apparently, such conflicts of interest were deemed irrelevant to the impartiality required to ensure the integrity of the entire vaccine approval process and the safety of millions of babies who would soon receive this new vaccine.

The new rotavirus vaccine:
On February 3, 2006, the U.S. Food and Drug Administration (FDA) approved a new live-virus, orally administered rotavirus vaccine—RotaTeq®—for infants under 32 weeks of age. Three weeks later, the CDC's Advisory Committee on Immunization Practices (ACIP) added it to its list of recommended childhood vaccines.[24] It is produced by Merck, designed to protect against four of the most common strains of rotavirus, and given as a three-dose series costing about $100 per dose, or $300 for the complete set.[25,26] Another live-virus, orally administered rotavirus vaccine—Rotarix®—developed by the British manufacturer GlaxoSmithKline, was licensed by the European Medicine Agency in 2006 and approved by the FDA in April of 2008. It is given in two doses, instead of three.[27]

How safe is the RotaTeq® rotavirus vaccine?
According to the vaccine manufacturer, the RotaTeq vaccine "contains 5 live reassortant rotaviruses. The rotavirus parent strains of the reassortants were isolated from human and bovine hosts." In addition, the reassortants are "propagated in Vero cells" (from the kidneys of African green monkeys). Each vaccine dose also contains sucrose, sodium citrate, sodium phosphate monobasic monohydrate, sodium hydroxide, polysorbate 80, cell culture media, "and trace amounts of fetal bovine serum."[28] (Fetal refers to fetus, and bovine pertains to a cow or calf. In 1981, Paul Offit discovered a unique rotavirus in a "calf" on a Pennsylvania farm. Since that time, researchers mixed some of the calf rotavirus genes with those from strains that infect humans to create the current vaccine.)[29]

Intussusception: According to the CDC, babies who received RotaShield—the initial rotavirus vaccine that was eventually withdrawn—were up to 30 times more likely to be stricken with intussusception within two weeks of the first dose.[30] Intussusception causes excruciating abdominal pain in babies. A portion of the intestinal wall telescopes in on itself. The wall of the intestine swells and bleeds. Soon, the baby gets weaker, may develop a fever and vomit bile. The baby's stools may contain blood and mucus. This is a medical emergency; without treatment, most children will die within a couple of days.[31]

The RotaTeq vaccine manufacturer warns parents to remain alert to the possibility of intussusception in their babies following use of this vaccine: "If your child develops sudden abdominal pain, vomiting, blood in their stools or other changes in their bowel movements, it may be a sign of a serious problem. You should call the doctor immediately."[32]

A study of this vaccine was recently published in the *New England Journal of Medicine*. Within this study, a safety substudy was conducted. One of the factors looked at was "potential cases of intussusception negatively adjudicated."[33] In other words, when babies in the study received either the rotavirus vaccine or placebo and were then suspected of being stricken with this serious intestinal ailment, a medical committee either confirmed or denied (negatively adjudicated) an intussusception diagnosis. When all of the denied cases were added up, babies who received the RotaTeq vaccine had a greater than threefold risk of hematochezia when compared to babies who received the placebo.[34] Hematochezia is the passage of bloody stools from the rectum, associated with lower gastrointestinal bleeding.[35]

The following reports of intussusception and/or hematochezia after receiving the RotaTeq vaccine were taken directly from the FDA's Vaccine Adverse Event Reporting System (VAERS).[36] They represent a very small sample of the reports.

▸ 268405: A 4-month-old baby developed intestinal obstruction 2 days after receiving the RotaTeq vaccine. Abdomen surgery revealed "intussusception with gangrenous ascending and transverse colon."

▸ 269344: A 4-month-old received the RotaTeq vaccine and subsequently developed intussusception and gastrointestinal necrosis. The infant required "surgery for resection at necrotic bowel."

▸ 266155: An 11-week-old female was vaccinated with RotaTeq and developed severe vomiting. The infant vomited so much that she was hospitalized. An ultrasound was performed and a diagnosis of intussusception was made.

▸ 266161: A 2-month-old baby received the RotaTeq vaccine and 6 days later was diagnosed with intussusception requiring surgical reduction.

▸ 279032: A 3-month-old started vomiting, and had bloody stools, after receiving RotaTeq. The infant was transferred from one hospital to another with symptoms of hematochezia, intussusception, and intestinal obstruction.

Seizures: A seizure is an abnormal electrical discharge in the brain. It may affect a small area of the brain or the entire organ. The body area affected by the seizure loses its regular function and may react uncontrollably. For example, if a seizure affects the entire brain, all of the extremities may shake wildly without restraint. Some seizures result in a glazed look (staring) and unresponsiveness. If a child has a febrile seizure, the risk for epilepsy doubles compared to the general population.[37] Epilepsy is a chronic neurological disorder characterized by recurrent, unprovoked, unpredictable seizures. Although some cases of epilepsy can be controlled with medication, currently there is no cure.

In placebo-controlled clinical trials of the new rotavirus vaccine, "seizures" and "seizures reported as serious adverse experiences" occurred at higher rates in vaccine recipients. For example, twice as many babies who received RotaTeq (as compared to babies who received placebo) had seizures within 7 days after any dose.[38] Seizures reported as serious adverse experiences occurred at a rate of 510 out of one million in the placebo group versus 750 out of one million in the vaccine group.[39] If 510 serious seizures out of one million babies is the normal base rate, then about 240 additional babies (the vaccinated ones) out of every one million (750 minus 510=240) will have an unfortunate—but avoidable! —serious seizure. Despite these revealing figures, the vaccine was licensed.[40]

Dermatitis: The *New England Journal of Medicine* safety substudy (noted earlier) also found that dermatitis occurred more often among vaccine recipients than among the group receiving placebo. Dermatitis, called eczema as well, is an inflammation of the skin. It is caused by an allergic reaction to specific allergens.[41]

Additional safety issues (RotaTeq): More than 71,000 infants were evaluated in three placebo-controlled clinical trials that were ultimately used to license this vaccine. Here is a summary of adverse reactions that occurred at a statistically higher rate among babies who received the RotaTeq vaccine when compared to babies who received a placebo. This list includes adverse events that occurred within 6 weeks of any dose (Figure 72):[42,43]

- Diarrhea. This is the most common symptom of rotavirus, the main reason to seek protection against this disease. However, in the studies used as a basis for licensing this vaccine, diarrhea occurred statistically more often in recipients of the vaccine than in babies who never received a single dose.
- Vomiting. Again, statistically more common in vaccine recipients.
- Otitis media. This is a painful inflammation or infection of the middle ear. Otitis media not only causes severe pain but may result in serious complications if it is not treated. An untreated infection can travel from the middle ear to the nearby parts of the head, including the brain. Although the hearing loss caused by otitis media is usually temporary, untreated otitis media may lead to permanent hearing impairment. Persistent fluid in the middle ear and chronic otitis media can reduce a child's hearing at a time that is critical for speech and language development. Children who have early hearing impairment from frequent ear infections are likely to have speech and language disabilities.[44]
- Bronchospasm. An abnormal constriction of the respiratory airway causing difficult and labored breathing. This condition is a chief characteristic of asthma and bronchitis. A cough and wheezing are common.
- Nasopharyngitis. This is a viral infectious disease of the upper respiratory system, often accompanied by a sore throat and runny nose.

In clinical trials used to evaluate this vaccine's safety, three doses were administered to *healthy* infants between 6 and 32 weeks of age.[45] Babies who are vaccinated when they are not healthy could react differently. Also, babies who received this vaccine in the clinical trials were not permitted to receive the oral polio vaccine.[46] Yet, babies throughout the world are vaccinated against polio precisely between 6 and 32 weeks of age. RotaTeq is a live viral vaccine that replicates in the small intestine. The oral polio vaccine contains live viruses as well. Babies who receive both vaccines near in time could react in ways not evaluated in the studies.

The long-term effects of this vaccine were not studied. With some drugs, unanticipated health problems take months or years to manifest. Afflictions could occur in the vaccinated individual or in the general population. For example, because this is a live virus vaccine, it sheds in the baby's stool for up to 15 days.[47] In fact, the vaccine manufacturer warns that there is a "theoretical" risk that the virus could be transmitted to non-vaccinated people.[48] Furthermore, "caution is advised when considering whether to administer RotaTeq to individuals with immunodeficient close contacts."[49] In other words, babies who are vaccinated against rotavirus could pass this infectious microbe on to other family members, such as parents, grandparents and people with weak immune systems. (This is more than a "theoretical" possibility; a precedent for this eventuality has already been established with other live-virus vaccines. For example, parents and grandparents of babies recently vaccinated against polio have been stricken with polio. This was one of the main rationales for removing the live-virus polio vaccine from the U.S. market.)[50-52]

The RotaTeq vaccine is recommended for babies at 2, 4 and 6 months of age.[53] However, the CDC already recommends that babies receive seven other vaccines at approximately 2, 4 and 6 months of age: hepatitis B, diphtheria, tetanus, pertussis (DTaP), haemophilus influenzae type B, pneumococcal and polio.[54] (The flu vaccine is also recommended starting at 6 months.)[55] Therefore, if parents follow official recommendations, their babies will receive a total of eight vaccines simultaneously on three separate occasions (nine vaccines at 6 months if the flu vaccine is included). As an adult, when was the last time that *you* took 8 drugs all at the same time? Would you trust your body to process all of them without incident, or would you be surprised if you did *not* have a bad reaction? (For more information, read the chapter on multiple vaccines administered simultaneously.)

Figure 72:

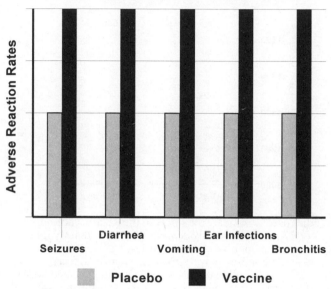

Rotavirus Vaccine *Increases* Adverse Reactions

Seizures, diarrhea, vomiting, ear infections, and upper respiratory disease all occurred at statistically higher rates among babies who received the RotaTeq vaccine when compared to babies who received a placebo. (Statistical differences are not drawn to scale.) Source: The vaccine manufacturer.

How safe is the Rotarix® rotavirus vaccine?

According to the vaccine manufacturer, the Rotarix vaccine is derived from "the human 89-12 strain...propagated on Vero cells." Each dose also contains calcium carbonate, calcium chloride, dextran, ferric (III) nitrate, magnesium sulfate, phenol red, potassium chloride, sodium hydrogenocarbonate, sodium phosphate, sodium L-glutamine, sodium pyruvate, sorbitol, sucrose and xanthan.[56] Clinical studies have found statistical correlations between this vaccine and higher rates of **death** (pneumonia-related), **convulsions** (epilepsy, grand mal, status epilepticus, and tonic), **bronchitis,** and **Kawasaki disease** (which often leads to heart disease and sudden death).[57-63] In addition, ten "non-pivotal" studies found that more parents of babies who received the vaccine (versus parents of babies in the placebo group) discontinued the study due to serious adverse events.[64] Yet, this vaccine was licensed as safe and is administered to millions of babies throughout the world every year.

Death: In the clinical studies used to evaluate the safety of the Rotarix vaccine, *vaccinated babies died at a much higher rate than non-vaccinated babies*—mainly due to a statistically significant increase in pneumonia-related fatalities: 68 deaths in the vaccinated group versus 50 deaths in the non-vaccinated group (a death rate of 18.5 versus 14.5 per 10,000).[65] In other words, for every one million babies who receive this vaccine, we can expect 1,850 to die. However, if we leave them unvaccinated, just 1,450 will die—400 babies per every million would be saved by *not* vaccinating them! (Figure 73) (As of April 2008, more than 25 million doses had already been distributed worldwide.)[66] In addition, twice as many vaccinated babies died from *diarrhea* when compared to the non-vaccinated babies.[67]

Figure 73:

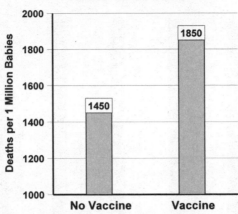

**Rotavirus Vaccine *Increases*
the Death Rate**

In the clinical studies used to evaluate the safety of the Rotarix vaccine, *vaccinated babies died at a much higher rate than non-vaccinated babies*—mainly due to a statistically significant increase in pneumonia-related fatalities: 68 deaths in the vaccinated group versus 50 deaths in the non-vaccinated group (a death rate of 18.5 versus 14.5 per 10,000). In other words, for every one million babies who receive this vaccine, we can expect 1,850 to die. However, if we leave them unvaccinated, just 1,450 will die—400 babies per every million would be saved by *not* vaccinating them! Source: The vaccine manufacturer.

Although babies who received the Rotarix vaccine were significantly more likely to contract pneumonia and die than babies who did not receive the vaccine, authorities tried to dismiss the results as implausible. In fact, the Independent Data Monitoring Committee (IDMC) commissioned to monitor the safety of the Rotarix vaccine development program, claimed that the disproportionate number of fatalities in the vaccinated babies "could be due to chance" or to "a spurious finding of statistical significance."[68] (It is not a scientifically acceptable practice to simply discount as a fluke undesirable study results.) The IDMC noted that "there is no known biological explanation for this observation. Natural rotavirus disease is not an established cause of mortality from non-diarrheal causes."[69]

The Rotarix manufacturer also sought to minimize the importance of the significantly greater number of pneumonia-related deaths following Rotarix vaccination by claiming there is no "causal relationship" between the events because "the existence of a rotavirus syndrome leading to lower respiratory tract infections has not been established."[70] However, Dr. Melinda Wharton, deputy director of the National Center for Immunization and Respiratory Diseases at the CDC, believes there may be a biologically plausible explanation: rotavirus disease, as developed in the placebo group, may actually *protect* against respiratory infection.[71]

A brief comment regarding placebos:
The composition of the placebo used in the RotaTeq vaccine safety trials was not revealed. However, the placebo used in the Rotarix vaccine safety trials "had the same constituents as the active vaccine" minus the vaccine virus.[72] (In other words, the placebo contained ferric (III) nitrate, magnesium sulfate, phenol red, etc.). This is not a true placebo, which should be a harmless substance. This deceptive tactic renders the "control group" counterfeit. When vaccines are compared to other substances that are capable of causing adverse reactions, the vaccine appears safer than it really is, and officially acknowledged adverse reactions to a vaccine may represent only a fraction of the true potential risks to the recipient.

How effective is the rotavirus vaccine?

The RotaTeq vaccine is designed to protect against four strains of rotavirus: serotypes G1-G4. Researchers would consider the vaccine a success if it could be proven "efficacious in preventing wild-type G1-G4 rotavirus gastroenteritis occurring 14 or more days after completion of the three-dose series through the first full rotavirus season after vaccination."[73] Using this definition, the vaccine was rated 74 percent effective "against any grade of severity" of rotavirus, and 98 percent effective against "severe" cases of the ailment.[74] (These figures are 87 percent and 96 percent, respectively, for Rotarix.)[75] In addition, the vaccine reduced hospitalizations "for rotavirus gastroenteritis caused by serotypes G1, G2, G3, and G4"—the strains included in the vaccine.[76]

Findings: Parents should realize that this vaccine will not protect against diarrhea caused by rotavirus strains not included in the vaccine. The vaccine is designed to protect against four strains of rotavirus, but several strains have been identified. In fact, the diversity of rotavirus strains is so great that up to 14 percent of them could not be typed.[77] Therefore, a child can receive the rotavirus vaccine and still become infected with rotavirus. In such cases, all of the symptoms of rotavirus, including severe diarrhea and dehydration, are possible.[78] Moreover, parents should know that children who are already infected with rotavirus, regardless of the strain, will not be protected by this vaccine.[79]

Diarrhea can also be caused by several different pathogens. For example, astrovirus infection occurs worldwide and is a significant cause of diarrhea. One study conducted in England showed that astroviruses were the most frequent viral cause of infectious intestinal disease.[80] Calicivirus infection is associated with diarrhea and vomiting lasting several days. Caliciviruses are very common, especially in children.[81] However, the rotavirus vaccine will not protect against diarrhea resulting from astroviruses, caliciviruses or the many other possible causes. It is only designed to protect against a limited number of rotaviruses (Figure 74).[82] In fact, the FDA and Merck believe that "Parental education on rotavirus gastroenteritis and on the vaccine will be essential to establish and maintain public confidence in this vaccine and to avoid confusion caused by cases of gastroenteritis in early childhood resulting from non-rotaviral etiologies and not preventable by rotavirus vaccine."[83] In other words, many parents will vaccinate their children with the rotavirus vaccine, subjecting them to all of the potential risks, in the hopes of preventing them from getting diarrhea. However, many of these vaccinated children will still get diarrhea from other causes, just not from one of the four rotavirus microbes included in the vaccine. When these vaccinated babies have diarrhea, the FDA and Merck don't want parents to think that their vaccine failed.

It is not possible to determine if a child has rotavirus without a positive identification. The standard protocol requires laboratory testing of the baby's stool for rotavirus using a commercial enzyme immunoassay kit.[84] Therefore, when babies are vaccinated against rotavirus and then have severe diarrhea days, weeks or months later, most parents will be unable to determine whether the vaccine failed, or worse, if it actually caused the disease.

The long-term efficacy of this vaccine has not been established. Most of the babies in the clinical trials were followed for just one full rotavirus season after vaccination. However, a single study found this vaccine to be 63 percent effective (against the rotavirus strains included in the vaccine) during a second rotavirus season.[85] If efficacy continues to wane through additional rotavirus seasons, authorities may recommend booster shots.

The new rotavirus vaccines were tested primarily in the U.S., Europe and Latin America. Authorities are not sure whether they will be as effective in poorer countries, claiming foreign children have different diets and are exposed to "a variety of health problems that can affect their ability to respond to some vaccines."[86] Actually, researchers are aware of a more likely reason their vaccine may fail with different groups of children: a multiplicity of circulating rotavirus strains—plus other diarrhea-causing viruses—that are not targeted by the vaccine. Researchers have previously admitted that "since reassortment vaccines were engineered to contain the most prevalent G antigens (G1-G4), these vaccines may protect less well against unusual strains circulating in other countries."[87]

Figure 74:

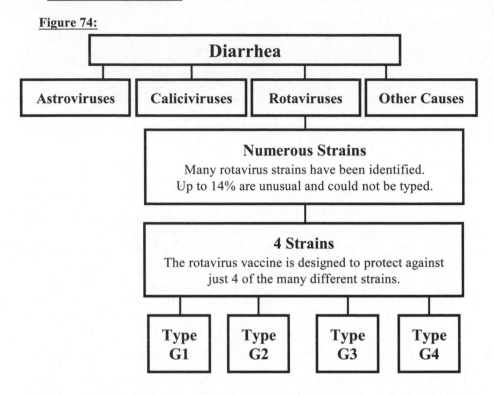

Diarrhea can be caused by astroviruses, caliciviruses, rotaviruses and other pathogens. Rotaviruses have many strains. The rotavirus vaccine is designed to protect against just 4 of the many different rotavirus strains capable of causing rotavirus infection. It will not protect against rotavirus strains not included in the vaccine, nor against diarrhea caused by astroviruses, caliciviruses and other pathogens. Source: The vaccine manufacturer.

© NZM

Are rotavirus vaccines necessary?

Some people don't think the rotavirus vaccine is necessary. For example: "They gave my son a new vaccine for diarrhea. Are you kidding me? They injected my 2-month-old with poison to prevent him from getting diarrhea? I was livid. And, of course, they told me that he might have diarrhea for the next 5-7 days! Can you believe that? I could've refused the shot and only risked a possibility of diarrhea instead of injecting him with something that will surely give it to him."[88]

In developed regions of the world, like the U.S. and Europe, most cases of rotavirus are mild enough that parents can care for their babies at home.[89] In poorer countries where diarrhea is the leading cause of child mortality, oral rehydration therapy (ORT) has proved to be quite successful. Case studies in Brazil, Egypt, Mexico and the Philippines confirm that increased use of ORT coincides with significant drops in mortality. In fact, according to a recent report on reducing deaths from diarrhea, published in the *Bulletin of the World Health Organization,* "With adequate political will and financial support, cost-effective interventions other than immunization can be successfully delivered by national programs."[90]

Human Papilloma Virus (HPV)
"Cervical Cancer Vaccine"

What is HPV?

Human Papilloma Virus (HPV) is a relatively common sexually transmitted disease passed on through genital contact, usually by sexual intercourse.

What are the symptoms of HPV?

There are more than 100 subtypes of HPV. Some forms of the virus can cause warts (papillomas), which may appear on a woman's cervix, vagina or vulva. Other forms of the virus can cause abnormal cell growth on the lining of the cervix—cervical dysplasia—that years later can turn into cancer. However, in more than 90 percent of cases the infections are harmless and go away without treatment. The body's own defense system eliminates the virus. Often, women experience no signs, symptoms or health problems.[1,2]

Who is most susceptible to HPV and cervical cancer?

People who begin having sex at an early age, who have many sex partners, or who have sex with somebody who has had many partners, are at greatest risk of contracting HPV.[3] In addition, U.S. black women have a 50 percent higher incidence rate than U.S. white women. Hispanic women in the United States have a 66 percent higher incidence rate when compared with non-Hispanic U.S. women.[4]

How prevalent and serious is cervical cancer?

The American Cancer Society (ACS) estimated that in 2007 about 11,150 cases of cervical cancer would be diagnosed in the United States (up 15 percent from the previous year) and about 3,670 women would die from the disease.[5] However, 2007 was an anomaly; cervical cancer incidence and death rates have consistently declined over the past 30 years. In 1975, 14.8 women (per 100,000 U.S. population) contracted the disease and 5.6 (per 100,000) died from it. By 2004, these figures had fallen by more than half: an incidence rate of 7.0 and a death rate of 2.4 (Figure 75).[6,7] These figures are even lower in women under 50 years of age: a 5.4 incidence rate and 1.3 death rate.[8] Some experts attribute this declining death rate to the widespread use of the Pap test which detects cervical abnormalities in the early stages. When detected at an early stage, invasive cervical cancer is one of the most successfully treated cancers.[9-11]

The median age of women when they are initially diagnosed with cervical cancer is 48 years.[12] About 85 percent of all new cases occur in women 35 years of age and older. More than half of all cervical cancer deaths occur in women 55 years of age and older. New cervical cancer cases and deaths are uncommon below the age of 35 and nearly nonexistent before the age of 20.[13,14]

The cervical cancer *incidence* rate begins to rise in women who are between 20 and 39 years of age, peaks at 40 to 69 years of age, then slightly tapers off in older age groups. For example, of all American women between the ages of 20 and 24, less than 2 per 100,000 are diagnosed with the disease. By contrast, of all U.S. women between the ages of 40 and 44, nearly 16 per 100,000 are diagnosed with cervical cancer. By 85 years of age, this figure drops to 11 per 100,000. The cervical cancer *death* rate is very low in younger age groups but steadily increases in older age groups. For example, cervical cancer deaths are virtually nonexistent in females less than 20 years of age. However, approximately 4 out of every 100,000 women between 45 and 49 years of age will die from the disease. This figure doubles by the time women reach their eighties.[15]

Cervical cancer is increasingly more prevalent in older age groups. Just 9 percent of all cases are in females less than 40 years of age. Only 1 percent of all cases are in females below 30 years of age. More than half of all cases are in women 60 years of age and older, while 73 percent of all cases are in women 50 years of age and older (Figure 76).[16]

Figure 75:

Declining Cervical Cancer
Incidence and Death Rates: 1975-2004

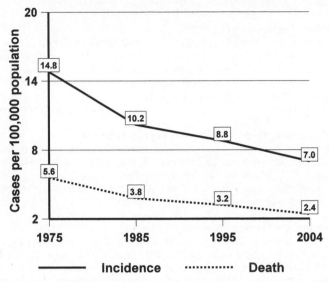

Cervical cancer incidence and death rates have consistently declined over the past 30 years. In 1975, 14.8 women (per 100,000 U.S. population) contracted the disease and 5.6 (per 100,000) died from it. By 2004, these figures had fallen by more than half: an incidence rate of 7.0 and a death rate of 2.4. Rates are even lower in women under 50 years of age: a 5.4 incidence rate and 1.3 death rate. Source: National Cancer Institute.

Cervical cancer is not as common as other cancers. In 2003, there were 14.4 cases of skin cancer per 100,000 population, nearly twice the rate of cervical cancer. Rates for colon cancer, lung cancer and breast cancer were even higher. In fact, women are nearly 15 times more likely to be stricken with breast cancer than cervical cancer (Figure 77).[17]

Does an HPV vaccine exist?
On June 8, 2006, the U.S. Food and Drug Administration (FDA) approved a new HPV vaccine—Gardasil® —for 9- to 26-year-old girls and women.[18] A few weeks later, the CDC's Advisory Committee on Immunization Practices (ACIP), which determines vaccine schedules in the U.S., voted to recommend that all girls ages 11 and 12 receive Merck's new vaccine.[19] This vaccine was licensed for boys, for genital warts, in 2009. Gardasil is designed to protect against four of the more than 100 different HPV strains (Figure 78).[20,21] It is given as a three dose series costing $120 per dose, or $360 for the complete set of shots.[22] Another HPV vaccine—Cervarix®—developed by a British manufacturer, was tested in older women and gained FDA approval in October 2009.[23] In 2014, the FDA licensed Gardasil 9, Merck's latest HPV vaccine.

How safe is the HPV vaccine?
According to the vaccine manufacturer, the HPV vaccine contains "virus-like particles of the major capsid protein of HPV Types 6, 11, 16 and 18." Each dose also contains 9.56mg of sodium chloride, .78mg of L-histidine, 50mcg of polysorbate 80, 35mcg of

Figure 76:

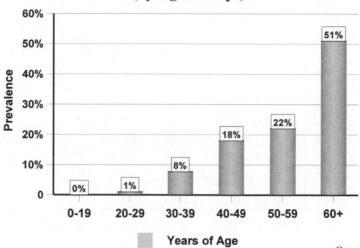

**Cervical Cancer Prevalence
(by Age Groups)**

Copyright © NZM

Cervical cancer is increasingly more prevalent in older age groups. Just 9 percent of all cases are in females less than 40 years of age. Only 1 percent of all cases are in females below 30 years of age. More than half of all cases are in women 60 years of age and older, while 73 percent of all cases are in women 50 years of age and older. Source: National Cancer Institute.

---

sodium borate, and "approximately 225mcg of aluminum (as amorphous aluminum hydroxyphosphate sulfate adjuvant)."[24] That's almost twice as much aluminum per dose as can be found in the pneumococcal vaccine.[25] Aluminum is neurotoxic—capable of damaging the nervous system—even in very small amounts, and has a long history of known and documented health hazards.[26,27] Studies have shown that aluminum in vaccines can enter the brain.[28,29] Aluminum may also cause inflammation at the injection site presaging chronic muscle fatigue and joint pain.[30,31] In fact, the American Academy of Pediatrics—the authoritative medical organization that promotes vaccines—recently acknowledged that "aluminum is now being implicated as interfering with a variety of cellular and metabolic processes in the nervous system and in other tissues."[32] (For more information about aluminum, read *Aluminum in Vaccines* on page 175, and see *Appendix II* on page 308.)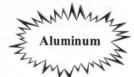

In clinical trials designed to test the safety and efficacy of the HPV vaccine, the FDA allowed the manufacturer to compare women who received the experimental vaccine (which contains aluminum) to women who received "placebo" injections containing aluminum. These aluminum-containing injections are not true placebos, which should be harmless substances. This tactic deceptively improves safety data by making the vaccine appear less reactive than it really is.[33] Nevertheless, 93 percent of the women who received the HPV vaccine reported one or more adverse events within 15 days of vaccination; just 7 percent of the vaccine recipients reported *no* adverse event.[34] Furthermore, a higher percentage of women in the vaccine group (versus those in the placebo group) "did not complete the vaccination series or withdrew shortly thereafter suggesting that the vaccine may have been associated with reduced tolerability."[35]

Figure 77:

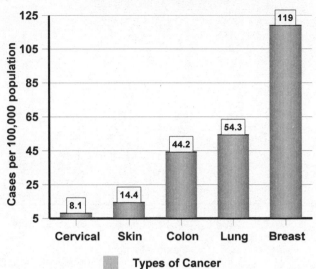

**Cervical Cancer Rates
Compared to Other Cancers**

Cervical cancer is not as common as other types of cancer. For example, in 2003 there were 14.4 cases of skin cancer per 100,000 population, nearly twice the rate of cervical cancer. Rates for colon cancer, lung cancer and breast cancer were even higher. In fact, women are nearly 15 times more likely to be stricken with breast cancer than with cervical cancer. Source: CDC—United States Cancer Statistics.

HPV vaccine and birth defects: In FDA documents that were released just three weeks before this vaccine was approved, it was discovered that five women who received the vaccine around the time of conception gave birth to children with birth defects. According to the manufacturer, "For pregnancies with estimated onset within 30 days of vaccination, 5 cases of congenital anomaly were observed in the group that received Gardasil compared to 0 cases of congenital anomaly in the group that received placebo. The congenital anomalies seen in pregnancies with estimated onset within 30 days of vaccination included pyloric stenosis, congenital megacolon, congenital hydronephrosis, hip dysplasia and club foot."[36-38]

HPV vaccine and breastfeeding: The vaccine manufacturer warns breastfeeding mothers that "it is not known whether vaccine antigens or antibodies induced by the vaccine are excreted in human milk. Because many drugs are excreted in human milk, caution should be exercised when Gardasil is administered to a nursing woman."[39] In fact, in pre-licensure trials of the HPV vaccine, nearly twice as many infants of mothers who received Gardasil and breastfed their babies had a "serious adverse experience" as compared to infants whose mothers received placebo. Three times as many breastfeeding infants whose mothers received Gardasil had "acute respiratory illnesses within 30 days post-vaccination of the mother" as compared to infants whose mothers received placebo.[40]

Additional pre-licensure safety issues: The FDA documents also revealed another concern: Women who are already infected by one of the four targeted HPV types when they're given the vaccine may have *greater* likelihoods of exhibiting precursors to cancer.[41] Yet, the FDA is not requiring vaccine providers to screen women for these viral infections

Figure 78:

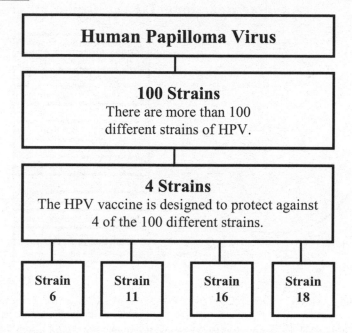

The HPV vaccine, Gardasil®, is designed to protect against 4 of the more than 100 different strains capable of causing HPV infection. Strains 6 and 11 are associated with genital warts; strains 16 and 18 are associated with pre-malignant lesions. Source: The vaccine manufacturer's package inserts.

prior to administering the shot. (This topic is covered in more detail in the section on HPV vaccine efficacy.) Pre-licensure studies of Gardasil also revealed that nine women who received the vaccine developed arthritis compared to only two cases among the placebo group. One woman who received the vaccine developed pancreatic cancer. There were 17 deaths during the clinical trials as well, but these were dismissed by clinical trial investigators as unrelated to the shots.[42]

Post-marketing Safety Issues

By February 13, 2017, ten-and-a-half years after the HPV vaccine was licensed in the U.S., 46,232 adverse reaction reports pertaining to Gardasil were filed with the federal government —an average of 11.8 reports per day. Nearly 30% of all reports required an emergency room visit, with thousands of teenage girls and young women needing to be hospitalized. The substance of these reports was made available through the Freedom of Information Act.[43-45] According to Tom Fitton of Judicial Watch, a government watchdog organization, they "read like a catalog of horrors."[46] In the case reports submitted to the FDA, 287 deaths were described due to blood clots, heart disease and other causes. In addition, many of the vaccine recipients were stricken with serious and life-threatening disabilities, including Guillain-Barré syndrome, myalgia, paresthesia, loss of consciousness, seizures, convulsions, swollen body parts, chest pain, heart irregularities, kidney failure, visual disturbances, arthritis, difficulty breathing, severe rashes, persistent vomiting, miscarriages, menstrual irregularities, reproductive system complications, genital warts, vaginal lesions and HPV infection—the main reason to vaccinate (Figure 79).[47]

<u>Figure 79:</u>

Adverse Reactions: HPV Vaccine

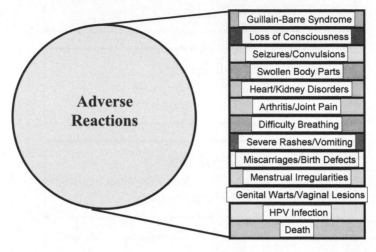

Between June 2006 and February 2017, the FDA received 46,232 adverse reaction reports pertaining to Gardasil. Many of the vaccine recipients were stricken with serious and life-threatening disabilities, including Guillain-Barré syndrome, myalgia, paresthesia, loss of consciousness, seizures, convulsions, swollen body parts, chest pain, heart irregularities, kidney failure, visual disturbances, arthritis, joint pain, difficulty breathing, severe rashes, persistent vomiting, miscarriages, menstrual irregularities, reproductive system complications, genital warts, vaginal lesions and HPV infection. Many of these teenage girls and young women were rushed to the hospital for debilitating ailments following their Gardasil shots; 287 deaths were recorded. (Although the reports appear to implicate the HPV vaccine in a variety of adverse reactions, definitive causation has not been established.) Source: FDA—Vaccine Adverse Event Reporting System (VAERS).

It should be noted that although the reports appear to implicate the HPV vaccine in a variety of adverse reactions, definitive causation has not been established. Conversely, it should also be noted that a confidential study conducted by a major vaccine manufacturer indicated that "a fifty-fold underreporting of adverse events" is likely.[48] In other words, perhaps only 2 percent of all adverse reactions are revealed. Thus, more than one million teens and young women could have been hurt by Gardasil during the ten-and-a-half year period between June 2006 and February 2017.

The case reports on the following pages were taken directly from the FDA's Vaccine Adverse Event Reporting System (VAERS).[49] They are organized by the type of debility sufferers experienced after their shots, and represent just a small sample of the potential HPV vaccine damage being inflicted on our young, vulnerable, female (and male) members of society. (Case numbers precede report summaries.)

Guillain Barré syndrome/myalgia/paresthesia: Guillain-Barré syndrome (GBS) is a serious disorder in which the body's immune system attacks the peripheral nervous system. Symptoms begin with tingling sensations in the legs, arms, and upper body. As the disease progresses, the muscles weaken or can no longer be used, there is a loss of mobility, and in severe cases, the individual may be paralyzed. Authorities have known for many years that vaccines can cause GBS.[50-52]

The technical definition of myalgia is muscle pain. However, when a person is "unable to sit up or walk," as described in case #276540 below, a diagnosis of myalgia may be incorrect and GBS could be the true infirmity. Paresthesia is an abnormal sensation, such as numbness, tingling or burning on the skin. The three seemingly separate terms may simply define gradations of a single, underlying neuromuscular debility. Several case reports in this category follow:

▶ 275639: A 9-year-old girl experienced bone pain, myalgia and tendonitis eight days after receiving her second dose of Gardasil. Emergency room care was required.

▶ 268143: A 13-year-old girl received the Gardasil vaccine and nine days later was hospitalized with "ascending weakness bilaterally, upper and lower extremities." She was diagnosed by a neurologist with Guillain-Barré syndrome.

▶ 276255: A 14-year-old teenager was vaccinated with Gardasil. According to her pediatric physician, she subsequently developed GBS and required hospitalization.

▶ 276540: A 15-year-old girl developed severe myalgia 11 days after receiving Gardasil. She was unable to sit up or walk. She also had a flushing rash, fever, nausea and diarrhea. Hospital care was required. Her condition was reported as serious and life-threatening.

▶ 276081: A 15-year old girl was vaccinated with Gardasil and developed "sciatic neuropathy." The physician noted that she had weakness in the left leg and loss of deep tendon reflex at the ankle. She also had sensory complaints, a limp and could no longer participate in physical activities. This was a permanent disability. Hospital care was required.

▶ 265839: A 16-year-old female was vaccinated with the first dose of HPV. She subsequently developed lower extremity weakness and was hospitalized with GBS.

▶ 277814: A 16-year-old teenager was vaccinated with Gardasil. The following day, she had "progressive bilateral numbness" and motor weakness. Her condition was reported as Guillain-Barré syndrome and hypoaesthesia.

▶ 277114: A 16-year-old teenager "collapsed, experienced weakness, sensory loss in extremities, and could not walk" after receiving Gardasil. Her adverse reaction was listed as a serious, permanent disability and required an extended hospital stay.

▶ 277667: Within a few hours after receiving her second dose of Gardasil, an 18-year-old female felt numbness and paralysis on the right side of her face. She was diagnosed with Bell's palsy. Emergency room care was required.

▶ 277106: Minutes after receiving Gardasil, an 18-year-old female experienced tingling and numbness on the left side of her face, reported as facial hypoaesthesia and paresthesia.

▶ 277584: An 18-year-old female received her first dose of Gardasil. Over the next several days and weeks, she developed muscle spasms, muscular weakness, musculoskeletal discomfort and pain.

▶ 276531: A 25-year-old woman developed Bell's palsy on the left side of her face after being vaccinated with Gardasil. Emergency room care was required.

▶ 278267: A 26-year-old woman was vaccinated with a second dose of Gardasil, immediately experienced left arm pain, nausea, dizziness, and loss of appetite. The following day, she had pain in her left arm that radiated down to her hand. Her fingers were weak and she was unable to use her hand. The pain radiated to her left leg and was disabling.

▶ 277130: A 26-year-old woman experienced myalgia seven days after receiving a second dose of Gardasil. The extreme pain in her muscle was described as a level 10 on a scale of 1 to 10. She required emergency room care.

Loss of consciousness/fainting/syncope: Many of the reports indicate that girls are fainting after receiving the shot. Some of them are losing consciousness and hitting their heads on tabletops and other nearby objects.

▶ 277597: An 11-year-old girl fainted in the doctor's office 10 minutes after receiving her first dose of Gardasil. She was taken to the emergency room.

▶ 274744: A 12-year-old girl received Gardasil and fainted as she was leaving the doctor's office. She hit her head when she fell and was taken to the hospital for a CAT scan because she was experiencing bad headaches.

▶ 262242: A 14-year-old girl received Gardasil, lost consciousness, fell and hit her nose on a drawer. She was transported to the hospital with a broken nose.

▸ 276064: A 15-year-old girl passed out in the hallway after receiving Gardasil.

▸ 277187: A 16-year-old teen received her first dose of Gardasil, fainted, fell to the floor, and hit her head causing an injury. She stopped hearing and saw everything white.

▸ 277498: A 16-year-old female received her HPV vaccine, lost consciousness and sustained a head injury. She was taken to the emergency room.

▸ 275993: A 16-year-old teenager was vaccinated with Gardasil. About 15 minutes later she felt dizzy, passed out, "hitting her face and head as she fell." She was rushed to the hospital for emergency care.

▸ 277669: After receiving her first dose of Gardasil, a 17-year-old teenager fainted. She felt tingling in her legs and arms, and was very dizzy. She was white in the face. The young lady was given smelling salts, and laid down for an hour, but complained of her legs feeling heavy. She had to be wheeled out to her car. The patient required an emergency room visit. Her adverse reaction was reported as paresthesia, syncope, dizziness and fatigue.

▸ 276220: A 17-year-old teenager developed a headache and fainted after being injected with her second dose of Gardasil. She was taken to the hospital.

▸ 276218: An 18-year-old female lost consciousness and hit her head after receiving her first dose of Gardasil. She was taken to the hospital.

▸ 275444: A 19-year-old girl passed out after receiving Gardasil. For 1½ hours, her blood pressure remained too low to get up off the floor.

▸ 275915: A 19-year-old student received her third dose of Gardasil, returned to her dorm, and lost consciousness in the dorm bathroom causing a head laceration. Emergency room care was required.

▸ 274598: A 21-year-old female received Gardasil, fainted, hit her head on the floor and suffered a concussion. She was rushed to an emergency room in an ambulance.

▸ 276042: A 22-year-old female passed out, fell and hit her head approximately 10 minutes after receiving Gardasil. About 20 minutes later, she became anxious and confused, and started crying. She was transported to the hospital with a possible concussion.

▸ 274582: A 25-year-old woman was vaccinated with Gardasil. Later that evening she passed out, fell to the floor and hit her head. Emergency room care was required.

Seizures/convulsions: A seizure is a neurological disorder with abnormal electrical impulses in the brain. There is often a loss of consciousness with twitching and shaking of the body. Staring spells and visual disturbances are common. Convulsions are a pathological condition causing the body to shake spasmodically and uncontrollably. The person's muscles violently contract and relax.

▸ 277575: A 13-year-old girl received her first dose of Gardasil, complained of an upset stomach, then passed out. Her eyes rolled back in her head and she began twitching. She would not regain consciousness nor respond to verbal stimulation. 911 was called and she was transported to the hospital. Her condition was labeled life-threatening.

▸ 275112: A doctor reported that his 13-year-old patient received Gardasil and within three minutes lost consciousness and experienced a seizure lasting two minutes.

▸ 276530: A 14-year-old girl fell to the floor in a seizure-like state after receiving the HPV vaccine. She was taken to the emergency room.

▸ 274941: A 15-year-old girl lost consciousness and had tonic convulsions approximately 5-10 minutes after receiving her first dose of Gardasil.

▸ 276314: A 16-year-old female received Gardasil and developed seizures within 15-20 minutes. 911 was called and the girl was taken to the hospital.

▸ 277665: A 16-year-old teenager had a seizure and lost consciousness after receiving her first dose of Gardasil.

▸ 277995: Approximately 5 minutes after receiving Gardasil, a 16-year-old girl fainted and had a seizure. It was reported as a convulsion.

▸ 277788: A 16-year-old teenager received her second dose of the HPV vaccine. Three days later, she had her first seizure and was taken to the emergency room. She was then admitted to the hospital that evening with a Grand Mal seizure.

▸ 277167: A physician reported that his female teen patient had a convulsion almost immediately after receiving Gardasil. She convulsed in front of the physician and her eyes rolled back. She required an emergency room visit. The doctor reported that another patient in the same age group also convulsed after receiving Gardasil.

▶ 277113: A 16-year-old female was vaccinated with Gardasil and immediately complained of pain and paresthesia in her arm. Ten minutes later, she experienced syncope with a tonic convulsion. She was hospitalized.

▶ 275798: A 19-year-old female received her first dose of Gardasil, lost consciousness "and had a seizure for about 10 minutes." She was rushed to the hospital in an ambulance.

▶ 277326: A 23-year-old female received her second dose of Gardasil. Three hours later, she fainted twice and had her first seizure. She had a second seizure 12 hours later.

▶ 275704: A 24-year-old woman was vaccinated with her first dose of Gardasil at 8:30 in the morning. A 7 o'clock that evening she had a seizure while driving. Emergency room care was required.

Swollen body parts/soreness:

▶ 277351: A 13-year-old girl received her first dose of Gardasil. A few hours later her entire arm, including the fingers, swelled up. She had not recovered two weeks later.

▶ 277000: Within one hour of receiving Gardasil, a 17-year-old teenage girl developed red and swollen hands and feet, lasting several hours.

▶ 277677: A 21-year-old female received the HPV vaccine. The next day, she awoke with a swollen, red face and red spots all over both legs. She was taken to the hospital.

▶ 276262: A 22-year-old woman developed severe urticaria (an allergic skin condition characterized by red, itchy, burning wheals) and experienced life-threatening angioedema of the throat starting 24 hours after receiving Gardasil. She had two hospital visits and needed high-dose steroids to control the adverse reaction. The problem lasted 10 days.

Chest pain/heart irregularities:

▶ 277813: A 16-year-old teenager received her first dose of Gardasil. Later that day, she experienced back pain, chest pain, a cardiac murmur, vertigo, nausea and difficulty breathing. She was taken to the hospital by ambulance.

▶ 276755: A 16-year-old teenager received Gardasil and developed a rapid heartbeat with dizziness and nausea.

▶ 274775: A 16-year-old teenager developed tachycardia (a racing heart) after receiving the HPV vaccine. She also experienced nausea, night sweats, insomnia, and missed several days of school due to her symptoms.

▶ 277776: A 17-year-old teenager experienced chest pain for four days, starting five days after Gardasil vaccination.

▶ 274972: A 17-year-old teenager developed chest pain a few hours after receiving her first dose of Gardasil. She required emergency room care.

Kidney failure:

▶ 277403: A 12-year-old girl had "a complete kidney failure" and was taken to the hospital a few days after receiving Gardasil.

▶ 275111: A 13-year-old girl developed blood in her stool approximately three days after receiving her second dose of Gardasil. She was admitted to the hospital where she was diagnosed with "acute kidney failure." Her condition was reported as a permanent disability that was immediately life-threatening.

Eye disorders:

▶ 275989: A 16-year-old teenager developed optic neuritis, blurred vision and double vision, ten days after receiving the HPV vaccine. She spent five days in the hospital under the care of a retinologist.

▶ 277994: One week after being vaccinated with Gardasil, a 17-year-old teenager developed bilateral uveitis.

▶ 274711: A registered nurse reported that her 17-year-old daughter developed uveitis with photosensitivity and an itchy rash on her arms, legs and trunk three weeks after receiving the HPV vaccine.

Arthritis/joint pain/arthralgia:

▸ 275151: A 16-year-old teenager was taken to the emergency room with juvenile rheumatoid arthritis after receiving Gardasil.

▸ 275250: A physician reported that his 18-year-old daughter received Gardasil. Three days later, her legs became sore and her knees and ankles began to hurt. She was unable to attend school because she could no longer walk normally, and was "walking like an old lady" with pain in her extremities. Her condition was reported as a serious and permanent disability that required hospital care.

▸ 277744: A 19-year-old female developed arthralgia of the hands and wrists, knee and ankle pain, fatigue, and flu-like symptoms, starting 2-3 weeks after HPV vaccination.

▸ 277430: A 22-year-old female developed joint pain and muscle aches starting two days after receiving her first HPV vaccine. The arthralgia and myalgia continued for at least six weeks. She was instructed not to receive additional doses of Gardasil.

▸ 277664: A physician's 23-year-old daughter experienced disabling joint pain and arthralgia in her knees and wrists after receiving the full series of Gardasil. The pain was causing the woman significant disability because she could not participate in former activities. Emergency room care was required.

▸ 276255: A 27-year-old woman developed arthralgia and neck pain after receiving her second dose of Gardasil. She refused to take the third dose.

▸ 277235: A 52-year-old woman received her second dose of Gardasil and needed to be taken to the emergency room with swollen joints in her hands, and extreme pain. She was diagnosed with rheumatoid arthritis.

Labored breathing/wheezing:

▸ 275584: A 16-year-old teenager received Gardasil. On the following day, she developed tightness in her chest and shortness of breath, along with swelling and pain at the injection site, and facial redness. The young lady was transported by ambulance to the emergency room where they administered oxygen, epinephrine and prednisone. Her reaction was reported as serious and life-threatening.

▸ 275510: A 17-year-old girl received her first dose of Gardasil. Fifteen minutes later, she had "an intense global feeling" in her throat and felt like she couldn't breathe. She was treated with corticosteroids and hospitalized for two days.

▸ 277657: An 18-year-old female could not swallow or breathe after receiving her first dose of Gardasil.

▸ 277402: A 21-year-old woman received her first dose of Gardasil and experienced tightness in her throat, difficulty swallowing, shortness of breath, diarrhea and headache. She required emergency room care.

▸ 277902: One day after a 22-year-old female received Gardasil, the injection site was red, swollen and puffy. Three days later, she called the doctor's office saying she had not felt good since the injection. Her throat was swollen and she was having trouble breathing. She complained of a stuffy nose, sore throat, ears aching and ringing in the ears. She wanted to "pull her hair out" because of the ringing in her ears. She was taken to the hospital. Her adverse reaction were disabling because she could not return to school or work. It was also reported as life-threatening. She had not recovered three weeks later.

▸ 276131: A physician reported that his female patient experienced shortness of breath and bronchospasm after being vaccinated with Gardasil.

Rashes/itching/hives:

▸ 277195: A 12-year-old girl developed hives on her arm and trunk 3 hours after receiving her second dose of Gardasil. It was reported as urticaria.

▸ 276135: A 13-year-old girl received her first dose of Gardasil and subsequently developed a rash on her arm and face that eventually spread to the rest of her body. She was diagnosed with allergic dermatitis and pityriasis rosea. Another female in her school class also experienced allergic dermatitis and pityriasis rosea after vaccination with Gardasil.

▸ 277112: A 17-year-old teenager received her second dose of Gardasil. She immediately had injection site swelling. Within two weeks, her arm became "scabby, scaly and bigger."

She then developed a severe rash with itching that spread to her whole body and face. The young lady visited a dermatology office where the nurse indicated that the rash "looked like a sunburn that had peeled, was swollen, flaked and scabbed." Hospital care was required. This adverse reaction was reported as serious and disabling.

▸ 276125: A 17-year-old teenager received her first dose of Gardasil. Four days later, she developed a red, itchy rash on the upper body, from the waist up. Emergency room care was required.

▸ 274732: A 17-year-old teenager developed red, painful lesions on her feet two days after HPV vaccination. Hospital care was required.

▸ 277458: A 21-year-old woman received the HPV vaccine. The following day, she developed itching and a rash on her chest. She was also nauseous, dizzy and fatigued. Emergency room care was required.

▸ 276349: A 21-year-old female broke out in an itchy rash on her arms, chest and neck three days after being vaccinated against HPV.

▸ 278066: A 24-year-old woman started itching on the buttocks after HPV vaccination. The itching spread to her abdomen and thighs.

▸ 276249: A couple of days after receiving Gardasil, a female patient developed "a flesh-colored, dry, flaky, itchy rash on her face" that lasted for five days.

▸ 276163: After her first and second doses of Gardasil, a female patient developed an extensive rash on her face. Emergency room care was required.

Severe vomiting:

▸ 276142: A 16-year-old female developed nausea and vomited for 14 hours after receiving her third dose of Gardasil. Emergency room care was required.

▸ 276134: A licensed practical nurse (LPN) reported that her 16-year-old daughter "experienced nausea and vomiting that lasted for several days" after her first and second doses of Gardasil.

▸ 276240: A 17-year-old teenager received her first dose of Gardasil. She experienced extreme nausea, diarrhea and dizziness after the injection. The young lady "was vomiting so hard that the blood vessels in her eyes broke." Emergency room care was required.

▸ 277751: A 25-year-old woman received the HPV shot and experienced persistent vomiting for several hours, requiring emergency room care.

Emotional/mood changes:

▸ 277305: A 17-year-old girl became agitated and emotional after receiving her second dose of Gardasil. She sobbed for nearly 3 hours.

▸ 277241: A 20-year-old female experienced a depressed mood and fatigue that lasted four days after receiving her first dose of Gardasil.

Miscarriages/abortion: Although Gardasil is not recommended for use in pregnant women, many pregnant women accidentally receive the shot. Some of these women have miscarriages shortly thereafter. Other women elect to have abortions. One wonders whether they have been counseled against giving birth due to the vaccine's possible association with birth defects.

▸ 274755: A 15-year-old girl was vaccinated with Gardasil during pregnancy and elected to have an abortion.

▸ 277668: A 16-year-old girl was vaccinated with Gardasil when she was 5 weeks pregnant. Seven weeks later she had a miscarriage.

▸ 278130: A 17-year-old girl was vaccinated with Gardasil when she was 18 weeks pregnant. She elected to have an abortion.

▸ 274219: A 17-year-old was vaccinated with Gardasil when she was about one week pregnant. A subsequent ultrasound revealed that the fetus was positive for neural tube defect (a serious birth defect of the brain and spinal cord).

▸ 277666: A 19-year-old female received her first and second doses of Gardasil when she was pregnant. She elected to have an abortion.

▸ 274942: A 19-year-old female was vaccinated with her first dose of Gardasil during

pregnancy and had a spontaneous abortion two weeks later.
  ▸ 274938: A 20-year-old female was vaccinated with her first dose of Gardasil during pregnancy and had a spontaneous abortion ten days later.
  ▸ 275779: A 23-year-old woman was vaccinated with Gardasil during pregnancy and had a miscarriage.
  ▸ 275630: A 24-year-old woman was vaccinated with Gardasil during pregnancy. After the shot, she had an appointment with her obstetrician/gynecologist who was unable to detect a fetal heartbeat. (The woman stated that her physician advised her to continue the injections with Gardasil, but she refused.)
  ▸ 277166: A 26-year-old woman received Gardasil when she was pregnant. Nine days later, she had a spontaneous abortion with an emergency D & C hemorrhage. She was hospitalized. This event was reported as life-threatening.
  ▸ 274754: A 26-year-old woman was vaccinated with her second dose of Gardasil during pregnancy and had a miscarriage.
  ▸ 275702: A physician reported that his teenage patient received Gardasil during pregnancy and had a spontaneous abortion.

Menstrual irregularities:
  ▸ 274718: A mother reported that after her 11-year-old daughter was vaccinated with Gardasil, her next menses was longer than usual, lasting six days (instead of three days). In addition, it was "very heavy and had a foul odor."
  ▸ 274291: A young girl received Gardasil and subsequently had her first menstrual cycle which was "extremely heavy." Emergency room care was required.
  ▸ 272865: A 13-year-old girl developed vaginal hemorrhage after Gardasil.
  ▸ 274738: A 13-year-old girl had a delayed menstruation after receiving Gardasil.
  ▸ 274573: A 13-year-old girl received Gardasil and developed vaginal bleeding that varied from light to heavy and has been continuous since the date of vaccine administration. Emergency room care was required.
  ▸ 274729: A 14-year-old girl experienced dizziness, anemia, and "heavy menstrual cycles" ever since receiving the HPV vaccine. Emergency room care was required.
  ▸ 276237: A 22-year-old female received her first dose of Gardasil. Subsequently, her menstrual cycle did not arrive on time. Her menstruation lasted for two weeks and was a heavier flow. Her menstrual cycle ended, then started again. After her second dose of the HPV vaccine, her menstrual cycle arrived on time but was a heavier flow. Emergency room care was required.

Reproductive system complications:
  ▸ 274612: A 12-year-old girl developed an ovarian cyst that ruptured ten days after receiving the first dose of Gardasil. Initially, the young lady started vomiting for a few days and then there was significant abdominal pain. Her condition was reported as a serious and permanent disability.
  ▸ 275701: A 13-year-old girl received Gardasil. Later that same month, she developed polycystic ovaries and a peritoneal abscess 10 centimeters in diameter. The condition was reported as serious and required hospitalization.
  ▸ 276564: A 17-year-old female developed "dysfunctional uterine bleeding" after receiving the HPV vaccine.

HPV/genital warts/vaginal lesions:
  ▸ 276147: A 15-year-old sexually *inactive* teenager developed "labia lesions" soon after receiving the HPV vaccine. This adverse reaction was reported as a "vulval disorder" and required emergency room care.
  ▸ 276165: A 16-year-old girl received her first dose of the HPV vaccine. Eleven days later, she was tested for HPV and the Pap smear results were positive for high-risk HPV. Emergency room care was required.
  ▸ 275705: A gynecologist reported that his 17-year-old patient developed "severe herpes simplex genitalis" and a "superinfection" after she received the HPV vaccine.

The patient experienced vulval pustules and vaginal inflammation. This condition was considered serious and the young lady was hospitalized.

▸ 276222: A pharmacist reported that his 19-year-old daughter received her first dose of the HPV vaccine. She then had a routine Pap test which revealed abnormal cells. Emergency room care was required.

▸ 274970: A 19-year-old female developed herpes simplex fever blisters in her mouth after receiving the HPV vaccine.

▸ 267418: A 22-year-old woman received all three doses of Gardasil and subsequently tested positive for high-risk HPV.

▸ 275392: A 23-year-old woman developed venereal warts in her rectal region within three weeks of being vaccinated with Gardasil. She had no exposure there.

▸ 276236: A 24-year-old woman received her first dose of the HPV vaccine. Ten days later, she developed lesions on her vagina, diagnosed as genital warts.

▸ 271148: A 25-year-old woman received her first dose of Gardasil. Four days later she developed painful genital warts requiring emergency room care.

▸ 276223: A physician reported that his female patient developed genital warts after receiving her second dose of the HPV vaccine.

▸ 276139: A physician reported that his female patient developed "herpetic lesions" around her genital region one week after receiving her second dose of Gardasil. She was diagnosed with a type 1 herpes virus infection.

Additional adverse reactions/multiple debilities:

▸ 276328: A 9-year-old girl received Gardasil. The next morning she awoke with acute torticollis (ironically, also referred to as "cervical dystonia," an extremely painful neurological disorder causing the head to lean to one side, often accompanied by tremors in the head or arms).

▸ 274663: A 9-year-old girl received Gardasil. Twelve days later she developed a fever, sore throat, rash, cyanosis (blue toes), and swollen joints (ankles, elbows, shoulders). She was unable to walk and required hospital care.

▸ 275992: A physician reported that an 11-year-old girl developed Stevens-Johnson syndrome (a potentially deadly skin disease) after Gardasil. She required hospital care.

▸ 276629: A 12 year-old girl became fatigued, nauseated and pallor less than two weeks after receiving Gardasil. Two weeks later, she developed acute onset hemolytic anemia requiring IV steroids and hospitalization. Her condition is serious and life-threatening.

▸ 275740: A 13-year-old girl developed pain in her groin, hip, knee and ankle after her first shot of Gardasil. These conditions severely worsened after her second shot. She also developed headaches, became lightheaded, blacked out in the shower and had episodes of blurred vision. She worked with a physical therapist and orthopedic doctor for six weeks, but had to stop because of her swollen knees and pain. Her next visit was with a rheumatologist. Hospital care was required.

▸ 272720: A 13-year-old girl experienced "internal bleeding throughout her body" after receiving Gardasil. She also had bruising and rectal bleeding. This was reported as a permanent disability, life-threatening, and required hospitalization.

▸ 276118: A 14-year-old girl developed a headache and her arm hurt really bad after being injected with Gardasil. Three days later "everything kind of hurt," she experienced fainting, dizziness, headaches, dehydration, and fluctuating blood pressure. Emergency room care was required.

▸ 276699: A 15-year-old girl received Gardasil and was hospitalized with thrombocytopenia (a blood disorder) two days later.

▸ 275812: A 15-year-old girl received Gardasil and 90 minutes later developed the "worst headache" she ever had, lasting several hours.

▸ 275251: One day after receiving Gardasil, a 17-year-old teenager developed twitching of her whole body that "looked as if she had Tourette's syndrome." As of two weeks post-vaccination there was no improvement. Her condition was reported as a serious and permanent disability requiring hospital care.

▸ 273514: An 18-year-old teenager received her first dose of Gardasil. Eight days later, she developed a mental disorder. She also became overtly sexual, had a "major psychiatric breakdown," and was hospitalized.

▸ 276146: A 21-year-old female received her first dose of Gardasil. Seven days later, she experienced abnormal dizziness, "fuzziness," nausea, and a sensation that she was spinning. She was seen by three doctors and underwent MRI. Her condition was reported as vertigo and required emergency room care.

▸ 276968: A 37-year-old woman developed flu-like symptoms after her first and second doses of Gardasil. She also had arthralgia, myalgia, insomnia, fever, nausea, vomiting, and diarrhea.

▸ 276138: A physician reported that his female patient developed neuropathy after receiving her first dose of Gardasil. She was referred to a neurologist.

▸ 276122: A pediatrician reported that his female patient was vaccinated with Gardasil and subsequently experienced muscle aches and hair loss. These adverse reactions were listed as myalgia and alopecia.

Death:

▸ 275428: A 12-year-old girl died six days after receiving Gardasil along with hepatitis A and chickenpox vaccines. The autopsy revealed myocarditis and ventricular tachycardia.

▸ 282372: A 17-year-old teenager was found unconscious (lifeless) during the evening of the same day that she received her first shot of Gardasil.

▸ 275438: A 19-year-old teenager collapsed and died two weeks after receiving the HPV vaccine. The autopsy revealed large blood clots in the heart.

▸ 275990: A physician's assistant reported that a female patient "died of a blood clot 3 hours after getting the Gardasil vaccine."

Gardasil co-administered with other vaccines: The FDA did *not* require Merck to evaluate the safety of co-administering Gardasil with other vaccines or prescription drugs (except the hepatitis B vaccine).[53] Yet, teenagers are often injected with several vaccines in conjunction with Gardasil. For example, in case #275823 below, the young girl received six vaccine/drugs simultaneously (TDaP is three vaccines). How often do we as adults take six different drugs simultaneously? Would we be more surprised if we did, or did not, have an adverse reaction? Girls who are injected with several vaccines during the same office visit appear to be especially susceptible to post-vaccinal ailments.

▸ 276351: An 11-year-old girl received Gardasil and Menactra (for meningococcal disease). She got down from the exam table, stood up and fell forward, hitting her forehead on the wall. The nurse pivoted her into a chair. The girl's eyes were open, her back was arched, arms straight and "posturing." When she came to, she continued to stare but was not alert. The young lady suffered a head injury.

▸ 275823: An 11-year-old girl received Gardasil along with TDaP, chickenpox and meningococcal vaccines. Nine days later, she developing a rash on the lips of her vagina.

▸ 274635: A 12-year-old girl was vaccinated with Gardasil along with TDaP. The TDaP was given first and the young lady appeared fine. HPV was then given "and within a minute or two, client's chin fell to chest while arm contracted at elbow up off lap. She did not respond to name or shaking of shoulders for approximately one minute, then became aroused, although very confused and unsure where she was. Called out for her mom and asked where she was and said she felt dizzy." She also complained of tingling lips, chills, a "heavy head," and paresthesia in her right arm, both hands and feet. Oxygen was given until the ambulance arrived and took her to the emergency room for additional care.

▸ 278268: A 12-year-old girl was vaccinated with Gardasil, hepatitis A, Hib and meningococcal. The next day, she returned to the doctor with groin pain. Five days later, she developed a headache and rash, and was hospitalized for herpes zoster and viral meningitis.

▸ 277319: A 12-year-old girl received Gardasil and hepatitis A vaccines. She became dizzy and lost consciousness twice within the next 5 minutes. She was taken to the hospital. The manufacturer assessed this case as "medically serious."

▸ 276541: A 12-year-old girl received Gardasil along with the meningococcal vaccine. Approximately 15 minutes later she collapsed and was hospitalized.

▸ 276442: A 13-year-old girl received Gardasil along with the meningococcal vaccine. She went to the waiting room where her brother and sister saw her fall to the floor hitting her head on a wooden play box. They said she just stared, and then her left arm and shoulder started twitching. She was pale, dizzy, and complained of a headache. She was transported to the emergency room in an ambulance.

▸ 277309: A 13-year-old girl received Gardasil along with chickenpox, hepatitis A and meningococcal vaccines. After the shots were given, she turned pale, rigid, and lost consciousness. When she came to, she had a blank stare and no response. She tried to walk, became limp, and needed to be lifted onto a resting platform.

▸ 277457: A 13-year-old girl received Gardasil along with meningococcal and TDaP vaccines. She had an anaphylactic reaction, developed a rash, started wheezing and had a difficult time breathing. She was taken to the hospital.

▸ 277385: A 13-year-old girl received Gardasil along with the hepatitis A and meningococcal vaccines. 17 days later, she was taken to the hospital with hematuria (red blood cells in the urine) and Henoch-Schonlein purpura.

▸ 275712: A 13-year-old girl received Gardasil along with the meningococcal vaccine. Within 10 minutes, she lost consciousness, fell backward and hit her head on the floor. She was hospitalized in intensive care with a "traumatic subarachnoid hemorrhage." Her adverse reaction was reported as life-threatening and required extended hospitalization.

▸ 274336: A 15-year-old teenager received Gardasil along with Menactra. The following day, she developed a headache, fever and vomiting. The second day after vaccination, her left foot became numb and her right hand developed tremors. She also had chest pain. Three days later, she was diagnosed with Guillain-Barré syndrome.

▸ 276352: A 16-year-old female received Gardasil along with the meningococcal vaccine. She left the exam room, then fell over, hit her head and had a tremor. Her eyes remained open with her head arched back and arms shaking.

▸ 276797: A 16-year-old teenager received Gardasil along with TDaP, chickenpox, and meningococcal vaccines. Within one week, the injection sites became red, swollen and painful. Within two weeks of injections, both lips swelled. Within four weeks of injections, her lips cracked, and by the fifth week after injection, she was hospitalized for stomatitis (inflammation of the mouth). She became dehydrated and needed I.V. care. The blister-type lesions spread to the back of the throat.

▸ 277390: A 16-year-old female received Gardasil along with TDaP, hepatitis A and meningococcal vaccines. One hour later, she developed a headache, tightness in her throat, and she started wheezing. In addition, her eyes were swollen and she developed a rash on both wrists. She was taken to the hospital.

▸ 277122: A 17-year-old teenager received Gardasil, along with hepatitis A and meningococcal vaccines. Shortly thereafter, she was found on the floor with clenched fists. When she came to, she complained of dizziness, nausea, and a headache. Her skin was cool and clammy. She began to vomit. When the young lady fell, she hit her head on a cabinet. She was transported to the hospital and diagnosed with a subdural hematoma.

▸ 277815: An 18-year-old received her first dose of Gardasil along with a meningococcal vaccine. She experienced weakness and tingling in her left arm, which spread over the entire length of her arm and also to her jaw. She experienced so much discomfort in her jaw that she had difficulty chewing. She was taken to the emergency room and was diagnosed with muscular weakness and paresthesia.

▸ 276634: An 18-year-old female received Gardasil along with TDaP and MMR vaccines. Within one day, her arm swelled to twice its normal size, she developed a high fever, chills, and hives, had trouble breathing, weakness and difficult ambulation, tachycardia, and severe dizziness.

▸ 276621: An 18-year-old female received Gardasil along with the meningococcal vaccine. The following morning, she started feeling sick. It started with a headache, neck and back pain. By that evening, she was running a high fever, hurting everywhere, with a severe headache. The shot site was about 4 inches in diameter. She was unable to walk without assistance because she was dizzy and lightheaded. She was unable to attend school or work. Her mother is aware of three other students who had reactions to Gardasil.

▸ 276602: An 18-year-old female received Gardasil along with TDaP, hepatitis A and meningococcal vaccines. Five minutes after receiving the HPV shot, she became pale and rigid, her eyes rolled back in her head, and she lost consciousness. When she came to, she had a blank stare.

▸ 274953: An 18-year-old female received Gardasil along with the meningococcal vaccine. She fainted at the clinic, then endured a back ache, headache, fever and "mental status changes." She was hospitalized with carpal pedal spasm, nystagmus, stridor, lack of spontaneous speech, bronchitis and disorders of the nervous system.

HPV vaccine mistakes: The HPV vaccine is often administered incorrectly, for example, during pregnancy. Here are a few other examples:

▸ 276238: A 4-month-old boy was given Gardasil instead of the Hib vaccine. The child experiencing diarrhea for over a week.

▸ 273751: A 4-month-old boy was administered Gardasil. He developed blotching of the skin, fever and vomiting.

▸ 277453: A 12-year-old girl was given two doses of Gardasil simultaneously, one dose in each arm.

▸ 276246: Gardasil was injected into the patient's buttocks, not the arm.

▸ 276152: A 64-year-old man was vaccinated with Gardasil instead of Zostavax (for shingles).

Refusing to report adverse reactions: As noted earlier, vaccine reactions are underreported. One of the main reasons for this is that many doctors refuse to file official adverse reaction reports even though they are legally required by federal law—the National Childhood Vaccine Injury Act of 1986—to do so. Doctors often subvert this law by merely claiming that they didn't feel the shot had anything to do with the injury. For example:

▸ 276124: Information has been received concerning a 15-year-old 'healthy individual' female who was vaccinated with Gardasil, first dose. After receiving the vaccine, the patient experienced swelling and hives in her extremities. The reporting physician's assistant did not want to be contacted for additional information because she does not treat this patient. The treating physician works in the same office as the reporting physician's assistant, but also did not want to be contacted for additional information because 'the physician did not feel the events were related.' The patient's swelling and hives persisted one week post-vaccination and required emergency room care.[54]

Gardasil overseas:
In Australia, Gardasil was given to schoolgirls starting in April of 2007. By the following month, it became evident that Australian teenage girls were being sickened and paralyzed from the shot just like American girls. For example, in one school alone, the Sacred Heart Girls' College, 26 girls were taken to the sick bay after injections. Seven girls were rushed to the hospital.[55] One student, Natasha D'Souza, collapsed and was left paralyzed for six hours. "I couldn't move at all," she said. "There were girls dropping like flies."[56] Other girls fainted, vomited, developed headaches, dizziness and skin rashes. The federal health minister, Tony Abbott, urged parents not to panic. Hospital staff denied that the girls' reactions were related to the shot. Australian Medical Association president, Mukesh Haikerwal, said it was important that girls continue to be vaccinated.[57]

How effective is the HPV vaccine?
Four studies were conducted to assess the efficacy of the HPV vaccine prior to its FDA approval. The first study consisted of 2,392 women 16 to 23 years of age. Approximately half of the women received three doses (at day 0, month 2, and month 6) of an HPV vaccine containing "40mcg of HPV-16 L1 virus-like particles formulated on 225mcg of aluminum adjuvant."[58] The others received three doses of an aluminum-containing placebo. The women were then scheduled for follow-up visits one month after the third vaccination (month 7), six months after the third vaccination (month 12), and every six months thereafter until month 48. (Some women were disqualified from the study much earlier; for example,

if they engaged in sexual intercourse within 48 hours before their month 7 follow-up. Other women withdrew from the program on their own.)[59]

The primary hypothesis stated that the HPV-16 vaccine would reduce HPV-16 infection when compared with the placebo injection. Thus, follow-up visits were designed to check for "persistent HPV-16 infection." A woman met this definition if she was negative for HPV-16 infection on day 0 and at month 7, then subsequently tested positive.[60]

Findings: Authors of the study reported no cases of HPV-16 infection in the group of women who received the vaccine versus 41 cases in the placebo group. As a result, they claimed a vaccine efficacy of 100 percent.[61] However, the primary rationale for vaccinating against HPV-16 infection is to prevent cervical cancer, yet half of all cervical cancers are *not* associated with HPV-16 infection.[62]

Of the 2,392 women enrolled in the study, only 768 of the women who received the vaccine were included in the "primary efficacy analysis." All women who received the entire series of HPV-16 vaccine (at day 0, month 2 and month 6) and then tested positive for HPV-16 infection at their month 7 follow-up *were excluded from the primary analysis.* Yet, the study neglects to tell us exactly how many women in each category (the vaccine group versus the placebo group) were excluded for testing positive at month 7.[63] If a significantly greater number of women who received the vaccine (versus women who received the placebo) were diagnosed with HPV-16 infection at month 7 and excluded from the "primary efficacy analysis" this would seriously compromise the study results. It might even indicate that the vaccine *causes* the disease.

The HPV-16 vaccine study followed women for "a median of 17.4 months" after completion of the vaccine regimen.[64] In other words, the 100 percent efficacy rate published by the study authors and touted by the vaccine manufacturer is predicated on just one-and-a-half years of review. This meager time frame is inadequate to determine a true efficacy rate. It takes many years for cancer to develop. Furthermore, if protection wanes because the HPV vaccine proves to be ineffective over time, booster shots may be recommended.[65]

Although women in the study were followed-up for a median of just 17.4 months, the vaccine manufacturer published altered data in its vaccine inserts, claiming "the median duration of follow-up was 4 years."[66] This is blatantly untrue according to the original study. Why would the vaccine manufacturer conduct such abbreviated follow-ups and then publish false information about it? There are several possibilities: 1) Many people know that short follow-up periods are insignificant and not credible, so the results needed to be "enhanced." 2) The manufacturer is afraid to conduct follow-ups of any significant length because vaccine potency may decline with time prohibiting future claims of "100 percent efficacy." 3) The vaccine manufacturer was in a race with another HPV vaccine manufacturer and rushed the results to be first to market. 4) It was an honest error that slipped past the FDA, CDC, authors of the vaccine study and officials representing the vaccine manufacturer. Clearly, the first three possibilities, with an implied monetary rationale, seem more likely. In fact, Merck said it has plans to lobby states to require the vaccine for all 12-year-old children before they can enter middle school. This will provide the pharmaceutical company with a guaranteed market for its product. According to Eliav Barr, Merck head of clinical development for the vaccine, "To have 100 percent efficacy is something that you have very rarely. We're breaking out the champagne."[67]

Other pre-licensure efficacy studies:

Three additional studies assessed the efficacy of the HPV vaccine against HPV strains 16 and 18 (which together may cause up to 70 percent of cervical cancers), as well as strains 6 and 11 (responsible for about 90 percent of genital wart cases).[68] Once again, the vaccine manufacturer claimed 100 percent efficacy in these studies—even though one of the vaccinated women became infected with high-grade HPV-16 disease, lowering the vaccine efficacy to 98 percent.[69,70] Of course, this high efficacy rate only applies to strains in the vaccine; Gardasil will not prevent infection with HPV types not contained in the vaccine. In fact, *during clinical trials of the vaccine, hundreds of women who received Gardasil contracted HPV disease.*[71,72] Furthermore, the drug maker warns women that "vaccination does not substitute for routine cervical cancer screening."[73]

Regarding the vaccine manufacturer's staggering claim of 100 percent efficacy, it is important to realize that *no actual cases of cervical cancer were prevented in any of the test subjects in any of the clinical studies of the HPV vaccine.* In fact, the FDA admits that "the study period was not long enough for cervical cancer to develop."[74] Instead, all claims for the effectiveness of this vaccine are based on an indirect analysis of efficacy. Scientists presume that certain "surrogate markers" or "precancerous lesions" (known as CIN-2, CIN-3, and AIS) precede cervical cancer. HPV vaccine researchers simply compared the number of these markers in women who received the vaccine to the number of these markers in women who received the placebo.[75] The prevention of these lesions is "believed" to result in the prevention of cervical cancer.[76] Again, no one actually contracted cervical cancer—not in the vaccine group or placebo group—and there is no actual proof to date that even one case of cancer has been, or will be, prevented by this vaccine.

When this vaccine was being assessed for approval, the FDA asked its panel of advisors to rule on whether Gardasil protected against HPV 16 and 18, not whether it specifically prevented cervical cancer.[77] In fact, during pre-licensure studies, *361 women who received at least one shot of Gardasil went on to develop precancerous lesions on their cervixes within three years,* just 14 percent fewer than in the placebo control group.[78] Scott Emerson, a professor of bio-statistics at the University of Washington, sat on the FDA advisory committee. He's not convinced the vaccine is worth the billions of dollars likely to be spent on it in the coming years. "I do believe that Gardasil protects against HPV 16 and 18, but the effect it will have on cervical cancer rates in this country is another question entirely. There is a leap of faith involved."[79]

The HPV vaccine and children:

Although efficacy of the HPV vaccine was evaluated in four clinical studies of women 16 to 26 years of age, the vaccine manufacturer and the FDA were especially interested in marketing this vaccine to young girls. They knew that "prior vaccination strategies have shown that the ideal time to administer any vaccine is before exposure to the infection."[80] With the HPV vaccine, this means that the vaccine should be given before females become sexually active. Furthermore, young girls are much more accessible than women, especially if the vaccine is mandated to enter the 6th or 7th grade. Therefore, in an attempt to "bridge the efficacy" of Gardasil from adult women to young girls, Merck evaluated "geometric mean titers" (GMTs) comparing "anti-HPV responses" in 16- to 23-year-old females with responses in 9- to 15-year-old girls.[81]

Although this "evaluation" or "study" cannot be found in any scientific or medical journal for independent review, one potentially significant observation can be made: 9- to 15-year-old vaccinated girls developed antibody responses to HPV-16 and HPV-18 that were *twice as high* as the levels found in older females.[82] Of course, little girls do not weigh as much as adult women, yet when they go to the doctor's office to receive their Gardasil shots, they will receive the same exact doses as larger women. (High titer levels can be dangerous. For example, in a peer-reviewed study published in *Lancet*, children who were vaccinated with high-titer measles vaccines had significantly higher infection rates—and mortality—than children who received the standard low-titer measles vaccine.)[83]

In this evaluation, the Gardasil manufacturer did not address the high-titer HPV levels but simply noted that 9- to 15 year-old girls developed "non inferior" immune responses when compared to older women, and made the following claim: "On the basis of this immunogenicity bridging, the efficacy of Gardasil in 9- to 15-year-old girls is inferred."[84] The FDA supports this contention by claiming that the vaccine should have similar efficacy in this younger age group.[85]

According to Barbara Loe Fisher, president of the National Vaccine Information Center (NVIC), "Merck and the FDA have not been completely honest with the people about the pre-licensure clinical trials."[86] The NVIC maintains that Merck's clinical trials "did not prove" the HPV vaccine is safe and effective for little girls.[87] In fact, it should be noted that, to date, no peer-reviewed studies have been conducted to determine the *safety* of this vaccine when administered to girls in this younger age group. Reliable statistical data is currently unavailable. The CDC, FDA and vaccine manufacturer will need to wait for *adverse reaction reports* from the parents of these young girls *after* they are injected with this new vaccine. Sadly, adverse reactions to the HPV vaccine in young girls (and females of all ages) are now being reported with great frequency.[88]

Post-marketing efficacy data:

A 2007 study published in the *Journal of the American Medical Association* found that nearly 27 percent of all females between the ages of 14 and 59 tested positive for the presence of human papilloma virus.[89] As a result, the media reported that about one-fourth of all women are infected with HPV and at risk of developing cervical cancer—unless they submit to the new HPV vaccine. However, infection with *high-risk* HPV strains is necessary for the development of cervical cancer. The study clearly noted that very few women are infected with the high-risk strains (16 and 18) included in the vaccine. In fact, the data revealed that just 1.5 percent of women were infected with HPV-16 and less than 1 percent (0.8 percent) were infected with HPV-18.[90] Furthermore, "most women with high-risk HPV on their cervix will not develop cervical cancer."[91] (The low-risk, wart-producing HPV strains 6 and 11, which are also included in the vaccine, were detected in just 1.3 and 0.1 percent of women, respectively.)[92]

Gardasil is being promoted as "100 percent effective." However, this is a deceptive assessment of its true ability to protect against cervical cancer. Early studies merely showed that Gardasil is effective against *just two strains of cancer-causing HPV* (the ones included in the vaccine).[93] Furthermore, the vaccine is only effective against these two strains *in women with no evidence of prior exposure to these two strains*.[94] When *all* of the women who were enrolled in the initial studies are included in the data (not just "virgins" or women with no evidence of prior exposure to HPV 16 and 18) the vaccine is only 44 percent effective against these two strains.[95,96] In another study, the vaccine's efficacy dropped to 39 percent in a population of women who had an average of only two lifetime sexual partners.[97] This vaccine has *no efficacy* in women who have already been exposed to the two cancer-causing strains included in the vaccine.[98] In fact, these women may have a *greater risk* of developing cervical cancer.[99]

Researchers have identified at least 15 cancer-causing HPV strains.[100] Gardasil is designed to protect against two of these (the ones included in the vaccine). Yet, a recent Merck-funded analysis—which cannot be located for peer review—warrants that Gardasil provides 38 percent "cross-protection" against ten other oncogenic HPV strains (types *not* included in the vaccine).[101,102] However, Merck's own product insert admits that "Gardasil does not prevent infection with HPV types not contained in the vaccine. Cases of disease due to non-vaccine types were observed among recipients of Gardasil."[103]

Surrogate markers and the FUTURE studies:

Gardasil's "efficacy" or "effectiveness" does *not* refer to the HPV vaccine's ability to prevent cervical cancer. The vaccine has never shown that it can prevent a single case of cervical cancer. Gardasil's efficacy only refers to its ability to prevent certain "surrogate markers" that could, under certain conditions, eventually lead to cervical cancer. These markers are "pre-malignant lesions" that often disappear or regress on their own.[104]

There are two main types of cervical lesions: cervical intraepithelial neoplasia (CIN) and adenocarcinoma in situ (AIS). CIN is further classified according to its level of advancement, or potential to become invasive and transmute from benign to malignant: CIN-1, CIN-2 and CIN-3. CIN-1 indicates the presence of HPV infection but is rarely problematic. It is not considered to be precancerous. In fact, current guidelines discourage treatment for this condition.[105] CIN-2, CIN-3 and AIS are considered by the FDA to be acceptable surrogate markers—even though CIN-2 lesions can also regress spontaneously.[106] Many researchers only consider CIN-3 and AIS to be appropriate surrogate markers. These lesions have the least likelihood of regression and the most potential to become invasive.[107]

In 2007, the *New England Journal of Medicine* published an analysis of two studies that assessed the efficacy of the HPV vaccine against *all* potentially oncogenic HPV types, not just the types found in the vaccine. Included were the ten non-vaccine strains that Merck declared Gardasil gives cross-protection against. This would provide a more honest assessment of the vaccine's likelihood to protect against cervical cancer. In the first study—the FUTURE I trial—the vaccine was shown to be just 20 percent effective. However, when the lesion types were analyzed, it was found that the vaccine was mainly reducing the number of CIN-1 lesions. The vaccine had *no efficacy* against higher-grade disease.[108] In the second study—the FUTURE II trial—the vaccine was shown to be just 17 percent effective at protecting against CIN-2, CIN-3 or AIS. However, when the lesion types were analyzed, it was found that the vaccine was only significant against CIN-2. The vaccine had *no efficacy* against CIN-3 or AIS (Figure 80).[109]

Sexually active females:
In the FUTURE II study, 93 percent of the females were non-virgins, more closely matching the real-life sexual backgrounds of teenagers and young women receiving Gardasil.[110] Sexually active females often harbor HPV infections without symptoms.[111] Yet, as previously noted, the vaccine is not effective in women who have already been exposed to the HPV strains included in the vaccine.[112] In the United States, 24 percent of females are sexually active by age 15 years, 40 percent by age 16, and 70 percent by 18 years of age.[113] Moreover, according to Diane Harper, a professor at Dartmouth Medical School and a longtime HPV researcher who was involved in Gardasil's clinical trials, as many as 10 percent of 11- and 12-year-old girls may already have HPV.[114] That could reduce the vaccine's efficacy. Even the American Cancer Society (ACS) does not agree with the CDC's recommendation to vaccinate older teens and young women. There is "insufficient evidence" that females 19 to 26 years of age will benefit from the vaccine because many have already been exposed to HPV.[115] In fact, a recent study found that 12 percent of all females 10 to 29 years of age tested positive for exposure to HPV-16, and 21 percent tested positive for at least one of the four HPV types included in the vaccine.[116] According to Dr. George Sawaya, who analyzed the FUTURE I and II studies, the benefits of the vaccine are modest. "The effect is fairly small." Therefore, "the recommendation for widespread vaccination of women after they become sexually active may need to be rethought."[117]

Can the HPV vaccine *increase* the risk of developing cervical cancer?
This vaccine is not only ineffective in women who have already been exposed to HPV-16 and HPV-18, but it may actually *increase* their likelihood of developing cervical cancer. When the FDA analyzed the clinical studies that Merck submitted for review in its application for a license to market Gardasil, one of its main concerns was "the potential for Gardasil to *enhance* cervical disease in subjects who had evidence of persistent infection with vaccine-relevant HPV types prior to vaccination."[118] In other words, women who are already infected with low-level HPV disease (strains 6,11,16 or 18) *before* they are vaccinated with Gardasil, are likely to have their infections exacerbated by the shot. In fact, the vaccine may cause relatively innocuous infections to develop into more severe, higher grade disease ("CIN-2, CIN-3 or worse"). In one study of women who tested positive for "vaccine-relevant HPV" prior to receiving Gardasil, the vaccine had an efficacy of negative 45 percent (-45%). These women were significantly *more likely* (than women in the placebo group) to develop high-grade markers for cervical cancer. In a gross understatement, the FDA concluded that "there is compelling evidence that the vaccine lacks therapeutic efficacy among women who have had prior exposure to HPV and have not cleared previous infection."[119]

Shortly after Gardasil was licensed, the FDA started receiving adverse reaction reports suggesting that women with HPV infection at the time of their HPV shot may be at increased risk of developing cervical cancer. The vaccine appears to aggravate or accelerate the cancer-causing potential of the virus. For example:

▸ 275991: After receiving Gardasil, a 19-year-old female with CIN 2 or 3 required a cone biopsy due to the rapid development of HPV. The doctor felt that her condition was aggravated by the vaccine. Her cervical dysplasia required hospital care.

▸ 277115: A 26-year-old woman previously diagnosed with cervical dysplasia and CIN-1 received Gardasil. One month later, she developed breast cancer. She received a second dose of Gardasil, and two months later a Pap smear confirmed that she was positive for HPV. Her condition was reported as "aggravated" and immediately life-threatening.[120]

Figure 80:

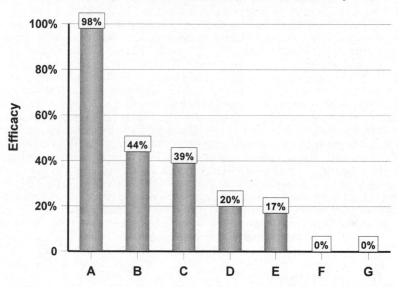

Efficacy of the HPV Vaccine
Using Various Definitions of Efficacy

A: 98% to 100% efficacy against 2 strains of HPV (16 and 18) in a population of women with no evidence of prior exposure to those strains. (This is the most widely-promoted efficacy figure despite its severely limited practicality.)

B: 44% efficacy against 2 strains of HPV (16 and 18) in a population of women with or without evidence of prior exposure to those strains.

C: 39% efficacy against 2 strains of HPV (16 and 18) in women with an average of just two lifetime sexual partners.

D: 20% efficacy against all low grade HPV infections (CIN-1) in women.

E: 17% efficacy against all mid-grade HPV infections (CIN-2) in women.

F: 0% efficacy against all high-grade infections (CIN-3 or AIS) in women.

G: 0% efficacy in women who have already been exposed to the two HPV strains included in the vaccine. (These women may have an *increased* risk of developing cervical cancer.)

Note: Efficacy does *not* refer to the HPV vaccine's ability to prevent cervical cancer. The vaccine has never shown that it can prevent a single case of cervical cancer. Gardasil's efficacy only refers to its ability to prevent certain "surrogate markers" that could, under certain circumstances, eventually lead to cervical cancer. These surrogate markers are "pre-malignant lesions" that often disappear or regress on their own. Source: Merck; FDA; *NEJM* (May 10, 2007); *CA Cancer J Clin* 2007(57).

"I do believe that Gardasil protects against HPV 16 and 18, but the effect it will have on cervical cancer rates in this country is another question entirely. There is a leap of faith involved."—Scott Emerson, FDA advisory committee member

Is the HPV vaccine causing "minor" HPV strains to flourish?

Research has shown that when vaccines only target a small number of strains capable of causing disease, less prevalent strains can replace the targeted vaccine strains. These less prevalent strains graduate from minor factors to major influences and may even become more virulent. For example, after the haemophilus influenzae type b vaccine (Hib) was introduced, the rate of invasive haemophilus influenzae type f disease (Hif) nearly quadrupled.[121] As another example, scientists have issued warnings that pneumococcal vaccines only targeting some strains of the disease "may increase carriage of and disease from serotypes not included in the vaccine."[122,123] Prevnar (the primary vaccine for pneumococcal disease) only targets 7 of the more than 90 different strains capable of causing the disease. When Prevnar was first licensed, just 35 percent of all cases of pneumococcal disease were caused by non-vaccine serotypes. Four years later, 73 percent of all cases were due to non-vaccine strains—and they have become more resistant to treatment![124]

Scientists are now concerned that Gardasil—which only targets two of at least 15 different cancer-causing HPV strains—might be allowing HPV strains previously considered minor to flourish and become major influences. Findings from the FUTURE II study on Gardasil show that "the contribution of nonvaccine HPV types to overall grade 2 or 3 CIN or AIS was sizable."[125] Even the FDA is worried that "other HPV types have the potential to counter the efficacy results of Gardasil."[126] In fact, in the FUTURE II study subjects, the overall incidence of HPV disease regardless of HPV type continued to increase, *raising the possibility that other oncogenic HPV types eventually filled the biological niche left behind after the elimination of HPV types 16 and 18.*[127] An analysis of data submitted to the FDA showed a disproportionate number of cases of grade 2 or 3 CIN that were related to *non-vaccine* HPV types among vaccinated women (Figure 81).[128]

Is the HPV vaccine mandatory?

Shortly after the new HPV vaccine was licensed for 9- to 26-year-old females, and recommended for all 11- and 12-year-old girls, Merck began lobbying individual states to require this vaccine for all girls before they can enter middle school. Merck also bankrolled Women in Government, a powerful advocacy group that exerts pressure on state legislators with regard to vaccine laws. A top official from Merck's vaccine division sits on Women in Government's business council.[129,130]

In February of 2007, Texas became the first state to compel 6th grade girls to receive three doses of Gardasil, a vaccine designed to prevent an infection that is not spread through casual contact but rather by way of sexual intercourse. Governor Rick Perry signed an executive order mandating the shots, bypassing the legislative process. According to Cathie Adams, president of Texas Eagle Forum, a political watchdog organization, Perry's decision "replaces the parent with the state. You're not only turning parents' rights upside down, but you're also subjecting children to an experimental vaccine. When that 12-year-old girl is expecting a baby [years later] and there's a birth defect, [we won't know] if those are related."[131]

Perry claimed it was important to protect girls from cervical cancer. However, Perry had several ties to Merck and Women in Government. For example, Perry's former chief of staff, Mike Toomey, was one of three lobbyists paid up to $250,000 and hired by Merck to petition Texas lawmakers on its behalf. State Representative Dianne White Delisi was a state director for Women in Government—and Perry's current chief of staff's mother-in-law. In addition, Perry received campaign donations from Merck during his re-election campaign.[132]

Merck's method of lobbying "is corrupt as far as I'm concerned," stated Adams. " Follow the money, it leads to Merck."[133,134] Dr. John Schiller, a National Cancer Institute scientist, was also uneasy with Merck's "heavy-handed" promotion of Gardasil. "When they do something, they spare no energy. It's the Merck way or the highway."[135] Schiller hopes it won't draw attention away from regular Pap screening, still the most important defense against cervical cancer. Another observer quipped that HPV really means Help Pay for Vioxx, a reference to Merck's dangerous pain-killing drug and subsequent lawsuits the drug giant underwent. Industry analysts calculated that Merck should make at least $1 billion per year on sales of Gardasil, and billions more if states mandate it.[136]

Figure 81:

Is the HPV Vaccine Causing "Minor" Cancer-Causing HPV Strains to Flourish?

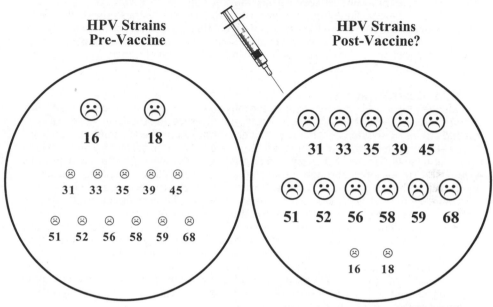

Scientists are concerned that Gardasil—which only targets two of at least 15 different cancer-causing HPV strains—might be allowing HPV strains previously considered minor to flourish and become major influences. Even the FDA is worried that "other HPV types have the potential to counter the efficacy results of Gardasil." In HPV study subjects, the overall incidence of HPV disease regardless of HPV type continued to increase, *raising the possibility that other oncogenic HPV types eventually filled the biological niche left behind after the elimination of HPV types 16 and 18.* An interim analysis of vaccine data submitted to the FDA showed a disproportionate number of cases of grade 2 or 3 CIN that were related to *non-vaccine* HPV types among vaccinated women! Source: FDA. Vaccines and Related Biological Products Advisory Committee Background Document (May 18, 2006). *New England Journal of Medicine* (May 10, 2007); 356:1991-93.

Three weeks later, Merck announced that it would stop its nationwide lobbying for states to mandate its new HPV vaccine because the company's profit motive, rather than public health, appeared to be guiding the debate.[137] However, just ten days later investigators discovered that a doctor who gets paid by Merck to promote Gardasil, helped Virginia lawmakers decide whether to mandate the vaccine for all 11-year-old girls in the state. Dr. Cecelia Boardman advised Virginia lawmakers about Gardasil without disclosing that she gives educational talks on the vaccine using Merck-supplied material.[138] According to John Abramson, a Harvard Medical School professor, Boardman should have disclosed her Merck relationship. Imagine a juror not disclosing financial ties to a corporation in whose judgment the juror was sitting. That would be unacceptable.[139]

In April of 2007, Texas legislators passed a bill reversing Governor Rick Perry's mandate that all preteen girls receive the HPV vaccine in order to enroll in 6th grade.[140] Several other states, including Michigan, Maryland, Mississippi, Colorado and New Mexico, also halted or vetoed proposed legislation to mandate Gardasil. However, other states were debating whether to mandate this vaccine.[141] It may be compulsory in your state by the time you read this. Of course, exemptions are possible.

Some doctors are not waiting for Gardasil to be mandated before compelling their female patients to receive it. Even more disturbing, underage girls are being vaccinated without their parent's knowledge or permission. For example: "Recently, during a routine exam for my 14-year-old daughter, I was asked to leave the room so the doctor could ask her some questions. When I returned, I was told that my daughter had just been given the HPV shot. I had not been given a chance to ask questions. I did not have a chance to decline. I was not told they were going to do it. Was it legal for them to give it to her without my verbal or written consent?"[142]

Ethical considerations:

The *New England Journal of Medicine* recently published a letter to the editor essentially arguing that because the HPV vaccine is effective (with respect to a small number of vaccine-related strains) it should be mandated.[143] (The author is a paid consultant to Merck.)[144] However, the legal justification for mandating vaccination is to protect the public health from contagious diseases that are spread through *casual* contact. The human papilloma virus (HPV) is *not* spread through casual contact; it is mainly transmitted through sexual intercourse. Thus, if 11- and 12-year-old girls are compelled to receive an STD vaccine, our society will have entered a new era of medical and pharmaceutical subjugation. It will be easy to rationalize mandating *any* new drug or vaccine—as long as it is "effective."

An editorial published in the *Journal of the American Medical Association* contends that "the rush to make HPV vaccination mandatory in school-aged girls presents ethical concerns and is likely to be counterproductive."[145] Several salient points were made:

- Given that the overall prevalence of HPV types associated with cervical cancer is relatively low and that the long-term effects are unknown, it is unwise to require a young girl with a very low lifetime risk of cervical cancer to be vaccinated without her assent and her parents' consent.
- Making the HPV vaccine mandatory contributes to long-standing parental concerns about the safety of school-based vaccinations. The use of compulsion, therefore, could have the unintended consequence of heightening parental and public apprehensions about childhood vaccinations.
- By making the vaccine mandatory, the state would probably complicate tort claims.... Ethically, if the state mandates an intervention, it should also provide a compensation system.
- Merck lobbied legislators to make the vaccine mandatory. Since the manufacturer stands to profit from widespread vaccine administration, it is inappropriate for the company to finance efforts to persuade states and public officials to make HPV vaccinations mandatory.
- In the absence of an immediate risk of serious harm, it is preferable to adopt voluntary measures....[146]

With regard to mandating Gardasil, Dr. Joseph Bocchini, chairman of the American Academy of Pediatrics, thinks "it would be wise to wait until we have additional information about the safety of the vaccine."[147] Dr. Harper is more candid. She said giving such a vaccine to 11-year-olds "is a great public health experiment."[148] Dr. Sawaya believes that "a cautious approach may be warranted in light of important unanswered questions about overall vaccine effectiveness, duration of protection, and adverse effects that may emerge over time."[149]

"It's the Merck way or the highway."
—Dr. John Schiller, National Cancer Institute scientist

The HPV vaccine and boys:

Although Gardasil was developed to prevent cervical cancer in women, researchers claimed that boys could be at risk for throat cancer if they have oral sex with girls who are infected with HPV. Therefore, "we would encourage industry and scientists to study the efficacy in boys and men so the vaccination program can be expanded."[150] This vaccine was eventually licensed for boys to combat genital warts. According to Barbara Loe Fisher, president of the National Vaccine Information Center (NVIC), "Merck and doctors in academia and research, who are developing and promoting widespread use of HPV vaccines, are going after the young boy market following a failure...to get HPV vaccine mandated for preteen girls in every state.... The call for all young boys to get a vaccine that was developed to prevent cervical cancer in women will help Merck out in its quest for the $3 billion dollar annual market it dreamed of when it tried to get the vaccine mandated for all young girls."[151] Another concerned observer believes that Merck's campaign to vaccinate boys with a shot designed to prevent cervical cancer in women, shows that the push to sell more vaccines has reached "a level of absurdity that should astonish any intelligent person.... What's next? Are they going to demand that all girls be vaccinated against prostate cancer?"[152]

Will this vaccine encourage sexual activity?

Some people are opposed to mandating this vaccine because it is designed to protect against a sexually transmitted disease and could send a subtle message condoning teenage sexual activity. For example, a survey of pediatricians indicates that many doctors think that vaccinating against a sexually transmitted disease "may encourage risky sexual behavior in my adolescent patients."[153] According to ACIP member, Dr. Reginald Finger, "There are people who sense that it could cause people to feel like sexual behaviors are safer if they are vaccinated, and may lead to more sexual behavior because they feel safe."[154] Gene Rudd, executive director of the Christian Medical Association, spoke with some of his associates who complained that "this is going to sabotage our abstinence message."[155] Rudd thinks that "Parents should have the choice. There are those who would say, 'We can provide a better, healthier alternative than the vaccine.'"[156]

What are the alternatives to this vaccine?

Numerous studies show convincing evidence that diet and nutritional factors can prevent many types of cancer, including cervical cancer, and even eliminate precursors to this disease. Fruits and vegetables, especially, have been shown to have beneficial effects against malignancies.[157-159] Among these nutritional factors, folate, or folic acid (a member of the B vitamins) has the most impressive record. Several studies show that low folate levels increase the effect of other risk factors for cervical cancer, including that of HPV infection. Conversely, high folate levels appear to be beneficial against HPV infection and other risk factors for cervical cancer. For example, in a recent study published in a leading journal on cancer, researchers found "evidence of a protective role of folate" with regard to pre-malignant lesions of the cervix.[160] Several studies also show that folic acid supplementation can reverse cervical dysplasia in patients using oral contraceptives —a known risk factor for this "pre-cancerous" condition. Patients with mild and moderate cervical dysplasia (CIN-1 and CIN-2) showed a full reversal of their condition in just three months following a diet rich with folic acid.[161-163] Other studies confirm these results.[164-176]

How much folic acid is sufficient?

Folic acid is critical to the synthesis of normal DNA. According to the CDC, childbearing women should take the recommended daily dosage of folic acid to reduce their baby's risk of birth defects—at least 400mcg.[177] During pregnancy, many doctors recommend at least 600mcg to 800mcg daily.[178,179] Cells that line the cervix replace themselves every 7 to 14 days, and must continuously manufacture DNA. Yet, many women consume less than 400mcg of folic acid per day. Therefore, ingesting a multiple vitamin containing recommended daily dosages of folic acid may be sufficient.[180] Other sources of this nutrient include dark, leafy green vegetables, lentils, chickpeas, asparagus, broccoli, and papaya.[181]

More nutrients to avert HPV and cervical cancer:

Insufficient vitamin A,[182-195] lycopene (found primarily in tomatoes),[196-201] riboflavin (B2),[202] pyridoxine (B6),[203] vitamin C,[204-208] glycoalkaloids (found primarily in potatoes),[209] other micronutrients,[210-222] antioxidants[223-231] and herbs[232-234] have all been associated with an increased risk of cervical cancer and its precursors. By increasing the amount of these nutrients in one's diet—or by applying some of these substances topically—cervical cancer risks may be reduced. In some instances, cervical dysplasia may even be reversed. For example, studies showed that up to 50 percent of women using vitamin A topically applied to the cervix had a complete reversal of cervical dysplasia.[235]

A study published in the *International Journal of Cancer,* found that 75 percent of women who ate the least amount of tomatoes had up to 4.7 times the risk for precancerous changes of the cervix (cervical intraepithelial neoplasia).[236] Another study measured and compared micronutrient levels in the blood of women with cervical cancer to micronutrient levels in the blood of non-cancerous women. The women with higher levels of lycopene and vitamin A consumed greater amounts of food with these substances and had one-third less chance of developing cervical cancer.[237] Another study, published in the *American Journal of Epidemiology,* concluded that "low vitamin C intake is an independent contributor to risk of severe cervical dysplasia."[238]

Summary:

- Cervical cancer is rare in younger females. Older women—*not* preteen and teenage girls—are most at risk of developing cervical cancer.
- Many of the women who develop cervical cancer did not have a Pap test. The Pap test detects cervical abnormalities in the early stages. When detected at an early stage, cervical cancer is one of the most successfully treated cancers.
- Cervical cancer is not as common as other types of cancer.
- The HPV vaccine contains a high concentration of aluminum, with many known and documented health hazards.
- The FDA has already received numerous reports of serious and life-threatening adverse reactions in recipients of the HPV vaccine. These include muscular paralysis, loss of consciousness, seizures, swollen body parts, severe rashes, heart irregularities, arthritis, wheezing and death.
- Some girls and young women developed genital warts, vaginal lesions and HPV infection after receiving the HPV vaccine.
- The vaccine may be linked with reproductive complications, including miscarriages, menstrual irregularities and birth defects.
- The vaccine's highly publicized 98% to 100% efficacy rate does *not* refer to its ability to prevent cervical cancer. The vaccine is only designed to prevent a limited number of "pre-malignant" lesions that often disappear or resolve on their own.
- The vaccine has never shown that it can prevent a single case of cervical cancer. It has little or no effect against higher grades of HPV infections.
- The vaccine is only designed to protect against 4 of the more than 100 different strains of HPV.
- The vaccine is only designed to protect against two of the more than 15 different HPV strains capable of developing into cervical cancer. Just a small percentage of women are infected with these strains.
- The vaccine does not directly target at least 13 different strains of cancer-causing HPV, so recipients of the shot may still develop cervical cancer.
- The vaccine has *no efficacy* in females who have already been infected with HPV strains included in the vaccine. In fact, these women may have a *greater risk* of developing cervical cancer.
- The vaccine might be allowing HPV strains previously considered minor to flourish and become major cancer-causing influences.
- Numerous studies show that women who make a few simple changes in their diet may be able to prevent cervical cancer, and even eliminate precursors to this disease.

Respiratory Syncytial Virus
(RSV)

What is RSV?
Respiratory syncytial virus (RSV) is the most common cause of bronchiolitis and pneumonia among infants and children under one year of age.[1] It also causes severe respiratory illness in the elderly.[2] RSV is very contagious. Symptoms are initially similar to the common cold, then worsen as the infected person develops fever, wheezing, and difficulty breathing. Most healthy children recover in one to two weeks.[3,4] However, during their first RSV infection, about one percent of infants will require hospitalization.[5] Treatment for severe RSV infection is mainly supportive: oxygen therapy, hydration, and nutrition.[6] Some people die from complications of the disease.[7]

How did RSV originate?
In 1956, respiratory syncytial virus (RSV) was discovered in chimpanzees.[8] According to Dr. Viera Scheibner, who studied more than 30,000 pages of medical papers dealing with vaccination, RSV viruses "formed prominent contaminants in polio vaccines and were soon detected in children." They caused serious cold-like symptoms in small infants and babies who received the polio vaccine.[9] In 1961, the *Journal of the American Medical Association* published two studies confirming a causal relationship between RSV and "relatively severe lower respiratory tract illness."[10,11] The virus was found in 57 percent of infants with bronchiolitis or pneumonia, and in 12 percent of babies with a milder febrile respiratory disease. Infected babies remained ill for three to five months.[12] RSV is communicable, and soon spread to adults where it has been linked to the common cold.[13]

Who is most at risk?
Today, children who are most at risk of serious complications from RSV include infants born prematurely (less than 35 weeks), and infants with chronic lung disease (broncho-pulmonary dysplasia), immune system problems, neuromuscular disorders, cystic fibrosis, congenital heart disease or other pre-existing conditions.[14]

Does an RSV vaccine exist?
An RSV vaccine does not yet exist. Researchers have been hampered by the mutable nature of the organism, and early attempts at developing an RSV vaccine actually made the disease worse on subsequent infection. In fact, during early clinical trials 80 percent of children who received an RSV vaccine were hospitalized, with some of the children dying.[15,16] However, two "preventive agents" were licensed by the FDA. In 1996, Respigam, an immune globulin treatment made from human plasma, became available.[17] In 1998, Synagis® —a "monoclonal antibody" produced in human and mouse genes—entered the market.[18,19] Synagis is indicated for the prevention of serious *lower* respiratory tract infections caused by RSV. It is given as a series of five monthly injections at the start of and during the RSV season (usually November to April). It is very expensive; each injection may cost $900 or more.[20] One mother reported being charged more than $7,000 for a single dose and $2600 for each subsequent dose. Her insurance did not pay.[21]

How safe is the RSV preventive agent?
In controlled clinical studies, Synagis was found to *increase* the likelihood of developing an upper respiratory tract infection, gastroenteritis, rhinitis, wheezing, otitis media (ear infection), and hernia (Figure 82).[22,23] Cyanosis and arrhythmia were also more likely in patients with congenital heart disease.[24] In addition, Synagis raised SGOT (serum glutamic-oxaloacetic transaminase) enzyme levels[25] —a possible sign of liver or heart damage.[26] Other adverse events reported in children receiving this "preventive" biotech commodity include: anaphylaxis, hypersensitive reactions, bronchiolitis, bronchitis, pneumonia, asthma, croup, respiratory failure, thrombocytopenia, hypotonia, unresponsiveness, fever, dyspnea,

Figure 82:

RSV Preventive Agent *Increases* the Risk of Upper Respiratory Disease, Ear Infections, and Other Ailments

Decreases Risk of...
Serious Lower
Respiratory Disease
Caused by RSV

Increases Risk of...
Upper Respiratory Disease,
Cyanosis, Otitis Media,
Rhinitis, and Hernia

Synagis® is indicated for the prevention of serious *lower* respiratory tract infections caused by RSV. In controlled clinical studies, Synagis was found to *increase* the risk of developing *upper* respiratory tract infections and other ailments. Source: The vaccine manufacturer; *Pediatrics* 1998;102:531-537.

sinusitis, apnea, diarrhea, vomiting, liver function abnormality, viral infection, fungal dermatitis, eczema, seborrhea, conjunctivitis, anemia, flu syndrome, and failure to thrive.[27]

How effective is the RSV preventive agent?

Studies show that Synagis reduced RSV hospitalization by approximately 50 percent. However, Synagis will not alter the incidence and mean duration of hospitalization for non-RSV respiratory illness nor will it prevent *upper* respiratory tract infections. In fact, babies receiving Synagis are *more likely* to experience upper respiratory tract infections than babies who do not receive it.[28] Furthermore, some babies will develop RSV despite having received Synagis. The data suggests that their illnesses will be no less severe than in babies who received a placebo.[29]

Anthrax

What is anthrax?
Anthrax is a severe bacterial disease that primarily affects warm-blooded animals, especially livestock. Humans can be infected as well. The disease is caused by the bacterium *Bacillus anthracis,* which produces spores that can remain dormant for years in soil and on animal products, such as hides, wool, hair or bones.[1]

How is anthrax contracted?
Animals get the disease by eating infected grass or carcasses, drinking infected water, or inhaling infected dust. They die suddenly with little or no symptoms.[2] *People* contract anthrax in one of three ways: 1) by coming into contact with the bacterium or infected animals or animal products, 2) by inhaling airborne particles, or 3) by eating undercooked meat from diseased livestock (Figure 83).[3]

How common is the disease?
Anthrax is rare; when it does occur, it is almost always an occupational hazard, contracted by those who sort wool or handle animal hides—farmers, butchers, and veterinarians. The disease is most often found in agricultural regions of South and Central America, eastern Europe, Asia, Africa, and the Middle East.[4] In the United States, during the early 1900s there were about 200 cases per year of the less threatening form in which the bacterium infects the skin.[5] In 1957, nine employees of a goat hair processing company became ill after handling a contaminated shipment from overseas.[6] In the 1970s, other cases occurred when contaminated goatskin drumheads were imported as souvenirs.[7] From 1900 to 1976, only 18 cases of the inhaled version were reported in the U.S.[8] However, in 2001 an unknown terrorist mailed anthrax to several media outlets and federal offices in the United States exposing numerous people to the disease.[9]

What are the symptoms of anthrax?
Symptoms usually appear within one week of exposure but vary depending upon how the disease is contracted:
Cutaneous anthrax is the most common, and mildest, form of the disease. This occurs through skin contact—when the bacteria enter a cut or wound. At first, an itchy raised area like an insect bite appears. Within one to two days, inflammation occurs and a blister forms around a black center of dying tissue. Other symptoms include shivering and chills. If bacteria spread to the nearest lymph gland, the disease can cause a form of blood poisoning that is fatal.
Inhalation or pulmonary anthrax occurs by inhaling the bacteria or bacterial spores. The disease begins with cold or flu-like symptoms—fever, fatigue, and headache—then progresses to bronchitis, pneumonia, and a state of shock. This rare form of anthrax is usually fatal.
Intestinal anthrax is caused by eating meat from an infected animal. The first signs are nausea and vomiting, loss of appetite, fever, and abdominal pain. It progresses to inflammation and ulcers of the stomach and intestines, vomiting of blood, and bloody diarrhea. This form of anthrax is also rare and often fatal.[10]

Is there a treatment for anthrax?
If caught early, anthrax is curable by administering high doses of penicillin.[11] Several antibiotics are effective against anthrax when it occurs naturally. Ciprofloxacin (Cipro) and Doxycycline (Doxy) have been licensed by the FDA for use against all forms of the disease.[12] However, moderate to severe side effects are possible.[13] For example, adverse reactions to Ciprofloxacin include nausea, diarrhea, vomiting, headache, stomach pain, skin rashes, mental confusion, tremors, seizures, hallucinations, and torn tendons. In one study, 16.5 percent of all Cipro recipients had adverse reactions. The drug had to be discontinued in 3.5 percent of the patients.[14] In a more recent study, 19 percent of all postal

Figure 83:

How is Anthrax Contracted?

Skin Contact	Inhalation	Intestinal

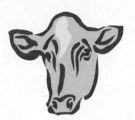 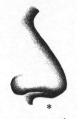 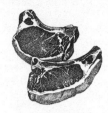

By coming into contact with the bacterium or infected animals	By inhaling airborne particles of anthrax	By eating undercooked meat from diseased livestock

© NZM

workers using "anti-microbial prophylaxis" for anthrax reported adverse reactions. Most were using Cipro. Eighty-two of the 3,863 people in the study group (2 percent) sought medical attention for symptoms of anaphylaxis, a potentially life-threatening allergic reaction. Eight percent of the Cipro recipients quit the medication.[15-17] Doxycycline is thought to be less reactive, but has been linked to nausea, vomiting, headache, chest pain, facial swelling, throat and tongue inflammation, genital and rectal itching, skin peeling, and hives.[18,19]

Although cutaneous anthrax may be cured following a single dose of an antibiotic, prolonged treatment is recommended. Victims of inhalation anthrax must take high doses of antibiotics for 60 days, starting immediately after exposure.[20] Some doctors use other regimens as well.

Anthrax is not considered contagious. There are no reports of the disease spreading from human to human. Thus, communicability is not likely when managing or visiting ill patients.[21] However, the prognosis for untreated anthrax is poor. About 20 percent of all unattended cutaneous cases will end in death. Most treated patients will recover.[22] All patients with inhalation anthrax will die if left untreated.[23] Only 10 percent will survive if treatment is postponed until symptoms appear and the spores have begun to release toxins.[24] Intestinal anthrax is fatal in about half the cases (Figure 84).[25]

Does an anthrax vaccine exist?

In 1863, anthrax became the first disease for which a causative agent—*Bacillus anthracis*—was isolated.[26] In 1881, Louis Pasteur developed the first anthrax vaccine for animals.[27] In 1935, a more virulent, live anthrax vaccine for animals was produced. However, goats, llamas, and other animals often died following vaccination.[28] By 1940, the Soviet Union developed the first anthrax vaccine for human use.[29] The United States and Great Britain produced human anthrax vaccines during the 1950s.[30]

The currently available U.S. human anthrax vaccine was formulated in the 1960s and licensed by the FDA in 1970, two years before efficacy data (scientific proof that it works) were required.[31,32] This vaccine—MDPH-PA (Protective Antigen) or MDPH-AVA (Anthrax Vaccine Adsorbed)—was produced until February 1998 by the Michigan Department of Public Health (MDPH) under contract with the Department of Defense (DoD). The business was sold in September 1998 and renamed Bioport.[33]

How safe and effective is the anthrax vaccine?

In 1954, researchers injected 25 rabbits with an anthrax vaccine. They were intentionally killed 23 days later so that researchers could perform autopsies on them, which revealed nothing unusual.[34] These same researchers studied short-term side effects to anthrax injections

Figure 84:

Prognosis for
Untreated Cases of Anthrax

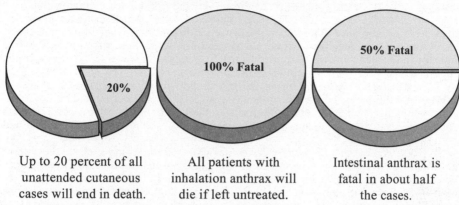

Up to 20 percent of all unattended cutaneous cases will end in death.	All patients with inhalation anthrax will die if left untreated.	Intestinal anthrax is fatal in about half the cases.

© NZM

in human subjects. They found a number of local and systemic reactions, including swelling at the injection site (up to 10cm in diameter), muscle aches, headaches, and mild-to-moderate malaise. Reaction rates increased with subsequent shots.[35]

In 1956, *Lancet* published a study that investigated the anthrax vaccine in both monkeys and humans. Some vaccine reactions were reported, but definitive conclusions could not be drawn because long-term follow-up of the study subjects was not conducted.[36]

In 1962, the *American Journal of Public Health* published the only randomized clinical study (Brachman, et al.) of a "protective-antigen anthrax vaccine."[37] Employees at four factories where anthrax-tainted goat hair was handled, were vaccinated. Although participants were only monitored for ill effects occurring within two days of each shot, and adverse reaction rates within this limited time frame were not recorded, some common adverse reactions were noted in several subjects, including "a ring of erythema" (greater than 5cm in diameter), nodules at the injection site (lasting several weeks), edema extending from the deltoid to the mid-forearm or wrist, and malaise.[38]

During the four year study period, there were 26 cases of anthrax (21 were cutaneous; 5 were inhalation). Three of these cases occurred in either partially or fully vaccinated recipients. The authors of the study concluded that the vaccine was 92.5 percent effective.[39] However, according to Dr. Meryl Nass, a recognized expert on anthrax and biological warfare, "the actual percent efficacy cannot be calculated due to the small number of cases...five inhalation cases do not permit any conclusion about vaccine efficacy with regard to inhaled organisms."[40] Also, according to a March 2000 investigative report issued by the Institute of Medicine (IOM), vaccine research was terminated at one of the four factories (the largest of the study sites) after the initial series of three injections. Data from this site is omitted from the study results, despite "a large number of systemic reactions."[41,42] The IOM report also noted that 81 subjects withdrew from the vaccine trials (at the other three factories) before completing the series of shots, yet data from these individuals was omitted from the study results as well.[43] Furthermore, the study fails to note whether the investigators were "blinded" or had knowledge (study bias) regarding who received the active vaccine or placebo.[44]

In 1962, and again in 1971, 76 employees at Fort Detrick, Maryland were tested to investigate the potential effects of intensive vaccination. Seventy-two of the 76 subjects had previously received the anthrax vaccine (plus other vaccinations). Although no clinical sequelae attributable to intense long-term immunization could be identified, there was evidence of a chronic inflammatory response, as shown by test abnormalities: elevated levels of hexosamine, an acute-phase reactant, and polyclonal elevations of gamma globulins.[45,46] However, no definitive conclusions can be drawn from these studies due to several shortcomings. According to the IOM report, "There was no comparison cohort and no random sampling of the employees. Therefore, the results may not apply to a broader population." Also, employees who left the study were excluded from the results.[47]

From 1986 to 1995, several studies tested the efficacy of the U.S. human anthrax vaccine on guinea pigs and mice. After the animals were vaccinated (typically with three shots, 2 to 3 weeks apart), they were exposed to several different strains of anthrax. Survival rates for vaccinated guinea pigs ranged from 0 percent to 100 percent.[48-55] Survival rates for vaccinated mice ranged from 0 percent to 10 percent.[56-58]

Several researchers also investigated the protective efficacy of a Russian anthrax vaccine, an English anthrax vaccine, a more virulent, live anthrax vaccine (Sterne), and experimental anthrax vaccines with the addition of novel adjuvants (antibody boosters). Most of these studies were conducted on guinea pigs and mice. The results were similar to those obtained from the U.S. vaccine.[59-62]

In 1993, the *Journal of Infectious Diseases* published a study in which monkeys were administered an anthrax vaccine shortly after being exposed to the disease. Survival rates were no better than in unvaccinated controls.[63] However, in 1996 U.S. army researchers published the results of a new study in which 25 adult rhesus monkeys received two injections of the human anthrax vaccine (two weeks apart). The monkeys were then exposed to the aerosolized spores of the Ames strain of anthrax at 8 weeks, 38 weeks, or 100 weeks. All of the vaccinated monkeys survived challenge at either 8 weeks or 38 weeks, and seven of eight monkeys survived challenge at 100 weeks.[64] Although the data in this study suggests that the U.S. human anthrax vaccine may protect adult rhesus monkeys against inhalation anthrax for up to two years, it is important to note that they were only exposed to a single strain of the disease. Researchers are currently aware of more than 1300 strains of anthrax.[65] The authors of this study also note that "immune mechanisms against inhalation anthrax may vary in different animal species." Thus, "these findings suggest...that the ability of the licensed human anthrax vaccine to stimulate cell-mediated immunity may be greater in some species than others."[66] Earlier studies using guinea pigs and mice already showed a wide variation of immune responses.[67] Furthermore, animals differ from humans in their immunological responses. No one knows how animal studies of vaccine efficacy can be extrapolated to people. In fact, the scientists who conducted the study admit: "There is currently no known surrogate marker or in vitro correlate of immunity that allows direct comparison of immunity in humans to that in monkeys."[68]

In 1998, U.S. army researchers published another study in which rhesus monkeys were exposed to inhalation anthrax six weeks after being vaccinated with either the U.S. human anthrax vaccine or with experimental anthrax vaccines. The data showed that one dose of each vaccine provided "significant protection."[69] Authors of this study also noted that "results of recent studies show that anthrax vaccines vary in their efficacy among different species."[70] Moreover, like the earlier primate study, the monkeys were only exposed to a single strain of anthrax. Researchers did not test their vaccines against any of the other hundreds of strains circulating across the globe.

An unpublished study conducted by the DoD in 1998 did test the U.S. human anthrax vaccine against more than 20 different strains from around the world. Guinea pigs were vaccinated prior to being exposed to each strain. Fourteen of the strains killed at least 75 percent of the vaccinated guinea pigs. Nine of the strains killed at least 85 percent of the rodents. Survival rates were even worse for strains found in Zimbabwe, Namibia and France (Figure 85).[71]

Summary:
The MDPH anthrax vaccine has several drawbacks:
- The only human field trial used to justify licensing the vaccine was conducted in the late 1950s and there were not enough cases of the disease to draw valid conclusions about vaccine efficacy.[72]

Figure 85:

U.S. Anthrax Vaccine:
Efficacy in Guinea Pigs
(Following Exposure to Geographically Diverse Anthrax Strains)

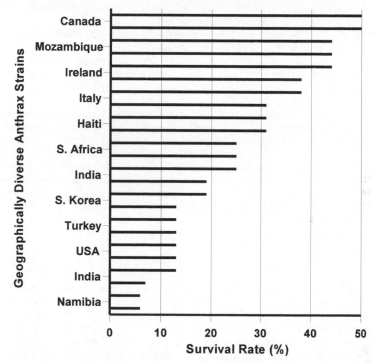

Guinea pigs were vaccinated prior to being exposed to one of more than 20 different anthrax strains from around the world. Fourteen of the strains killed at least 75 percent of the vaccinated guinea pigs. Nine of the strains killed at least 85 percent of the rodents. Survival rates were even worse for strains found in Zimbabwe, Namibia, and France. Source: DoD; presented at the International Anthrax Conference (September 1998).

- The vaccine was licensed for occupational use—mainly for veterinarians and other persons "engaged in diagnostic or investigational activities"—not as a prophylactic against inhalation anthrax.[73]
- This vaccine is "not highly effective... a number of people who were vaccinated subsequently developed anthrax."[74]
- No controlled clinical trials in humans were ever conducted, and there are no peer-reviewed published studies warranting its safety.[75,76]
- It contains several potentially toxic substances, including aluminum hydroxide (see *Appendix II*), benzethonium chloride, and formaldehyde.[77]
- About 20 percent of those vaccinated develop chronic medical problems.[78]
- The vaccine formulation has been changed; the current vaccine contains about five times more PA (bacterial matter) than the earlier vaccine.[79]
- Potency varies from lot to lot.[80]
- Full coverage requires six injections during 18 months, plus annual booster shots.[81]
- It is not licensed for children.[82]
- No one knows the effect on pregnant women or reproductive capacity.[83]

A new anthrax vaccine:

In October 2002, the U.S. government awarded two competing companies —Avecia (located in the U.K.) and VaxGen, Inc. (of California)—contracts to produce a new human anthrax vaccine "suitable for civilian populations."[84] The new vaccine must be produced "with recombinant DNA technology" and be able to provide immunity to inhalation anthrax in three or fewer doses within six months (unlike the current vaccine which uses older technology and requires six shots over 18 months).[85]

In September of 2006, Avecia, working with a $71 million contract, announced that its Phase I trial of a new human anthrax vaccine involving 111 healthy adults appeared safe and showed signs that vaccinated people were developing immunity to anthrax. However, early results indicated that this vaccine may be weaker or less effective than the currently licensed anthrax vaccine. According to one anthrax expert, "the implication...is that the immune response was not as good."[86]

Meanwhile, VaxGen, working with an $877 million contract, missed several important deadlines, and by November 2006 it was behind schedule and appeared to be in violation of its agreement.[87-90] In fact, it received a "clinical hold notification" from the FDA postponing the company's second Phase II trial of the vaccine. The FDA called a halt to further testing "in response to questions about the drug's reliability."[91] Two weeks later, the FDA announced that it would postpone a decision on whether to permanently cancel the program. Instead, VaxGen was given one month "to meet with the FDA...and try to find a pathway forward."[92] Vaccine delivery was pushed back until at least 2008.[93]

Anthrax Vaccines Within the U.S. Military

Thousands of U.S. military personnel who served in the Persian Gulf War were incapacitated from "unknown" causes. Their debilitating ailments ranged from bleeding rashes, gums and sinuses, to muscle aches, swollen joints, chronic fatigue, diarrhea, hair loss, severe headaches, and memory loss. Over time, their symptoms became more acute. Many vets are now confined to wheelchairs and hospital beds.[94,95] For example, after one veteran returned from his stint of duty as an army platoon leader, his health began to deteriorate. "The trouble started with spots on his [legs], which soon spread to other parts of his body. Then, his eyes swelled shut and his lips bloated till the skin split. When his skin cleared up, his joints [ached]."[96]

After returning from the Gulf War, another veteran "developed [flu-like] symptoms, with fever, aching joints, and swollen lymph nodes. During the next three years [his health deteriorated]. He became unsteady on his feet and increasingly tired. He suffered frequent headaches and often became disoriented, losing his way home.... Today, he uses a wheelchair, can't work, drive, open a soft drink can, or stay awake long enough to read a book."[97]

Although speculation on the cause of this dilemma ranged from pesticides and burning oil wells to undetected Iraqi nerve gases, on May 6, 1994 the truth was told. On that day, Senator John D. Rockefeller IV held a congressional hearing to determine if mandatory vaccines damaged veterans' health. He also released a report summarizing the results of a six-month investigation into the roots of the problem. Here are some excerpts:[98,99]

★ Congressional Hearing: May 6, 1994 ★
Is Military Research Hazardous to Veterans' Health?
Chairman John D. Rockefeller IV

A few months ago, Americans were shocked to learn that our government intentionally exposed thousands of U.S. citizens to radiation without their knowledge or consent. Although many of us expressed horror at the apparently unethical behavior of our government, we were all relieved to hear that such experiments had been stopped long ago. We'd like to think that these kinds of abuses are a thing of the past, but the legacy continues. During the Persian Gulf War, hundreds of thousands of soldiers were given experimental vaccines and drugs, and today we will hear evidence that these medical products could be causing many of the 'mysterious illnesses' those veterans are now experiencing.

The results of our investigation showed a reckless disregard that shocked me, and I think they will shock all Americans. The use of investigational drugs in the Persian Gulf is especially troublesome. The Pentagon...threw caution to the winds, ignoring all warnings of potential harm, and gave these drugs to hundreds of thousands of soldiers with virtually no warnings and no safeguards. If that wasn't bad enough, they administered these drugs and vaccines in such a way that there is a very good chance they wouldn't have even worked for the intended purpose. They would not have protected most soldiers from chemical or biological warfare. Most Americans would agree that the use of soldiers as guinea pigs in experiments that were designed to harm them...is not ethical. These experiences put hundreds of thousands of U.S. troops at risk, and may have caused lasting harm to many individuals.

In this report, we will examine how decisions made by DoD regarding the use of investigational drugs and vaccines in the Persian Gulf War were based on inadequate information and in some cases by ignoring evidence that soldiers would be harmed unnecessarily. We will also discuss how the DoD's failure to provide medical treatment or information to soldiers was unjustifiable, unethical, sometimes illegal, and caused unnecessary suffering. In addition, information about the use of these investigational drugs and vaccines, and adverse reactions that resulted, usually were not included in soldiers' medical records. As a result, veterans who became ill following the use of these medical products are often unable to prove that their illness or disability was related to their military service.

Forced anthrax vaccines:
Thousands of Gulf War veterans were forced to take an anthrax vaccine. Eighty-two percent received no written or verbal information about it; 76 percent could not refuse it; 42 percent reported side effects after receiving it (Figure 86).[100] Here are a few typical comments by Gulf War veterans:

  ‣ I passed out after the anthrax shot.
  ‣ We were told not to tell we got anthrax shots because there wasn't enough for British and French troops.
  ‣ I could refuse the shot if I wanted court martial.
  ‣ I don't have a spleen, and wonder if I should have taken those drugs and vaccines. I want my health back.[101]

Despite the many lessons to be learned from the compulsory vaccine program inflicted on Gulf War veterans, on December 15, 1997, Secretary of Defense William S. Cohen announced a new plan to vaccinate all active duty personnel against anthrax. This "medical force protection effort" is called the Anthrax Vaccine Immunization Program (AVIP).[102] Shortly after it was instituted, veterans began complaining about debilitating illnesses following their shots. They were unable to decline the vaccine and authorities refused to document adverse reactions. Eventually, the soldiers' complaints reached Congress, and from March 1999 through October 2000 several hearings were held—presided over by Congressmen Christopher Shays, Steven Buyer and Dan Burton—to investigate the safety and efficacy of the DoD's AVIP. (Excerpts from these hearings are posted on the *Thinktwice Global Vaccine Institute* website: www.thinktwice.com/military.htm)

Afghanistan and Iraq:
Although thousands of Gulf War veterans and other military personnel experienced adverse reactions to mandatory anthrax vaccines, and congressional leaders held several hearings in an attempt to remedy the military's flawed vaccine policy, few changes were made. In fact, anthrax vaccines remained mandatory for U.S. military personnel serving in Afghanistan and Iraq. This section contains a few of their unsolicited emails sent to the *Thinktwice Global Vaccine Institute* (www.thinktwice.com):[103]
  ‣ "I am a veteran who just got out of the U.S. Navy. I was forced against my will to receive the anthrax and smallpox vaccines. My only other option was DISHONORABLE discharge which would take away every benefit of being a veteran, making my service pointless. When I was vaccinated with anthrax I started going bald, my eyesight went

Figure 86:

Gulf War Veterans and the Mandatory Anthrax Vaccine

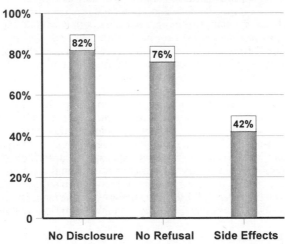

Gulf War vets were forced to take an anthrax vaccine. 82 percent received no written or verbal information about it; 76 percent could not refuse it; 42 percent reported side effects after receiving it. Source: U.S. Senate (May 6, 1994).

---

from 20/30 to 20/80 (in two months) and I started getting severe stomach cramps and migraine headaches.... I have always been in great health and standing until then."

▸ "I went to medical to submit an adverse event form and I was told I cannot. I was told my hair fell out because it was genetic (note: this occurred when I was 22 and nobody on either side of my family is bald). I was told my eyesight changed because I work with computers, and I was told that my headaches were from stress and my stomach aches were from the change to Navy food on a daily basis. (All this occurred in a few months' time span.) They said I could NOT submit an adverse reaction form. The only place I could note this was when I separated from the military, and I put all this information in my medical separation page. This comes as little consolation to me as my hair has continued to thin, my eyes have worsened, I still have migraine headaches, and my stomach still hurts constantly."

▸ "I did some research and you cannot vaccinate against airborne anthrax. Nobody has or can create a vaccine for the lungs, and inhalation anthrax is why we received the vaccine. I am only protected from ingestion (which would imply food poisoning), or cutaneous, which if I stay within the ship, a missile with anthrax couldn't infect me there. So using common sense, they weren't worried about Saddam launching a missile; they were worried about food poisoning or on-board terrorism. Also, I learned that many people on the ship that were 'buddy-buddy' with the doc onboard didn't have to get anthrax or smallpox vaccines. Surely the doc with an MD would not put his friends at risk like this unless he knew it wasn't necessary! I smell the stink of government conspiracy all over these vaccinations."

▸ "To sum it up, I would rather have received a DISHONORABLE discharge than poison. I would have outlet to the media in my home state (MN) and made a spectacle, then got my benefits reinstated. Currently, no employer has asked to see my DD-214 which proves my honorable discharge. I bought a house but the VA load was worse off than a regular 30-year fixed loan so I didn't use the benefits there, and my current work gives tuition reimbursement so I don't even need my GI bill for college. My benefits are worthless to me, and now I am stuck with the side effects of poison because I placed my trust in man and not God. I would encourage all people in the military to not get the shot, get the dishonorable discharge, petition for reinstatement. They tell you you'll be McDonald's bound, but my current employer only knows that I served for 5 years, not what type of discharge I received. How many employers are not going to hire you because you didn't want anthrax in your body? They will ALL still hire you. It's not like you were kicked out of the military for insubordination, assault, robbery, disorderly conduct...you refused poison, they'll understand! Don't listen to the scare tactics that you'll be flippin' burgers for the rest of your life because of your dishonorable discharge. If it's because of refusal to take poison, they'll understand."

▸ "I am in the Army and I am currently refusing the anthrax vaccine. I don't feel it has been proven safe. I need any information that may help put a shred of doubt into my battalion commander's head so he will not order me held down and forcefully injected. Please help by providing information. Thank you."

▸ "My husband plans to disobey a lawful order and pay the price since he will be ordered to take the anthrax vaccine. We feel the government is NOT giving all the facts, and there are so many unknown facts about the side effects and infertility. It's sad to say, but with the vaccine coming up so close, today was the first and only educational class that the Marines attended. It also bothers me a great deal that there was no formal or informal invitation for the families of the servicemen and women to attend. Unfortunately, almost everything is written by the Department of Defense, so we will be fighting this alone. If there is any information on this topic that you can forward to us, it would be greatly appreciated. Thank you."

▸ "My son is active duty in the U.S. Marine Corp, stationed in California. He called this evening with a concern about the mandatory anthrax vaccine to be given soon. I'm looking for possible side effects, such as infertility (he's only 19). Any concrete information? Thank you."

▸ "I was phoned by a couple whose children are my clients. I am to be seeing the older boy sometime this week because he is coming home on leave this evening. This boy had one anthrax vaccine and was not happy with the way he felt afterwards. His parents told their son that he could refuse the vaccine. He tried to explain this to his superiors. They called it 'insubordination' and told him that they would opt him out of the service with a cut in rank and pay over the next 5 months. He said that he understood. Then they explained that he would not be happy at all about the way he will be treated until he is discharged. He said that he understood. He would not be getting the $25,000 that was promised him for college, either. He said that this was a small price to pay for his health. All of this was told to him over several days of having to come in to speak with this superior officer, and then his leave was canceled and then delayed. Back and forth and back and forth—playing head games with him. He would have a scheduled appointment to see the officer and then would hang around for 30 to 45 minutes waiting for him, only to be told that he could not see him today, reschedule for the following day. This went on for several more days. Then, when he finally got to see him, the officer asked if he had reconsidered accepting the vaccine. When he told him that he had not changed his mind, the officer threatened him with court martial, saying that he would spend the rest of his ten months of service in the brig and that he would be forcibly vaccinated with the anthrax vaccine anyway. The boy asked for a paper that stated that he was forcibly vaccinated against his will with the anthrax. They refused to give him anything but the vaccination and the court martial. They gave him his leave and told him to think about it and have an answer when he returned to duty after the vacation. His sister, who is also in the service and gave birth to her first child 3 weeks ago, told him that she had been vaccinating service personnel for the past 3 months. Whenever anyone refused the anthrax or any other vaccine, they were forcibly held down and vaccinated anyway. She said that they had two large servicemen standing by just for that purpose. Those who refused were kicked or struck, and were screaming and kicking. But they were vaccinated nonetheless. She said that there was no way to get out of it. I thought that I would share this with you. Thanks for all of your help."

Postscript: On December 22, 2003 federal Judge Emmett Sullivan ruled that the DoD anthrax vaccine program was illegal and issued a temporary injunction against the DoD. According to Sullivan, "The women and men of our armed forces put their lives on the line every day to preserve and safeguard the freedoms that all Americans cherish and enjoy. Absent an informed consent or presidential waiver, the United States cannot demand that members of the armed forces also serve as guinea pigs for experimental drugs."[104]

On October 27, 2004 federal Judge Emmett Sullivan again ruled that the DoD anthrax vaccine program was illegal and issued a another injunction against the DoD. According to Sullivan: "The men and women of our armed forces deserve the assurance that the vaccines our government compels them to take into their bodies have been tested by the greatest scrutiny of all—public scrutiny. This is the process the FDA in its expert judgment has outlined, and this is the course this Court shall compel FDA to follow.... Accordingly, the involuntary anthrax vaccination program, as applied to all persons, is rendered illegal absent informed consent or a presidential waiver...."[105]

Despite these injunctions, in October of 2006 the DoD announced that compulsory anthrax vaccination of military personnel serving in Iraq, Afghanistan and South Korea will resume within the next 30 to 60 days. According to William Winkenwerder Jr., Assistant Secretary of Defense for Health Affairs, the vaccine is safe and effective. It only causes minor side effects, such as "swelling, redness, flu-like symptoms, some pain and malaise." Dr. Meryl Nass, Director of the Military and Biodefense Vaccine Project disagrees. She asserts that "America's military service members deserve to be fully informed about the deaths, chronic illness and disabilities that many soldiers have experienced following anthrax vaccination.... They are suffering with crippling, life-altering illnesses that are being swept under the rug. We know the anthrax vaccine is reactive, and we suspect it is especially risky for those with hereditary and other risk factors that DoD refuses to investigate or acknowledge."[106]

On July 26, 2007 Congress held another hearing on the anthrax vaccine and Gulf War illnesses (GWI).[107] In testimony presented by Dr. Meryl Nass, it was revealed that the DoD funded research "that was carefully designed to create a smokescreen around both GWI and anthrax vaccine injuries, presumably to deflect culpability...."[108] In fact, of 300 studies investigating potential causes of GWI, *none* looked specifically at the anthrax vaccine.[109] In non-DoD studies, it was found that British anthrax vaccinations increased the risk of chronic GWI by as much as 230 percent.[110-112] As of June 26, 2007, the Vaccine Adverse Event Reporting System (VAERS) received 5,359 adverse event reports associated with the anthrax vaccine. The FDA designated 12.5 percent of these "serious" with 44 deaths.[113,114] Meanwhile, government officials who supported and expanded anthrax vaccinations while in office are now on the payroll of the vaccine manufacturer, or companies with government contracts related to anthrax vaccine. This includes two former Secretaries of the U.S. Department of Health and Human Services (HHS).[115]

On October 1, 2008 Mike Leavitt, Secretary of the Department of Health and Human Services, declared a seven-year "anthrax emergency" through the end of 2015. Authorities sought to increase the U.S. stockpile of anthrax vaccine *for use in civilian populations*—despite persistent doubts about its safety—while providing manufacturers and government planners with blanket immunity from liability.[116]

Herpes Zoster
(Shingles)

What is Herpes zoster?
Herpes zoster (HZ), commonly known as shingles, is a reactivation of the chickenpox virus (varicella zoster). HZ can only occur in people who were previously infected with chickenpox. Although most people regain their health several days after contracting chickenpox, the virus that caused the illness never leaves the body. It lies dormant in a group of nerve cells (the dorsal root ganglion) near the spine. As people age, it is possible for the virus to become active again and reappear in the form of shingles.[1,2]

What are the symptoms of shingles?
Shingles appears as a rash, or cluster of blisters, on one side of the body. The rash is itchy, burning, tingling and painful. It usually lasts for two to four weeks. However, once this initial phase is over, some people are stricken with post herpetic neuralgia (PHN)—severe and debilitating nerve pain that may persist for weeks, months or years. It can seriously disrupt one's quality of life.[3,4]

Treatment
Episodes of shingles resolve on their own without intervention. However, some treatments may reduce the extent and duration of symptoms as well as the likelihood of developing post herpetic neuralgia. Cool water compresses, lotions and topical analgesics are often recommended to ease the discomfort. Antiviral agents may be prescribed as well.[5]

Is shingles contagious?
Although people with shingles cannot transmit the ailment to other people—you get shingles from your own dormant chickenpox virus—people who have not had chickenpox can get chickenpox if they come in close contact with a person who has shingles.[6]

Who is most susceptible to shingles?
Shingles can occur in people of all ages (provided they have already had chickenpox at some time in their life) but is more common after the age of 50.[7] The risk increases with advancing age.[8] At one time, researchers believed that the elderly were more susceptible to shingles because their immune systems weaken with age, allowing the dormant chickenpox virus to reactivate as shingles. However, many experts now realize that the elderly may be more susceptible to shingles simply because they tend to have less contact with young children who are infected with chickenpox.[9,10] Apparently, when adults who had chickenpox at some previous time in their life come into contact with young children infected with chickenpox, their immunity to varicella is naturally and asymptomatically (without symptoms) boosted, protecting them from shingles.[11] According to one study: "The peculiar age distribution of zoster may in part reflect the frequency with which the different age groups encounter cases of varicella."[12] When these periodic encounters occur, antibody protection is boosted and attacks of HZ are postponed.[13] It should also be noted that people who have been *vaccinated* against chickenpox are susceptible to shingles as well.[14]

How common is shingles?
The rate of contracting shingles has increased dramatically since 1995 when the U.S. government recommended—and many states mandated—that all children receive Varivax, Merck's new chickenpox vaccine. Prior to the widespread use of the chickenpox vaccine, there were about 500,000 cases of shingles annually in the United States.[15] However, from 1998 to 2003 (during a period of increasing varicella vaccination) HZ incidence among adults increased by 90 percent.[16] The number of shingles cases in 2002 was 33 percent higher than in 2001 and 56 percent higher than in 2000.[17] Apparently, there is a societal benefit when chickenpox remains endemic. When the wild-type varicella virus

273

is permitted to circulate naturally throughout society, adults receive beneficial periodic exposures to the virus boosting their immune systems and helping to suppress the reactivation of herpes zoster. However, as more and more children are vaccinated with the synthetic or manufactured chickenpox virus, the natural virus becomes less pervasive and there are fewer opportunities for adults to receive these periodic boosts. This has led to much higher rates of shingles in Americans.[18] The FDA, CDC and vaccine manufacturer have traded a relatively mild childhood disease—chickenpox—for a much more serious ailment that affects adults.[19-21] In fact, shingles causes five times as many hospitalizations and three times as many deaths as chickenpox.[22,23]

Dr. Gary Goldman, an expert varicella research analyst, was hired by the CDC in 1995 to collect data and monitor trends associated with the newly introduced chickenpox vaccine. Goldman elaborates on this issue: "Due to the universal varicella vaccination program whereby every healthy child is vaccinated at age 12 months, there are no longer the seasonal outbreaks of varicella that occurred in schools and communities. These annual outbreaks and exposures (called exogenous exposures) played a significant role in boosting cell-mediated immunity to help suppress the reactivation of herpes zoster among children and adults who had a previous history of natural or wild-type varicella."[24] Consequently, "the universal varicella vaccination program in the United States...will leave our population vulnerable to shingles epidemics."[25] In fact, "there appears to be no way to avoid a mass epidemic of shingles lasting as long as several generations among adults."[26] Goldman estimates that it will take more than 50 years before the shingles epidemic will begin to subside. He calculates that in this time period there will be an additional 14.6 million shingles cases among adults less than 50 years old, presenting society with an additional medical cost burden of $4.1 billion—$82 million annually.[27]

A shingles vaccine:

The CDC is fully aware of the link between their own national chickenpox vaccine campaign and skyrocketing cases of shingles. Epidemiologists from the CDC are apparently hoping that "any possible shingles epidemic associated with the chickenpox vaccine can be offset by treating adults with a shingles vaccine."[28] Therefore, on May 25, 2006, the U.S. Food and Drug Administration (FDA) licensed Zostavax® for use in people who are 60 years of age and older.[29] This vaccine, designed to reduce the risk of shingles, is manufactured by Merck, the same company that developed Varivax, the chickenpox vaccine whose very "success" may be *causing* epidemics of shingles (Figure 87).[30]

Dr. Goldman is unequivocal regarding the use of new vaccines to treat problems created by old vaccines. He asserts that "the shingles vaccine serves as a vaccine to offset the initial deleterious effects associated with the similar and related varicella vaccine. It will be difficult to replicate the protection against shingles that existed naturally in the community when incidence of chickenpox was high."[31] Goldman believes that "using a shingles vaccine to control shingles epidemics in adults would likely fail because adult vaccination programs have rarely proved successful. There appears to be no way to avoid a mass epidemic of shingles lasting as long as several generations among adults."[32]

How safe is the new shingles vaccine?

The new shingles vaccine, Zostavax, is at least 14 times more potent than Varivax, Merck's chickenpox vaccine. According to the vaccine manufacturer, Zostavax contains a "live, attenuated varicella-zoster virus initially obtained from a child with naturally occurring varicella, then introduced into human embryonic lung cell cultures, adapted to and propagated in embryonic guinea pig cell cultures and finally propagated in human diploid cell cultures" (fetal tissue). Each dose also contains sucrose, hydrolyzed porcine (pig) gelatin, sodium chloride, monosodium L-glutamate (MSG), sodium phosphate dibasic, potassium phosphate monobasic, potassium chloride, and "residual components of MRC-5 cells including DNA and protein, and trace quantities of neomycin (an antibiotic) and bovine calf serum."[33] (For more information about vaccines cultured from human fetal tissue, and to read a summary of common ingredients in vaccines, see *Appendices III* and *IV* on pages 309-310.)

Figure 87:

Chickenpox Vaccine ➡ Shingles ➡ Shingles Vaccine

New Vaccine

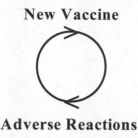

Adverse Reactions

The chickenpox vaccine may be causing epidemics of shingles, a condition now being treated with a shingles vaccine. New vaccines cause adverse reactions which health authorities attempt to rectify with new vaccines. Source: *International Journal of Toxicology* 2005; 24:205-213. *Vaccine* (May 9, 2005): 3349-3355.

Adverse reactions:

In the main clinical study used to justify licensing the new shingles vaccine, adverse reactions and "serious" adverse reactions were reported with significantly greater frequency in recipients of the vaccine than in recipients of a placebo.[34] "Systemic" adverse events also occurred more frequently among vaccine recipients. For example, more vaccine recipients had "cardiovascular events," including congestive heart failure and pulmonary edema.[35] Respiratory infection, respiratory disorder, skin disorder, flu syndrome, rhinitis, asthenia (weakness) and diarrhea all occurred with greater frequency in the vaccine group as well (Figure 88).[36] In addition, "the overall incidence of vaccine-related injection-site adverse experiences was significantly greater for subjects vaccinated with Zostavax versus subjects who received placebo."[37] Vaccinees had more pain, tenderness, itching and swelling at the injection site. They also experienced more headaches.[38]

Many people in the study—both vaccine recipients and recipients of a placebo—contracted shingles. Some of these people had HZ-related complications. Although fewer vaccine recipients contracted shingles when compared to recipients of a placebo (see efficacy data in the following section), among all of the people in the study who had HZ-related complications, a higher percentage of vaccine recipients were stricken with sensory loss and ophthalmic zoster[39] (a herpes zoster rash that infects the eye and can cause inflammation, scarring and visual impairment).

In an additional clinical study, a higher potency Zostavax was compared to a lower potency Zostavax (similar to potencies studied in the primary study). Serious adverse events among recipients of this vaccine included cases of angina pectoris, coronary artery disease, enteritis (inflammation of the intestine) and depression.[40] "Severe injection-site reactions" were also more common.[41]

The vaccine manufacturer warns that Zostavax may result in "a more extensive vaccine-associated rash or disseminated disease in individuals who are immunosuppressed."[42] Also, "post-marketing experience with varicella vaccines suggests that transmission of vaccine virus may occur between vaccinees...and susceptible contacts."[43] In other words: a) people with weak immune systems may have more severe reactions to the vaccine, and b) healthy people who elect to receive this vaccine should be aware that they can spread the live virus to other members of society, with potentially drastic consequences.

Figure 88:

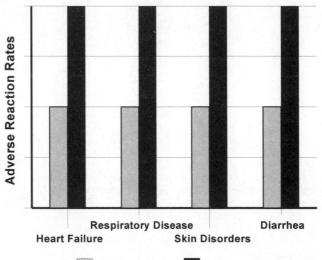

Shingles Vaccine *Increases* Adverse Reactions

Adverse reactions and "serious" adverse reactions, including congestive heart failure, respiratory infections, skin disorders, and diarrhea all occurred with greater frequency in recipients of the shingles vaccine when compared to adults who received a placebo. (Statistical differences are not drawn to scale.) Source: *New England Journal of Medicine* (June 2, 2005);352, No.22: 2271-84. The vaccine manufacturer.

Adverse Reaction Reports

The following case reports were taken directly from the FDA's Vaccine Adverse Event Reporting System (VAERS).[44] They represent just a small sample of the vaccine damage possibly linked to the shingles vaccine.

▸ 269160: A physician reported that his 20-year-old daughter caught chickenpox after her mother received the shingles vaccine. The vaccinated mother also broke out with "itchy unilateral lesions."

▸ 269643: Three days after receiving the shingles vaccine, a 60-year-old woman experienced numbness in her legs, lips and around her mouth. She could not walk and was sent to a neurologist to determine if she developed Guillain-Barré syndrome.

▸ 269157: A physician reported that his 60-year-old wife received the shingles vaccine and broke out in "itchy lesions" two weeks later.

▸ 269135: A 60-year-old woman received the shingles vaccine. That same day, she developed a painful "atypical shingles rash" requiring emergency care.

▸ 266376: A 60-year-old man had a stroke after receiving the shingles vaccine.

▸ 266040: An elderly woman had a stroke 24-48 hours after getting a shingles vaccine.

▸ 269127: An elderly woman received the herpes zoster vaccine and three days later developed herpes genitalis and herpes labialis.

▸ 269133: A 63-year-old man received the shingles vaccine and two hours later developed an itchy "maculopapular rash" on his head, body and extremities. Emergency care was required.

▸ 269155: A 64-year-old woman developed "chickenpox" after receiving the shingles vaccine. Emergency care was required.

▸ 278808: A 64-year-old woman developed outbreaks of shingles that were "significant and painful" after receiving a shingles vaccine.

▸ 262880: An elderly woman developed a painful case of shingles a few days after her husband received the shingles vaccine.

▸ 269115: A 67-year-old woman received the shingles vaccine and three days later developed a painful rash and blisters.

▸ 269458: A 72-year-old woman developed herpes zoster in the perineum one day after receiving the herpes zoster vaccine. Emergency care was required.

▸ 267061: A 72-year-old woman received the shingles vaccine and developed shingles two days later, with pain radiating from her back to her breast.

▸ 279024: A 79-year old-woman received the shingles vaccine and three days later had overall body pain, weakness, with tingling in her feet and arm. She was hospitalized for several days with a tentative diagnosis of Guillain-Barré syndrome.

▸ 267069: The day after an 89-year-old woman received the shingles vaccine she awoke with excruciating body pain, burning and throbbing of ears, pressure in her head, stomach pain, severe headache, neck pain, and paresthesia.

How effective is the new shingles vaccine?

According to the vaccine manufacturer, Zostavax is 51 percent effective at reducing the risk of developing herpes zoster in adults 60 years of age or older when compared with a placebo. However, among seniors 70 to 79 years of age, efficacy drops to 41 percent. Efficacy plummets to 18 percent among seniors 80 years of age and older (Figure 89).[45]

Authors of the HZ vaccine study also evaluated the "duration of pain" in study subjects who contracted shingles after being vaccinated with Zostavax. On average they were in pain for 20 days versus 22 days of pain for study subjects who developed shingles after receiving a placebo.[46,47] In addition, researchers measured how effective the HZ vaccine was at reducing the "burden of illness." (The precise way in which "burden of illness" was defined and the statistical methods for analyzing this designation were developed by Merck, the HZ vaccine manufacturer.) Published results show that the vaccine reduced the burden of illness due to herpes zoster among people 60 years of age or older by 61 percent, and reduced the incidence of post herpetic neuralgia by 67 percent.[48]

The HZ vaccine was mainly tested on white people. It is common knowledge that minorities have varying immune systems and that they often react differently to medical substances. Therefore, published HZ vaccine efficacy figures may not apply to people from different races or cultures.[49]

People who participated in the HZ vaccine study were monitored for herpes zoster for a mean duration of 3.12 years.[50] In other words, vaccine "efficacy" is predicated on approximately 37 months of surveillance. The vaccine manufacturer acknowledges that "duration of protection after vaccination with Zostavax is unknown.... The need for revaccination has not been defined."[51]

Conflicts of interest?

The HZ vaccine manufacturer, Merck, "participated in the organization of oversight activities and monitored the progress" of the primary study used to justify licensing this vaccine.[52] In addition, several leading authors of this study received consultation fees, lecture fees, or honoraria from Merck.[53,54] Others received grant support from Merck or owned stock in Merck—all while concurrently overseeing important aspects of the study requiring complete objectivity.[55] Two of the researchers were actively involved in this study while having "partial interests in relevant patents."[56] Still others were employees of Merck.[57]

Important healthcare branches of the U.S. government that are designed to protect the public—the FDA and CDC—are riddled with conflicts of interest as well. For example, the FDA compromised its integrity by claiming there is no evidence the shingles vaccine is to blame for the significantly higher number of serious adverse reactions in recipients

Figure 89:

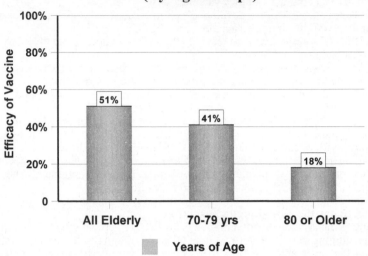

Efficacy of the Shingles Vaccine
(By Age Groups)

The shingles vaccine, Zostavax, is 51 percent effective at reducing the risk of developing herpes zoster in adults 60 years of age or older when compared with a placebo. Among seniors 70 to 79 years of age, efficacy drops to 41 percent. Efficacy plummets to 18 percent among seniors 80 years of age and older. Source: The vaccine manufacturer.

---

of the vaccine when compared to recipients of a placebo.[58,59] This is an absurd assertion considering that the primary shingles study that the FDA used to license this vaccine was specifically designed to provide the clinical evidence of the vaccine's safety profile. If the safety data of this study can be arbitrarily discounted by the FDA simply because the results did not conform to preconceived or desired expectations, then the entire study can be rejected on the same basis. However, that would be unprecedented, especially since Dr. Ann Arvin, a paid consultant to Merck, "praised the size and design of the study, saying its results were not open to much doubt."[60]

Finally, at least one member of the CDC's Advisory Committee on Immunization Practices (ACIP), Dr. William Schaffner, received financial payment from Merck to discuss Zostavax with reporters.[61] This questionable practice lowers public confidence in the high ethical standards that should be required and are expected from the custodians of our healthcare system. It also encourages public cynicism toward media coverage of all vaccine-related news. How can we trust *any* claim pertaining to vaccine safety and efficacy when custodians of our healthcare system are receiving money from the drug companies they are commissioned to oversee? The FDA and CDC appear to be mere sycophants to the pharmaceutical industry. A functional system of healthcare checks and balances is imperative.

> "The universal varicella vaccination program in the United States...will leave our population vulnerable to shingles epidemics. There appears to be no way to avoid a mass epidemic of shingles lasting as long as several generations among adults."
> —Gary Goldman, PhD, expert varicella research analyst

Pneumonia
Pneumococcal disease (in adults)

What is pneumococcal pneumonia?
Pneumococcal pneumonia is the most common type of pneumonia, a potentially serious ailment characterized by inflammation or infection of the lungs.[1] A bacterium called *streptococcus pneumoniae* causes pneumococcal pneumonia. This same microorganism can also cause bacteremia (an infection of the blood) and meningitis (inflammation of the brain and spinal cord).[2]

How prevalent is pneumococcal pneumonia?
Pneumococcal pneumonia can occur after an upper respiratory tract infection such as the flu, especially in people with preexisting health problems and the elderly.[3] Some authorities estimate that 500,000 cases of pneumococcal pneumonia occur annually in the United States.[4] About 5 percent of people who get pneumococcal pneumonia will die from it.[5]

Who is most susceptible to pneumococcal pneumonia?
The risk of getting pneumonia from any source (bacterial or viral) increases after age 40 and doubles after age 60.[6] People with chronic ailments, such as heart or lung disease, kidney failure, alcoholism, diabetes, HIV infection and certain types of cancer, are more likely to get pneumococcal disease. They are also more likely to die from the disease.[7]

Does a pneumococcal pneumonia vaccine exist?
Two vaccines for pneumococcal disease have been available since the 1970s: 1) Pneumovax® by Merck, and 2) Pnu-Immune® by Wyeth. They are "polysaccharide" vaccines designed to protect against 23 of the approximately 90 different pneumococcal strains capable of causing bacterial disease.[8,9] These two vaccines are mainly recommended for seniors and high risk children over 2 years of age.[10] They are not recommended for younger children. (A pneumococcal vaccine is available for younger children. For more information, turn to page 205.)

How safe is the pneumococcal pneumonia vaccine?
According to the vaccine manufacturer, the following adverse reactions have been reported during clinical trials of the shot and/or in post-marketing experience: Guillain-Barré syndrome, radiculoneuropathy, paresthesia, arthritis, arthralgia, myalgia, lymphadenopathy, thrombocytopenia, anaphylactoid reactions, cellulitis, serum sickness, headache, rash, nausea, vomiting, chills, fever and fatigue.[11] In addition, local and systemic adverse reaction rates are high. For example, in persons 65 years of age or older, local adverse reactions (such as pain at the injection site, swelling, and decreased limb mobility) occurred in 53 percent of vaccine recipients. Systemic adverse reactions (such as headaches, muscle aches, and fatigue) occurred in 22 percent of the vaccine recipients. Adverse reaction rates were even higher in persons 50 to 64 years of age: 73 percent experienced local reactions, while 36 percent had systemic experiences.[12] Revaccination with a booster dose 3 to 5 years later resulted in even higher adverse reaction rates than during receipt of the primary shot. For example, in persons 65 years of age or older, 53 percent experienced local adverse reactions after the 1st dose while 79 percent experienced these debilities after the 2nd dose.[13]

The CDC's Advisory Committee on Immunization Practices (ACIP) states that the pneumococcal vaccine may be administered at the same time as the influenza vaccine (by separate injection in the other arm).[14] However, some people have reported serious reactions after receiving both shots simultaneously. For example: "I had the pneumonia and flu vaccines given to me. About 20 minutes after the shots, I was in excruciating pain. It was so bad that I went to the emergency room the next day. They tried to find out which arm had which shot, but that information was not recorded. The pain went on and on. Today, over 6 months later, I still only have partial use of my arm, and still have pain associated with certain movements. I have numbness in both arms and hands. My nails are beginning to come off my fingers. I am very concerned that I may have Guillain-Barré syndrome. I would like to add that the hospital in Pittsburgh that administered the shots wants nothing to do with helping me."[15]

How effective is the pneumococcal pneumonia vaccine?

Several studies have shown that the pneumococcal vaccine is ineffective; it does not work.[16-25] Apparently, its poor efficacy is related to "rapid antibody washout" and other causes.[26] Some authorities have noted that "those at highest risk of infection and complications, such as the immunocompromised and aged, benefit least from the vaccine."[27] In 2007, researchers working for *The Cochrane Collaboration*—an objective, independent well-respected source of scientific evidence—published the results of their thorough assessment of every significant study throughout the world (from 1954 through 2003) pertaining to the polysaccharide pneumococcal vaccine. The authors of the review found that the vaccine is 53 percent effective against invasive pneumococcal infection. However, they also made the following conclusion: "The combined results from the randomized studies fail to show that the polysaccharide pneumococcal vaccine is effective in preventing either pneumonia or death."[28] In fact, it does not matter whether vaccine recipients are middle-aged or elderly (55 years and above), with or without chronic illness; the "pneumonia" vaccine does not reduce the incidence of pneumonia or death.[29]

It is also important to note that the pneumococcal pneumonia vaccine will not protect against pneumococcal infections caused by strains not included in the vaccine. It is only designed to prevent disease caused by the limited number of strains included in the vaccine (23 of approximately 90 different strains).[30] In addition, this vaccine will not protect against bacterial infections caused by haemophilus influenzae type b or meningococcus.[31] Thus, vaccinated adults may still contract bacterial disease, including meningitis, blood infections and pneumonia.

Travel Vaccines

This chapter contains information on several vaccines that are often recommended by the authorities when traveling overseas.

Tuberculosis

What is tuberculosis?
Tuberculous (TB) is a serious infectious disease caused by *Mycobacterium tuberculosis,* a bacterium. It usually affects the lungs but can attack other parts of the body, such as the bones or brain. Symptoms include fever, night sweats, loss of appetite, weight loss, chest infection, coughing, blood in sputum, and constant fatigue.[1,2] In earlier times, tuberculosis was known as consumption because victims were "consumed" by the disease and dwindled away.[3]

Tuberculosis is linked to poor living conditions, cramped housing, inadequate ventilation, and social deprivation.[4] It is much more common in urban environments.[5] Tuberculosis is spread through the air when infected people cough or sneeze, though it usually requires spending a long time in the company of someone who has the disease.[6,7] In most cases, newly infected people have no symptoms; only about 10 percent of people infected with tuberculosis actually develop the disease.[8]

How prevalent is TB?
Tuberculosis has infected and killed millions of people worldwide—especially Western Europeans—at least since the 1500s.[9] Large sanatoriums were built to treat victims (and remove them from society lessening their chances of infecting others).[10] Today, the disease is still problematic in some parts of the world, with about 8 million new cases diagnosed each year.[11] In 2005, the TB rate in Africa was 343 cases per 100,000 people.[12] In both 2005 and 2006, the TB rate in the United States was less than 5 cases per 100,000 people.[13]

Who is most at risk of contracting TB?
Some groups are more likely than others to become infected with TB. These include: people with HIV or other immune system weaknesses; people in close contact with someone who has TB; homeless people or anyone who lives in slums; people from countries where TB is common; people in nursing homes or prisons; people who inject drugs; and people with certain medical conditions, such as diabetes or cancer.[14]

Can tuberculosis be treated?
In most cases, tuberculosis can be cured. Treatment mainly consists of taking antibiotics and other anti-TB drugs. Full recovery could take several months.[15]

Is a TB vaccine available?
In 1921, two French scientists working at the Pasteur Institute, Albert Calmette and Camille Guérin, introduced the first tuberculosis vaccine—BCG—which was named after them (Bacillus-Calmette-Guérin).[16] Today, the BCG vaccine is used in many countries with high rates of TB. However, it is not recommended for general use in the U.S. because the risk of TB infection is low, the vaccine has "variable effectiveness," and it interferes with tuberculin skin test results.[17] (Also, it is manufactured in France.) New TB vaccines are under development.[18,19]

How safe is the BCG (TB) vaccine?
In 1930, the BCG vaccine was procured from France and given to 251 children in a German clinic; most of these children became ill and 77 died. The German people were outraged and blamed France. The doctor who administered the vaccine was tried in court and sentenced to prison.[20]

Today, the BCG vaccine is known to cause adverse events. The shot produces a pimple at the site of injection and enlarges the lymph nodes in the surrounding area. After a few weeks, the pimple bursts and releases pus, leaving a keloid, or large, ugly scar. The vaccine may also cause abscesses on the groin lymph nodes, usually 3-7 months later. Lymph node abscesses may also develop in the armpit or hollow above the collar bone. Some people develop bone or joint inflammation, skin infection, or "generalized BCG infection" —vaccine-induced tuberculosis. These serious adverse reactions occur on average 14 months after vaccination and may persist as "permanent functional disorders."[21] Musculo-skeletal lesions and "fatal disseminated lesions" have also occurred after BCG vaccination.[22]

How effective is the BCG vaccine?

A long-term study conducted in the United States showed that the BCG vaccine has an efficacy of just 14 percent.[23] Another study conducted in Britain claimed an efficacy of 77 percent.[24] However, in 1968 the World Health Organization (WHO) conducted the world's largest field study of the BCG (tuberculosis) vaccine. The entire population of 364,000 people (except for babies under the age of one month) living in the province of Madras, India were injected with the BCG vaccine. At the same time, a second district with a similar population was used as a control, where nobody was given the vaccine. In 1979, eleven years after the study was initiated, WHO presented its findings: "The field trial, conducted under optimal conditions, did not demonstrate any effectiveness of the BCG vaccine."[25] This was a gross understatement; in actuality, the vaccinated population had a considerably greater number of TB cases than the unvaccinated population.[26]

In 1980, *Lancet* acknowledged that "the history of immunization against tuberculosis is a story of setback, controversy and surprise."[27] In 1993, the *British Medical Journal* reported that all 62 employees of a French hospital who contracted tuberculosis had been vaccinated against the disease.[28] In 1996, *Lancet* published the results of a long-term, placebo-controlled BCG efficacy study carried out on more than 66,000 citizens of Malawi. Researchers concluded that "there was no evidence that any of the trial vaccines contributed to protection against pulmonary tuberculosis."[29] In fact, "the rate of diagnostically certain tuberculosis was higher among...individuals who received a second BCG than among those who received placebo."[30] In 1998, the German vaccination commission (STRIKO) published the following statement in *Der Kinderarzt*, a prestigious medical journal, retracting its endorsement of the TB vaccine: "In view of the epidemiological situation in Germany, the lack of evidence for the effectiveness of the BCG vaccine, and the not uncommon severe, undesired side effects of the BCG vaccine, the STRIKO can no longer support the recommendation for this vaccine."[31] In 1999, new research confirmed that the BCG vaccine does not work.[32] In 2007, researchers found that newer TB vaccines currently in use may be less immunogenic than the older ones.[33]

Tuberculin Skin Test

What is a tuberculin skin test?

A tuberculin skin test aids in the diagnosis of tuberculosis (TB), an infectious disease that affects the lungs. The test is done by inserting a small amount of TB toxins (tuberculin) under the top layer of skin on the inner forearm. If the person being tested has ever been exposed to tuberculosis, their skin will react to the toxins by developing a firm red bump at the site within two days. The most commonly used tuberculin skin test is the Mantoux skin test, which contains fixed amounts of TB antigens called purified protein derivative (PPD). Although the Mantoux TB test is not a vaccine, TB antigens are placed in a syringe and injected under the skin.[1,2]

How safe is the TB test?

The most widely used Mantoux skin test is Tubersol®, produced by Aventis Pasteur. According to the manufacturer, the product is "...obtained from a human strain of *mycobacterium tuberculosis*." In addition, it contains Tween 80 as a stabilizer; phenol is added as a preservative.[3] Tween 80 is a trade name for polysorbate 80, which may contain 1,4-dioxane—a suspected carcinogen and known liver and kidney toxicant.[4,5] Phenol is a suspected liver, kidney, respiratory, cardiovascular, and central nervous system toxicant.[6]

How effective is the TB test?
Many factors can influence test results. Thus, false negatives and false positives are relatively common. For example, a New York woman, Maureen Ryan, recently spent two months confined to her home, taking large doses of antibiotics, after she was misdiagnosed with TB. She was frightened that she had spread the disease to her children and grandchildren. In May of 2007, she was compensated $75,000 for the ordeal.[7] Viral infections, viral vaccines, malnutrition, leukemia, and the use of immunosuppressant drugs can cause a false negative tuberculin reaction.[8] False positives can result from a prior tuberculosis vaccination (the BCG vaccine) or from non-tuberculosis infections. (Ms. Ryan had been struggling with a bronchitis-like illness.)[9] Furthermore, health practitioners who are responsible for interpreting test results by measuring the size of the firm red bump, often misdiagnose.[10,11] Additional tests, such as a chest X-ray or sputum culture may be requested.[12]

Is the TB test mandatory?
Health care workers, college students and some school-age children who are presumed to be at greater risk of contracting tuberculosis are expected to submit to the tuberculin skin test every year. It may be a mandatory requirement to procure or retain a job.[13] For example, here is an unsolicited letter regarding this topic: "I'm looking for guidance regarding mandatory annual TB testing in hospitals because I consider a TB skin test to be on par with an unwanted immunization. As you know, a TB skin test requires that a small amount of the tuberculosis germ be injected into your body. The hospital where I work is forcing every employee, regardless of their health or job duties, to have an *annual* TB test. This policy is in direct opposition to OSHA regulations, which specifically state that only hospital or healthcare workers who have direct contact with high-risk populations need to be tested annually. I do not have direct contact with any patient population and have very limited contact with any medical staff. But because I am paid from a certain accounting code, I've been targeted for this program. I'm concerned about the long-term health effects of an *annual* TB test program. Can you provide any guidance. The hospital administration has been very aggressive in their efforts to implement this program and they have stated that it is a law that I be tested, and if I refuse I may be placed on unpaid leave."[14]

Some institutions accept vaccine exemptions. If you are opposed to the TB test, read your state vaccine laws to explore options. If an exemption is not obtainable, a non-invasive, FDA-approved Meridian Stress Assessment can scan your body for viruses, bacteria and other pathogens. A computer printout of the results might be accepted by authorities.[15,16]

Yellow Fever

What is yellow fever?
Yellow fever is a viral disease that is transmitted to humans through the bite of an infected mosquito (the female *Aedes aegypti* or *Haemgogus*). The illness cannot be spread directly from person to person. Once bitten by an infected mosquito, the incubation period is 3 to 6 days. The onset of disease is sudden, with flu-like symptoms, including fever, chills, headache, pain in the lower back, loss of appetite, nausea and vomiting. Most cases are mild, last less than a week, and the person makes a full recovery.[1,2] People who recover from the disease gain lifelong immunity against reinfection. In about 15 percent of cases, the disease progresses to jaundice, internal bleeding, plus liver, kidney and other organ system failures. Liver failure causes yellowing of the skin, giving the disease its name. From 20 to 50 percent of patients with liver and kidney failure will die, usually within 1 to 2 weeks.[3-5]

How prevalent is yellow fever?

The World Health Organization (WHO) *estimates* that there are 200,000 cases of yellow fever per year worldwide[6]—despite official WHO statistics through 2004 showing an average of less than 1,000 cases per year for the past 35 years (Figure 90).[7] About 90 percent of cases occur in rural sub-Sahara Africa near the equator (between 15 degrees latitude north and 10 degrees latitude south). The remaining cases occur in tropical South America.[8] During inter-epidemic periods, which may last years or even decades, transmission levels in many countries are often undetectable.[9] Nigeria, the country with the greatest number of recorded cases since 1950, had just 49 cases from 1995 through 2004, with 11 deaths.[10] Ghana had 13 deaths attributed to yellow fever during this same 10-year period.[11]

Who is most at risk of contracting yellow fever?

In rural West Africa, infants and children are at greatest risk of infection, especially during the late rainy and early dry seasons (July-October). In South America, the disease occurs most often in young men working in forested areas, especially during the rainy season (January-March). Urban transmission is less likely; yellow fever has not occurred in South American towns and cities for many years.[12] Foreign travelers to rural regions of countries in the midst of yellow fever outbreaks may be at increased risk as well. (From 1996-2002, there were a total of five yellow fever fatalities among all American and European travelers.)[13]

Is a yellow fever vaccine available?

Two live-virus yellow fever vaccines have been available since the 1930s. YF-Vax® by Sanofi Pasteur "is prepared by culturing the 17D-204 strain of yellow fever virus in living avian leukosis virus-free chicken embryos." The vaccine also contains sorbitol and gelatin. A booster dose is required after 10 years.[14] This vaccine is not available at the doctor's office; it is only given at approved vaccination centers. Recipients of the shot are provided with an International Certificate of Vaccination that is valid for 10 years.[15]

How safe is the yellow fever vaccine?

Yellow fever vaccines have been linked to multiple organ system failure (vaccine-associated viscerotropic disease), virtually identical to severe and fatal cases of yellow fever caused by the wild-type of yellow fever virus. The vaccine may also cause profound nervous system reactions, including Guillain-Barré syndrome and neurotropic disease (previously named post-vaccinal encephalitis).[16-18] Curiously, the vaccine manufacturer suggests that victims of the shot only had themselves to blame; their adverse reactions were more than likely "due to undefined host factors, rather than to intrinsic virulence of the 17DD vaccine viruses."[19] Other adverse reactions associated with this vaccine include asthma, life-threatening allergic reactions, and systemic reactions, such as fever, headache, muscle ache, weakness and malaise, that often persist for up to ten days.[20] In one study, 72 percent of vaccine recipients experienced "non-serious" (but in some cases severe) adverse events, and up to 30 percent had systemic reactions.[21]

Serious adverse reactions: As early as 1960, *Pediatrics* wrote about the yellow fever vaccine causing inflammation of the brain.[22] In 1970, German researchers documented chromosomal changes following yellow fever vaccination.[23] In 1990, the *Journal of Infection* confirmed encephalitis after the shot.[24] In 1994, researchers documented several cases of severe post-vaccination reactions to the yellow fever vaccine: "The patients presented with rapidly progressing swelling of the left arm with associated fever and other constitutional symptoms a few hours after inoculation with the vaccine. Some of the patients developed gangrene of the affected limb, five of them went into coma and died."[25] In 1995, researchers once again documented coma after yellow fever vaccination.[26] In 1997, *Lancet* reported on hemorrhagic disease after the shot.[27] In 1999, the *Journal of Allergy and Clinical Immunology* documented 22 cases of anaphylactic reactions caused by the shot.[28] In 2001, the *Canadian Medical Association Journal* analyzed seven cases of multiple organ system failure linked to the vaccine.[29] That same year, the CDC also reviewed cases of multiple

Figure 90:

Yellow Fever Cases
(Worldwide)

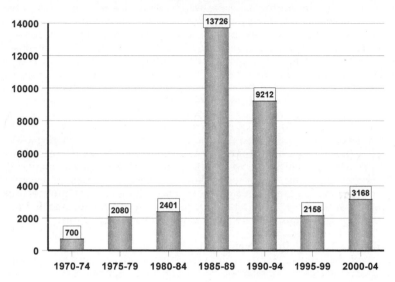

From 1970 through 2004, there was a worldwide average of less than 1,000 reported cases of yellow fever per year. About 90 percent of all cases occur in rural sub-Sahara Africa near the equator. The remaining cases occur in tropical South America. Source: WHO.

---

organ system failure (vaccine-associated viscerotropic disease) caused by the vaccine.[30] Also in 2001, *Lancet* reported on two cases of severe reactions following the shot: "The first case, in a 5-year-old white girl, was characterized by sudden onset of fever accompanied by headache, malaise, and vomiting three days after receiving yellow fever and measles-mumps-rubella vaccines. Afterwards, she decompensated with icterus and hemorrhagic signs and died after a 5-day illness. The second patient—a 22-year-old black woman —developed a sore throat and fever accompanied by headache, myalgia, nausea, and vomiting four days after yellow fever vaccination. She then developed icterus, renal failure, and hemorrhagic diathesis, and died after six days of illness."[31] In a separate paper, *Lancet* also published the following report: "We describe a man vaccinated with the 17D204 strain of yellow fever virus, who subsequently died of yellow fever. Severe, rapidly progressive, and ultimately fatal disease can follow use of the 17D204 vaccine strain. There is need for renewed discussion as to the safety of the vaccine and the indications for its use."[32] Another *Lancet* paper reported that the CDC "was notified of three patients who developed severe illnesses days after yellow fever vaccination. The clinical presentations were characterized by fever, myalgia, headache, and confusion, followed by severe multi-systemic illnesses."[33] The three patients died. Several other papers published in 2001 and 2002 also documented cases of severe illness and death following yellow fever vaccination.[34-38] A report published in a 2002 edition of the CDC's *Morbidity and Mortality Weekly Report (MMWR)* discussed two cases of multiple organ system failure, and four separate cases of neurotropic disease, following yellow fever vaccination.[39] All of the cases of multiple organ system failure led to respiratory breakdown, lymphocytopenia, thrombocytopenia, hypotension and renal malfunction. Sixty-seven percent of these and earlier documented cases were fatal.[40] In 2004, *Epidemiology and Infection* wrote about four fatal adverse events in Brazil following yellow fever vaccination.[41] That same year, an Australian journal reported on "six deaths internationally, including one from Australia, plus other cases of severe systemic adverse events following yellow fever vaccination."[42] These reactions "have raised concern about the safety of the yellow fever vaccine, particularly among older vaccinees."[43] Also in 2004, *Vaccine* noted that "Yellow fever vaccine-associated viscerotropic and neurotropic diseases have been recently identified in various countries. Previously, post-vaccination multiple organ system failure was recognized as a rare serious adverse event of yellow fever vaccination, and 21 cases of post-vaccinal encephalitis had been recorded."[44] In 2005, *Southern Medical Journal* described "a case of yellow fever vaccine-associated viscerotropic disease that occurred after vaccination in a 22-year-old female. Our patient presented with a clinical syndrome of fever, headache, nausea, and vomiting, which quickly progressed to multi-organ failure and ultimately death on hospital day four."[45] In 2006, the *Journal of Clinical Virology* described another case of vaccine-associated viscerotropic disease in a young woman "who died after vaccination with 17D-204 strain."[46] Also in 2006, researchers noted that "during 1996 through 2004, 29 cases of yellow fever vaccine-associated viscerotropic disease have been reported worldwide; 17 were fatal."[47] In 2007, the *Journal of Travel Medicine* wrote about a 64-year-old woman who "presented with brachial herpes zoster infection three days after vaccination against yellow fever."[48] That same year, researchers analyzed 15 cases of encephalitis, encephalomyelitis, and Guillain Barré syndrome either "definitely" or "probably" caused by the yellow fever vaccine.[49] In another 2007 paper, researchers documented 12 cases of aseptic meningitis "temporally" linked to yellow fever vaccinations.[50]

How effective is the yellow fever vaccine?
To determine the yellow fever vaccine's efficacy, researchers use a surrogate method adopted by the World Health Organization. They calculate the number of virus-neutralizing antibodies found in the vaccine recipient's blood ten days after injection. If this antibody titer level matches previously established standards "shown to protect 90 percent of monkeys from lethal intracerebral challenge," the vaccine is considered effective. By this measure, "the seroconversion rate was greater than 91 percent in all but two studies and never lower than 81 percent."[51]

Is the yellow fever vaccine mandatory for travel overseas?
The yellow fever vaccine is recommended for persons 9 months of age or older traveling to or living in areas of Africa or South America where yellow fever infection is officially reported at the time of travel.[52] Some countries require a valid International Certificate of Vaccination if the individual has been in countries (even if only in transit) either known or thought to harbor the yellow fever virus. Some countries may waive the requirements for travelers staying less than two weeks that are coming from areas where there is no current evidence or significant risk of contracting yellow fever.[53] For more information about exemptions, contact the embassy of the country or countries that you plan to visit.

Supplementary safety measures:
Regarding diseases transmitted by mosquitos, authorities recommend applying reliable insect repellant on skin and clothing. Other precautions include remaining in air-conditioned or well-screened areas and wearing clothes that cover most of the body.[54]

Typhoid Fever

What is typhoid fever?
Typhoid fever, also known as enteric fever, is a serious intestinal illness caused by the *Salmonella typhi* bacterium. Symptoms appear one to two weeks after exposure and include a sustained fever as high as 104° F (40°C), malaise, loss of appetite, profuse sweating, stomach cramps, headache, diarrhea, rose-colored spots on the trunk, and an enlarged liver and spleen. Complications are possible, and may involve bleeding in the lower gastrointestinal tract, encephalitis or cardiac failure. Without treatment, symptoms may persist for weeks or months and could lead to death.[1-4]

How is typhoid fever contracted?

Persons with typhoid fever carry the bacteria in their intestinal tract and bloodstream. Typhoid germs are spread by eating food or drinking beverages handled by a person who is shedding the disease in their feces, especially in areas of the world where hand washing is uncommon. The disease can also be contracted if sewage contaminated with *S. typhi* gets into the water that is used for drinking or washing food. More rarely, insects feeding on feces may transfer the bacteria, especially in regions of the world where public sanitation is poor.[5]

How is typhoid fever treated?

Standard treatment involves the administration of antibiotics. The case-fatality rate is less than one percent with antibiotic treatment.[6]

How prevalent and risky is typhoid fever?

Typhoid fever is very rare in the industrialized regions of the world such as the United States, Canada, western Europe, Australia and Japan.[7] This disease is common in countries with low levels of hygiene and in regions of the world with poor water and sanitation systems.[8,9] In the United States, only about 300 cases occur each year; about 75 percent of these are acquired through international travel.[10] Travelers from the United States to the Indian subcontinent, Asia, Africa and Latin America have a greater risk. In the developing world, typhoid fever affects approximately 21 million people each year.[11]

How can travelers protect against typhoid fever?

Travelers to areas where typhoid fever is possible should observe the following precautions:
• Drink only water that is boiled or treated with chlorine. Bottled beverages with no ice are usually safe. Bottled carbonated water is safer than uncarbonated water.
• Eat only foods that have been thoroughly cooked and are still hot.
• Avoid raw fruits that cannot be peeled; peel them yourself.
• Make sure all vegetables are cooked; avoid salads.
• Avoid foods and beverages from street vendors.[12]

Is a typhoid fever vaccine available?

In 1896, Sir Almroth Edward Wright, a British immunologist, developed the first vaccine against typhoid fever.[13] In 1909, Frederick Fuller Russell, a U.S. Army physician, developed the first American typhoid fever vaccine.[14] In 1911, the entire U.S. army received this prophylactic shot.[15] Today, two typhoid fever vaccines are available: Typhim Vi, a capsular polysaccharide vaccine given by injection, and Vivotif Berna (Ty21a), a live-attenuated, oral vaccine.[16] A third typhoid fever vaccine, Ty800, is in clinical trials and could become available very soon.[17]

How safe is the typhoid fever vaccine?

The following adverse reactions have been reported following receipt of the typhoid fever vaccine: injection site pain, fever, headache, rash, dizziness, myalgia, nausea, abdominal pain, diarrhea, vomiting, anaphylaxis, facial edema, throat swelling, transverse myelitis, polyarthritis, Guillain-Barré syndrome and cerebral herniation leading to death.[18] In a recent analysis of the FDA's Vaccine Adverse Event Reporting System (VAERS), published in a February 2004 issue of *Clinical Infectious Diseases,* of all reports pertaining to both the injectable and oral typhoid fever vaccines, 7.5 percent and 5.5 percent , respectively, described hospitalization, life-threatening illness, permanent disability or death.[19]

How effective is the typhoid fever vaccine?

According to the CDC, typhoid fever vaccines "are not completely effective."[20] The injectable vaccine is believed to be 55 percent effective three years after vaccination of children 5 to 16 years of age. The oral vaccine has shown an efficacy of 62 percent for seven years after the last dose.[21] As a result, the New York Department of Health issued a report stating that strict attention to food and water precautions while traveling to developing countries where significant exposure to typhoid may occur "is the most effective preventive method."[22]

Is the typhoid fever vaccine recommended?
Typhoid fever is rare in the United States. Therefore, the Advisory Committee on Immunization Practices (ACIP) only recommends this vaccine for travelers to endemic areas, persons with intimate exposure to an *S. typhi* carrier, and microbiology/laboratory personnel who work frequently with the disease.[23]

Cholera

What is cholera?
Cholera is an acute intestinal illness caused by the *Vibrio cholerae* bacterium. The infection is often mild or without symptoms, although sometimes it can be severe. The disease is characterized by profuse, watery diarrhea, vomiting, thirst, dry mucous membranes, and muscle cramps. If left untreated, rapid loss of body fluids can lead to dehydration, shock and death.[1,2]

How is cholera contracted?
A person may get cholera by drinking water or eating food contaminated with the cholera bacterium.[3]

How is cholera treated?
Cholera is mainly treated by oral rehydration. Fluids and salts lost through diarrhea should be quickly replaced. Intravenous fluids and electrolytes are sometimes necessary. With prompt rehydration, death is unlikely.[4]

How prevalent and risky is cholera?
In 2005, there were about 132,000 cases reported to the World Health Organization. Nearly 95 percent of reported cases were from Africa. Cholera has been very rare in industrialized nations for the last 100 years. In the United States, cholera has been virtually eliminated by modern sewage and water treatment systems; it is not a major threat.[5]

How can travelers avoid getting cholera?
Cholera is easily prevented. The risk of contracting the disease is very low, even for travelers visiting areas with known cases of cholera. Travelers to areas where cholera has occurred should observe the following precautions:
- Drink only water that is boiled or treated with chlorine. Bottled beverages with no ice are usually safe.
- Eat only foods that have been thoroughly cooked and are still hot.
- Avoid eating risky foods, especially fish and shellfish.
- Make sure all vegetables are cooked; avoid salads.[6]

Is a cholera vaccine available?
Although two oral cholera vaccines are available, neither is licensed in the United States.[7] In June of 2007, Japanese researchers created an edible cholera vaccine "embedded in a specially developed strain of rice."[8]

How safe is the cholera vaccine?
Common side effects include gastrointestinal symptoms: abdominal pain, cramps, diarrhea and vomiting. Arthralgia, paresthesia, rash and flu-like symptoms are also likely.[9] In addition, the medical literature contains several studies linking the cholera vaccine to more serious adverse reactions, including liver failure, heart ailments, skin disorders and neurological complications. For example, studies document the following ailments after cholera vaccination: acute renal failure, myocarditis, ventricular tachycardia, cutaneous

lesions, leuko-encephalomyelitis, transverse myelitis, nerve paralysis, and neuropsychiatric complications.[10-17]

How effective is the cholera vaccine?
The cholera vaccine provides a "brief and incomplete immunity."[18] Trials of an early cholera vaccine showed a 50 percent efficacy rate after three years.[19]

Is the cholera vaccine recommended?
U.S. travelers have a low risk of contracting cholera. Therefore, the CDC does *not* recommend this vaccine. Furthermore, most countries do not require this vaccine as a condition of entry, although some local authorities may request documentation of cholera vaccination. In such instances, the traveler may request a medical waiver. Many travel clinics offer a medical waiver written on physician stationery.[20]

Japanese Encephalitis

What is Japanese encephalitis?
Japanese encephalitis is a viral infection (caused by an arbo-flavivirus) that is spread to humans by infected mosquitoes in Asia. Domestic pigs and wading birds are reservoirs for the virus. A specific mosquito, *Culex tritaeniorhynchus,* that lives in rural rice-growing and pig-farming regions, can spread the virus from the pig or bird to a human. The disease cannot be spread from person to person.[1-3]

Symptoms of the disease usually appear 6 to 8 days after the bite of an infected mosquito. Most infected people have mild symptoms or none at all. However, in people who develop a more severe case of the disease (about 1 of every 250 people who are infected) Japanese encephalitis starts as a flu-like illness, with fever, chills, tiredness, headache, nausea and vomiting. The disease can progress to neck rigidity, disorientation, neurological sequelae and inflammation of the brain (encephalitis). Death is possible.[4]

How is Japanese encephalitis treated?
There is no specific treatment for Japanese encephalitis. Antibiotics are not effective against viruses. Care of patients is limited to treatment of symptoms and complications of the disease.[5]

Who is most at risk for Japanese encephalitis?
People who live in rural areas where the disease is common are most at risk. In Asia, 30,000 to 50,000 cases are reported each year. Japanese encephalitis is a seasonal disease that occurs in the summer and fall in temperate regions of China, Japan and Korea. Outbreaks have also occurred in Taiwan, Thailand, Vietnam, Cambodia, Myanmar, India, Nepal and Malaysia.[6,7]

Japanese encephalitis is very rare in U.S. travelers to Asia. The chance of getting this disease is very small because, a) only a certain species of mosquito can spread Japanese encephalitis, b) in areas infested with mosquitoes, only a small number are infected with the virus, and c) among all persons who are infected by a mosquito bite, very few will develop an illness. Less than one case per year is reported in U.S. civilians and military personnel traveling to and living in Asia.[8]

Does a Japanese encephalitis vaccine exist?
There is a vaccine designed to protect against Japanese encephalitis—JE-VAX®, manufactured by Aventis Pasteur, Inc.[9] It is prepared by injecting the Japanese encephalitis virus into the brains of mice. The infected mouse brains are then "harvested and homogenized" in phosphate buffered saline, then inactivated with formaldehyde. Thimerosal (a mercury derivative) is added as a preservative (see *Appendix I*). Other ingredients include gelatin and polysorbate 80. The final product also contains "mouse serum protein."[10] (China produces a live-virus Japanese encephalitis vaccine for India, Nepal, Sri Lanka and South Korea.[11] Other Japanese encephalitis vaccines using new technologies are under development.[12])

How safe is the Japanese encephalitis vaccine?

According to the vaccine manufacturer, the following side effects have been reported following receipt of the Japanese encephalitis vaccine: flu-like symptoms, including fever, headache, malaise, rash, chills, dizziness, myalgia, nausea, vomiting and abdominal pain. Other reported reactions include: hives and facial swelling, joint swelling, generalized itching, respiratory distress, Guillain-Barré syndrome, renal failure, seizures, encephalitis, encephalopathy, transverse myelitis, optic neuritis, cranial nerve paresis, cerebellar ataxia, Bell's palsy, fatal myocarditis and sudden death. Some of these reactions occurred following receipt of the Japanese encephalitis vaccine concurrent with other vaccines. According to the manufacturer, "the relationship of JE-VAX to the etiology of these adverse events is unknown."[13]

How effective is the Japanese encephalitis vaccine?

The efficacy of the vaccine was tested in Thai children. Researchers claimed that a two-dose regimen provided 91 percent efficacy. However, the CDC conducted a "controlled immunogenicity trial" on U.S. military personnel and showed that "neutralizing antibody was produced in fewer than 80 percent of vaccinees following two doses of the vaccine in U.S. travelers."[14] In addition, antibody levels declined substantially in most recipients of the shot within six months. In fact, the vaccine manufacturer acknowledges that "long-term protection, as demonstrated by persistence of neutralizing antibody for more than two years, has not yet been shown."[15] Today, a three-dose regimen is advocated, with booster doses every two years.[16]

Is the Japanese encephalitis vaccine recommended?

This vaccine is licensed for use in U.S. travelers to rural areas where the disease is common. However, JE-VAX is *not* recommended for all persons traveling to or residing in Asia. This vaccine is mainly recommended for persons spending a month or longer in epidemic or endemic areas during the transmission season, especially if travel will include rural areas. This vaccine is also recommended for laboratory workers at risk of exposure to the Japanese encephalitis virus.[17-19]

Other precautions:

According to the CDC, the Japanese encephalitis vaccine "is not 100 percent effective and is not a substitute for mosquito precautions."[20] Thus, travelers should take steps to avoid mosquito bites:

- Wear clothes that cover most of the body.
- Use an effective mosquito repellant on skin and clothes.
- Stay in air-conditioned or well-screened rooms.
- Use a bednet and aerosal room insecticide.
- Minimize outdoor activities during mosquito feeding times, mainly during the cooler hours at dusk and dawn.[21,22]

Rabies

What is rabies?

Rabies is a serious disease caused by a *lyssa* virus.[1] The virus exists in the saliva of infected mammals.[2] Such animals may exhibit unusual or aggressive behavior.[3] ("Lyssa," the term used to describe the rabies virus, is a Greek word meaning madness. "Rabies" comes from the Latin "rabiere," meaning to rage or become violent.)[4] Humans get rabies when they are bitten by an infected bat, skunk, raccoon, dog, cat, monkey, fox or other infected animal.[5]

This disease has a long incubation period. Initially, there may be no symptoms. However, weeks, months or even a year after a bite rabies can cause irritability, pain, fatigue, insomnia, hypersalivation (foaming at the mouth), headaches and fever. (Symptoms usually appear 20 to 60 days after exposure.) In addition, victims often suffer from thirst but experience excruciating pain when swallowing liquids. Many develop hydrophobia, or fear of water. The rabies virus attacks the nervous system and brain. Encephalitis, seizures, hallucinations, loss of consciousness and paralysis soon follow. Left untreated, rabies is almost always fatal.[6-8]

How common is rabies?

In the United States, Canada and Europe, cases of rabies in humans are extremely rare.[9] For example, in the United States from 1990 through 2005, there were only 39 cases diagnosed.[10] However, several thousand people are treated each year for possible exposure to rabies after being bitten by an animal.[11] More than 99 percent of all human deaths from rabies occur in Africa, Asia, South America and India, reporting 30,000 rabies deaths annually.[12]

Does a rabies vaccine exist?

In 1885, Louis Pasteur and Emile Roux developed the first rabies vaccine. This vaccine was harvested from infected rabbits and successfully tested on Joseph Meister, a 9-year-old boy who was mauled by a rabid dog.[13] Since 1967, rabies vaccines have been made in human diploid cells.[14] Some rabies vaccines are also made in fetal rhesus monkey lung cells or chicken embryo fibroblasts.[15] Other ingredients may include human albumin, processed bovine gelatin, potassium glutamate, sodium EDTA, and the antibiotics neomycin, chlortetracycline, and amphotericin B.[16] In addition, b-propiolactone, a suspected cancer-causing agent, is used to inactivate the live rabies viruses included in the vaccine.[17,18]

Who should get the rabies vaccine?

Pre-exposure vaccination: Authorities recommend the rabies vaccine for persons in high-risk groups, such as veterinarians and other animal handlers, or people who are likely to come into contact with potentially rabid animals. This vaccine is not routinely recommended for the general population.[19,20]

Post-exposure treatment: The rabies vaccine is recommended for anyone who has been bitten by an animal that could be harboring the rabies virus.[21] (However, if the animal is a dog, cat or ferret, appears healthy, and is available for 10 days of observation, prophylaxis should not begin "unless animal develops clinical signs of rabies.")[22] The purpose of this vaccination is to overtake the virus during the incubation period of the disease. Five doses are given over a 28-day period, plus a shot of rabies immune globulin is given at the same time as the first dose.[23]

How safe is the rabies vaccine?

The rabies vaccine has a high rate of side effects. For example, up to 74 percent of recipients will experience soreness, itching and swelling at the injection site. Up to 40 percent will develop headaches, muscle aches, nausea, dizziness and abdominal pain. About six percent will develop hives, fever and joint pain.[24] According to the manufacturer, "neurological and neuroparalytical events" have been reported following administration of the rabies vaccine.[25] The rabies vaccine manufacturer also publishes the following warning in its inserts: "Anaphylaxis, encephalitis including death, meningitis, neuroparalytic events such as encephalitis, transient paralysis, Guillain-Barré syndrome, myelitis, retrobulbar neuritis, and multiple sclerosis have been reported to be temporally associated with the use of [the rabies vaccine]."[26] The manufacturer also lists other adverse events following receipt of this vaccine, including swollen lymph nodes, pain in limbs, gastrointestinal complaints, severe headache, flu-like symptoms, arthralgia, myalgia, rash, circulatory reactions, sweating, chills, monoarthritis, allergic reactions, transient paresthesias, urticaria, bronchospasm, visual disturbances, palpitations, vertigo, hot flushes and extensive limb swelling.[27]

The rabies vaccine is made with live rabies viruses that are inactivated with b-propiolactone, a "probable human carcinogen" according to the Environmental Protection Agency (EPA).[28] If the viruses are not adequately disabled, recipients of the vaccine could contract the disease. This possibility is very real. For example, in April of 2004, Aventis Pasteur issued a recall of four lots of its rabies vaccine after it identified the presence of non-inactivated (live) rabies virus in its product. Three of the four potentially dangerous lots were distributed in the United States and internationally for more than six months before the recall was initiated.[29]

How effective is the rabies vaccine?

According to the vaccine manufacturer, modern day prophylaxis has proven "nearly 100 percent successful."[30] In clinical studies that evaluated pre-exposure vaccination, when the rabies vaccine was given according to the recommended immunization schedule, "100 percent of subjects attained a protective titer."[31] In studies that evaluated post-exposure treatment, the rabies vaccine "provided protective titers of neutralizing antibody in 158 of 160 patients within 14 days and in 215 of 216 patients by day 28 to 38."[32]

RhoGAM®
for Hemolytic Disease of the Newborn (HDN)

What is Hemolytic Disease of the Newborn?

Some people are born without a certain protein on the surface of their red blood cells. These people are considered Rh-negative. Everyone else is Rh-positive. If you are Rh-negative and pregnant with a baby who is Rh-positive—and if your blood and the baby's blood mix—your immune system may develop antibodies against the baby's blood cells. These antibodies are usually not dangerous to the first child because they rarely have time to grow in strength and number. However, if you become pregnant again, and your next child is also Rh-positive, he or she could develop Hemolytic Disease of the Newborn (HDN). This is a condition whereby your body misinterprets the fetus' red blood cells as foreign, vigorously attacking them; a miscarriage or stillbirth are possible. Conversely, the child could be born with jaundice, anemia, or develop other health problems.[1] Most babies born with HDN will be cured, but it is a grave condition requiring intensive care.[2]

Who is Rh-negative?

About 15 percent of Caucasian women are Rh-negative. Eight percent of African-America and Hispanic women are Rh-negative. Just 1 percent of Asian and Native American women are Rh-negative. The condition is genetic, like being born with a certain eye color.[3]

How are babies protected from HDN?

In 1968, researchers introduced RhoGAM, an immune globulin designed to protect babies from HDN. It is usually administered as an injection to Rh-negative pregnant women at 28 weeks gestation. If the newborn is Rh-positive, another shot is given to the mother within 72 hours after giving birth. It is given to the mother to stop her from producing antibodies that might attack the red blood cells of any additional Rh-positive babies she may have in the future if she becomes pregnant again.[4]

How safe is the RhoGAM shot?

Incredibly, until just a few years ago the Rhogam shot contained mercury. Mercury in a mother's body can be passed to her fetus.[5] Millions of pregnant women received these mercury-containing Rhogam injections.[6] Research conducted by Dr. F. Edward Yazbak showed that women who received mercury-laden Rhogam shots during pregnancy had higher rates of autism in their children than women who did not receive these shots.[7] Dr. Stephanie Cave also observed that many of the mothers of autistic children in her practice are Rh-negative.[8] Despite the evidence linking mercury-containing Rhogam injections with higher rates of autism, in 2007 researchers *surveyed* 214 mothers and concluded there is no link between mercury-Rhogam shots and autism. Curiously, the authors of this alleged objective "study" declared: "We hope this report...will offset some of the decreased compliance with immunization recommendations."[9,10]

The Rhogam shot contains immune globulin produced from human plasma. The blood from thousands of donors is pooled together, then filtered for viruses and other infectious agents.[11,12] Despite this filtration process, the manufacturer's product insert includes a warning that because RhoGAM is made from human blood, it "may carry a risk of transmitting infectious agents, e.g., viruses, and, theoretically, the Creutzfeldt-Jakob disease (CJD) agent.... There is also the possibility that unknown infectious agents may be present..."[13]

The final product contains glycine, sodium chloride, and polysorbate 80—a possible carcinogen.[14-16] Documented allergic reactions include tightness of the chest, wheezing, hives, hypotension, and anaphylaxis.[17] Fever, chills, headache and fatigue are also possible.[18] In addition, some people who receive RhoGAM may experience severe joint pain or rheumatoid arthritis. For example, here is an unsolicited adverse reaction report provided by an unhappy recipient of the injection: "I have been suffering debilitating arthritis ever since shortly after receiving the shot, but I was told that it is not related. They will not

293

report it to the Adverse Reactions office, and the office will not accept my own report without the judgment of my doctor."[19]

Is the RhoGAM shot mandatory?

Some Rh-negative pregnant women are uncomfortable receiving a prenatal injection at 28 weeks gestation, especially when their baby's blood type is unknown. Doctors used to wait until the baby was born and administered the shot to the mother only if the baby was confirmed Rh-positive. However, some women refused the shot after giving birth because it is produced from other people's blood, and they feared it could be tainted with unknown viruses. This placed all subsequent pregnancies by these women at potentially greater risk (if the babies are Rh-positive), so doctors started requiring a prophylactic shot prenatally.[20]

Despite standard policy, most healthy Rh-negative pregnant women may decline a prenatal Rhogam injection.[21] However, during pregnancy some conditions could arise whereby the baby's blood begins to mix with the mother's blood (for example, following amniocentesis or an injury to the abdomen).[22] If this occurs, doctors will insist upon administering the shot. In addition, Rh-negative women who do not receive a prenatal Rhogam shot, for whatever reason, will be expected to receive it within 72 hours postpartum if the baby is born Rh-positive.[23]

Options for a healthy pregnancy and birth:

There are things a pregnant woman can do to reduce the likelihood that her blood will mix with her baby's blood. For example, a good prenatal diet with lots of blood-building foods such as beets, dark leafy greens, and sea vegetables will help the baby and placenta develop properly. Drinking lots of red raspberry leaf tea, citrus juices, and eating foods rich in vitamin C will tone the uterus for labor, keep the placenta healthy, and help reduce blood loss during and after birth. The umbilical cord should stop pulsing before it is cut. Strong contractions will help the placenta to separate safely from the uterus. A natural birth with few interventions could reduce the risk of maternal and fetal blood mixing.[24]

Vitamin K

What is vitamin K?

People need vitamin K for blood clotting. Without enough vitamin K, small cuts can result in severe bleeding. Most older children and adults manufacture vitamin K naturally in their guts, and receive supplemental vitamin K from the food they eat. However, newborn babies have very little vitamin K in their bodies at birth. It may take several weeks for their guts to start making it. With low levels of vitamin K, some babies develop hemorrhagic disease—a rare bleeding disorder of the brain.[1] The problem of bleeding into the brain occurs mainly from 2 to 6 weeks after birth.[2] Without vitamin K supplementation at birth, approximately 1 of every 20,000 babies could develop this condition.[3,4]

Who is most at risk of vitamin K deficiency?

Breastfed newborns are at greater risk of vitamin K deficiency than babies who are formula-fed because baby food is supplemented with unnaturally high levels of vitamin K—10 times the U.S. recommended daily allowance per liter of formula—and there is little vitamin K in breast milk.[5-7] Nevertheless, most, if not all, babies who develop late onset hemorrhagic disease—the most serious form of intracranial bleeding—have grave underlying ailments, such as hepatitis, cystic fibrosis or celiac disease.[8]

Does a vitamin K shot exist:

In 1985, the American Academy of Pediatrics decided that since some newborns need vitamin K, it would be okay to give it to every newborn. A national policy requiring all babies to receive an injection of vitamin K shortly after birth was enacted—despite a prominent refutation of routine vitamin K injections that was previously published in *Lancet,* a well-respected medical journal. Researchers concluded that "healthy babies, contrary to current beliefs, are not likely to have a vitamin K deficiency.... The administration of vitamin K is not supported by our findings."[9] Today, several nations mandate a prophylactic strategy of routinely injecting vitamin K in all newborns. (Note: the vitamin K shot is not a vaccine.)

How safe is the vitamin K shot?

The active ingredient in the vitamin K shot is phytomenadione—a synthetic chemical derived from "2-methyl-3-phytyl-1, 4-napthoquinone."[10] In the United States, Merck produces it under the trade name AquaMephyton®; in Australia, Roche manufactures it as Konakion®.[11,12] The U.S. brand also contains benzyl alcohol added as a preservative. Benzyl alcohol has been associated with toxicity in newborns.[13] The Australian brand contains glycholic acid, hydrochloric acid and sodium hydroxide.[14] In addition, some sources claim that polysorbate 80 and phenol, possible carcinogens, were also used in manufacturing this product (although they are not listed by either manufacturer).[15-17]

Merck's current product insert includes a graphic warning with regard to the intravenous use of its product.[18] Merck also lists adverse reactions that have been reported following the parenteral (injectable) administration of its product, including difficulty in swallowing, troubled breathing, dizziness, rapid and weak pulse, low blood pressure, profuse sweating, lightheadedness or fainting, tightness in the chest, anaphylactoid reactions, swelling of the eyelids, face or lips, hypotension, scleroderma-like lesions that have persisted for long periods, cyanosis (bluish discoloration of the skin caused by lack of oxygen in the blood), hemolysis (destruction of red blood cells), hyperbilirubinemia (an excess of bilirubin, or bile pigment, in the blood), jaundice, and death.[19]

Vitamin K injections and leukemia:

In 1990, the *British Journal of Cancer* published a study concluding that vitamin K shots administered to newborns doubles their risk of developing leukemia before the age of 10, with a peak incidence occurring before the age of 5.[20] In 1992, the *British Medical Journal* published another study that reinforced the findings of the previous one. Researchers found that vitamin K injections given to newborns also increased their chances of developing other forms of cancer—not just leukemia. There was no increase in cancer rates when babies did not receive vitamin K or when they received oral vitamin K in place of a vitamin K injection. The authors of the study provided the following understated warning: "The only two studies so far to have examined the relation between childhood cancer and intramuscular vitamin K have shown similar results, and the relation is biologically plausible. The prophylactic benefits against hemorrhagic disease are unlikely to exceed the potential adverse effects from intramuscular vitamin K."[21] The authors urged exclusive use of oral vitamin K.

In 1993, the American Academy of Pediatrics convened a task force to investigate "Controversies Concerning Vitamin K and the Newborn." The task force concluded that "since parenteral vitamin K prevents a life-threatening disease of the newborn and the risks of cancer are unproven and unlikely..." vitamin K injections should continue to be given to all babies.[22] In other words, the previous studies showing correlations between vitamin K injections and higher rates of cancer should be disregarded. The task force did, however, recommend that an oral dose form of vitamin K be developed and licensed.

In 1998, the *British Medical Journal* published two additional studies that weighed in on the controversy concerning vitamin K shots and cancer. In the first study, researchers noted that "the possibility that there is some risk cannot be excluded."[23] Furthermore, "even a 10 percent increase would imply that prophylaxis using the commonly recommended 1mg intramuscular dose should be restricted to babies at particularly high risk of vitamin K deficiency bleeding; alternately, a lower dose might be given to a larger proportion of those at risk."[24] The second study concluded that "it is not possible, on the basis of currently published evidence, to refute the suggestion that neonatal intramuscular vitamin K administration increases the risk of early childhood leukemia."[25]

What are the alternatives to a vitamin K shot?

According to Dr. Sherri Tenpenny, "It seems to be incongruous that babies of well fed, well nourished mothers are born with a deficiency of an essential vitamin and require an injection at birth for supplementation."[26] Tenpenny believes that a better way for infants to get enough vitamin K at birth is to ensure that their mothers eat large quantities of food containing natural forms of vitamin K—such as alfalfa, brussels sprouts, cabbage, cauliflower, spinach, broccoli, asparagus, and green tea—prior to delivery and during the time they are nursing.[27] Dr. Randall Neustaedter notes that since vitamin K injections may be associated with an increased risk of cancer, and since vitamin K given within 12 hours of birth can reduce the risk of vitamin K deficiency bleeding, "it seems prudent to give an oral dose of 1-2mg."[28] Dr. Linda Palmer recommends that nursing infants "be supplemented with several low oral doses of liquid vitamin K. Alternately, the nursing mother can take vitamin K supplements daily or twice weekly for 10 weeks."[29] (If nursing moms choose oral vitamin K for their newborns, authorities emphasize that repeat doses are necessary.[30,31] The recommended frequency and potency of doses might vary by product manufacturer or other circumstances.)

Is the vitamin K shot mandatory?

Doctors and nurses routinely administer vitamin K shots to all newborns because hospitals are mandated by state law to provide the injection. However, the shot may be declined. Parents who wish to refuse the shot are encouraged to do so in writing prior to the birth of their baby.[32] Oral vitamin K may be accepted or declined as well.

Multiple Vaccines
(Administered Simultaneously)

The current schedule of CDC-recommended vaccines is so crowded that doctors administer several shots during a single office visit (Figure 91), often with disastrous results. For example, infants receive eight vaccines during their two-month visit to the doctor: diphtheria, tetanus and pertussis (DTaP), polio, hepatitis B, Hib, pneumococcal and rotavirus. This regimen is repeated at four months, and again at six months.[1] (The flu vaccine may also be given at six months—nine chemical and pathogenic substances at one time!)[2] Parents—and doctors—often forget that vaccines are drugs. How often do we, as adults, ingest (or receive by injection!) nine drugs at the same time? Would we be more surprised if we did or did not have an adverse reaction?

Why are so many vaccines given at the same time?
Several vaccines are administered simultaneously for convenience, not safety. In fact, there are few studies supporting the practice. Vaccine manufacturers are not required to test their products in all of the combinations that they are likely to be used. For example, teenage girls may be injected with the HPV shot, along with tetanus, diphtheria and pertussis (TDaP), hepatitis A and meningococcal vaccines[3]—even though this combination of drugs was never tested for safety (or efficacy). Adults might receive hepatitis A, B, measles, mumps and rubella (MMR), polio, tetanus and diphtheria (DT) vaccines during the same doctor appointment.[4] Seniors could be simultaneously injected with flu, pneumonia, shingles, tetanus and diphtheria (TD) vaccines.[5] Many of these vaccine recipients are also taking medications for other ailments. Although recipients of multiple vaccines are rarely screened for possible drug interactions, there is ample evidence showing that when two or more drugs are taken together, this could magnify the potential for a serious adverse reaction.

Figure 91:
Crowded Vaccine Schedule

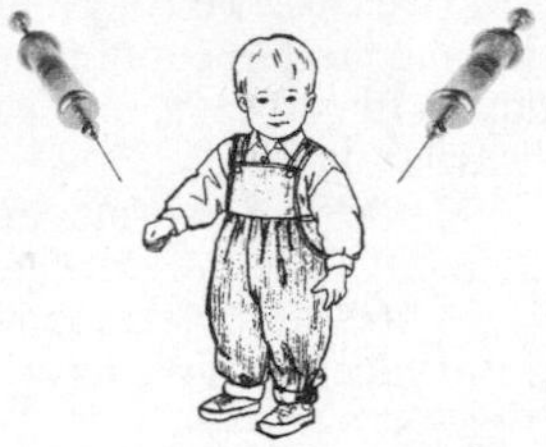

Toxic synergy:
Dr. Russell Blaylock has studied the "science of toxic synergy." He notes that when two weakly toxic pesticides are used alone, neither causes Parkinson's syndrome in experimental animals. However, when they are combined, they can cause the full-blown disease quite rapidly. He likens this to multiple vaccines administered simultaneously: "Vaccinations, if too numerous and spaced too close together, act like chronic illness."[6] Two recent studies have confirmed that sudden infant death is possible following inoculation with multiple vaccines in a single shot.[7,8] Drs. Andrew Wakefield, Robert Sears, and Stephanie Cave have suggested spacing some vaccines apart.[9-11] However, it's important to understand that this strategy will not guarantee protection against serious—or even fatal—side effects. Every "body" is different; no two people react the same way. *Single vaccines administered separately can, and often do, cause adverse reactions*. Still, if vaccines must be given, common sense alone tells us that several vaccines administered together are likely to be more problematic than individual shots spaced apart over a period of time.

International vaccine schedules:
A recent study, published in *Human and Experimental Toxicology,* found that nations requiring the most vaccines for their infants tend to have the worst infant mortality rates. For example, the United States requires infants to receive 26 vaccines (the most in the world) yet more than 6 U.S. infants die per every 1000 live births. In contrast, Sweden and Japan administer 12 vaccines to infants, the least amount, and report less than 3 deaths per 1000 live births. Evidence linking vaccines to SIDS is also discussed in this study.[12]

Adverse Reaction Reports

Vaccine Adverse Event Reporting System (VAERS): In 1986, Congress passed the *National Childhood Vaccine Injury Act*. The "safety" provisions of this law required the government to monitor adverse reactions to vaccines. To satisfy this requirement, the FDA and CDC jointly developed the Vaccine Adverse Event Reporting System (VAERS), a federal database where doctors, nurses and concerned parents could report suspected reactions to vaccines. (Parents can file a report by calling 1-800-822-7967.) VAERS became available in the 1990s and immediately provided evidence of harm. Despite resistance from doctors, who often unlawfully refuse to report suspected vaccine reactions, to date more than 300,000 reports have been filed.[13,14] These reports include people (mostly children) who have been permanently damaged or killed after receiving one or more vaccines. In fact, many of the serious adverse reactions—tens of thousands of them—occurred after receiving multiple vaccines simultaneously. The following reports, taken directly from VAERS, represent a very small number of cases:[15]

▶ 164271: A one-month-old female infant received DTaP, Hib, hepatitis B and inactivated polio vaccines. Ten days later she had a seizure and was admitted to the hospital. The following day she had three more seizures. The seizures increased in frequency to more than 12 per day. After 60 days, she was diagnosed with convulsions, grand mal seizures, and mental retardation.

▶ 98498: A two-month-old male infant received DTaP, Hib and inactivated polio vaccines. Two days later he developed intestinal bleeding and was hospitalized.

▶ 102563: A two-month-old male infant received DTaP, hepatitis B, Hib, and inactivated polio vaccines. Two days later he was found lifeless and cyanotic, but responded to rescue breaths.

▶ 175725: A four-month-old female received DTaP, Hib, pneumococcal and inactivated polio vaccines. The following day she went into respiratory distress. After being hospitalized for 18 days, she had not recovered.

▶ 269344: A four-month old male received DTaP, hepatitis B, pneumococcal, inactivated polio, and rotavirus vaccines. The infant experienced vomiting, developed gastrointestinal necrosis, intussusception, and required surgery for resection at necrotic bowel.

▶ 253421: A one-year-old male received DTaP, Hib, hepatitis B, MMR, pneumococcal, and inactivated polio vaccines. Four weeks later he developed thrombocytopenic purpura, a serious blood disorder.

▶ 231779: A five-year-old female received DTaP, MMR and inactivated polio vaccines. The following day she developed severe seizures and irregular brain patterns, with limited ability to speak and function.

▶ 156056: A 15-year-old female became incoherent and developed seizures three days after receiving hepatitis A and tetanus-diphtheria vaccines.

▶ 233038: A 21-year-old male received hepatitis A, B, inactivated polio, meningococcal, tetanus-diphtheria, and MMR vaccines. One month later he developed headache, amnesia, vomiting, myelitis, paralysis from the chest down, inability to void the bowels, and encephalitis with lesions on the brainstem and spinal cord. After being hospitalized for six months, he had not recovered.

▶ 245210: A 21-year-old male received flu, meningococcal and tetanus-diphtheria vaccines. Six weeks later, he developed Guillain-Barré syndrome, facial paralysis and blurred vision. After being hospitalized for 26 days, he had not recovered.

▶ 236182: A 23-year-old male received meningococcal, MMR, smallpox and tetanus-diphtheria vaccines. Three days later his throat swelled shut and he became unconscious for three days. He developed a fever and broke out with sores over his shoulders, neck, face and scalp. After being hospitalized for seven weeks, he had not recovered.

▶ 233585: A 36-year-old female received the pneumococcal and meningococcal vaccines. Three days later she started to develop numbness in her lower back and legs. She was diagnosed with Guillain-Barré syndrome, incontinence, myasthenia and cellulitis. After being hospitalized for 20 days, she had not recovered.

Thinktwice Global Vaccine Institute (www.thinktwice.com): In 1996, *Thinktwice* was established to provide parents and other concerned people with educational resources enabling them to make more informed vaccine decisions. *Thinktwice* encourages an uncensored exchange of vaccine information, and supports every family's right to accept or reject vaccines. This section contains unsolicited reports of adverse reactions following the administration of several vaccines simultaneously. These reports are typical, and represent a very small sample of the daily emails received by the *Thinktwice Global Vaccine Institute:*[16]

▸ "My son was born premature, just three pounds, three ounces at birth. At his two-month check the nurse said he needed his shots. I argued with her but she gave him four shots. I will never forget the scream he let out. Less than 24 hours later he died—and I was accused of his death!"

▸ "Our beautiful daughter was born in February and died in April. On the day that she died, I had taken her to the military base hospital for her two-month checkup. The doctor told me that she was just perfect. Then the doctor said that she needed four shots. She assured me that it was completely normal and that it was better to give her all at such an early age (because she wouldn't remember the shots). That evening after feeding her, we laid her down to sleep and checked on her 45 minutes later. She was dead. I told the police, coroner and investigators that I thought it was the shots because she was perfectly fine that day before the shots. But after three weeks we finally got an answer from the autopsy that it was SIDS. To this day I believe that it was the shots and no one can convince me otherwise."

▸ "I had a baby girl on June 3 and she passed away on August 5, two days after she got her shots. They told me it was SIDS, but I don't believe that. A healthy happy-go-lucky baby doesn't just pass away."

▸ "I almost killed my own daughter by allowing her pediatrician to give her shots. At birth, my baby could already hold her head up and look around. She displayed numerous signs of being a gifted child. She scored a 10 on the Apgar test. When she was two months old, we took her to her checkup. What happened there I will never forget, and I will tell everyone I know for the rest of my life to inform them of the dangers of these immunizations. The first thing they did to my poor baby was give her a polio vaccine, then they jabbed a needle in her right leg, and then jabbed another needle in her left leg. She screamed like never before. Sure, needles hurt, and she will cry, but this cry was much different than any cry she has ever had before. We took her home believing what the doctor had told us. Later that night, she began to act so much different than normal. Her high-pitched screams shrieked so painfully, and her little tears could have made a river rise. Her breathing was shallow, she could only pant, unable to catch her breath. We called the 'doctor' (I use that term lightly), and we were told that this was normal, and that we would have to call back during normal office hours because they were closing. Let me just say this, we are lucky that our daughter is still here with us, where she belongs. Needless to say, I am now well informed on 'immunizations,' and will never allow another doctor to jeopardize her precious life. I hope every parent will study all materials on this subject to make an informed decision."

▸ "My baby developed gastro-esophageal reflux disease, ear infections, stopped nursing and sleeping, started regressing, losing weight and interest in the world, to name a few horrors that she's been through. She was on three to four medicines a week. It all started at two months old after all her shots were administered."

▸ "Our son had his first round of vaccines at two months and was hospitalized for 21 days at Oakland Children's Hospital. There he had to have blood transfusions, many, many tests, and several other medicines to save his life. Funny, all those doctors won't step up and say it was a reaction to the shots. They tell us he is allergic to eggs, which are in the shots, but they won't say he almost died from them! No more vaccines for him."

▸ "When my son was three months old I received a letter to have him inoculated. My gut response was a strong 'No!' Unfortunately, I was then married to a very dominant man, and after a month I was persuaded to have him inoculated after all. The vaccine was a combination of diphtheria, whooping cough, tetanus and polio. They also included a vaccine called Hib. An hour after we were home, my baby started stiffening up. His crying was unlike anything I had ever heard—an extremely high-pitched type of wailing that had me going stark raving mad. There was nothing I could do. He didn't want to be comforted, no breastfeeding, no touching, nothing! All he did was lie on the bed, staring straight ahead, screeching like a jet engine. When I called my doctor, he told me it was very likely our boy had 'brain irritation,' judging by that odd crying. He advised me NOT to take him to the hospital, as anything that would be done to him would probably aggravate the obvious state of severe shock he was in. Taking his advice, I darkened the room, keeping away as much visual and auditory input from my son as possible. Finally, after about three hours of constant high-pitched crying, he seemed to 'get back to earth' and actually was aware of his surroundings. After breastfeeding him, he fell into a very deep sleep and slept for 10 hours straight. I don't need to tell you that I have NEVER, ever let my children be vaccinated afterwards! My son still has the high-pitched wailing whenever he gets hurt or when he has an intense emotional shock. People will literally cover their ears because it hurts to hear him cry. When I contacted the Health Service about his reaction, they told me it was nothing to worry about, and that more children had those types of adverse side effects from vaccinations. I had stood at the brink of losing my son and they called it a 'normal' reaction. Now I tell as many people as possible that there are alternatives to allopathic inoculations."

▸ "After my son received his diphtheria, tetanus, pertussis, Hib, polio, and hepatitis B shots, he developed a persistent cough, then pneumonia and an ear infection. This 'ear infection' has lasted almost six weeks."

▸ "IS OUR GOVERNMENT KILLING OUR CHILDREN? This is a subject that has touched my own family. My brother and sister-in-law had a baby recently. This baby had his vaccine shots at three months. The mother was never informed about the possible side effects. I got a call from the mother three days after the vaccines. He was vomiting, extremely irritable, had not slept for three days, screaming, whining, having right-sided convulsions, and refusing to drink the mother's breast milk. I asked only two questions: Was he vaccinated, and when? She said, 'He had polio, meningitis, hepatitis B and DPT. Immediately after, all the symptoms started to develop. On the third day the violent seizures started.' I told her to take the baby to the emergency hospital. I met them there; the doctor on staff recorded the vaccines the baby had on hospital files. Tests were done (blood, urine, and a CAT scan). The brain scan showed a cerebral hemorrhage the size of a golf ball. All doctors at both hospitals (the Medical Center and Children's Hospital) denied the brain damage was from the vaccines, claiming he was born with it! They wanted to do brain surgery ASAP. All of this was happening so fast! When you held this little baby you could feel the violent contractions in his tiny body and the pain he was going through. His body felt like it was short-circuiting itself, like something very powerful had invaded his entire body. I am a homeopath. The only thing that saved this baby's life were a few remedies. I didn't let the hospital know what I was doing, but had the permission of both parents to administer the homeopathic remedies. Within 20 minutes we witnessed a remarkable change. The baby fell into a deep sleep (after convulsing 24 hours). When he woke, all was fine. CAT scans were done to prove the cerebral hemorrhage had stopped. Allopathic MD's will all play dumb when it comes to the relationship between vaccines and seizures. My wish is to tell as many parents as possible."

▸ "This is the most difficult letter I have ever had to write, and yet I feel that if I don't write it someone else's baby could be at risk. My emotions at the moment are of anger, confusion, and most of all disgust at the medical profession who took the oath to save, not destroy, a human being, let alone a baby. My granddaughter was born in August, a special blessing to my son and daughter-in-law, and myself. I was so overwhelmed the night she was born; I cut her cord and held her and thanked the good Lord above for this wonderful gift he has blessed us all with. She was a happy little girl and healthy—everything a grandmother could wish for. I will never, ever forget the telephone call I received on December 6 from my son, so hurt, so confused and scared, telling me 'Mom, I have some dreadful news.' I still choke up now when I think about it. My daughter-in-law had dutifully taken her to the doctor for her four-month-old shots just as they recommend, and to whom we are to believe in (or so we are told). The next day she was gone from our lives. Parents, I beg you from the bottom of my heart, THINK TWICE. Maybe, just maybe, we can all save another baby's life. For me and my family, it's too late, but you still have a choice to do something."

▶ "I lost my son on October 23. The afternoon before, he had gone in for his four-month well-baby checkup, which included vaccines. Seventeen hours later I found him lifeless. His body was still warm. I know that it hadn't been that long. During those last hours, he wasn't himself. I thought it was a normal reaction. He would not eat and he was sleeping way more than usual. When he would wake up, he would let out this unnerving shrill noise. It was terrifying. When the paramedics arrived I had given them a copy of his shot records. There was nothing that the doctors could do. I don't know what made me ask for a copy of those records when I was at the office. I had a bad feeling going in. The doctor reassured me that it was routine and everything was going to be fine. When the detective contacted them, they assured him that it was not the shots. He had six vaccines that day. We are still waiting for the toxicology report. The agony of knowing that this could have been prevented and that the public is not aware is unbearable. Our baby will forever be remembered in our hearts: June 26—October 23."

▶ "My daughter was fine until she had her second Hib and DT vaccines. She became ill after this and was unable to grasp anything. She went from a very vocal, social five-month-old to a withdrawn silent seven-month-old who failed her checkup on all counts."

▶ "After my baby had her six-month shots (DTaP, polio, and Hib) she had what the emergency room doctor considered a febrile seizure. She was fine until then. Three days later the doctor said she had streptococcal pneumonia. When she is not sleeping, she wriggles and cries like she is in pain."

▶ "My son received EIGHT vaccines on February 13, 2007. They were DTaP (diphtheria, tetanus, pertussis), IPV, Hib, Hep B, Prevnar and RotaTeq. He was six months old. One week later he was inconsolable and lethargic. Another three days later he presented with seizures and suffered a significant stroke. Two-thirds of his right brain is permanently damaged. I am not sure what his future holds."

▶ "Our son received his vaccines at six months. His older sister had adverse reactions [to DPT] of high fever and high-pitched screaming, so his doctor recommended pediatric DT. I was reassured that there was no reason to be concerned. Within six hours after his dose of Hib and DT, our son was not himself. I laid him down for a nap because he looked pale and his skin felt cold and clammy. Something told me to check on him moments after I laid him down. He was in his crib, blue, with his eyes rolling back, then fixed in a strange stare, rigid limbs, foaming at the mouth, and his chest appeared to be laboring to breathe. My husband and I raced him to the emergency room which, thank God, was just down the street. I had to stimulate him by calling his name and gently shaking him. He stared in a strange way that I had never seen, and he was barely breathing. Everything seemed surreal. My husband and I were so scared. We did not know if he would make it to the hospital. When we arrived, seconds later they quickly grabbed him out of my arms. They did not know his name and did not have time to ask. They called him Charlie Brown. They suctioned out his throat, but of course nothing was blocking his airway; it was just closing on it's own. As quickly as this started, he spontaneously came out of it. He was smiling up at the doctors and nurses who were trying to save him. Everyone applauded and laughed. We were just lucky. Our son is now two years old and there appears to be no permanent damage. I always wonder what damage occurred that I am not aware of yet. My precious son almost died in my arms. Needless to say, I never vaccinated him again. I pray for those who don't know the dangers, as well as for those who were not as lucky as we were."

▶ "My normal, healthy 12-month-old daughter was vaccinated with hepatitis B, polio, and varicella. The next day she began to vomit and did not stop for two hours. She became completely lethargic and ended up in the emergency room with IV fluid pumping through her to keep her alive. All the medical staff told me this could not be a reaction to her vaccinations. What do you think?"

▶ "My son received his DTaP shot and Prevnar. The following morning he had seven seizures. He would go ghost-white and throw out his arms. They would be rigid and jerking. He stared straight ahead and didn't breathe. He used to say mama and dada [before the shots]. Now he only babbles. He is far behind in all areas tested."

▶ "My son had five seizures since his last shots (DTaP, Hib and MMR). He was sick at the time. They gave him his shots anyway, telling me it didn't matter. What can I do?"

▸ "At 14 months, my daughter received her MMR and chickenpox shots. Six days later she developed a fever. I did not think much of it as she has reacted with a small fever after some of her other shots. That next morning she woke up crying and had a high fever and quickly stiffened up, eyes rolled back, and passed out. We rushed her to the emergency room. The doctor said she had a febrile seizure. She continued to have a fever for three more days, then developed a cough and wheezy breathing. Our doctors do not think it is from the vaccine, even though I know it is. It is so obvious; she was in perfect health. We're praying that she returns to her old self completely."

▸ "I am the mother of a two-year-old with autism. His symptoms began almost immediately following his series of immunizations at 14 months [when nine drugs were introduced into his tiny body—for measles, mumps, rubella, diphtheria, pertussis, tetanus, polio, varicella, and Hib]. Our lives have literally been turned upside down by the fact that our son who was healthy previous to his immunizations now has asthma, celiac disease, and autism. As soon as his first diagnosis was handed down I hit the internet looking for any information on this disease and what I could do to help him. So far, he is in occupational, speech, and toddler play group therapy. Next week he begins music therapy, and the following week he will start behavioral therapy. My son has chronic vomiting and diarrhea that are attributable to his celiac disease (vomiting up to five days a week, often more than once a day), and has regressed in his development. He lost the use of language. Last weekend I heard the word 'Mama' for the first time in nine months! And I ache for my husband who hasn't heard 'Daddy' from his little boy in a year. I am infuriated at the medical establishment for what they have done to my son, especially because there is little way to prove what is obvious. They can always claim that my son's autism was inborn, though he developed NORMALLY for the first 14 months of life!"

▸ "My daughter who is three years old received MMR, Hib, hepatitis B, and polio vaccinations on June 21, 2007. On June 27-30 she had fevers at night up to 104 degrees. On July 12, she had a seizure in the car lasting 15 minutes. She was pushing her finger into her eye, staring straight ahead. I asked her why she was doing this but got no response. She was also making a chewing motion with her mouth. On July 14, she had another seizure lasting two minutes, making noises with her lips, staring, and not responsive. My primary care physician and ER doctors say this is not related to the vaccines. I am scared that they are lying to me."

▸ "My niece got her shots for kindergarten last week and had a scary reaction to them. After leaving the health office and going to the car she told her mother that she felt sick to her stomach and then passed out. She stopped breathing and wet her pants. Her body started jerking. Her mother ran into the office and they couldn't find a pulse. They were getting ready to start CPR and had called 911. Then she woke up. Her speech was not right at first and her heartbeat was irregular. They took her to the hospital and said that she was just afraid of the shots."

▸ "I experienced an acute reaction to several vaccines I received (MMR, hepatitis A, hepatitis B, and yellow fever) prior to leaving the country. I still suffer every day from these ill effects: fatigue, joint pain, restlessness, and cognitive dysfunction."

▸ "My dearest son died 10 hours after receiving his fourth dose of diphtheria, tetanus, pertussis, Hib and polio vaccines. He was 20 months old. I knew he was dead when I heard my husband wailing like an animal. I grabbed Spencer's stiff and lifeless body and screamed, 'God, No, Not My Baby! He Can't Be Dead!' I administered CPR for 15 minutes, pounded on his chest, and yelled, 'Come Back, Come Back, Come Back!' Then I heard my father say over the phone to 911, 'We've got a dead baby here.' Realization hit. I opened his eyes, and he was dead. I then hugged his stiff body and emitted sounds I didn't know any human being was capable of making. I cannot adequately express my horror, anger, and ultimate suffering. My life turned upside down in one day, and each day that goes by I look at as one day closer to death, one day closer to my baby. Why? Because they told me the benefits outweigh the risks. What does that really mean, and why are these people allowed to play God?"

New Vaccines

The vaccines reviewed in previous chapters represent just a few of the many that already exist or are in developmental stages. For example, medical scientists are working on several "therapeutic" vaccines to treat different types of cancer. They are also developing vaccines against AIDS, addiction, hepatitis E, venereal disease, venoms, environmental toxins, and even the common cold. Scientists are also experimenting with a vaccine against pregnancy, vaccines crossbred into our food supply, and a time-released "supervaccine."[1-3]

If the principles behind the theory of vaccinations are flawed, future vaccines may be doomed to failure as well. For example, according to Dr. Richard Moskowitz, the people that need an AIDS vaccine the most are already seriously immunocompromised. Giving a suppressive vaccine to everyone would increase the odds of developing AIDS in people who are already at high risk. It would weaken the general population as well.[4,5] In fact, Merck recently announced that it was halting its international study of an experimental AIDS vaccine when 24 of its volunteers who received the shot became infected with HIV, the virus that causes AIDS.[6] Although industry insiders consider this a major setback, it won't end the search for an AIDS vaccine. According to one analyst, the company that comes up with the first successful AIDS vaccine would have "a license to print money. You're talking about a Carl Sagan kind of number—billions and billions of dollars."[7]

In the following section, new vaccines against swine flu, avian flu, and ear infections are summarized. Animal vaccines are reviewed as well.

Swine flu vaccine:

Swine flu is similar to seasonal flu. The virus is spread when infected people cough or sneeze. Symptoms include a fever, headache, sore throat, aches and chills. Vomiting and diarrhea may occur as well. In April 2009, a new strain of swine flu (A/California/04/2009 —H1N1) was detected. It contained a unique mix of genetic material from human, bird, and pig viruses. Six of the eight genes came from swine flu H1N2 viruses circulating in the United States from 1999-2001. The other two genes came from swine flu viruses circulating in Europe from 1985-1998. No one knows when, where, or how they were mixed together and mutated to form the current H1N1 virus.[8]

The 2009 swine flu infection was passed from person to person around the world. However, according to Dr. Thomas R. Frieden, director of the CDC, "The overwhelming majority of people with [swine] flu are going to do just fine. They won't need testing and they won't need treatment."[9] In fact, most of the 36 U.S. children who died from swine flu during the Spring and Summer of 2009 had underlying medical problems: neurodevelopmental and respiratory disorders.[10] More than half of the adults who died from swine flu had an underlying chronic illness or medical condition, such as asthma, diabetes, immune deficiency, or morbid obesity.[11] Most of the people who became ill recovered without requiring medical treatment. Nevertheless, on June 11, 2009 the World Health Organization (WHO) declared a pandemic due to the rapid spread of the virus.

Although swine flu can be treated with antiviral medicine, authorities initiated a campaign to develop several new swine flu vaccines and inoculate the population. This also occurred in 1976, when the CDC made up a false tale of deadly swine flu epidemics sweeping the nation if mass vaccinations were not quickly instituted. U.S. citizens were systematically vaccinated, and several weeks later hundreds were stricken with the crippling Guillain-Barré syndrome; several of the vaccinated people died.[12,13]

During the summer of 2009, several vaccine manufacturers raced to develop and test new swine flu vaccines hoping to make them available by the Fall of 2009. However, according to Margaret Chan, head of WHO, "Having a vaccine available is not the same as having a vaccine that is proven safe."[14] In fact, the "informed consent" form given to people brave enough to test the new vaccines excluded a list of ingredients. Dr. Barbara Mulach, with the National Institutes of Health, explained: "Because the product is still not licensed, we are evaluating this vaccine under the Investigational New Drug (IND) statute. Under this statute, the information about composition is considered proprietary."[15]

Additional research revealed that some of the new vaccines would be conventional flu shots while others would be live-virus vaccines squirted up the nose. About 80 percent of the new swine flu vaccines contained mercury.[16] Two manufacturers, Novartis and GlaxoSmithKline, experimented with squalene,[17] a controversial adjuvant (immune stimulant) which was used in anthrax vaccines and may be associated with Gulf War Illness.[18] Another company, Protein Sciences, developed a swine flu vaccine using insect cell technology. This was done by infecting fall armyworm (caterpillar) cells with a baculovirus carrying the gene for hemagglutinin, a molecule on the surface of the H1N1 virus.[19]

In June of 2009, Kathleen Sebelius, Secretary of the Department of Health and Human Services, invoked the little-known 2006 Public Readiness and Emergency Preparedness Act (PREPA), giving legal immunity to swine flu manufacturers for injuries stemming from the use of swine flu vaccines and "any associated adjuvants" (such as squalene).[20] Nevertheless, authorities were determined to give one or more doses of these vaccines to millions of pregnant women, children, caretakers of children, young adults, healthcare workers, military personnel, and older people with chronic illness.[21,22] Healthcare workers who refused the vaccine risked losing their jobs.[23] Other people who refused the vaccine could be quarantined, as permitted by federal law.[24]

Avian flu vaccine:
In Asia and Africa, epidemics of a bird flu (influenza A virus H5N1) have infected and killed poultry. Occasionally, the disease spreads from chickens to people. Scientists are concerned that if the virus mutates, it will not only spread from poultry to people, but from person to person. This could potentially cause a worldwide pandemic. In April of 2007, the FDA approved for human use, a bird flu vaccine developed by Sanofi-Aventis, "despite concerns it might not be that effective at protecting people against avian influenza."[25] The vaccine is being stockpiled by the U.S. government in case the bird flu virus mutates and rapidly spreads among people.[26] The vaccine is produced in chicken eggs with the H5N1 bird flu virus. Aluminum is added to stimulate antibody production. Common side effects include fever, headache, muscle ache, fatigue, nausea, arthralgia and diarrhea.[27]

Ear infection vaccine:
Scientists have developed a new vaccine against middle-ear infections, for use in children under two years of age. The vaccine contains proteins from 11 different strains of streptococcus pneumonia bacteria attached to a strain of haemophilus influenzae bacteria.[28] According to Dr. Anthony Tucker, an ear, nose and throat surgeon, "only a proportion of ear infections are caused by bacteria, and only some of those by these bacteria."[29] Furthermore, "the suggestion here is giving a vaccination against something that isn't life-threatening."[30] Although ear infections are not fatal, researchers believe that we are in a new era where vaccines will be designed to prevent "nuisance illnesses."[31]

Animal vaccines:
Veterinary vaccines, like shots for humans, can be harmful. They have been linked to autoimmune and neurological disorders, including cancer, diabetes, arthritis, tumors, seizures, allergies, digestive problems, organ failure, and other serious ailments. For example, Waylon, a Brindle Great Dane, developed repetitive and destructive behavior patterns (similar to vaccine-induced autism in children) after his shots. Bean, a domestic short hair, had recurring injection-site tumors (cancer) after her annual feline leukemia vaccines.[32]

Although the rabies vaccine may be the only one that is legally required, many veterinarians no longer support annual revaccination—an arbitrary recommendation which leads to unnecessary risks through *over*-vaccination. Others refuse to use certain vaccines because the disease is either so benign or rare that the risk of vaccination outweighs the potential benefits. There are efficacy problems with canine and feline vaccines as well. For example, puppies are susceptible to canine parvovirus during the same period when maternal antibodies neutralize vaccines.[33] According to Catherine Diodati, author of *Vaccine Guide for Dogs and Cats: What Every Pet Lover Should Know,* "natural healthcare modalities offer your pet viable alternatives to vaccines and conventional drugs."[34]

Laws, Options and More

This chapter briefly addresses a few common questions and concerns pertaining to vaccine laws, misconceptions, reversing damage, and health alternatives.

Are vaccines mandatory?

Manufacturers produce vaccines for the FDA to license and regulate. The CDC establishes a recommended schedule. State legislators then write the laws dictating who must be vaccinated within their state (usually children) and how often. Schools and other institutions enforce the laws. However, vaccines are not legally required under several circumstances.

Young children: In many states, young children are not legally required to be vaccinated. Babies born at hospitals may be subjected to a hepatitis B vaccine within hours of birth. However, this is a hospital policy, not a state law. Parents can withhold consent. (If parents reject the shot, they must never let the baby out of eyesight until they leave the hospital because medical personnel have been known to surreptitiously vaccinate newborns against the parents' wishes.)[1]

Children taken to the doctor for well-baby visits will be subjected to a cocktail of vaccines. However, these are merely recommended by the CDC and enforced by the pediatrician. Unless the state you live in mandates these vaccines for infants, they are not legally required. If parents object to the shots, doctors may resort to scare tactics by lecturing them with horror stories about unvaccinated children contracting diseases and dying. They may also challenge the parents' competence or even threaten to call Social Services for child neglect. Many quit their patients, refusing to see them again.[2] Parents should be thankful that this dysfunctional relationship with their health care practitioner has been terminated. Naturopathic doctors may be an option and can be found in the local telephone book.

Public institution: State vaccine laws are generally written to regulate enrollment in public institutions. Vaccines may be required to enter daycare, public school or college. However, all states offer legal exemptions to "mandatory" vaccines. (For an explanation on why schools should NOT mandate vaccines, visit: www.thinktwice.com/school.htm) If you do not wish to vaccinate your child but would still like to enroll your child in a public school, acquire a copy of your state vaccine laws to determine which exemptions are permitted. All states permit medical waivers if a doctor will certify that vaccines might hurt the child. (Doctors rarely provide a medical waiver. When they are willing to write one, it's usually to exempt just one or two vaccines that caused a serious reaction on a previous dose.) Most states also offer a religious exemption, but each state has a different way of defining it. Again, acquire a copy of your state law to determine precise requirements. (Contrary to popular belief, religious exemptions do not have to be written by the head of a church.) Some states also offer a philosophical exemption. For example, Arizona, California, and Colorado allow parents to enroll their children in public school without vaccines if they sign a letter indicating that they have "beliefs" opposed to vaccines. The law does not require parents to elaborate upon their beliefs. Several other states also permit philosophical exemptions. Simply sign the vaccine waiver and submit it. Authorities are legally obligated to honor the exemption.

Private institution: Private schools, daycares and colleges are not obligated to honor religious or philosophical exemptions, although many choose to accept non-vaccinated children. Be sure to call the private school, daycare or college prior to beginning the application process to ascertain their vaccine policy. Otherwise, your child may be removed from the institution after he or she has been enrolled.

Employer: Owners of private businesses may institute policies requiring vaccines. For example, hospital workers may be expected to receive an annual flu shot, plus rubella and hepatitis B vaccines. Some employers may accept an exemption. Others will issue an ultimatum: get the shots or find another job.

Foreign travel: Vaccines are often recommended but rarely required for travel from the United States to foreign countries. For more information, contact the embassies of the countries that you plan to visit. Vaccines are rarely required to enter the United States from another country. The U.S. State Department provides a waiver for applicants who object to the shots on religious or moral grounds.

Can an unvaccinated child spread disease to vaccinated children?

Doctors often claim that unvaccinated children are "disease carriers" who could infect vaccinated children. They use this as a rationale to force-vaccinate all children. This is an illogical argument because an unvaccinated child cannot put vaccinated children at risk if the vaccines are effective. *Vaccinated* children may spread disease. For example, the oral polio vaccine was discontinued in the U.S. because the live polio virus was shedding in the stools of vaccinated babies. When parents changed the baby's diapers, they were exposed to the disease; some were crippled by vaccine-associated polio.[3] This vaccine is still used in Third World countries. In Nigeria, 69 people were recently paralyzed by this vaccine.[4]

Can vaccine damage be corrected or reversed?

Enlightened health practitioners are more aware than ever before of the link between vaccines, autoimmune ailments and neurological disorders. Some people who are hurt by vaccines can be helped. Each condition is unique and requires professional analysis. An individualized therapeutic regimen can then be established.

What are the options to non-vaccination?

Dr. Robert Mendelsohn was a pediatrician for 30 years. He originally recommended vaccines until he discovered that they were damaging his young patients. He stopped recommending vaccines and began speaking out against them. He also believed that there are very few conditions that warrant medical attention; allopathic intervention may do more harm than good.[5] Parents who choose not to vaccinate their children may wish to investigate naturopathic physicians and alternative health practitioners. They can be found in the local telephone book.

Where can I get more information about vaccines?

For official information about vaccines, contact vaccine manufacturers, the FDA, CDC or World Health Organization. For uncensored vaccine information, the *Thinktwice Global Vaccine Institute* (www.thinktwice.com) provides many valuable resources, including links to several other important vaccine websites.

Appendices

This section contains three tables and a glossary that summarize some of the more shocking ingredients included in vaccines. Appendix I is a list of vaccines that contain mercury. Appendix II is a list of vaccines that contain aluminum. Appendix III is a list of vaccines that contain viruses cultured from aborted human fetuses. (For some people this causes a profound moral dilemma.) Appendix IV describes other unusual substances that may be found in vaccines, such as fetal bovine (calf) serum, MSG, porcine (pig) gelatin, phenol, ammonium sulfate, hydrochloric acid and formaldehyde.

Appendix I:
Vaccines that Contain Mercury

Some vaccines contain thimerosal, which is approximately 50 percent mercury by weight. Thimerosal is added to vaccines as an anti-bacterial preservative, especially when the vaccine is distributed in multi-dose vials. Some vaccines are labeled as 'preservative-free' indicating that no preservative (thimerosal or otherwise) is used in the vaccine; however, traces used during the manufacturing process may be present in the final formulation. In other words, *some vaccines that are 'preservative-free' may contain traces of thimerosal.* Similarly, the term 'thimerosal-reduced' usually indicates that thimerosal is not added as a vaccine preservative, but trace amounts may remain from use in the manufacturing process. The following vaccines contain mercury:

Vaccine	Product Name	Mercury per Dose
DTaP	Tripedia TriHIBit	.3mcg .3mcg
DT	Sanofi Pasteur	.3mcg/25mcg*
Td	Decavac Mass. Public Health	.3mcg 8.3mcg
Tetanus	Aventis Pasteur	.3mcg/25mcg*
Hepatitis A/B	Twinrix	1mcg
Influenza	Afluria Fluarix Fluzone FluLaval Fluvirin	24.5mcg* 1mcg 25mcg* 25mcg* 1mcg/25mcg*
Meningococcal	Menomune	25mcg*
J. Encephalitis	JE-VAX	17.5/35mcg–child/adult

*Represents mercury content for each single dose extracted from a multi-dose vial.

Source: The vaccine manufacturers' product inserts. (Note: This list is intended as a general guide and does not include all vaccines that may contain mercury. For accurate, up-to-date information, contact the individual manufacturers.)

Appendix II:
Vaccines that Contain Aluminum

Some vaccines contain aluminum salts, which are added as adjuvants to help the vaccine stimulate a stronger immune response and increase efficacy. There are three types of aluminum-containing adjuvants used in vaccines: 1) aluminum hydroxide, also referred to as aluminum hydroxy-phosphate sulfate (AH), 2) aluminum phosphate (AP), and 3) aluminum potassium sulfate (APS). The following vaccines contain aluminum:

Vaccine	Product Name	Aluminum per Dose
Polio (IPV)	Pediarix (IPV, DTaP, Hep B) Pentacel (IPV, DTaP, Hib) Quadracel (IPV, DTaP)	850mcg (AH,AP) 330mcg (AP) 330mcg (AP)
DTaP	Pediarix (DTaP,Hep B, IPV) Pentacel (DTaP, IPV, Hib) Quadracel (DTaP, IPV) TriHIBit (DTaP, Hib) Daptacel (DTaP) Tripedia (DTaP) Infanrix (DTaP) Boostrix (Tdap) Adacel (Tdap)	850mcg (AH,AP) 330mcg (AP) 330mcg (AP) 170mcg (APS) 330mcg (AP) 170mcg (APS) 625mcg (AH) 390mcg (AH) 330mcg (AP)
Tetanus/DT/Td	Tetanus/Lederle (TT) Tetanus/A. Pasteur (TT) Tet-Dip/S. Pasteur (DT) Decavac (Td) Tenivac (Td)	800mcg (AP) 250mcg (APS) 170mcg (APS) 280mcg (APS) 330mcg (AP)
HPV	Gardasil Cervarix	225mcg (AH) 500mcg (AH)
Hepatitis A	Vaqta (Hep A) Havrix (Hep A) Twinrix (Hep A & B)	225/450mcg–child/adult (AH) 250/500mcg–child/adult (AH) 450mcg (AH,AP)
Hepatitis B	Pediarix (HepB, DTaP, IPV) Comvax (Hep B, Hib) Twinrix (Hep A & B) Recombivax (Hep B) Engerix-B (Hep B)	850mcg (AH,AP) 225mcg (AH) 450mcg (AH,AP) 250/500mcg–child/adult (AH) 250/500mcg–child/adult (AH)
Hib	Pentacel (Hib, DTaP, IPV) TriHIBit (Hib, DTaP) Comvax (Hib, Hep B) PedvaxHib (Hib)	330mcg (AP) 170mcg (APS) 225mcg (AH) 225mcg (AH)
Pneumococcal	Prevnar 13	125mcg (AP)
Anthrax	BioThrax	600mcg (AH)

Source: The vaccine manufacturers' product inserts. (Note: This list is intended as a general guide and does not include all vaccines that may contain aluminum. In addition, some forms of aluminum may be more persistent at triggering a macrophagic immune response or over-activation of the immune system. For accurate, up-to-date information regarding aluminum content in vaccines, contact the individual manufacturers.)

Appendix III:
Vaccines that Contain Viruses
Cultured from Aborted Human Fetuses

A virus must be given a medium in which to propagate, or reproduce itself. Although several vaccines contain viruses that were bred in animal cells, some vaccines contain viruses grown in human cells. The most common human cell lines used in vaccines are MRC-5, RA27/3, and WI-38, cultured from aborted human fetuses. The following vaccines were produced from these human fetal cell lines:

Vaccine	Product Name	Fetal Cell Line
Polio	Poliovax, IPV, Pentacel, Quadracel, Td Polio Adsorbed, Infanrix Hexa	MRC-5
DTaP	Pentacel, Quadracel, Infanrix Hexa	MRC-5
MMR	MMR-II, Priorix, ProQuad/MMRV, MR Vax, Eolarix, Biavax-II, Meruvax-II	RA 27/3, WI-38, MRC-5
Hepatitis A	Vaqta, Havrix, Avaxim, Epaxal, Twinrix, Vivaxim	MRC-5
Hepatitis B	Twinrix, Infanrix Hexa	MRC-5
Hib	Pentacel, Infanrix Hexa	MRC-5
Chickenpox	Varivax, Varilrix, ProQuad/MMRV	RA 27/3, WI-38, MRC-5
Shingles	Zostavax	WI-38, MRC-5
Rabies	Imovax	MRC-5

Source: The vaccine manufacturers' product inserts. (Note: Some vaccines under development —including shots for influenza, avian flu, HIV, and rheumatoid arthritis—use less common human fetal cell lines: PER.C6, HEK-293, WI-26, and VA4.)

> *"There is a grave responsibility to use alternative vaccines and to make a conscientious objection with regard to those which have moral problems.... Cooperation [in the vaccine program] occurs in a context of moral coercion. Parents are forced to act against their conscience...."*
> —Summary of an official Vatican statement[†]

[†]"Moral reflections on vaccines prepared from cell lines derived from aborted human fetuses." *Pontifical Academy for Life* (June 9, 2005). [An English translation of a commentary which appeared in the Italian scholarly journal, *Medicina e Morale*.]

Appendix IV:
Common Ingredients in Vaccines

Vaccines contain antigens, preservatives, adjuvants, stabilizers, antibiotics, buffers, diluents, emulsifiers, and inactivating chemicals. They also contain residue from animal and human growth mediums. Here is a partial list of vaccine ingredients, with brief comments:

ANTIGENS: The main component of any vaccine, designed to induce an immune response. These are either weakened germs or fragments of the disease organism: **viruses** (*polio*), **bacteria** (*Bordetella pertussis*), and **toxoids** (*Clostridium tetani*) are examples.

GROWTH MEDIUMS: Viruses require a medium in which to propagate. Common broths include chick embryo fibroblasts; chick kidney cells; mouse brains; African green monkey kidney (Vero) cells; and human diploid (fetal) cells (MRC-5, RA 27/3, WI-38).

PRESERVATIVES: Are used to stop microbial contamination of vaccines. **Thimerosal (mercury)** is a recognized developmental toxin and suspected immune, kidney, skin and sense organ toxin. **Benzethonium chloride** is a suspected endocrine, skin and sense organ toxin. **2-phenoxyethanol** is a suspected developmental and reproductive toxin; chemically similar to antifreeze. **Phenol** is a suspected blood, developmental, liver, kidney, neuro, reproductive, respiratory, skin and sense organ toxin.

ADJUVANTS: Are used to enhance immunity. **Aluminum salts** are the most common. **Squalene** has been added to anthrax vaccines, and may be linked to Gulf War illnesses.

STABILIZERS: Inhibit chemical reactions and prevent vaccine contents from separating or sticking to the vial. **Fetal bovine (calf) serum** is a commonly used stabilizer. **Monosodium glutamate (MSG)** helps the vaccine remain unchanged when exposed to heat, light, acidity, or humidity. **Human serum albumin** helps stabilize live viruses. **Porcine (pig) gelatin,** which protects vaccines from freeze-drying or heat, can cause severe allergic reactions.

ANTIBIOTICS: Prevent bacterial growth during vaccine production and storage. **Neomycin** is a developmental toxin and suspected neurotoxin. **Streptomycin** is a suspected blood, skin and sense organ toxin. **Polymyxin B** is a suspected liver and kidney toxin.

ADDITIVES (Buffers, diluents, emulsifiers, excipients, residuals, solvents, etc.): Some of these, such as **sodium chloride**, are probably benign. **Egg proteins** and **yeast** can cause severe reactions. **Ammonium sulfate** is a suspected liver, neuro and respiratory toxin. **Glycerin** is a suspected blood, liver and neuro toxin. **Sodium borate** is a suspected blood, endocrine, liver and neuro toxin. **Polysorbate 80** (Tween 80) is a suspected skin and sense organ toxin. **Hydrochloric acid** is a suspected liver, immune, locomotor, respiratory, skin and sense organ toxin. **Sodium hydroxide** is a suspected respiratory, skin and sense organ toxin. **Potassium chloride** is a suspected blood, liver and respiratory toxin.

INACTIVATING CHEMICALS: These kill unwanted viruses and bacteria that could contaminate vaccines. **Formaldehyde** (or **formalin**) is a known carcinogen and suspected liver, immune, neuro, reproductive, respiratory, skin and sense organ toxin; used in embalming fluids. **Glutaraldehyde** is a suspected developmental, immune, reproductive, respiratory, skin and sense organ toxin. **Polyoxyethylene** is a suspected endocrine toxin.

CONTAMINANTS: Vaccines may also contain dangerous, unintended substances, such as SV-40 found in some polio vaccines, and HIV discovered in early hepatitis B vaccines.

Source: The vaccine manufacturers' product inserts; Chemical profiles: www.scorecard.org

Notes

Introduction

1. Ioannidis, J. "Contradicted and initially stronger effects in highly cited clinical research." *JAMA* (July 13, 2005):218-28.
2. Roderick, M., et al. "Should the UK introduce varicella vaccine?" *Archives of Disease in Childhood* (November 2007).
3. Riaza Gómez, M., et al. "Complications of varicella in children." *Anales españoles de pediatria* (March 1999);50(3):259-62. [Spanish.]
4. Institute of Medicine. "Vaccine safety committee proceedings." (*National Academy of Sciences:* Washington, DC, May 11, 1992):40-41.
5. Kessler, DA. "Introducing MEDWatch: a new approach to reporting medication and device adverse effects and product problems." *JAMA* (June 2, 1993):2765.
6. Miller, NZ., et al. "Infant mortality rates regressed against number of vaccine doses routinely given: is there a biochemical or synergistic toxicity?" *Hum Exp Toxicol* (May 4, 2011). Published online: www.het.sagepub.com
7. Dworkin, MS., et al. "The changing epidemiology of invasive haemophilus influenzae disease, especially in persons ≥65 years old." *Clinical Infectious Diseases* 2007;44:810-816.
8. Unsolicited correspondence received by the author.
9. "The global vaccine market—evaluation of past, current and future market trends." *Genetic Engineering and Biotech News* (June 19, 2007).
10. University of Pennsylvania. "World vaccines market: vaccine segments analysis, vaccine cases and future forecast." *Center for Vaccine Ethics and Policy* (March 27, 2011).
11. See Notes 9 and 10.
13. Unsolicited correspondence received by the author.

Smallpox

1. *World Book Encyclopedia,* Vol 17 "Smallpox." (1994):513.
2. Maltin, LJ. "What is smallpox?" *WebMD* (2001).
3. *Microsoft Encarta Online Encyclopedia,* "Smallpox." (Oct 26, 2001).
4. Seercom. "Smallpox: treatment." www.seercom.com
5. McKendrick, GD. "Exanthematic virus infections." In: Scott, RB., ed. *Price's Textbook of the Practice of Medicine.* (London: Oxford University Press, 1973):159-169.
6. Dixon, C. *Smallpox* (London: Churchill, 1962).
7. See Note 3.
8. WHO. "Fifty years of the World Health Organization in the Western Pacific region—report of the regional director to the regional committee, Western Pacific: chapter 27, Smallpox."
9. Fenner, F., et al. *Smallpox and Its Eradication* (Geneva: WHO, 1988).
10. Hopkins, DR. *Princes and Peasants: Smallpox in History* (Chicago: University of Chicago Press, 1983).
11. Chase, A. *Magic Shots: A Human and Scientific Account of the Long and Continuing Struggle to Eradicate Infectious Diseases by Vaccination* (NY: William Morrow and Co., 1982).
12. McNeill, WH. *Plagues & Peoples.* (Anchor Press, 1976).
13. Cerny, J. "Egypt: From the Death of Ramses II to the End of the 21st Dynasty." In: Edwards, I.E., ed. *The Cambridge Ancient History* (Cambridge University Press, 1975):606-657.
14. Littman, RJ., et al. "Galen and the antonine plague." *American Journal of Philology* 1973;94:243-55.
15. Stearn, EW., et al. *The Effect of Smallpox on the Destiny of the Amerindian* (Boston: Humphries, 1945).
16. Zinsser, H. *Rats, Lice, & History* (Little, Brown..., 1935).
17. Ruffer, MA. "Pathological note on the royal mummies of the Cairo Museum." In: Moodie, RL., ed. *Studies in the Palaeopathology of Egypt* (U. of Chicago Press, 1921):175-76.
18. Ruffer, MA., et al. "Note on an eruption resembling that of variola in the skin of a mummy of the 20th Dynasty (1200-1100 BC)." *Journal of Pathology and Bacteriology* 1911;15:1-4.
19. Barquet, N., et al. "Smallpox: The triumph over the most terrible of the ministers of death." *Annals Internal Med* (Oct 15, 1997);127:635-42.
20. Edwardes, EJ. *A Concise History of Small-pox and Vaccination in Europe* (London: H.K. Lewis, 1902).
21. Fenner, F. "Nature, nurture and my experience with smallpox eradication." *eMJA* 1999;171:638+. www.mja.com.au
22. See Note 2.
23. Koplow, DA. *Smallpox: The Fight to Eradicate a Global Scourge* (University of California Press, 2003):24.
24. WHO. "The global eradication of smallpox: final report." *Global Commission for the Certification of Smallpox Eradication* (Geneva, 1980).
25. See Note 21.
26. See Note 8.
27. As documented by the CDC and WHO.
28. Tandy, EC. "The regulation of nuisances in the American colonies." *Amer J of Public Health* (Oct 1923);13(10):810-813.
29. See Note 11.
30. Bayne-Jones, S. *Evolution of Preventive Medicine in the United States Army, 1607-1939* (Washington, DC: Office of the Surgeon General, Dept. of the Army, 1968):21.
31. McBean, E. *The Poisoned Needle* (Mokelumne Hill, CA: Health Research, 1974):12.
32. See Note 19.
33. Hume, EH. *The Chinese Way of Medicine* (Baltimore: Johns Hopkins University Press, 1940).
34. See Note 4.
35. Ibid.
36. White, W. *The Story of a Great Delusion: In a Series of Matter-of-Fact Chapters* (London: EW. Allen, 1885): xi.
37. Martin, GJ. *Immunology: From Pasteur to the Search for an AIDS Vaccine* (NY: Venture Books, 1989).
38. Parish, HJ. *History of Immunization* (UK: E & S Livingstone, 1965).
39. Hale, AR. *Medical Voodoo* (NY: Gotham House, 1935):66.
40. See Note 11, p. 44.
41. Fox, R. *Great Men of Medicine* (Random House, 1947):85.
42. See Notes 19, 37, and 38.
43. See Note 36, p. xiii.
44. Levin, NA., et al. "Human cowpox infection," *eMedicine Journal* (October 24, 2001);2(10). www. emedicine.com
45. Crookshank, EM. *History and Pathology of Vaccination, Volume 1: A Critical Inquiry* (London: H.K. Lewis, 1889).
46. Moore, J. *The History and Practice of Vaccination* (London: J. Callow, 1817).
47. See Note 36, p. xiii.
48. Harding Rains, AJ. *Edward Jenner and Vaccination* (East Hussex, England: Wayland Publishers, 1974):59.
49. Jenner, E. *An Inquiry into the Causes and Effects of the Variolae Vaccinae, a Disease Discovered in Some of the Western Counties of England* (London: Printed for the Author, 1798).
50. Ibid., pp. 2-7.
51. See Note 36, pp. xiv-xv.
52. Ibid., p. xvi.
53. Ibid, pp. xi-xii.
54. Ibid., pp. xv-xvi.
55. Miller, G., ed., *To Doctor Alexander J. G. Marcet, London, 11 November 1801, Letters of Edward Jenner and Other Documents Concerning the Early History of Vaccination* (London, England: The Johns Hopkins Press, 1983):13.
56. See Note 49, p. 74.
57. Ibid., p. 29.
58. See Note 36, pp. xvi-xvii.
59. See Note 49, p. 66.
60. Ibid., pp. 60-61.
61. See Note 36, p. xviii.
62. Ibid., p. xxviii.
63. Ibid., p. xxxi.
64. Ibid., p. xxxii.
65. Ibid.
66. Ibid., p. xxxv.
67. See Note 31, p. 72.
68. Ibid., p. 64.
69. See Note 38.
70. See Note 31, p. 33.
71. Official statistics, England. Reported in *Vaccine & Serum Evils* by Shelton, HM. (San Antonio: Health Research, 1966):23.
72. Allen, H. *Don't Get Stuck! The Case Against Vaccinations and Injections* (Tampa, Florida: Natural Hygiene Press, 1975):32.
73. See Note 31, p. 27.
74. Ibid., p. 13.
75. Ibid.
76. Koren, T. "Tedd Koren's 2nd November 2001 newsletter," *Koren Publications, Inc.* (November 9, 2001).
77. Ibid.
78. See Note 31, p. 16.
79. "Vaccination in Italy," *NY Med J* (July 22, 1899).
80. Ibid.
81. Shelton, HM. *Vaccine and Serum Evils* (San Antonio, Texas: Health Research, 1966):20-21.
82. Ibid., pp. 21-22.
83. See Note 72, p. 36.
84. 1920 Report of the Philippine Health Service. As reported in *Vaccine and Serum Evils* by Shelton, HM. (San Antonio: Health Research, 1966):21.
85. See Note 36, p. xxi.
86. Official statistics from England and Wales. As reported in *Vaccine and Serum Evils* by Shelton, HM. (San Antonio, Texas: Health Research, 1966), pp. 23-24.
87. See Note 72, pp. 36-37.
88. Gandhi, MK. *Gandhi an Autobiography: Story of my Experiments with Truth* (Boston: Beacon Pr., 1957).
89. See Note 72.
90. Hume, MC. *150 Reasons for Disobeying the Vaccination Law by Persons Prosecuted Under It* (Cheltenham, Eng, 1878).
91. Ibid.
92. Sinclair, I. "Smallpox." www.whale.to
93. See Note 90.
94. *The Vaccination Inquirer and Health Review, Volume V: April 1883 to March 1884* (London: The London Society for the Abolition of Compulsory Vaccination, 1884).
95. Ibid., see title page.
96. *New York Press* (January 26, 1909).
97. See Note 31, pp. 21-24; 42, 72.
98. Garrow, RP. "Fatality rates of small-pox in the vaccinated and unvaccinated," *British Med J* (January 14, 1928):74.
99. Parry, LA. "Fatality rates of small-pox in the vaccinated and unvaccinated," *British Med J* (January 21, 1928):116.
100. In a congressional statement by Senator Dolliver, United States Senate (February 25, 1909).
101. U.S. Dept. of Agriculture. *Farmer's Bulletin* (April 22, 1915):15.
102. Report of the Andrews Committee (May 1925). Report of the Rolleston Committee (Feb 1928). See Note 81, p. 14.
103. *New York State Journal of Medicine* (May 15, 1926).
104. *J of the American Medical Association* (July 1926).
105. *Lancet* (September 4, 1926).
106. *Lancet* (October 9, 1926).
107. See Notes 98 and 99.
108. Health Organization of the League of Nations: Geneva. "Report of the Commission of Smallpox and Vaccination," (August 27, 1928).
109. Ibid.

110. *The International News Service* (February 27, 1930).
111. *J of the American Medical Association* (April 5, 1930).
112. Office of Vital Statistics: Washington, DC.
113. *Lancet* (December 6, 1952).
114. *Vaccination at Work*, p. 47 (see Note 31, p. 82).
115. DeVries, E. *Postvaccinal Perivenous Encephalitis* (Amsterdam: Elsevier Publishing Company, 1959).
116. Dick, GWA. "Scientific Proceedings; Symposium on Virus Diseases. 13th Annual Meeting of the British Medical Association, Belfast." *British Medical Journal*, 1962;2:319.
117. Dixon, CW. *Smallpox.* (London: J & A Churchill, 1962).
118. Spillane, JD., et al. "The neurology of Jennerian vaccination—a clinical account of the neurological complications which occurred during the smallpox epidemic in South Wales in 1962." *Brain*, 1964;87:1-44.
119. Miller, H., et al. "Multiple sclerosis and vaccination." *British Medical Journal* (April 22, 1967): 210-213.
120. Neff, JM., et al. "Complications of smallpox vaccination, United States, 1963. II. Results obtained by four statewide surveys." *Pediatrics* 1967;39:916-923.
121. Lane, MJ. "Complications of smallpox vaccination," *New England J of Medicine* 1968;281(22):1201-08.
122. Carnahan, S. and Rinpoche, LK. *In the Presence of My Enemies: Memoirs of Tibetan Nobleman Tsipon Shuguba.* (Santa Fe, New Mexico: Clear Light Publishers, 1995):8.
123. Elben. *Vaccination Condemned* (Los Angeles: Better Life Research, 1981):1-15.
124. See Note 31, pp. 72-84.
125. Redfield, R., et al. "Disseminated vaccinia in a military recruit with human immunodeficiency virus (HIV) disease." *New England Journal of Medicine* (March 12, 1987):673.
126. Wright, P. "Smallpox vaccine 'triggered AIDS virus.'" *London Times* (May 11, 1987).
127. Rappoport, J. "Smallpox vaccine as AIDS trigger." *L. A. Weekly* (June 5-11, 1987):8.
128. See Note 126.
129. Franks, G. *AIDS and Vaccinations: The London Times Reports* (Denton, TX: Pure Water Products, 1988):21-23.
130. See Note 126.
131. Ibid.
132. Ibid.
133. "Monkeypox," *British Med J* (January 6, 1973):3-4.
134. Baxby, D. "Smallpox-like viruses from camels in Iran." *Lancet* (November 18, 1972):1063-1065.
135. Gispen, R., et al. "Monkeypox-specific antibodies in human and simian sera from the Ivory Coast and Nigeria." *Bull WHO* 1976;53:355-360.
136. "Monkeypox." www.justice.loyola.edu
137. Ibid.
138. Marennikova, SS. "Field and experimental studies of poxvirus infection in rodents." *Bull WHO* 1979; 57(3):461-464.
139. Bedson, HS. "Enzyme studies for the characterization of some orthopoxvirus isolates." *Bull WHO* 1982; 60(3):377-380.
140. Barrett, J. "Monkeypox," *Gale Encyclopedia of Medicine.*
141. See Note 134.
142. Radio National. "The health report: monkeypox." *Australian Broadcasting Corporation* (September 1, 1997).
143. WHO. "Fact sheet No. 161: monkeypox." (Dec. 1997).
144. American Veterinary Medical Assoc. "Largest outbreak of monkeypox reported." *J of the AVMA* (Mar 15, 1998).
145. See Note 143.
146. See Note 142.
147. Fenner, F., et al. "Smallpox and its eradication." (Geneva, 1988).
148. Mahy, BW., et al. "The remaining stocks of smallpox virus should be destroyed." *Science* 1993;262:1223-24.
149. Joklik, WK., et al. "Why the smallpox virus stocks should not be destroyed." *Science* 1993;262: 1225-26.
150. "Another reprieve for smallpox virus." *Lancet* 1993; 342:505-506.
151. Voelker, R. "Scientists still debate the fate of smallpox virus." *JAMA* 1993;270:2908.
152. "End of line for smallpox virus?" *Nature* 1993; 336:711.
153. WHO. "Destruction of variola virus: memorandum from a WHO meeting. *Bulletin of the WHO* 1994;72:841-844.
154. Marwick, C. "Smallpox virus destruction delayed yet again." *J of the American Medical Association* 1995;273:446.
155. Maurice, J. "Smallpox virus wins stay of execution." *Science* 1995;267:450.
156. WHO Press Release. "WHO executive board recommends destruction of smallpox virus." (January 25, 1996).
157. See Notes 3, 8, and 19.
158. Miller, J. "U.S. set to retain smallpox stocks." *The New York Times* (November 16, 2001).
159. See Notes 21 and 158.
160. Bazell, R., et al. "Anthrax fears close Senate offices." *MSNBC* (October 16, 2001). www.msnbc.com
161. Associated Press. "Congress closes for anthrax sweep." *The Santa Fe New Mexican* (October 18, 2001):A1.
162. Bazell, R., et al. "Anthrax strains in 3 attacks linked." *MSNBC* (October 19, 2001). www.msnbc.com
163. Check, E., et al. "Bioterrorism: bracing for the worst." *Newsweek* (October 29, 2001):41.
164. Neergaard, L. "Health officials review smallpox plan." *Associated Press* (October 19, 2001).
165. Cohen, J., et al. "Vaccines for biodefense: a system in distress." *Science* (October 19, 2001):500.
166. Rosenthal, SR., et al. "Developing new smallpox vaccines." *Emerging Infec Dis, CDC* (Nov-Dec 2001);7(6).
167. Stolberg, SG. "Immunization: vast uncertainty on smallpox vaccine." *New York Times* (October 19, 2001).
168. Greenberg, M. "Complications of vaccination against smallpox." *Am J Dis Child* 1948;76:492-502.
169. Cangemi, VF. "Acute pericarditis after smallpox vaccination." *N Engl J Med* 1958;258:1257-9.
170. Copeman, PWM., et al. "Eczema vaccinatum." *British Medical Journal* 1964;2:906-8.
171. Neff JM., et al. "Complications of smallpox vaccination —United States, 1963. II. Results obtained by four statewide surveys." *Pediatrics* 1967;39:916-23.
172. Neff, JM., et al. "Complications of smallpox vaccination. I. National survey in the U.S., 1963." *NEJM* 1967;276:125-32.
173. Fulginiti, VA., et al. "Progressive vaccinia in immuno-logically deficient individuals." (NY: The National Foundation-March of Dimes, Birth Defects, Original Article Series, Immunologic Deficiency Diseases in Man, 1968);4:129-45.
174. Marmelzat, WL. "Malignant tumors in smallpox vaccination scars." *Arch Dermatol* 1968;97:406.
175. Lane, JM., et al. "Routine childhood vaccination against smallpox reconsidered." *NEJM* 1969;281:1220-4.
176. Lane, JM., et al. "Complications of smallpox vaccination, 1968. National surveillance in the U.S." *NEJM* 1969; 281:1201-8.
177. Holtzman, CM. "Postvaccination arthritis." *NEJM* 1969; 280:111-2.
178. Lane, JM., et al. "Complications of smallpox vaccination, 1968: ten statewide surveys." *J Infect Dis* 1970; 122: 303-9.
179. Lane, JM., et al. "Deaths attributable to smallpox vaccination, 1959 to 1966, and 1968." *JAMA* 1970; 212:441-4.
180. DeNoon, D. "Smallpox vaccine key defense against attack." *WebMD* (November 8, 2001).
181. See Note 8.
182. Neff, JM., et al. "Complications of smallpox vaccination: 1968 surveillance in a comprehensive care clinic." *Pediatrics* 1972;50:481-3.
183. Rowland, R. "U.S. trying to boost smallpox vaccine supply." *CNN, Atlanta* (October 24, 2001). www.cnn.com
184. Stephenson, J. "Researchers launch a web-based resource for smallpox research." *JAMA* (February 21, 2001).
185. See Notes 142, 164, 166, 167, and 179.
186. Miller, J., et al. "September 11 attacks led to push for more smallpox vaccine." *New York Times* (October 22, 2001).
187. Center for Strategic and International Studies. "Dark Winter: A Bioterrorism Exercise." *Johns Hopkins Center for Civilian Biodefense Studies; Anser Institute for Homeland Security* (June 2001). www.hopkins-biodefense.org
188. Ibid.
189. Meltzer, MI., et al. "Modeling potential responses to smallpox as a bioterrorist weapon—Appendix I: A mathematical review of the transmission of smallpox." *Emerging Infec Dis, CDC* (Nov-Dec 2001);7(6).
190. Milloy, S. "Smallpox attack exaggerated." *Fox News* (October 5, 2001). www.foxnews.com
191. See Note 186.
192. Ibid.
193. See Note 183.
194. See Note 165, p. 499; Note 166; and Note 167.
195. Orent, W. "The smallpox wars: biowarfare vs. public health." *The American Prospect* 1999;10(44).
196. Sepkowitz, KA. "How contagious is vaccinia?" *New England J of Medicine* (January 30, 2003);348:5.
197. See Note 165, p. 499.
198. See Note 142.
199. See Note 167.
200. See Note 165, p. 500.
201. See Note 158.
202. Connolly, C. "Smallpox vaccine reactions jolt experts." *Washington Post* (December 5, 2002). www.washingtonpost.com
203. Schwenk, TL. "A look back at the recent smallpox vaccination program." *Journal Watch* (January 10, 2006).
204. Reuters. "U.S. probes death of nurse vaccinated for smallpox." (March 26, 2003). www.alertnet.org
205. Meckler, L. "Woman vaccinated against smallpox dies." *Star Tribune* (March 25, 2003). www.startribune.com
206. Connolly, C. "Reactions may be linked to vaccine: three workers report serious side effects." *Wash. Post* (Feb 28, 2003).
207. See Note 31, pp. 42, 72 and 83.
208. CDC. "Smallpox vaccine and heart problems: information for people who have recently received the smallpox vaccine." (March 31, 2003).
209. Casey, CG., et al. "Adverse events associated with smallpox vaccination in the United States, January— October 2003. *JAMA* (December 7, 2005);294:2734-43.
210. Sejvar, JJ., et al. "Neurologic adverse events associated with smallpox vaccination in the United States, 2002-2004." *JAMA* (December 7, 2005);294:2744-50.
211. See Note 203.
212. Manier, J. "Smallpox shot infects soldier's toddler son: boy critically ill; mom stricken." *Chicago Trib* (March 17, 2007).
213. Nuzzo, J. "FDA advisory committee unanimously recommends approval of ACAM2000." *Center for Biosecurity* (May 18, 2007). www.upmc-biosecurity.org
214. "ACAM2000 clinical trials update." *Acambis* (April 13, 2004). www.acambis.co.uk
215. "Smallpox vaccine gets good FDA reviews." *USA Today* (May 15, 2007). www.usatoday.com
216. Wyeth Laboratories. "Dryvax (Smallpox vaccine, dried, calf lymph type)." Product insert from the vaccine manufacturer (reproduced by the FDA). Updated: November 6, 2002.
217. See Note 164.
218. Ibid.
219. See Note 167.
220. Gostin, LO. "Model State Emergency Health Powers Act." Prepared by The Center for Law and the Public's Health at Georgetown and Johns Hopkins Universities for the CDC. (As of October 23, 2001):1-40. www.publichealthlaw.net
221. Ibid., pp. 28-29.
222. Ibid., pp. 16-18; Sections 303: Effect of declaration, and 304: Enforcement.
223. Knight Ridder News. "Health agency proposes quarantine plan for states." *Santa Fe New Mexican* (Oct. 2001):A1+.
224. See Note 220, p. 39; Section 807: Repeals.

225. Richardson, D. "Danger: forced vaccination for all under CDC's proposal." *PROVE newsletter* (November 2, 2001).
226. See Note 220.
227. DiPentima, MC., et al. "Pediatricians knowledge, views, and perspectives on smallpox and smallpox vaccine." *Clinical Pediatrics* (March 2006);45(2):165-72.
228. Wortley, PM., et al. "Healthcare workers who elected not to receive smallpox vaccination." *Am J Prev Med.* (March 2006);30(3):258-65.
229. See Note 206.
230. U.S. Department of Health and Human Services. "HHS issues final rule for smallpox vaccine injury compensation program." Press release: June 16, 2006. www.hhs.gov
231. See Notes 213 and 215.
232. Associated Press. "U.S. buys new smallpox vaccine." *CBS News* (June 5, 2007). www.cbsnews.com

Polio

1. Okonek, BM., et al. "Development of polio vaccines." *Access Excellence* (Feb 16, 2001):1. www.accessexcellence.org
2. Volk, WA., et al. *Basic Microbiology, 4th edition.* (Philadelphia, PA: J.B. Lippincott Co., 1980):455.
3. Physician's Desk Reference (PDR); 55th edition. (Montvale, NJ: Medical Economics, 2001):778.
4. Burnet, M., et al. *The Natural History of Infectious Disease* (New York, NY: Cambridge University Press, 1972):16.
5. See Note 3.
6. Neustaedter, R. *The Vaccine Guide* (Berkeley, California: North Atlantic Books, 1996):107–8
7. See Note 3.
8. Baby Center. "The polio vaccine (0-12 months)."
9. Moskowitz, R. "Immunizations: the other side. *Mothering* (Spring 1984):36.
10. Houchaus. "Ueber poliomyelitis acuta." *Munch Med Wochenschr* 1909;56:2353–55.
11. Lambert SM. "A yaws campaign and an epidemic of poliomyelitis in Western Samoa." *J Trop Med Hyg* 1936;39:41–6.
12. Lindsay, KW., et al. *Neurology and Neurosurgery Illustrated.* (Edinburgh/London/New York: Churchill Livingston, 1986)·100, Figure I5.2. From National Morbidity Reports.
13. McCloskey, BP. "The relation of prophylactic inoculations to the onset of poliomyelitis." *Lancet* (April 18, 1950):659–63.
14. Geffen, DH. "The incidence of paralysis occurring in London children within four weeks after immunization." *Med Officer* 1950;83:137–40.
15. Martin, JK. "Local paralysis in children after injections." *Arch Dis Child* 1950;25:1–14.
16. Hill, AB., et al. "Inoculation and poliomyelitis. A statistical investigation in England and Wales in 1949." *BMJ* 1950;ii:1–6.
17. Medical Research Council Committee on Inoculation Procedures and Neurological Lesions. "Poliomyelitis and prophylactic inoculation." *Lancet* 1956;ii:1223–31.
18. Sutter, RW., et al. "Attributable risk of DTP (diphtheria and tetanus toxoids and pertussis vaccine) injection in provoking paralytic poliomyelitis during a large outbreak in Oman." *J of Infectious Diseases* 1992; 165:444–9.
19. Ibid., p. 444.
20. Strebel, PM., et al. "Intramuscular injections within 30 days of immunization with oral poliovirus vaccine—a risk factor for vaccine-associated paralytic poliomyelitis." *NEJM* (February 23, 1995):500+.
21. Editorial. "Provocation paralysis." *Lancet* 1992;340:1005.
22. Wyatt, HV. "Provocation poliomyelitis: neglected clinical observations from 1914-1950." *Bull Hist Med* 1981;55:543–57.
23. Townsend-Coles, WF., et al. "Poliomyelitis in relation to intramuscular injections of quinine...drugs." *Trans R Soc Trop Med Hyg* 1953; 47:77–81.
24. Guyer, B., et al. "Injections and paralytic poliomyelitis in tropical Africa." *Bull WHO* 1980;58:285–91.
25. Bodian, D. "Viremia in experimental poliomyelitis. II. Viremia and the mechanism of the 'provoking' effect of injections of trauma." *Amer J Hyg* 1954;60:358–70.
26. Wyatt, HV. "Incubation of poliomyelitis as calculated from time of entry into the central nervous system via the peripheral nerve pathways." *Rev Infect Dis* 1990;12:547-56.
27. Wyatt, HV., et al. "Unnecessary injections and paralytic polio in India." *Trans R Soc Trop Med Hyg* 1992;86: 546–9.
28. See Note 21.
29. See Note 21, p. 1006 and Note 27.
30. Chandra, RK. "Reduced secretory antibody response to live attenuated measles and poliovirus vaccines in malnourished children." *British Medical Journal* 1975;ii:583–5.
31. McBean, E. *The Poisoned Needle* (Mokelumne Hill, California: Health Research, 1957):116.
32. Ibid.
33. Sandler, B. *American J of Pathology* (January 1941).
34. Sandler, B. *Diet Prevents Polio* (Milwaukee: Lee Foundation for Nutritional Research, 1951).
35. Allen, N. *Don't Get Stuck: The Case Against Vaccinations* (Oldsmar, Florida: Natural Hygiene Press, 1985):166.
36. See Note 33, pp. 116-118 and p. 146.
37. Ibid., p. 146.
38. See Note 31, p. 146 and Note 35. Data taken from North Carolina State Health Department figures.
39. Ibid.
40. Harry, NM. "The recovery period in anterior poliomyelitis." *British Medical Journal* 1938;1:164–7.
41. Sharrard, W. "Muscle recovery in poliomyelitis." *J Bone Joint Surgery* 1955; 37B:63–79.
42. Affeldt, JE., et al. "Functional and universal recovery in severe poliomyelitis." *Clin Orthop* 1958;12:16–21.
43. Hollenberg, C., et al. "The late effects of spinal poliomyelitis." *Can Med Assoc J* 1959;81:343–6.
44. Ramlow, J., et al. "Epidemiology of the post-polio syndrome." *American Journal of Epidemiology* 1992;136:783.
45. See Notes 40-44.
46. See Note 6, p. 108 and Notes 40-44.

47. "A Science Odyssey: People and Discoveries. Salk produces polio vaccine." www.pbs.org
48. Offit, P. *The Cutter Incident* (Yale University Press, 2005).
49. Offit, P. "The Cutter Incident: 50 Years Later." *New England Journal of Medicine* 2005;352:1411-1412.
50. See Note 1.
51. See Notes 1 and 47.
52. Ibid.
53. Ibid.
54. Strebel, PM., et al. "Epidemiology of polio in U.S. one decade after the last reported case of indigenous wild virus associated disease." *Clin Infec Dis,* CDC (Feb 1992):568–79.
55. Gorman, C. "When the vaccine causes the polio." *Time* (October 30, 1995):83.
56. Shaw, D. "Unintended casualties in war on polio." *Philadelphia Inquirer* (June 6, 1993):A1.
57. See Notes 1 and 47.
58. CDC. *MMWR* 2000;49:1–22.
59. Reuters Medical News. "CDC publishes updated polio prevention recommendations for the U.S." (May 22, 2000).
60. The Associated Press. "Polio cases caused by vaccine." *The Santa Fe New Mexican* (January 31, 1997).
61. See Note 31, p. 140. From government statistics, as reported in Associated Press, from Boston (Aug 30, 1955).
62. See Note 35, p. 146.
63. See Note 31, p. 142.
64. Ibid.
65. Ibid., p. 140.
66. Ibid.
67. See Note 31, p. 144. As reported by Saul Pett in an Associated Press dispatch from Pittsburgh (October 11, 1954).
68. See Note 31, pp. 142-45.
69. *Washington Post* (September 24, 1976).
70. American Academy of Pediatrics, *Report of the Committee on Infec Dis: 1986* (Elk Grove Village, Illinois: AAP):284–5.
71. See Note 54.
72. Aventis Pasteur, Inc. "Polio Vaccine Inactivated, Ipol®." Product insert from the vaccine manufacturer, April 2005.
73. See Note 54.
74. Institute of Medicine. "An evaluation of poliomyelitis vaccine policy options." *IOM Publication 88-04* (Washington DC: National Academy of Sciences, 1988)
75. Vaccine Adverse Event Reporting System VAERS. Rockville, MD.
76. IOS. "The Polio vaccine coverup—OPV Vaccine Report: Document #14." www.ios.com/~w1066/poliov6.html
77. See Note 54, p. 568.
78. See Notes 55, 56 and 72.
79. From an unsolicited email received by the *Thinktwice Global Vaccine Institute.* www.thinktwice.com
80. CDC. "Polio: what you need to know." *U.S. Dept. of Health and Human Services* (October 15, 1991):3.
81. See Note 72.
82. Ibid.
83. Ibid.
84. See Note 3, p. 780 and Note 72.
85. Mendelsohn, R. *How to Raise a Healthy Child...In Spite of Your Doctor* (Ballantine Books, 1984):231.
86. Alderson, M. *International Mortality Statistics* (Washington, DC: Facts on File, 1981):177–8.
87. Ibid.
88. See Note 85.
89. Hearings Before the Committee on Interstate and Foreign Commerce, House of Representatives, 87th Congress, 2nd Session on HR 10541 (May 1962):94–112.
90. Los Angeles County Health Index: Morbidity and Mortality, Reportable Diseases.
91. See Note 89, pp. 96-97.
92. O'Hern, M. *Profiles: Pioneer Women Scientists.* Bethesda, MD: National Institutes of Health.
93. Curtis, T., et al. "Scientist's polio fear unheeded: how U.S. researcher's warning was silenced." *The Houston Post* 1992: A1 and A12.
94. Sweet, BH., Hilleman MR. "The vacuolating virus: SV-40." As cited in: "The polio vaccine and simian virus 40," by Moriarty, TJ. www.chronicillnet.org/online/bensweet.html
95. See Note 93.
96. Moriarty TJ. "The polio vaccine and simian virus 40." *Online News Index.* www.chronicillnet.org/online/bensweet.html
97. Shah, K., et al. "Human exposure to SV40." *American Journal of Epidemiology* 1976;103:1-12.
98. Curtis, T. "The origin of AIDS: A startling new theory attempts to answer the question 'Was it an act of God or an act of man?'" *Rolling Stone* (March 19, 1992):57.
99. Bookchin, D., et al. "Tainted polio vaccine still carries its threat 40 years later. *The Boston Globe* (January 26, 1997).
100. See Notes 97 and 98.
101. Innis, MD. "Oncogenesis and poliomyelitis vaccine." *Nature* 1968;219:972–3.
102. Soriano, F., et al. "Simian virus 40 in a human cancer." *Nature* 1974;249:421–4.
103. Weiss, AF., et al. "Simian virus 40-related antigens in three human meningiomas with defined chromosome loss." *Proceedings of the Nat Academy of Science* 1975;72(2):609–13.
104. Scherneck, S., et al. "Isolation of a SV-40-like papovavirus from a human glioblastoma." *Internat J Cancer* 1979;24:523–31.
105. Stoian, M., et al. "Possible relation between viruses and oromaxillofacial tumors. II. Research on the presence of SV-40 antigen and specific antibodies in patients with oromaxillofacial tumors." *Virologie* 1987;38:35–40.
106. Stoian, M., et al. "Possible relation between viruses and oromaxillofacial tumors. II. Detection of SV40 antigen and of anti-SV40 antibodies in patients with parotid gland tumors." *Virologie* 1987;38:41–6.
107. Bravo, MP., et al. "Association between the occurrence of antibodies to simian vacuolating virus 40 and bladder cancer in male smokers. *Neoplasma* 1988;35:285–8.
108. O'Connell, K., et al. "Endothelial cells transformed by

SV40 T-antigen cause Kaposi's sarcoma-like tumors in nude mice." *American Journal of Pathology* 1991;139(4):743–9.

109. Weiner, LP., et al. "Isolation of virus related to SV40 from patients with progressive multifocal leukoencephalopathy." *New England Journal of Medicine* 1972;286:385–90.

110. Tabuchi, K. "Screening of human brain tumors for SV-40-related T-antigen." *International J of Cancer* 1978;21:12–7.

111. Meinke, W., et al. "Simian virus 40-related DNA sequences in a human brain tumor." *Neurology* 1979;29:1590–4.

112. Krieg, P., et al. "Episomal simian virus 40 genomes in human brain tumors." *Proceedings of the National Academy of Science* 1981;78:6446-50.

113. Krieg, P., et al. "Cloning of SV40 genomes from human brain tumors." *Virology* 1984;138:336–40.

114. Geissler, E. "SV40 in human intracranial tumors: passenger virus or oncogenic 'hit-and-run' agent?" *Z Klin Med* 1986;41: 493–5.

115. Geissler, E. "SV40 and human brain tumors." *Progress in Medical Virology* 1990;37:211–22.

116. Bergsagel, DJ., et al. "DNA sequences similar to those of simian virus 40 in ependymomas and choroid plexus tumors of childhood." *NEJM* 1992;326:988–93.

117. Martini, M., et al. "Human brain tumors and simian virus 40." *J of the National Cancer Institute*, 1995;87(17):1331.

118. Lednicky, JA., et al. "Natural simian virus 40 strains are present in human...tumors." *Virology* 1995;212(2):710–7.

119. Tognon, M., et al. "Large T antigen coding sequence of two DNA tumor viruses, BK and SV-40, and nonrandom chromosome changes in two gioblastoma cell lines." *Cancer Gen and Cytogenics* 1996;90(1): 17–23.

120. Vilchez, RA., et al. "Association between simian virus 40 and non-hodgkin lymphoma." *Lancet* (Mar 9, 2002):817–23.

121. See Notes 109-120.

122. Carbone, M., et al. "SV-40-like sequences in human bone tumors." *Oncogene* 1996;13(3):527–35.

123. Pass, HI., Carbone, M., et al. "Evidence for and implications of SV-40-like sequences in human mesotheliomas." *Important Advances in Oncology* 1996:89-108.

124. Rock, A. "The lethal dangers of the billion dollar vaccine business." *Money* (December 1996):161.

125. Ibid.

126. Carlsen, W. "Rogue virus in the vaccine: Early polio vaccine harbored virus now feared to cause cancer in humans." *San Francisco Chronicle* (July 15, 2001):7. Research by Susan Fisher, epidemiologist, Loyola University Medical Center.

127. NIH. Zones of contamination: Globe staff graphic.

128. Bookchin, D., et al. "Tainted polio vaccine still carries its threat 40 years later." *The Boston Globe* (January 26, 1997).

129. "SV-40 contamination of polio vaccine." *Well Within Online* (February 3, 2001). www.nccn.net/~wwithin/ polio.htm

130. Rosa, FW., et al. "Absence of antibody response to simian virus 40 after inoculation with killed-poliovirus vaccine of mother's offspring with...tumors." *NEJM* 1988;318:1469.

131. Rosa, FW., et al. "Response to: Neurological tumors in offspring after inoculation of mothers with killed poliovirus vaccine." *New England Journal of Medicine* 1988;319:1226.

132. See Note 98, p. 58.

133. Martini, F., et al. "SV-40 early region and large T antigen in human brain tumors, peripheral blood cells, and sperm fluids from healthy individuals." *Cancer Research* 1996;56(20):4820–5.

134. See Note 124, p. 163.

135. See Note 133.

136. Ibid.

137. Fisher, B. "Vaccine safety consumer group cites conflict of interest in government report on cancer and contaminated polio vaccine link." *NVIC* Press Release (January 27, 1998).

138. See Note 126, p. 10.

139. Ibid., pp. 10 and 13.

140. National Cancer Inst (June 2001). See Note 126, p.11.

141. See Note 56, pp. 57-58.

142. Koprowski, H. "Tin anniversary of the development of live virus vaccine." *JAMA* 1960;174:972–6.

143. Hayflick, L., Koprowski, H., et al. "Preparation of poliovirus vaccines in a human fetal diploid cell strain." *American J Hyg* 1962;75:240–58.

144. Koprowski, H. In a letter sent to the Congressional Health and Safety Subcommittee, April 14, 1961.

145. Ibid.

146. See Note 124, p. 159.

147. Ibid.

148. Ibid.

149. Curtis, T. "Expert says test vaccine: backs check of polio stocks for AIDS virus." *Houston Post* (Mar 22, 1992):A21.

150. See Note 126, p. 5, and Note 149.

151. Essex, M., et al. "The origin of the AIDS virus." *Scientific American* 1988;259:64–71.

152. Karpas, A. "Origin and spread of AIDS." *Nature* 1990; 348:578.

153. Kyle, WS. "Simian retroviruses, poliovaccine, and origin of AIDS." *Lancet* 1992;339:600–1.

154. Elswood, BF., Stricker, RB. "Polio vaccines and the origin of AIDS." *Medical Hypothesis* 1994:42:347–54.

155. Myers, G, et al. "Emergence of simian/human immunodeficiency viruses." *AIDS Res Human Retro* 1992:8: 373–86.

156. "Workshop on simian virus-40 (SV-40): A possible human polyomavirus." *NVIC* (Jan 27-28, 1997). www.909shot.com. (Includes a summary of evidence presented at the Eighth Annual Houston Conference on AIDS.)

157. Martin, B. "Polio vaccines and the origin of AIDS: the career of a threatening idea." *Townsend Letter for Doctors* (January 1994):97–100.

158. Curtis, T. "Did a polio vaccine experiment unleash AIDS in Africa?" *The Washington Post* (April 5, 1992):C3+.

159. See Note 98, pp. 54+.

160. See Note 149, and Notes 151-154.

161. World Health Organization. "T-lymphotropic retroviruses of nonhuman primates. WHO informal meeting." *Weekly Epidemiology Records* 1985;30:269–70.

162. See Note 154.

163. See Notes 152 and 154.

164. See Notes 154 and 161.

165. Ohta, Y., et al. "No evidence for the contamination of live oral poliomyelitis vaccines with simian immunodeficiency virus." *AIDS* 1989;3:183–5.

166. Ibid.

167. Huet, T., et al. "Genetic organization of a chimpanzee lentivirus related to HIV-1." *Nature* 1990;345:356–9.

168. Desrosiers, RC. "HIV-1 origins: A finger on the missing link." *Nature* 1990;345:288–9.

169. Sabin, AB. "Properties and behavior of orally administered attenuated polio-virus vaccine." *JAMA* 1957;164:1216–23.

170. Plotkin, SA., Koprowski, H., et al. "Clinical trials in infants of orally administered polio viruses." *Pediatrics* 1959; 23:1041–62.

171. Barin, F., et al. "Serological evidence for virus related to simian T-lymphotropic retrovirus III in residents of West Africa." *Lancet* 1985;ii:1387–9.

172. See Note 98, pp. 106+.

173. Hirsch, VM., et al. "Simian immunodeficiency virus infection of macaques: End-stage disease is characterized by widespread distribution of proviral DNA in tissues." *Journal of Infectious Disease* 1991;163(5): 976–88.

174. See Note 3 and Note 98, p. 60.

175. Bohannon, RC., et al. "Isolation of a type D retrovirus from B-cell lymphomas of a patient with AIDS." *J of Virology* 1991;65(11):5663–72.

176. Khabbaz, RF., et al. "Simian immunodeficiency virus needlestick accident in a lab worker." *Lancet* 1992;340: 271–3.

177. Gao, F., et al. "Human infection by genetically diverse SIVsm-related HIV-2 in West Africa." *Nature*, 1992;358:495–9.

178. See Note 155.

179. Giunta, S., et al. "The primate trade and the origin of AIDS viruses." *Nature* 1987;329:22.

180. Seale, J. "Crossing the species barrier—viruses and the origins of AIDS in perspective." *J R Soc Med* 1989;82: 519–23.

181. Lecatsas, G. "Origin of AIDS." *Nature* 1991;351:179.

182. Gilks, C. "Monkeys and malaria." *Nature* 1991;354:262.

183. See Notes 98, 126, 149, 151-154, and 156-158.

184. Grmek, MD. *History of AIDS: Emergence and Origin of a Modern Pandemic.* (Princeton, NJ: Princeton U Pr, 1990).

185. See Note 154.

186. Koprowski, H. "Historical aspects of the development of live virus vaccine in poliomyelitis." *BMJ* 1960;ii:85–91.

187. Ibid.

188. See Note 98, p. 59.

189. Lebrun, A., et al. "Vaccination with the CHAT strain of type I attenuated poliomyelitis virus in Leopoldville, Belgian Congo." *Bulletin of the WHO* 1960;22:203–13.

190. See Note 186.

191. See Note 157, p. 98.

192. Klein, A. *Trial by Fury.* (Charles Scribner's Sons, 1972).

193. Sabin, AB. "Present position of immunization against poliomyelitis with live virus vaccines." *BMJ* 1959;i:663–80.

194. Mahmias, AJ., et al. "Evidence for human infection with an HTLV III/LAV-like virus in Central Africa, 1959." *Lancet* 1986;i:1279–80.

195. Huminer, D., et al. "AIDS in the pre-AIDS era." *Rev Infect Dis* 1987:9:1102–8.

196. Corbitt, G., et al. "HIV infection in Manchester, 1959." *Lancet* 1990;ii:51.

197. Cohen, J. "Debate on AIDS origin: Rolling Stone weighs in—controversial article angers vaccine experts by claiming AIDS could have been spread by polio vaccines in Africa." *Science* (March 1992):1505.

198. Hooper, E. "Sailors and star-bursts, and the arrival of HIV." *British Medical Journal* 1997;315:1689-1691.

199. Vandamme, A., et al. "Tracing the origin and history of the HIV-2 epidemic." *PNAS*, Vol. 100, No. 11 (May 27, 2003).

200. Kanabus, A., et al. "The origins of HIV and the first cases of AIDS." *Avert.* www.avert.org/origins.htm

201. See Note 154.

202. See Notes 158 and 186.

203. Hrdy, DB. "Cultural practices contributing to the transmission of human immunodeficiency virus in Africa." *Rev Infect Dis* 1987; 9:1109–19.

204. See Note 98, p. 60.

205. Ibid.

206. Ibid.

207. See Note 154.

208. Ibid.

209. Sonnet, J., et al. "Early AIDS cases originating from Zaire and Burtundi (1962-1976)." *Scan J Infec Dis* 1987;19:511–7.

210. See Note 98, pp. 106+.

211. Ibid.

212. See Note 98, p. 59.

213. Ibid., p. 60.

214. Ibid., p. 106+.

215. Ibid.

216. Gallo, R. *Virus Hunting.* (NY: HarperCollins, 1991).

217. See Note 98, p. 108.

218. [Koprowski eventually filed a lawsuit against Tom Curtis and *Rolling Stone* (see Note 98) for "...the destruction of (his) professional and personal reputation, for mental and emotional suffering, and for...humiliation and embarrassment...." *Rolling Stone* paid one dollar in symbolic compensation to Koprowski and printed a "clarification" stating that the mass polio vaccination campaign conducted in the Belgian Congo from 1957-1960 using a vaccine developed by Koprowski was only "one of several disputed and unproven theories" about how AIDS might have originated. ("'Origin of AIDS' Update." *Rolling Stone*, Dec 9, 1993: 39.) For more info: *The Seeds of Doom* by C. Biasco, 2005.]

219. Tager, A. "Preliminary report on the treatment of recurrent herpes simplex with poliomyelitis vaccine (Sabin's)." *Dermato logica* 1974;149:253–5.

220. See Note 98, Note 126, and Notes 151-158.

221. See Note 153.

222. See Note 154.

223. "Centers for Disease Control Task Force on Karposi's Sarcoma and Opportunistic Infections. Epidemiological aspects of the current outbreak of Kaposi's sarcoma and opportunistic infections." *New England Journal of Medicine* 1982;306:252.
224. See Note 153.
225. Ibid.
226. Korn, P. "The new AIDS mystery." *Redbook* (July 1994);82.
227. Ibid.
228. Painter, K. "Usual routes of infection ruled out: 12-year-old's parents blame polio vaccine, but scientists discount that theory." *USA Today* (March 8, 1994);A1.
229. Extracted from a copy of the civil tort claim (U.S. District Court, New Jersey).
230. See Note 226, p. 106.
231. Ibid.
232. See Note 226.
233. Seven percent of AIDS in Michigan have no identifiable cause. As reported to the *Thinktwice Global Vaccine Institute*.
234. See Note 226.
235. Cowley, G. "Cannibals to cows: the path of a deadly disease." *Newsweek* (March 12, 2001);53.
236. Center for Biologics Evaluation and Research. "Bovine spongiform encephalopathy (BSE)." *FDA* (January 23, 2001).
237. Ibid. "What is BSE?"
238. See Note 236, "Does BSE...occur in humans?"
239. See Note 236, "What is the new variant form of CJD that the experts in the U.K. believe might be related to the BSE outbreak in cattle?"
240. See Note 235, p. 54.
241. *Nature* 1996;381:743-4.
242. *Nature* 1996;383:685-690.
243. *Nature* 1997;389:498-501.
244. *PNAS* 1999;96:15137-242.
245. *Lancet* 1996;347:921-5.
246. See Note 235, p. 56.
247. See Note 236, "How did people get new variant of CJD?"
248. Mad Cow Homepage. "Two million children inoculated with BSE vaccines." *Daily Express* (May 2, 2000).
249. Marwick, C. "FDA calls bovine-based vaccines currently safe." *JAMA* (September 13, 2000). www.jama.ama-assn.org
250. Mercola, J. "U.K. recalls polio vaccine over 'Mad Cow' fears." (October 29, 2000). www.mercola.com
251. See Note 236, "If vaccines are safe, why did the U.K. recall their polio vaccine?"
252. See Notes 3 and 72.
253. See Note 236, "Which bovine-derived materials are used in vaccine manufacture?"
254. See Note 248.
255. Ibid.
256. Hawkes, N. "BSE fears over polio vaccinations." *The Times* (October 21, 2000). www.thetimes.co.uk
257. Figures taken from Department of Health Reports, U.K. (October 2, 2000). www.doh.gov.uk/cjd
258. Meikle, J. "Vaccine fiasco exposes loopholes." *Guardian Newspapers Unlimited* (Oct 21, 2000). guardianunlimited.co.uk
259. See Note 236, "If vaccines are safe, why did the U.K. recall their polio vaccine?"
260. See Note 250.
261. FDA. "Points to consider in the characterization of cell lines used for the production of biologics." *The Center for Biologics Evaluation and Research* (December 1993).
262. See Note 236, "What measures has the FDA taken to ensure that people are not exposed to the BSE agent in vaccines?"
263. See Note 249.
264. Ibid.
265. Wilcox, G. "Farm Sanctuary. Proposed rule to ban substances in animal food [Docket No. 96-N-0135]," (May 15, 1999). In a letter to the FDA.
266. Ibid.
267. Marsh, R. *Dev Biol Stand* 1993;80:111-8.
268. Cutlip, RC. *J of Infectious Diseases* 1994;169:814-20.
269. See Note 265.
270. See Note 236, "When will vaccine manufacturers finish replacing cow-derived materials in vaccines with materials obtained from countries free of BSE?"
271. See Note 249.
272. See Note 124, p. 161.
273. Rustigan, R., et al. "Infection of monkey kidney cultures with virus-like agents." *Proc Soc Exp Biol Med* 1955;88: 8-16.
274. See Note 157, p. 100.
275. Morris, JA., et al. "Recovery of cytopathogenic agent from chimpanzees with coryza (22538). *Proc Soc Exp Biol Med* 1956;92;544-9.
276. Scheibner, V. *Vaccination: 100 Years of Orthodox Research... Medical Assault on the Immune System.* (Blackheath, NSW, Australia: Scheibner Publications, 1993):153.
277. Ibid.
278. Parrot, RH., et al. "II. Serological studies over a 34-month period in children with bronchiolitis, pneumonia and minor respiratory diseases." *JAMA* 1961;176(8):653-57.
279. Chanock, RM., et al. "Respiratory syncytial virus." *JAMA* 1961;176(8):647-53.
280. Ibid.
281. Hamparian, V., et al. "Recovery of new viruses (coryza) from cases of common cold in human adults." *Proc Soc Exp Med Biol* 1961;108:444-53.
282. CDC. "Respiratory syncytial virus," (June 21, 1999).
283. Public Health Laboratory Service, "Seasonal diseases: respiratory syncytial virus," (March 16, 2000). www.phls.co.uk
284. The Triplet Connection. "RSV—a serious subject," 2000. www.tripletconnection.com
285. Applied Genetics News. "Eat your vaccine." (Aug 2000).
286. See Note 276.
287. See Note 124, pp. 159-161.
288. Martin, J., et al. "African green monkey origin of the atypical cytopathic 'stealth virus' isolated from a patient with chronic fatigue syndrome." *Clin Diag Virology* 1995;4:93-103.

289. Fisher, B. "Did the first oral polio vaccine lots contaminated with monkey viruses create a monkey-human hybrid called HIV-1?" *The Vaccine Reaction* (April 1996);3.
290. Eighth Annual Houston Conference on AIDS..., 1996.
291. *American Journal of Hygiene* 1958;68:31-44.
292. See Note 289, p. 1.
293. Urnovitz, HB., et al. "Urine antibody tests: new insights into dynamics of HIV-1 infection." *Clin Chem* 1999;45: 1602-13.
294. See Note 289, pp. 1-4.
295. World Health Organization, "Problems with eradicating polio," *Science News* (November 25, 2000):348.
296. Reuters Health. "Polio outbreak in Dominican Republic and Haiti caused by vaccine-derived virus." *Reuters Medical News* (December 4, 2000). www.id.medscape.com
297. Crainic, R., et al. "Polio virus with natural recombinant genomes isolated from vaccine associated paralytic poliomyelitis. *Virology* 1993; 196:199-208.
298. Yoshida, H., et al. *Lancet* (October 28, 2000).
299. See Note 295.
300. See Note 296.
301. Ibid.
302. Ibid.
303. "Update on vaccine-derived polioviruses." *Medscape* (November 13, 2006). [See also: *MMWR* 2005;55(40:1093-97.]
304. Ibid., Table 1: Outbreaks of circulation vaccine-derived polioviruses—Worldwide, 1988-2006.
305. Pallansch, MA., et al. "The eradication of polio—progress and challenges." *NEJM* (Dec 14, 2006);355(24):2508-2511.
306. Ibid.
307. Ibid.
308. See Notes 3 and 72.
309. Sanofi Pasteur. "IPV (Diploid cell origin)." Product insert.
310. See Note 137.
311. Associated Press, "Monkey virus debate: should animals be used to produce vaccines?" *CNN Interactive* (Jan 29, 1997).
312. Ibid.
313. See Note 99.
314. In a presentation at a Vaccine Safety Forum Workshop: Institute of Medicine (November 1995).
315. See Note 289, pp. 4-5 and Note 290.
316. Ibid.

Influenza

1. National Institute of Allergy and Infectious Diseases. "Flu fact sheet." *Nat. Institutes of Hlth* (Last updated: Nov 17, 2006.)
2. U.S. Department of HHS. "Inactivated influenza vaccine: what you need to know—2006-07." *CDC* (June 30, 2006).
3. U.S. Department of HHS. "Live, intranasal influenza vaccine: what you need to know—2006-07." *CDC* (June 30, 2006).
4. Keep Kids Healthy. *Influenza.* www.keepkidshealthy.com
5. CDC. "Vaccine Info: Influenza Vaccine." www.cdc.gov
6. WHO Press Release, "Experts decide content of 1999-2000 Northern Hemisphere influenza vaccine," (February 17, 1999).
7. FDA. "Influenza virus vaccine 2006-2007 season: influenza vaccine lot release status." www.fda.gov See also: FDA, "Additional influenza vaccine approved for upcoming flu season." *FDA News* (Sep 28, 2007).
8. MedImmune Vaccines, Inc. "Influenza Virus Vaccine Live, Intranasal FluMist: 2006-2007 Formula." Product insert.
9. WHO. "Recommended composition of influenza virus vaccines for use in the 2016-2017 northern hemisphere influenza season." www.who.int
10. CDC. "Prevention and control of influenza: recommendations of the ACIP, 2007." *MMWR* (July 13, 2007); 56(RR06):1-54. See also: CDC. "2007-08 influenza prevention & control recommendations for using TIV and LAIV during the 2007-08 influenza season." www.cdc.gov (October 26, 2007).
11. Ibid.
12. Sanofi Pasteur, Inc.—Fluzone®; GSK— Fluarix®. ID Biomedical Corp.—FluLaval®. Influenza virus vaccine 2008-2009 formulas. Product inserts from the vaccine manufacturers.
13. CSL, Ltd.—Afluria®; Sanofi Pasteur, Inc.—Fluzone®; ID Biomedical Corp.—FluLaval®; Novartis—Fluvirin®. Influenza virus vaccine 2008-2009 formulas. Product inserts.
14. Ibid.
15. Institute for Vaccine Safety. "Thimerosal content in some U.S. licensed vaccines." *Johns Hopkins Bloomberg School of Pub Hlth* (Aug 6, 2008). www.vaccinesafety.edu/thi-table.htm
16. FDA. "Thimerosal in vaccines: Table3." (Updated: Sept. 6, 2007.) www.fda.gov/CBER/vaccine/thimerosal.htm
17. See Note 13, See also: ID Biomedical—Fluarix; MedImmune— FluMist®. Influenza virus vaccine 2008-2009 formulas. Product inserts.
18. Connaught Laboratories. "The making of a flu vaccine." *LA Times* (Reprinted in the *Kansas City Star*, Feb. 24, 1993).
19. See Notes 2, 3, and 5.
20. See Note 3.
21. Meadows, M. *FDA Consumer Mag.* (Sept-Oct, 2003).
22. "What's up with FluMist?" *Hlth Serv Columbia U.* 2010. www.goaskalice.columbia.edu
23. *The Daily Mail.* "Flu vaccines 'not worth the bother' says expert." www.dailymail.co.uk (October 27, 2006).
24. Ibid.
25. See Note 5, pp. 2-3. See also Notes 8 and 17.
26. National Vaccine Information Center (NVIC). "The flu and the flu vaccine." www.909shot.com/flufax.htm
27. Hurwitz, ES., et al. "Guillain-Barré syndrome and the 1978-79 influenza vaccine." *NEJM* 1981;304:1557-61.
28. Kaplan, JE., et al. "Guillain-Barré syndrome in the United States, 1978-1981: Additional observation from the national surveillance system." *Neurology.* 33:633-37.
29. Scheibner, "Flu vaccination: is it safe?" *Natural Health* (June/July 1993):19-21.
30. Lohse, A., et al. "Vascular purpura and cryoglobulinemia after influenza vaccination. Case-report and literature review. *Rev Rhum Engl Ed.* (June 1999);66(6):359-60.
31. Schmutz, JL., et al. "Does influenza vaccination induce

bullous pemphigoid?" *Ann Dermatol Vernereol.* (Oct 1999); 126(10):765. [French.]

32. Cummins, D., et al. "Haematological changes associated with influenza vaccination in people aged over 65: case report and study." *Clin Lab Haematol* (Oct 1998);20(5): 285-7.

33. Downs, AM., et al. "Does influenza vaccination induce bullous pemphigoid?" *Br J Dermatol* (Feb 1998);138(2):363.

34. Kawasaki, A., et al. "Bilateral anterior ischemic optic neuropathy following influenza vaccination." *J Neuroophthalmol* (Mar 1998);18(1):56-9.

35. Lasky, T., et al. "The Guillain-Barré syndrome and the 1992-1993 and 1993-1994 influenza vaccines." *NEJM* (Dec 1998);339(25):1797-802.

36. Park, CL, et al. "Does influenza vaccination exacerbate asthma?" *Drug Saf.* (August 1998);19(2):83-8.

37. Ramakrishnan, N, et al. "Thrombotic thrombocytopenic purpura following influenza vaccination—a brief case report." *Conn Med.* (October 1998);62(10):587-8.

38. Selvaraj, N., et al. "Hemiparesis following influenza vaccination." *Postgrad Med J.* (October 1998);74 (876):633-5.

39. Confino, I., et al. "Erythromelalgia following influenza vaccine in a child." *Clin Exp Rheumatol* (Jan-Feb 1997):111-3.

40. Desson, JF., et al. "Acute benign pericarditis after anti-influenza vaccine." *Presse Med.* (Mar 22, 1997):415. [French.]

41. Hull, TP., et al. "Optic neuritis after influenza vaccination." *Am J Ophthalmol* (Nov1997);124(5):703-4.

42. Kelsall, JT., et al. "Microscopic polyangitis after influenza vaccination." *J Rheumatol.* (June 1997);24(6):1198-1202.

43. Owensby, JE., et al. "Cellulitis and myositis caused by Agrobacterium radiobacter and Haemophilus parainfluenzae after influenza virus vaccine." *S. Med J.* (July 1997);90(7):752-4.

44. Bernad Valles, M., et al. "Adverse reactions to different types of influenza vaccines." *Med Clin (Barc).* (Jan 13, 1996);106(1):11-4. [Spanish.]

45. Fournier, B., et al. "Bullous pemphigoid induced by vaccination." *Br J Dermatol.* (July 1996);135(1):153-4.

46. Honkanen, PO., et al. "Reactions following administration of influenza vaccine along or with pneumococcal vaccine to the elderly." *Arch of Internal Med* (Jan 22, 1996); 156(2):205-8.

47. Lear, JT., et al. "Bullous pemphigoid following influenza vaccination." *Clin Exp Dermatol.* (Sep 1996); 21(5):392.

48. Ray, CL., et al. "Bilateral optic neuropathy...with influenza vaccination." *J Neuroophthalmol.* (Sep 1996); 16(3):182-4.

49. Antony, SJ., et al. "Postvaccinial (influenza) disseminated encephalopathy (Brown-Sequard syndrome)." *J Natl Med Assoc* (Sep 1995);87(9):705-8.

50. Cambiaghi, S., et al. "Gianotti-Crosti syndrome in an adult after influenza virus vaccine." *Derm* 1995; 191(4):340-1.

51. Herdderschee, D., et al. "Myelopathy following influenza vaccination." *Ned Tijdschr Geneeskd* (October 21, 1995); 139(42):2152-4. [Dutch.]

52. Biasi, D., et al. "A case of reactive arthritis after influenza after influenza vaccination." *Clin Rheum* (Dec 1994); 13(4)645.

53. Blanche, P., et al. "Development of uveitis following vaccination for influenza." *Clin Infect Dis* (Nov 1994); 19(5):979.

54. Bodokh, I., et al. "Reactivation of bullous pemphigoid after influenza vaccine." *Therapie.* (Mar-Apr 1994):154. [French.]

55. Brown, MA., et al. "Rheumatic complications of influenza vaccination." *Aust N Z J Med.* (October 1994); 24(5):572-3.

56. Beijer, WE., et al. "Polymyalgia rheumatica and influenza vaccination." *Dtsch Med Wochenschr.* (Feb 5, 1993);118(5): 164-5. [German.]

57. Boutros, N., et al. "Delirium following influenza vaccination." *Am J Psychiatry.* (Dec 1993);150(12):1899.

58. Mader, R., et al. "Systemic vasculitis following influenza vaccination—report of 3 cases and literature review." *J Rheumatol* (August 1993);20(8):1429-31. Review.

59. Robinson, T., et al. "Side effects of influenza vaccination." *Br J Gen Pract.* (Nov 1992);42(364):489-90.

60. Ward, DL. Re: "GBS & influenza vaccination in the US Army, 1980-1988." *Am J Epidem* (Aug 1, 1992);136(3):374-6.

61. Young, G. "Side effects of influenza immunization." *Br J Gen Pract* (March 1992);42(356):131.

62. Roscelli, JD., et al. "Guillain-Barré syndrome and influenza vaccination in the US Army, 1980-1988." *Am J Epidemiol* (May 1, 1991);133(9):952-5.

63. Molina, M., et al. "Leukocytoclastic vasculitis secondary to flu vaccination." *Med Clin (Barc).* (June 9, 1990):78. [Spanish.]

64. Pelosio, A., et al. "Influenza vaccination and poly-radiculoneuritis of the GBS type." *Medicina (Firenze)* (Apr-Jun 1990);10(2):169. [Italian.]

65. Buchner, H., et al. "Polyneuritis cranialis? Brain stem encephalitis and myelitis following preventive influenza vaccination." *Nervenarzt* (Nov 1988);59(11):679-82. [German.]

66. Gnanasekaran, SK., et al. "Influenza vaccination among children with asthma in Medicaid managed care." *Ambulatory Pediatrics* 2006;6:1-7.

67. Jefferson, T., et al. "Assessment of the efficacy and effectiveness of influenza vaccines in healthy children: systematic review." *Lancet* 2005;365(Feb. 26):773-80.

68. Napoli, M. "Doubts about safety of flu vaccine in kids." *Center for Med Consumers* (Oct 2005). medicalconsumers.org

69. See Note 8.

70. Paddock, C. "FluMist effective for kids under 5 but still under review says FDA." *Medical News Today* (May 15, 2007).

71. FDA. "FluMist® live, attenuated influenza vaccine briefing document: prior approval supplemental BLA, indication extension to include children less than 5 years of age." (Confidential document.) *FDA Vaccines and Related Biological Products Advisory Committee* (April 19, 2007).

72. Ibid.

73. Peck, P. "FDA okays nasal spray flu vaccine for younger kids." *Medpage Today* (Sep 20, 2007). www.medpagetoday.com

74. Dorsett, A. "Boy's illness a mystery." *Express news, San Antonio* (March 10, 2005). www.mysanantonio.com

75. Unsolicited flu vaccine queries and comments received by the *Thinktwice Global Vaccine Institute.* www.thinktwice.com

76. See Notes 2 and 3.

77. Digitized Editorial Research Reports by *Congressional Quarterly, Inc.,* 1986. (Wikipedia article on H3N2.)

78. See Notes 2 and 3.

79. CDC. "Deaths: final data for 2003." *U.S. Department of HHS, National Vital Statistics Reports* (Apr 19, 2006); 54(13).

80. Ibid.

81. CDC. "Deaths: final data for 2002." *U.S. Department of HHS, National Vital Statistics Reports* (Oct 12, 2004);53(5).

82. CDC. "Deaths: final data for 2001." *U.S. Department of HHS, National Vital Statistics Reports* (Sep 18, 2003);52(3).

83. Ibid.

84. Ibid.

85. McKeever, TM., et al. "Vaccination and allergic disease: a birth cohort study." *Amer J Pub Health* (Jun 2004);94(6):985-9.

86. Farooqi, IS., et al. "Early childhood infection and atopic disorder." *Thorax* 1998;53:927-932.

87. Nilsson, L., et al. "A randomized controlled trial of effect of pertussis vaccines on atopic disease." *Archives of Pediatric and Adolescent Medicine* (August 1998);152(8):734-8.

88. Kemp, T., et al. "Is infant immunization a risk factor for childhood asthma or allergy?" *Epidemiology* 1997;8:678-80.

89. Odent, MR., et al. "Pertussis vaccination and asthma: is there a link?" *JAMA* 1994;272:592-93.

90. Cortiel, P. "Fragebogen zu meinem ungeimpften kind." A German survey of parents taken Mar 2001 through Apr 2004.

91. CDC. "Deaths: final data for 1999." *U.S. Department of HHS, National Vital Statistics Reports* (Sep 21, 2001);49(8).

92. CDC. "Deaths: final data for 2000." *U.S. Department of HHS, National Vital Statistics Reports* (Sep 16, 2002);50(15).

93. See Notes 79, 81, and 82.

94. CDC. "Deaths: preliminary data for 2004." *U.S. Department of HHS, National Vital Statistics Reports* (Jun 28, 2006);54(19).

95. Thompson, WW., et al. "Mortality associated with influenza and RSV in the United States." *JAMA* 2003;289:179-186.

96. Merck & Co., Inc. "Pneumovax®23 (Pneumococcal vaccine polyvalent)." Product insert (March 2007).

97. See Notes 79 and 81.

98. American Association for Justice. "Chiron's contaminated vaccine production facility." www.atla.org (December 9, 2005).

99. Frankel, G., et al. "Britain: U.S. told of vaccine shortage." *Washington Post* (October 9, 2004):A1.

100. Roos, R. "Officials urge high-risk groups to get flu shots soon." *Center for Infectious Disease Research and Policy* (Sep 14, 2005). www.cidrap.umn.edu

101. Simonsen, L., et al. "Impact of influenza vaccination on seasonal mortality in the U.S. elderly population." *Archives of Internal Medicine* 2005;165:265-72.

102. See Notes 79 and 94.

103. Summary of the "2004 National Influenza Vaccine Summit Invitees" roster.

104. Nowak, G. "Planning for the 2004-2005 influenza vaccination season: a communication situation analysis." *U.S. Department of HHS.*

105. Ibid.

106. Doshi, P. "Are U.S. flu death figures more PR than science?" *BMJ* (December 10, 2005);331:1412.

107. See Note 5, p. 1.

108. Ibid.

109. Ibid.

110. See Note 26.

111. Brammer, TL. "Surveillance for Influenza—U.S.: 1994-95, 1995-96, and 1996-97 seasons." *MMWR: CDC* (April 28, 2000).

112. See Note 26.

113. See Note 111.

114. Norton, A. "Flu shots cut misery, but not costs." *Reuters.* www.dailynews.yahoo.com

115. CDC. "Update: influenza activity—United States and worldwide, 2003-04 season, and composition of the 2004-05 influenza vaccine." *MMWR* 2004;53:547-52.

116. CDC. "Preliminary assessment of the effectiveness of the 2003-04 inactivated influenza vaccine—Colorado, December 2003." *MMWR,* 2004;53:8-11.

117. Fisher, BL. "Informed consent advocate says government and industry should release flu vaccine effectiveness data." Press release. *Nat Vaccine Information Center* (Dec 10, 2003).

118. Fisher, BL. "Flu vaccine: missing the mark." *The Vaccine Reaction,* National Vaccine Information Center (Spring 2004).

119. See Note 5, pp. 3 and 7.

120. See Note 67.

121. Ibid.

122. Roos, R. "Efficacy of flu shots in children under 2 questioned." *Center for Infectious Disease Research and Policy* (Feb 25, 2005). www.cidrap.umn.edu

123. See Notes 67 and 122.

124. Smith, S., et al. "Vaccines for preventing influenza in healthy children." *The Cochrane Collaboration: Cochrane Database of Systematic Reviews* (John Wiley & Sons, Ltd.), 2006(1). Art. No. CD004879.

125. Alliance for Human Research Protection. "Oxford study—no evidence flu vaccine works in infants: USA and Canada's flu vaccination programmes for children based on little evidence," (Feb 25, 2005). www.ahrp.org

126. Szilagyi, PG., et al. "Influenza vaccine effectiveness among children 6 to 59 months of age during 2 influenza seasons." *Arch Pediatr Adol Med* 2008;162(10)943-51.

127. Rivetti, D., et al. "Vaccines for preventing influenza in healthy adults." *The Cochrane Collaboration: Cochrane Database of Systematic Reviews* (John Wiley & Sons, Ltd.), 2004(3). Art. No. CD001269.

128. Rivetti, D., et al. "Vaccines for preventing influenza in the elderly." *The Cochrane Collaboration: Cochrane Database of Systematic Reviews* (John Wiley & Sons, Ltd.), 2006(3). Art. No. CD004876.

129. Ibid.

130. Kuhle, CL., et al. "An influenza outbreak in an immunized nursing home population: inadequate host response or vaccine failure?" *Annals of Long-Term Care* 1998;6[3]:72.

131. Ibid.

132. Thomas, RE., et al. "Influenza vaccination for healthcare workers who work with the elderly." *Cochrane Collaboration: Cochrane Database of Systematic Reviews* (John Wiley & Sons), 2006(3). Art. No. CD005187.

133. Ibid.

134. See Note 101.

135. Manning, A. "Flu shot's effectiveness in elderly is questioned." *USA Today* (Feb 14, 2005). www.usatoday.htm

136. Geier, BA., et al. "Influenza vaccine: review of effectiveness of the U.S. immunization program, and policy considerations." *J Am Phys Surg* 2006;11(3):69-74.

137. Jefferson, T. "Influenza vaccination: policy versus evidence." *British Medical Journal* 2006; 333:912-915.

138. Ibid.

139. BBC News. "Winter flu jab's evidence queried." www.newsvote. bbc.co.uk (October 26, 2006).

140. Cates, CJ., et al. "Vaccines for preventing influenza in people with asthma." *The Cochrane Collaboration: Cochrane Database of Systematic Reviews* (John Wiley & Sons, Ltd.), 2007(2). Art. No. CD000364.

141. Bhalla, P., et al. "Vaccines for preventing influenza in people with cystic fibrosis." *The Cochrane Collaboration: Cochrane Database of Systematic Reviews* (John Wiley & Sons, Ltd.), 2007(2). Art. No. CD001753.

142. See Note 139.

143. See Note 137.

144. King, Jr., JC., et al. "Effectiveness of school-based influenza vaccination." *NEJM* 2006; 355:2523-32.

145. Bodewes, R., et al. "Yearly influenza vaccinations: a double-edged sword?" *The Lancet* (December 2009);9(12):784-88.

146. Bodewes R., et al. "Vaccination against human influenza A/H3N2 virus prevents the induction of heterosubtypic immunity against lethal infection with avian influenza A/H5N1 virus." *PLoS One* 2009;4(5):e5538.

147. Bridges, CB., et al. "Effectiveness and cost-benefit of influenza vaccination of healthy working adults." *J of the Amer Medical Association* (Oct 4, 2000);285:1655-1663.

148. Fox, M. "Study: giving flu vaccine doesn't save money." *Reuters*. www.dailynews.yahoo.com See also Note 114.

149. Advisory Committee on Immunization Practices. "Prevention and control of influenza: recommendations of the ACIP." *MMWR* 1996;45:1-24. See also Notes 2 and 3.

150. From an unsolicited email received by the *Thinktwice Global Vaccine Institute*. www.thinktwice.com

151. Ibid.

152. See Notes 128, 130, and 132.

153. CDC, ACIP. "Prevention and control of influenza, pt. I: recommendations of the ACIP." *MMWR* 1993;42 (RR-6):1-13.

154. Alling, DW., et al. "A study of excess mortality during influenza epidemics, US: 1968-1976." *Am J Epid* 1981;113:30-43.

155. Eickhoff, TC., et al. "Observations of excess mortality associated with epidemic influenza." *JAMA* 1961;176:776-782.

156. Woodman, R. "UK offers free flu vaccinations to elderly, but millions might not take advantage." *Reuters Medical News* (September 26, 2000).

157. CDC. www.cdc.gov/nip/Q&A/genqa/thimerosal.htm

158. See Note 117.

159. "Childhood influenza-vaccination coverage—United States, 2002-03 influenza season." *JAMA* 2004;292: 2074-75.

160. AAP News. "Flu vaccine extended to kids 6-23 months." *American Acad. of Pediatrics* (August 2002).

161. See Note 159.

162. Consumer Affairs. "Expanded flu shot recommendations for children." www.consumeraffairs.com (Feb 23, 2006.)

163. See Notes 2 and 3.

164. Ibid.

165. Vaccine Ethics. "Flu vaccine recommendation expanded through age 18." www.VaccineEthics.org (Feb 27, 2008)

166. See Note 91.

167. See Notes 81, 82 and 92.

168. See Note 160.

169. See Note 79.

170. Johns Hopkins. "Johns Hopkins flu expert calls for mandatory vaccination of healthcare workers; view is subject to debate." www.hopkinsnet.jhu.edu (November 2005).

171. Woolhandler, S., et al. "Influenza vaccination and health care workers in the U.S." *J General Internal Med* (Feb 6, 2006).

172. Recer, P. "Study: health workers major sources of flu in old-age homes." *Associated Press* (October 9, 1997).

173. See Note 170.

174. Ibid.

175. Medical News Today. "Mandatory flu shot not justified for healthcare workers" (Sep 13, 2006).

176. Flores, D. "Flu shots mandatory for all New Jersey preschoolers." *The Philadelphia Inquirer* (August 19, 2008).

177. Sena, J. "Santa Fe schools trying out new flu mist vaccine." *The New Mexican* (October 16, 2008).

178. Cannell, JJ., et al. "Epidemic influenza and vitamin D." *Epidemiology and Infection* (Dec 2006);134(6):1129-40.

179. Totheroh, G. "What's the real story on vitamin D? *CBN News Science and Medical Reporter* (November 17, 2007).

180. Schor, J. "Vitamin D and influenza." *Naturopathy Digest* (October 17, 2008). www.naturopathydigest.com

Tetanus

1. *The World Book Encyclopedia,* Volume 19 (1994):182.

2. Frick, L. "Tetanus." *Gale Encyclopedia of Alternative Medicine* (2001). www.find articles.com

3. Skudder, PA., et al. "Current status of tetanus control: importance of human tetanus-immune globulin." *Journal of the American Medical Association* 1964;188:625-627.

4. Mortimer, E. "Immunization against infectious disease." *Science* (May 26, 1978); Volume 200:905.

5. Moskowitz, R. "Immunizations: the other side." *Mothering Magazine* (Spring 1984):36.

6. Neustaedter, R. *The Vaccine Guide*. (Berkeley, California: North Atlantic Books, 1996):100.

7. Dunavan, CP. "Blindsided by tetanus." *Discover/The Gale Group and LookSmart* (January 2000). www.findarticles.com

8. CDC. Figures extracted from several *Morbidity and Mortality Weekly Reports (MMWR)*, including: "Notifiable diseases/deaths in selected cities weekly information: Table 1." *MMWR* (January 5, 2007);55(52). "Summary of notifiable diseases—United States, 2005." *MMWR* (March 30, 2007);54(53). "Summary of notifiable diseases—United States, 2004." *MMWR* (June 16, 2006);53(53). "Summary of notifiable diseases—United States, 2003, Table 8." *MMWR* (April 22, 2005);52(54). "Summary of notifiable diseases, United States, 1999." *MMWR* 1999 (April 6, 2001);48(53):84-90.

9. Mackay, I. "Tetanus." *Virology Down Under* 2001. www.uq.edu.au

10. National Advisory Committee on Immunization. *Canadian Immunization Guide* (Ottawa: Canada Communication Group Publishing, 1993):116.

11. CDC. "Tetanus: U.S., 1985-86. *MMWR* 1987;36:477-481.

12. CDC. "Tetanus: U.S., 1987-88. *MMWR* 1990;39:37-41.

13. Oxygen Media. "Drugs: tetanus antitoxin (systemic)." *ThriveOnline* 2001. www.thriveonline.oxygen.com

14. See Note 9.

15. CDC. Figures extracted from several *MMWR's*.

16. CDC. "Summary of notifiable diseases, United States, 1999." *MMWR* 1999 (April 6, 2001);48(53):84-90.

17. Currently available from Aventis Pasteur for children 7 years of age or older, and adults. For booster use only. (Not for primary immunization.) Contains thimerosal (25µg mercury per dose). Contact the manufacturer for more information.

18. Currently available from Aventis Pasteur for infants and young children. Sanofi Pasteur produces a booster vaccine for children 7 years of age or older, and adults.

19. Currently available from Aventis Pasteur (Tripedia and Daptacel) or GlaxoSmithKline (Infanrix) for infants and young children. GlaxoSmithKline also produces Boostrix for adolescents. Sanofi Pasteur produces Adacel for adolescents and adults. Contact the manufacturers for more information.

20. Currently available from Sanofi Pasteur (TriHIBit).

21. Currently available from GlaxoSmithKline (Pediarix).

22. McComb, JA., et al. "Passive-active immunization with tetanus immune globulin (human)." *NEJM* 1963;268:857-862.

23. Medline. "Tetanus immune globulin (systemic)." www.nlm.nih.gov (Accessed November 14, 2006.)

24. Aventis Pasteur, Inc. "Diphtheria and Tetanus Toxoids and Acellular Pertussis Vaccine Adsorbed—Tripedia." Product insert, December 2003.

25. RXList. "Diphtheria and Tetanus Toxoids and Acellular Pertussis Vaccine Adsorbed — Tripedia." Product description extracted from Aventis Pasteur, Inc., Data on File. www.rxlist .com/cgi/generic2/tripedia.htm (Updated June 6, 2006.)

26. Aventis Pasteur, Inc. "Tetanus Toxoid Adsorbed USP." Product insert as of April 1999.

27. RXList. "Tetanus Toxoid for Booster Use Only." Product description extracted from Aventis Pasteur, Inc., Data on File. www.rxlist.com (Updated June 6, 2006.)

28. Aventis Pasteur, Inc. "Tetanus and Diphtheria Toxoids Adsorbed for Adult Use—Decavac." Product insert from the vaccine manufacturer. Product information as of Dec 2005.

29. RXList. "Tetanus and Diphtheria Toxoids Adsorbed for Adult Use—Decavac." Product description from Aventis Pasteur, Inc., Data on File. www.rxlist.com (June 3, 2006.)

30. Physician's Desk Reference (PDR); 55th edition. (Montvale, NJ: Medical Economics, 2001):878.

31. Sisk, CW., et al. "Reactions to tetanus-diphtheria toxoid (adult)." *Archives of Environmental Health* 1965;11:34-36.

32. Jacobs, RL., et al. "Adverse reactions to tetanus toxoid." *Journal of the American Medical Association* 1982;247(1):40-42.

33. Myers, MG., et al. "Primary immunization with tetanus and diphtheria toxoids." *JAMA* 1982;248(19):2478-2480.

34. Deacon, SP., et al. "A comparative clinical study of adsorbed tetanus vaccine and adult-type tetanus-diphtheria vaccine." *Journal of Hygiene* (Cambridge: 1982);89:513-519.

35. White, WG., et al. "Reactions to tetanus toxoid." *J of Hygiene* 1983; 71:283-297.

36. Fawcett, HA., et al. "Injection-site granuloma due to aluminum." *Arch Dermatol* 1984;120:1318-1322.

37. Macko, MB., et al. "Comparison of the mortality of tetanus toxoid boosters with tetanus-diphtheria toxoid boosters." *Annals of Emerging Medicine* 1985;14(1):33-35.

38. Church, JA., et al. "Recurrent abscess formation following DTP immunizations: association with hypersensitivity to tetanus toxoid." *Pediatrics* 1985;75:899-900.

39. Unpublished data on file; Lederle Laboratories. As reported in Note 30, pp. 1683-1684.

40. Blumstein, GI., et al. "Peripheral neuropathy following tetanus toxoid administration." *JAMA* 1966;198:1030-1031.

41. Wilson, GS. "Allergic manifestations: post-vaccinal neuritis." *Hazards of Immunization* 1967:153-156.

42. Tsairis, P., et al. "Natural history of brachial plexus neuropathy." *Archives of Neurology* 1972;27:109-117.

43. Schlenska, GK. "Unusual neurological complications following tetanus toxoid." *J Neur* 1977;215:299-302.

44. Pollard, JD., et al. "Relapsing neuropathy due to tetanus toxoid." *Journal of Neurological Science* 1978; 37:113-125.

45. Quast, U., et al. "Mono- and polyneuritis after tetanus vaccination." *Devel Bio Stand* 1979;43:25-32.

46. Eibl, M., et al. "Abnormal T-lymphocyte subpopulations in healthy subjects after tetanus booster immunizations," *New England Journal of Medicine* (November 26, 1981):1307-1313.

47. Buttram, H., et al. "Bringing vaccines into perspective," *Mothering Magazine* (Winter 1985):30.

48. Reinstein, L., et al. "Peripheral neuropathy after multiple tetanus...injections." *Arch Phys Med Rehab* 1982;63:332-34.

49. Fenichel, GM. "Neurological complications of tetanus toxoid." *Archives of Neurology* 1983;40:390.

50. Holliday, PL., et al. "Polyradiculoneuritis secondary to immunization with tetanus and diphtheria toxoids." *Archives of Neurology* 1983;40:390.

51. Rutledge, SL., et al. "Neurologic complications of immunizations. *Journal of Pediatrics* 1986;109:917-924.
52. CDC. "Adverse events following immunization." *MMWR* 1985; 34(3):43-47.
53. CDC. "Recommendations of the immunization practices advisory committee (ACIP): diphtheria, tetanus and pertussis: guidelines for vaccine prophylaxis and other preventive measures." *MMWR* 1985;34:405-426.
54. CDC. "Update: vaccine side effects, adverse reactions, contraindications, and precautions." *MMWR* 1996;45:22-31.
55. Kroger, G., et al. "Tetanusimpfung: Vertraglichkeit und Vermeidung von Nebenreaktionen." [Tetanus vaccination: tolerance and avoidance of adverse reactions.] *Klininische Wochenschrift* 1986;64:767-775.
56. Newton, N., et al. "Guillain-Barré syndrome after vaccination with purified tetanus toxoid." *S Med J* 1987;80:1053-1054.
57. Schwartz, G., et al. "Acute midbrain syndrome as an adverse reaction to tetanus immunization." *Inten Care Med* 1988;15:53-4.
58. Jawad, AS., et al. "Immunisation triggering rheumatoid arthritis?" *Annals of Rheumatic Disease* 1989; 48:174.
59. Read, SJ., et al. "Acute transverse myelitis after tetanus toxoid vaccination." *Lancet* 1992;339:1111-1112.
60. Topaloglu, H., et al. "Optic neuritis and myelitis after booster tetanus toxoid vaccination." *Lancet* 1992; 339:178-179.
61. Institute of Medicine. *Adverse Events Associated with Childhood Vaccines: Evidence Bearing on Causality.* (Washington, DC: National Academy Press, 1994).
62. Ibid.
63. Regamey, RH. Die Tetanus-Schutzimpfung. [Tetanus immunization in *Handbook of Immunization.*] In: Herrlick, A., ed. *Handbuch Schutzimpfungen* (Berlin: Springer, 1965).
64. Staak, M., et al. Zur problematik anaphylaktischer Reaktionen nach aktiver Tetanus-Immunisierung. [Anaphylactic reaction following...tetanus immunization.] *Deutsche Medizinische Wochenschrift* 1973; 98:110-11.
65. See Note 61.
66. Kemp, T., et al. "Is infant immunization a risk factor for childhood asthma or allergy?" *Epidem* 1997;8(6):678-680.
67. Hurwitz, EL., et al. "Effects of diphtheria-tetanus-pertussis or tetanus vaccination on allergies and allergy-related respiratory symptoms among children and adolescents in the United States." *J of Manipulative and Physiological Therapeutics* 2000;23:1-10.
68. See Note 26.
69. Recommendations of the Immunization Practices Advisory Committee (ACIP). "Diphtheria, tetanus, and pertussis: recommendations for vaccine use and other preventive measures." *MMWR* 40: No. RR-10, 1991.
70. See Note 26.
71. See Notes 26 and 61.
72. See Notes 28 and 61.
73. See Notes 26 ad 51.
74. See Note 26, and Notes 40-42.
75. See Notes 24 and 61.
76. Ibid.
77. See Notes 24 and 28.
78. These personal stories are typical of the unsolicited emails received by the *Thinktwice Global Vaccine Institute.*
79. CDC. "Recommended immunization schedule for persons aged 0-6 Years—United States, 2011." *Department of HHS.* www.cdc.gov
80. Mendelsohn, R. *But Doctor, About That Shot...The Risks of Immunizations and How to Avoid Them.* (Evanston, IL: The People's Doctor Newsletter, Inc., 1988):4.
81. Berger, SA., et al. "Tetanus despite preexisting anti-tetanus antibody." *JAMA* 1978;240;769-770.
82. Passen, EL., et al. "Clinical tetanus despite a 'protective' level of toxin-neutralizing antibody." *Journal of the American Medical Association* 1986;255:1171-1172.
83. Vieira, BI., et al. "Cephalic tetanus in an immunized patient." *Medical Journal of Australia* 1986;145:156-157.
84. Mortimer, E. "Immunization against infectious disease." *Science* (May 26, 1978):905.
85. "Can modified tetanus occur?" *NEJM* 1962;266:1117-18.
86. Edsall, G. "Modified tetanus." *NEJM* 1962;276:520.
87. Katz, KC., et al. "Postoperative tetanus: a case report." *Canadian Medical Association Journal* 2000; 163(5):571-573.
88. See Note 30, p. 1683.
89. Burns, EA., et al. "Specific humoral immunity in the elderly: in vivo and in vitro response to vaccination." *Journal of Geriatric Ontology* 1993;48(6):B231-B-236.
90. Murphy, SM., et al. "Tetanus immunity in elderly people." *Age and Aging* 1995;24(2):99-102.
91. Kishimoto, S., et al. "Age-related decline in the in vitro and in vivo syntheses of anti-tetanus toxoid antibody in humans." *Journal of Immunology* 1980;125(5):2347-2352.
92. Meydani, SN., et al. "Vitamin E supplementation and in vivo immune response in healthy elderly subjects. A randomized controlled trial." *JAMA* 1997;277(17):1398-1399.
93. "Clinical profile...studies on four women immunized with Pr-hCG-TT," *Contraception* (Feb 1976):253-68.
94. "Observations on the antigenicity and clinical effects of a candidate antipregnancy vaccine: B-subunit of human chorionic gonadotropin linked to tetanus toxoid." *Fertility and Sterility* (October 1980):328-335.
95. "Phase I clinical trials of a World Health Organization birth control vaccine," *Lancet* (June 11, 1988):1295-98.
96. "Vaccines for fertility regulation," *Research in Human Reproduction, Biennial Report: 1986-87* (Geneva: Who Special Programme of Research, Development and Research Training in Human Reproduction, 1988); chapter 11, pp. 177-198.
97. "Anti-hCG vaccines are in clinical trials." *Scandinavian Journal of Immunology* 1992;36:123-126.
98. Anderson, K., et al. *Mosby's Medical, Nursing, and Allied Health Dictionary* (St. Louis, MO: Mosby-Year Book, Inc., 1994):326, 684.
99. See Notes 93-97.
100. Ibid.
101. Talwar, GP., et al. "Prospects of an anti-hCG vaccine inducing antibodies of high affinity..." *Reproductive Technology 1989* (Amsterdam; NY: Elsevier Science Publishers, 1990):231.
102. "Abortifacient vaccines loom as new threat." *HLI Reports* (Gaithersburg, MD: Human Life International, Nov 1993):1-2.
103. Miller, J. *HLI Reports* (Gaithersburg, MD: Human Life International, June/July 1995):13(8).
104. WHO. "Prevent 565,000 children from dying of neonatal tetanus every year." *Expanded Programme on Immunization* (Geneva, 1991):1.
105. "Case definitions: neonatal tetanus." *Epidemiological Bulletin* (Pan American Health Organization, March 2000);21(1).
106. See Note 7.
107. Wassilak, S., et al. "Tetanus toxoid," in *Vaccines,* ed. Plotkin, S., et al. (Philadelphia: W.B. Saunders, 1994):66.
108. CDC. "Neonatal tetanus—Montana, 1998." *MMWR* (November 6, 1998);47(43).
109. See Note 7.
110. WHO. "Vaccines, immunization and biologicals—Tetanus toxoid controversy, Philippines." *WHO Internat.* www.who.int
111. See Notes 103 and 110.
112. Ibid.
113. Ibid.
114. Manila regional trial court case: Borlongan, MB (March 19, 1995):11. As quoted in Note 110.
115. See Note 110.
116. See Notes 103 and 110.
117. In an interview with Sr. Pilar Verzosa. As quoted in Note 110.
118. See Note 110.
119. See Note 103.
120. Lancet (June 11, 1988):1296. As quoted in Note 103.
121. "Three DOH vaccines untested by BFAD." *The Philippine Star* (April 4, 1995):1, 12.
122. See Note 78.
123. See Note 23.
124. "Tetanus shots in short supply." *New Mexican* (June 22, 2001):B-4.

Diphtheria

1. *The World Book Encyclopedia,* Volume 5 (1994):215-216.
2. Ibid.
3. Elben. *Vaccination Condemned,* (Los Angeles: Better Life Research, 1981):57. Data taken from government statistics in NY and Massachusetts.
4. New York Health Bulletin (February 1924).
5. Dublin, L., et al. *Twenty-Five Years of Health Progress* (New York: Metropolitan Life Insurance Company, 1937):60.
6. Physician's Desk Reference (PDR); 55th edition. (Montvale, NJ: Medical Economics, 2001):787.
7. CDC. Data published in several *MMWRs.*
8. CDC. "Summary of notifiable diseases, 1992." *MMWR* 1993;41(55).
9. CDC. "Reported cases, deaths, vaccine preventable diseases, US, 1950-2005." *Pink Book* (Dec 13, 2006). www.cdc.gov
10. CDC. "Summary of notifiable diseases, 1999." *MMWR* (April 6, 2001);48(53):84-90.
11. CDC. "Notifiable diseases/deaths in selected cities weekly information." *MMWR Weekly* (Jan 5, 2001);49(51):1167-1174.
12. See Note 3, pp. 40-90.
13. Mackay, I. "Diphtheria: antitoxin." *Virology Down Under* 2001. www.uq.edu.au/vdu/diphth.htm
14. Mortimer, EA., et al. "Immunization against infectious disease." *Science* 1978;200:902.
15. See Note 6., pp. 785-787.
16. See Note 3, p. 58. Government statistics in England and Wales.
17. See Note 4.
18. See Notes 3 and 4.
19. See Note 3. Data taken from Biggs, JT: "Annual report: sanitation vs. vaccination."
20. Alderson, M. *International Mortality Statistics* (Washington, DC: Facts on File, 1981):61-162.
21. See Note 5, p. 56.
22. *Journal of the American Medical Association* (February 1, 1919: January 9, 1926; April 3, 1926; April 16, 1927).
23. Wilson, SG. *The Hazards of Immunization* (London: The Athlone Press, 1967):21-22.
24. *J of the American Medical Association* (Nov 1919).
25. See Note 3, pp. 71-77.
26. *Times Herald* (Nov 29, 1919).
27. *J of the American Medical Association* (April 8, 1922).
28. *J of the American Medical Association* (Nov 4, 1922).
29. *J of the American Medical Association* (April 15, 1924).
30. *British Medical Journal* (September 26, 1925).
31. See Note 3, p. 59. Date taken from a government Report of the Royal Commission of Inquiries.
32. *J of the American Medical Association* (March 16, 1929).
33. See Note 3, pp. 40-41. As reported in *The Golden Calf,* p. 127.
34. *Daily Telegraph* (March 28, 1934).
35. *British Medical Journal* (June 8, 1935).
36. *Lancet* (January 1938).
37. See Note 3, p. 67.
38. *The Vaccination Inquirer* (September 1947).
39. See Note 23, p. 38.
40. *Mercury Magazine* (April 11, 1950).
41. McCloskey, BP. "The relation of prophylactic inoculations to the onset of poliomyelitis." *Lancet* (April 18, 1950):659-63.
42. Geffen, DH. "The incidence of paralysis occurring in London children within four weeks after immunization." *Med Officer* 1950;83:137-40.
43. Martin, JK. "Local paralysis in children after injections." *Arch Dis Child* 1950:25:1-14.
44. Hill, AB., et al. "Inoculation and poliomyelitis. A statistical investigation in England and Wales in 1949." *BMJ* 1950;ii:1-6.
45. Bodian, D. "Viremia in experimental poliomyelitis. II. Viremia and the mechanism of the 'provoking' effect of injections

of trauma." *Amer J Hyg* 1954;60:358-70.
46. Medical Research Council Committee on Inoculation Procedures and Neurological Lesions. "Poliomyelitis and prophylactic inoculation." *Lancet* 1956;ii:1223-31.
47. Guyer, B., et al. "Injections and paralytic poliomyelitis in tropical Africa." *Bull WHO* 1980;58:285-91.
48. Wyatt, HV. "Provocation poliomyelitis: neglected clinical observations from 1914-1950." *Bulletin of Historical Medicine* 1981;55:543-57.
49. Sutter, RW., et al. "Attributable risk of DTP (diphtheria and tetanus toxoids and pertussis vaccine) injection in provoking paralytic poliomyelitis during a large outbreak in Oman." *J Infectious Diseases* 1992; 165:444-9.
50. Wyatt HV., et al. "Unnecessary injections and paralytic polio in India." *Trans R Soc Trop Med Hyg* 1992;86:546-49.
51. Editorial. "Provocation paralysis." *Lancet* 1992;340:1005.
52. Strebel, PM., et al. "Intramuscular injections within 30 days of immunization with oral poliovirus vaccine—a risk factor for vaccine-associated paralytic poliomyelitis." *NEJM* (February 23, 1995):500+.
53. Mendelsohn, R. *How to Raise a Healthy Child...In Spite of Your Doctor.* (Ballantine Books, 1984):245.
54. Ibid.
55. Bureau of Biologics. "Minutes of the 15th meeting of the panel of review of bacterial vaccines and toxoids with standards and potency." *FDA* (November 20-21, 1975).
56. See Notes 6 and 10.
57. Hardy, IR., et al. "Current situation and control strategies for resurgence of diphtheria in newly independent states of the former Soviet Union." *Lancet* 1996;347:1739-1744.
58. Prospero, E., et al. "Diphtheria: epidemiological update and review of prevention and control strategies." *European J Epidem* 1997;13:527-34.
59. Vellinga, A. "Response to diphtheria booster vaccination in healthy adults: vaccine trial." *BMJ* (Jan 22, 2000);320:217.
60. Associated Press and Reuters. "FDA recalls diphtheria vaccine found to be too weak." *CNN Interactive* (January 29, 1999). www.cnn.com
61. Ibid.

Pertussis (DTaP)

1. Coulter, HL. and Fisher, BL. *A Shot in the Dark: Why the P in DPT Vaccination May be Hazardous to Your Child's Health* (Garden City Park, NY: Avery Pub Group, 1991):4-6.
2. CDC. "Summary of notifiable diseases, United States, 2003." *MMWR* (April 22, 2005);52 (54):78; Table 12: Deaths from selected notifiable diseases—United States, 1996-2001.
3. Cave, S. *"What your Doctor May Not Tell You About Children's Vaccinations,* (New York: Warner Books, 2001):138.
4. Ibid., p. 139.
5. CDC. "Notice to readers recommended childhood immunization schedule—United States, 1997." *MMWR* (January 17, 1997);46(02).
6. Aventis Pasteur, Inc. "Diphtheria and tetanus toxoids and acellular pertussis vaccine adsorbed—Tripedia." Product insert.
7. Ibid.
8. GlaxoSmithKline. "Pediarix [Diphtheria and tetanus toxoids and acellular pertussis adsorbed, hepatitis B (recombinant) and inactivated poliovirus vaccine combined]." Product insert as of October 2008.
9. "Mercury in medicine: are we taking unnecessary risks?" *Government Reform Committee Hearing,* Washington, DC. (July 18, 2000.)
10. See Note 1, p. 11.
11. Ibid., pp. 13-14.
12. Ibid., pp. 32-34.
13. *Whooping Cough, the DPT Vaccine and Reducing Vaccine Reactions* (Vienna, VA., National Vaccine Information Center 1989):10-16.
14. *Immunization: Survey of Recent Research* (United States Department of Health and Human Services, April 1983):76.
15. "Nature and the rates of adverse reactions associated with DTP and DT immunizations in infants and children," *Pediatrics* (November 1981); Volume 68, No. 5.
16. See Note 6.
17. See Notes 6 and 8.
18. Aventis Pasteur, Inc. "Diphtheria and tetanus toxoids and acellular pertussis vaccine adsorbed—Daptacel." Product insert from the vaccine manufacturer. Product information, March 2003.
19. GlaxoSmithKline. "Infanrix—Diphtheria and tetanus toxoids and acellular pertussis vaccine adsorbed." Product insert from the vaccine manufacturer. Product info as of Aug 2003.
20. GlaxoSmithKline. "Boostrix (Tetanus toxoid, reduced diphtheria toxoid and acellular pertussis vaccine, adsorbed)." Product insert from the vaccine manufacturer. Product information as of March 2003.
21. Madsen, T. "Vaccination against whooping cough." *J of the American Medical Association* 1933; 101(3):187-88.
22. Byers, RK., et al. "Encephalopathies following prophylactic pertussis vaccine." *Pediatrics* 1948;1(4):437-57.
23. Anderson, IM., et al. "Encephalopathy after combined diphtheria-pertussis inoculation." *Lancet* (Mar 25, 1950):537-39.
24. Low, NL. "Electroencephalographic studies following pertussis immunizations." *Journal of Pediatrics* 1955;47:35-39.
25. Baird, HW., et al. "Infantile myoclonic seizures." *J of Pediatrics* 1957;50:332-39.
26. Berg, JM. "Neurological complications of pertussis immunization." *British Medical Journal* (July 5, 1958):24-27.
27. Kulenkampff, M., et al. "Neurological complications of pertussis inoculation." *Arch of Dis in Children* 1974;49:46-49.
28. Dick, G. "Convulsive disorders in young children." *Proceedings of the Royal Society of Med* 1974;67:371-72.
29. Ehrengut, W. "Convulsive reactions after pertussis immunization." *Deutsche Medizinische Wochenschrift* 1974;99:2273-79. [German.]
30. Stewart, GT. "Vaccination against whooping cough: efficacy vs. risks." *Lancet* (January 29, 1977):234-37.
31. Ibid.
32. Hennessen, W., et al. "Adverse reactions after pertussis vaccination. International Symposium on Immunization: Benefit vs. Risk Factors, Brussels." *Developments in Biological Standardization* 1979;43:95-100.
33. Miller, DL., et al. "Pertussis immunisation and serious neurological illness in children." *BMJ* 1981;282:1595-99.
34. Alderslade, R., et al. "The National Childhood Encephalopathy Study, whooping cough: reports from the Committee on Safety of Medicines and the Joint Committee on Vaccination and Immunisation." *London Department of Health and Social Security* 1981:79-154.
35. Cody, CL., et al. "Nature and rates of adverse reactions associated with DTP and DT immunization in infants and children." *Pediatrics* 1981:68:650-60.
36. Pollock, TM., et al. "A 7-year survey of disorders attributed to vaccination in NW Thames region." *Lancet* 1983;1:753-57.
37. Miller, D., et al. "Pertussis immunisation and serious acute neurological illnesses in children." *BMJ* 1993;307:1171-76.
38. Strom, J. "Further experience of reactions, especially of a cerebral nature in conjunction with triple vaccination." *BMJ* 1967;4:320-323.
39. Wilson, J. "Proceedings: Neurological complications of DPT inoculation in infancy." *Arch Dis Child* 1973 Oct; 48(10):829-830.
40. Cupic, V., et al. "Role of DTP vaccine in the convulsive syndromes in children." *Lijec Vjesn* (June 1978); 100(6):345-348. [Serbo-Croatian.]
41. Pokrovskaia, N. "Convulsive syndrome in DPT vaccination (a clinico-experimental study)." *Pediatriia* (May 1983);(5):37-39. [Russian.]
42. Prensky, AL., et al. "History of convulsions and use of pertussis vaccine." *J of Pediatrics* 1985 Aug;107(2):244-255.
43. Walker, AM. "Neurologic events following diphtheria-tetanus-pertussis immunization." *Pediatrics* (March 1988);81(3):345-349.
44. Baraff, LJ. "Infants and children with convulsions and hypotonic-hypo-responsive episodes following diphtheria-tetanus-pertussis immunization: follow-up evaluation." *Pediatrics* (June 1988);81(6):789-794.
45. Shields, WD. et al. "Relationship of pertussis immunization to the onset of neurologic disorders: a retrospective epidemiologic study." *J of Pediatrics* (November 1988);113(5):801-805.
46. Jacobson, V. "Relationship of pertussis immunization to the onset of epilepsy, febrile convulsions and central nervous system infections: a retrospective...study." *Tokai J Exp Clin Med* 1988;3 Suppl: 137-142.
47. Griffin, MR., et al. "Risk of seizures and encephalopathy after immunization with the diphtheria-tetanus-pertussis vaccine." *JAMA* (March 23-30, 1990);263(12):1641-1645.
48. Ehrengut, W. "Bias in evaluating CNS complications following pertussis immunization." *Acta Paediatr Jpn* (August 1991);33(4):421-427.
49. Blumberg, DA. "Severe reactions associated with diphtheria-tetanus-pertussis vaccine: detailed study of children with seizures, hypotonic-hypo-responsive episodes, high fevers, and persistent crying." *Pediatrics* (June 1993);91(6):1158-1165.
50. Cherry JD., et al. "Pertussis immunization and characteristics related to first seizures in infants and children." *Journal of Pediatrics* (June 1993);122(6):900-903.
51. Steinman, WL., et al. "Pertussis toxin is required for pertussis vaccine encephalopathy." *Proceeds of the National Acad of Sciences* 1982:8733-36.
52. Osvath, P., et al. "IgE levels of infants with complications after pertussis vaccination." *Allergologia et Immunopathologia* 1979;7:111-114.
53. See Note 36.
54. Werne, J., et al. "Fatal anaphylactic shock occurrence in identical twins following second injection of diphtheria toxoid and pertussis antigen." *JAMA* 1946;131(9):730-35.
55. Galazka, A., et al. "Complication and reactions after vaccination against pertussis." *Epidem Review* 1972;26:411-24.
56. Leung, A. "Anaphylaxis due to DPT vaccine." *Journal of the Royal Society of Medicine* 1985;78:175.
57. Ovens, H. "Anaphylaxis due to vaccination in the office." *Canadian Medical Association Journal* 1986; 134:369-70.
58. Jacob, J., et al. "Increased intracranial pressure after diphtheria, tetanus, and pertussis vaccine." *Am J Dis Child* (Feb 1979);133(2):217-18.
59. Mathur, R., et al. "Bulging fontanel following triple vaccine." *Indian Pediatr* (June 1981);18(6):417-418.
60. Iwasa, S., et al. "Swelling of the brain in mice caused by pertussis: quantitative determination and the responsibility of the vaccine." *Jpn J Med Sci Biol* 1985;38(2):53-65.
61. Shendurnikar, N. "Bulging fontanel following DPT" *Indian Pediatr* (November 1986);23(11):960.
62. Gross, TP., et al. "Bulging fontanelle after immunization with diphtheria-tetanus-pertussis vaccine and diphtheria-tetanus vaccine." *J Pediatr* (March 1989);114(3):423-425.
63. Facktor, M., et al. "Hypersensitivity to tetanus toxoid." *Journal of Allergy and Clinical Immunology* 1973;52:1-12.
64. Zupanska, B., et al. Autoimmune haemolytic anaemia in children." *British Journal of Haematology,* 1976;34:511-20.
65. Haneberg, B., et al. "Acute hemolytic anemia related to diphtheria-pertussis-tetanus vaccine." *Acta Paediatrica Scandinavica* 1978;67:345-50.
66. Odent, M., et al. "Pertussis vaccination and asthma: is there a link?" *JAMA* (August 24/31, 1994):592-93.
67. Kemp, T., et al. "Is infant immunization a risk factor for childhood asthma or allergy?" *Epidemiology* 1997;8:678-80.
68. Farooqi, IS., et al. "Early childhood infection and atopic disorder." *Thorax* 1998;53:927-932.
69. Hurwitz, EL., et al. "Effects of diphtheria-tetanus-pertussis or tetanus vaccination on allergies and allergy-related respiratory symptoms among children and adolescents in the United States." *J of Manipulative and Physiological Therapeutics* 2000;23:1-10.
70. McDonald, KL., et al. "Delay in diphtheria, pertussis, tetanus vaccination is associated with a reduced risk of childhood

asthma." *J Allergy Clin Immunology* 2008;121(3):626-31.

71. Bernsen, R., et al. "Reported pertussis infection and risk of atopy in 8- to 12-yr-old vaccinated and non-vaccinated children." *Pediatric Allergy and Immunology* 2008;19(1):46-52.

72. Coulter, HL. *Vaccination, Social Violence, and Criminality: The Medical Assault on the American Brain,* (Berkeley, CA: North Atlantic Books, 1990):50.

73. Kalokerinos, A. *Every Second Child Was Doomed to Death—Unless One Dedicated Doctor Could Open His Colleagues' Eyes and Minds* (New Canaan, CT: Keats Publishing, Inc., 1974).

74. Noble, GR., et al. "Acellular and whole-cell pertussis vaccines in Japan: report of a visit by U.S. scientists." *JAMA* 1987;257:1351-56.

75. Cherry, JD., et al. "Report of the task force on pertussis and pertussis immunization." *Pediatr* (Jun 1988);81(6):933-84.

76. Scott, J. "Report: U.S. slips in fight to cut infant mortality." *Press & Sun Bulletin* (extracted from the *Los Angeles Times,* March 1, 1990).

77. Bernier, RH., et al. "Diphtheria-tetanus toxoids-pertussis vaccination and sudden infant deaths in Tennessee." *Journal of Pediatrics* 1982;101(5):419-21.

78. Hutcheson, R. "DTP immunization and sudden infant death— Tennessee." *MMWR* 1979;28:131-35.

79. Baraff, L., et al. "Possible temporal association between diphtheria-tetanus toxoid-pertussis vaccination in sudden infant death syndrome." *J of Pediatric Infectious Diseases* 1983;2:7.

80. Roberts, SC. "Vaccination and cot deaths in perspective." *Archives of Disease in Childhood* 1987;62:754-59.

81. Walker, AM., et al. "Diphtheria-tetanus-pertussis immunization and sudden infant death syndrome." *Am J Public Health* (August 1987); 77(8):945-51.

82. Fine, PE and Chen, RT. "Confounding in studies of adverse reactions to vaccines." *American Journal of Epidemiology* 1992;136(2):121-35.

83. Scheibner, V. *Vaccination: 100 Years of Orthodox Research Shows that Vaccines Represent a Medical Assault on the Immune System.* (Blackheath, NSW, Australia: Scheibner Publications, 1993):59-70;225-235.

84. Karlsson, LG and Scheibnerova. "Evidence of the association between non-specific stress syndrome, DPT injections and cot death." Pre-print of a study…2nd National Immunisation Conference in Canberra (May 1991).

85. Scheibner, V. "'Evidence of the association between non-specific stress syndrome, DPT injections and cot death." Proceedings of the 2nd National Immunisation Conference in Canberra (May 27-29, 1991).

86. Scheibnerova, V. *Cot Death as Due to Exposure to Non-Specific Stress and General Adaption Syndrome: Its Mechanisms and Prevention* (NSW, Australia: Association for Prevention of Cot Death, October 1990).

87. See Note 83, p. 262, and Notes 84-86.

88. Torch, WC. "DPT immunization: A potential cause of the sudden infant death syndrome (SIDS)." Amer Acad of Neur, 34th Annual Meet, Apr 25-May 1, 1982. *Neur* 32(4):pt. 2.

89. Ibid.

90. "Vaccine Injury Compensation." *Hearing Before the Committee on Labor and Human Resources;* 98th Congress, 2nd Session (May 3, 1984).

91. These stories were emailed to the *Thinktwice Global Vaccine Institute.* www.thinktwice.com

92. Leviton, R. "Shot in the Dark," *Yoga J* (May/June, 1992):112-14.

93. Bannister, R. *Brain's Clinical Neurology,* 5th Ed. (Oxford: University Press, 1978):409.

94. See Note 72, pp. xiii-xiv; Chapters 1-5.

95. See Note 72, p. xiv.

96. Ibid., p. 103.

97. Merritt, HH. *Textbook of Neurology,* 6th Ed. (Philadelphia, PA:Lea and Febiger, 1979):104.

98. Neal, JB. *Encephalitis: A Clinical Study,* (New York: Grune and Stratton, 1942):378-379.

99. See Note 97, pp. 102-103.

100. Ford, F.R. *Diseases of the Nervous System in Infancy, Childhood, and Adolescence,* (Springfield: C.C. Thomas, 1937):349.

101. Lurie, et al. "Late results noted in children presenting post-encephalitic behavior," *Amer J of Psychiatry* 1947;104:178.

102. Baker, AB. "The central nervous system in infectious diseases of childhood." *Postgraduate Medicine* 1949;5:11.

103. Annell, AL. "Pertussis in infancy—a cause of behavioral disorders in children," *Acta Societatis Medicorum Upsaliensis,* XVIII, Supplement 1, (1953):17,33.

104. See Notes 97 and 98.

105. See Note 72, pp. 120-121.

106. Ross, DM., et al. *Hyperactivity: Research, Theory, and Action,* (New York: John Wiley, 1982).

107. Cowart, VS. "Attention-deficit hyperactivity disorder: physicians helping parents pay more heed," *Journal of American Medical Association* (May 13, 1988);259(18):2647.

108. Long, K., et al. "Detection and treatment of emotionally disturbed children in public schools: problems and theoretical perspectives," *J of Clinical Psychology* (January 1984);40(1):378.

109. See Note 107.

110. Healy, JM. *Endangered Minds: Why Our Children Don't Think* (New York: Simon & Schuster, Inc., 1990):13-15.

111. Ibid.

112. Ibid., pp. 17-18.

113. Ibid., pp. 27-35.

114. See Note 72, pp. 61-62.

115. Ibid., p. 112.

116. "Vaccine fund needs booster shot." *Common Cause Magazine* (May/June, 1991):10.

117. "Congress votes help to youngster hurt by vaccine," *Tucson Citizen* (May 9, 1990):1-2A.

118. See Note 72, p. 113.

119. Ibid., p. 112.

120. See Note 72, pp. 179-181.

121. Bond, ED., et al. *The Treatment of Behavior Disorders Following Encephalitis,* (NY: The Commonwealth Fund, 1931): 14-15.

122. Elliott, FA. "Biological roots of violence," *Proceedings of the American Philosophical Society,* (1983);127(2): 84-93.

123. See Note 72, pp. 171-241. See also: *The New York Times* (December 5, 1987): B1.

124. Rimland, B., et al. "The manpower quality decline: an ecological perspective," *Armed Forces and Society,* (Fall 1981);8(1):56.

125. See Note 72, pp. 186-187.

126. This unsolicited personal story was received via email by the *Thinktwice Global Vaccine Institute.* www.thinktwice.com

127. Ibid.

128. Lewis, D. *Vulnerabilities to Delinquency* (NY: SP Medical and Scientific Books, 1981):28.

129. Hollander, HE., et al. "Characteristics of incarcerated delinquents: relationship between development disorders, environmental and family factors, and patterns of offense and recidivism," *J of American Child Psychiatry* 1985;24(1):225.

130. See Note 107.

131. Moyer, KE. *The Psychobiology of Aggression* (New York: Harper and Row, 1976):36.

132. "Plan for a Nationwide Action on Epilepsy." *Commission for Control of Epilepsy* 1977. (Unpublished material cited in Note 69, pp. 197-198.)

133. *The New York Times* (September 17, 1985):C1+.

134. See Note 110, p. 140.

135. Lidsky, TI., et al. "Are movement disorders the most serious side effects of maintenance therapy with antipsychotic drugs?" *Biological Psychiatry* 1981;16(12):1189-1194.

136. Cowart, VS. "The ritalin controversy: what's made this drug's opponents hyperactive?" *Journal of the American Medical Association* (May 6, 1988);259(17):2522.

137. Workman-Daniels, et al. "Childhood Problem Behavior and Neuropsychological Functioning in Persons at Risk for Alcoholism," *J of Studies on Alcoholism* 1987;48(3):187-193.

138. Sarason, IG., et al. *Abnormal Psychology,* Sixth Edition, (Englewood Cliffs, NJ: Prentice Hall, 1989):433.

139. See Note 91.

140. See Note 1, pp. 208-210.

141. See Note 75.

142. See Note 83, pp. 46-47.

143. Cherry, J.D. "The future use of acellular pertussis vaccines in the U.S." *Vaccine Bulletin* (January 1987):2.

144. See note 74.

145. Tompson, M. As quoted in: *But Doctor, About That Shot…The Risks of Immunizations and How to Avoid Them,* by Mendelsohn, RS. (Evanston, IL: The People's Doctor Newsletter, Inc., 1988):96.

146. Storsaeter, J., et al. "Mortality and morbidity from invasive bacterial infections during a clinical trial of acellular pertussis vaccines in Sweden." *Pediatric Infectious Disease Journal* 1988;7:637-45.

147. Blennow, M., et al. "Adverse reactions and serologic response to a booster dose of acellular pertussis vaccine in children immunized with acellular or whole-cell vaccine as infants." *Pediatrics* 1989;84:62-67.

148. *AAP News Release* (April 15, 1992).

149. Fisher, BL. *The Consumer's Guide to Childhood Vaccines.* (Vienna, VA: National Vaccine Information Center, 1997):37.

150. See Notes 6, 8, 18, 19 and 20.

151. See Note 91.

152. Moskowitz, R. "Immunizations: The Other Side." *Mothering* (Spring 1984):36.

153. Alderson, M. *International Mortality Statistics* (Washington, DC: Facts on File, 1981):164-65.

154. Halperin, et al. "Persistence of pertussis in an immunized population: results of the Nova Scotia enhanced pertussis surveillance program," *Journal of Pediatrics* (Nov. 1989):686-693.

155. See Note 75.

156. Pichichero, ME., et al. "Diphtheria-Pertussis-Tetanus vaccine: reactogenicity of commercial products," *Pediatrics* (Feb. 1979):256-260.

157. Lambert, H. "Epidemiology of a small pertussis outbreak in Kent County, Michigan." *Pub Health Report* 1965;80:365-69.

158. "Placebo-controlled trial of two acellular pertussis vaccines in Sweden—protective efficacy and adverse events." *Lancet* 1988;I:955-60.

159. "License application for pertussis vaccine withdrawn in Sweden." *Lancet* 1989; I:114.

160. Ibid.

161. Liese, JG., et al. "Efficacy of a two-component acellular pertussis vaccine in infants." *Journal of Pediatric Infectious Disease* 1997;16:1038-44.

162. Vickers, D., et al. "Whole-cell and acellular pertussis vaccination programs and rates of pertussis among infants and young children." *Canadian Med Assoc J* 2006;175(10):1213-17.

163. Edelman, K., et al. "Immunity to pertussis 5 years after booster immunization during adolescence." *Clinical Infectious Diseases* (May 15, 2007);44:1271-77.

164. U.S. Department of Health and Human Services. *20th Immunization Conference Proceedings, Dallas, Texas, May 6-9 1985* (October 1985):83-84.

165. CDC. "Current trends pertussis surveillance—United States, 1986-1988. *MMWR* (Feb 2, 1990);39(4);57-58,63-66.

166. *Vaccine Bulletin* (February 1987):11.

167. Christie, DC., et al. "The 1993 epidemic of pertussis in Cincinnati: resurgence of disease in a highly immunized population of children," *NEJM* (July 7, 1994):16-20.

168. Ewanowich, CA., et al. "Major outbreak of pertussis in Northern Alberta, Canada." *Journal of Clinical Microbiology* (July 1993):1715-25.

169. CDC. "Pertussis outbreak—Vermont, 1996." *MMWR* (September 5, 1997);46(35): 822-26.

170. Ibid.

171. DeMelker, HE., et al. "Reemergence of pertussis in the highly vaccinated population of the Netherlands: observations

on surveillance data." *Emerging Infectious Diseases* (July/August 2000);6(4):348-57.
172. Ibid.
173. Theodoridou, M., et al. "Pertussis outbreak detected by active surveillance in Cyprus in 2003." *Euro Surveillance* (May 2007);12(5).
174. Ibid.
175. Moerman, L., et al. "The re-emergence of pertussis in Israel." Israel Vaccine Research Initiative. *Israel Med Assoc J* (May 2006);8:308-311.
176. Ibid.
177. Ibid.
178. CDC. "Recommended immunization schedule for persons aged 0-6 years—United States, 2011."
179. National Institutes of Health. "Diphtheria immunization." *Medline Plus Med Encyclopedia.* www.mlm.nih.gov
180. See Note 6.
181. Cherry, JD. "Immunity to pertussis." *Clinical Infectious Diseases* (May 15, 2007);44:1278.
182. Sanofi Pasteur Limited. "Tetanus toxoid, reduced diphtheria toxoid and acellular pertussis vaccine adsorbed—Adacel." Product insert from the vaccine manufacturer. Product information as of January 2006.

Measles

1. Fisher, BL. *The Consumer's Guide to Childhood Vaccines.* (Vienna, VA: National Vaccine Information Center, 1997):18.
2. Moskowitz, R. "Immunizations: the other side." *Mothering* (Spring 1984):34.
3. *The World Book Encyclopedia,* Volume 13 (1994):345.
4. Krishnamurthy, KA., et al. "Measles a dangerous disease: a study of 1000 cases in Madurai." *Indian Pediatr* 1974:267-71.
5. See Note 1.
6. Ibid., pp. 17 and 18.
7. CDC. U.S. "Measles, mumps, and rubella: what you need to know," *Dept of Health and Human Serv* (Oct 15, 1991):1.
8. Mendelsohn, R. *How to Raise a Healthy Child...In Spite of Your Doctor.* (Ballantine Books, 1987):236-37.
9. Neustaedter, R. *The Vaccine Guide.* (North Atlantic Books, 1996):142.
10. *Clinical Infectious Diseases* (September 1994):493.
11. Oomen, APC. "Clinical experience of hypovitamine A." *Fed Proc* 1958;17:111-124.
12. Wilson, D., et al. "Infection and nutritional status. III. The effect of measles on nitrogen metabolism in children." *American Journal of Clinical Nutrition* 1961;9:154-58.
13. Sommer, A., et al. "Increased risk of respiratory disease and diarrhea in children with pre-existing mild vitamin A deficiency." *American Journal of Clinical Nutrition* 1984;40:1090-95.
14. Sommer, A., et al. "Impact of vitamin A supplementation on childhood mortality: a randomized clinical trial." *Lancet* 1986;1:1169-73.
15. Barclay, AJG., et al. "Vitamin A supplements and mortality related to measles: a randomised clinical trial." *BMJ* (January 31, 1987):294-96.
16. Keusch, GT. "Vitamin A supplements—too good to be true." *New England Journal of Medicine* (October 4, 1990):986.
17. Frieden, TR., et al. "Vitamin A levels and severity of measles: New York City." *Am J Dis Child* 1992; 146:182-86.
18. Ibid.
19. *Pediatric Nursing* (September/October 1996).
20. See Notes 3 and 4.
21. Morley, D. "Severe measles: some unanswered questions." *Reviews of Infectious Diseases* (May/June 1983):460-62.
22. Scheibner, V. *Vaccination: 100 Years of Orthodox Research Shows that Vaccines Represent a Medical Assault on the Immune System.* (Blackheath, NSW, Australia: Scheibner Publications, 1993):92.
23. Witsenburg, BC. "Measles mortality and therapy," pp. 26-27. From an abstract of a 1967-1968 measles epidemic study conducted in Ghana.
24. Ibid.
25. Ahmady, AS., et al. "The adverse effects of antipyretics in measles." *Indian Pediatrics* (January 1981):49-52.
26. Buttram, Harold. In a foreword to *Vaccines: Are They Really Safe and Effective?* by Neil Z. Miller. (Santa Fe, New Mexico: New Atlantean Press, 2008):10.
27. See Note 25, p. 52.
28. Ibid.
29. See Note 8, pp. 80-81.
30. Schulz, G. "Verhütet Fieber Karzinome?" *Münchn Med Wschr* 1969;18:1051-52.
31. Abel, U. "Die Antineoplastische Wirkung Pyrogener Bakterientoxine." *Disser Tumorzentrum Heidelberg* 1986:1-16.
32. See Note 22, p. 90.
33. Chase, A. *Magic Shots: A Human and Scientific Account of the Long and Continuing Struggle to Eradicate Infectious Diseases by Vaccination.* (NY: William Morrow & Co., 1982):311.
34. Ibid.
35. Ibid., p. 312.
36. See Note 3, p. 346.
37. Markowitz, L. and Katz, S. "Measles Vaccine," *Vaccines,* edited by Plotkin, SA. and Mortimer, EA. (Philadelphia: W.B. Saunders, 1994):232.
38. See Note 3, p. 346.
39. Diodati, C. *Immunization: History, Ethics, Law and Health.* (Windsor, Ontario, Canada: Integral Aspects Inc., 1999):11.
40. Physician's Desk Reference (PDR); 55th edition. (Montvale, NJ: Medical Economics, 2001):1884.
41. Ibid.
42. Schneck, S.A. "Vaccination with measles and central nervous system disease." *Neurology* 1968;18 (part 2):79-82.
43. Institute of Medicine. *Adverse Events Associated with Childhood Vaccines: Evidence Bearing on Causality.* (Washington, DC: National Academy Press, 1994).
44. Jabbour, JT., et al. "Epidemiology of subacute sclerosing panencephalitis (SSPE)." *JAMA* 1972;220:959-62.

45. Belgamwar, RB., et al. "Measles, mumps, rubella vaccine induced subacute sclerosing panencephalitis." *Journal of the Indian Medical Association* 1997;95(11):594.
46. National Institutes of Health. "The search for health: eliminating measles." *U.S. Department of Health and Human Services* (April 1983).
47. Landrigan, PJ., et al. "Neurological disorders following live measles-virus vaccination." *JAMA* 1973;223(13):1459-62.
48. Miller, CL. *Lancet* (September 17, 1983).
49. Beale, AJ. "Measles vaccines." *Proceedings of the Royal Society of Medicine* 1974;67:1116-1119.
50. Roden, AT. "Fits following immunization." *Proceedings of the Royal Society of Medicine* 1974; 67:24.
51. Jagdis, F., et al. "Encephalitis after administration of live measles vaccine." *Journal of the Canadian Medical Association* (April 19, 1975);112(8):972-75.
52. Hirayama, M. "Measles vaccines used in Japan." *Reviews of Infectious Diseases* 1983;5:495-503.
53. Pollock, TM., et al. "A 7-year survey of disorders attributed to vaccination in NW Thames Region." *Lancet* 1983;1:753-57.
54. Jorch, G. et al. "Coincidence of virus encephalitis and measles-mumps vaccination." *Monatsschr Kinderheilkd* 1984; 132(5):299-300.
55. Martinon-Torres, F., et al. "Self-limited acute encephalopathy related to measles component of viral triple vaccine." *Rev Neurol* (May 1-15, 1999);28(9):881-82.
56. Grose, C., et al. "Guillain-Barré syndrome following administration of live measles vaccine." *American Journal of Medicine* 1976;60:441-43.
57. Norrby, R. "Polyradiculitis in connection with vaccination against morbilli, parotitis and rubella." *Lakartidningen* 1984;81:1636-37.
58. Morris, K., et al. "Guillain-Barré syndrome after measles, mumps, and rubella vaccine." *Lancet* 1994; 343:60.
59. See Note 43.
60. Vaccine Adverse Event Reporting System VAERS. Rockville, MD.
61. Oski, FA., et al. "Effect of live measles vaccine on the platelet count." *New England J of Medicine* 1966;265:352-56.
62. Böttiger, M., et al. "Swedish experience of two dose vaccination programme aiming at eliminating measles, mumps, and rubella." *British Medical Journal* 1987;295:1264-67.
63. Koch, J. et al. "Adverse events temporally associated with immunizing agents—1987 report." *Canada Diseases Weekly Report* 1989;15:151-58.
64. Fescharek, R., et al. "Measles-mumps vaccination in the FRG: an empirical analysis after 14 years of use. II. Tolerability and analysis of spontaneously reported side effects." *Vaccine* 1990;8:446-56.
65. Nieminen, U., et al. "Acute thrombocytopenic purpura following measles, mumps and rubella vaccination: A report on 23 patients." *Acta Paediatrica* 1993;82:267-70.
66. Farrington, P., et al. "A new method for active surveillance of adverse events from diphtheria/tetanus/pertussis and measles/mumps/rubella vaccines." *Lancet* 1995;345: 567-69.
67. Jonville-Bera, AP., et al. "Thrombocytopenic purpura after measles, mumps, and rubella vaccination: a retrospective survey by the French Regional Pharmacovigilance Centres and Pasteur-Merieux Serums et Vaccins." *Pediatr Infect Dis J* 1996;15:44-48.
68. See Note 43.
69. Beeler, J. et al. "Thrombocytopenia after immunization with measles vaccines: review of the Vaccine Adverse Events Reporting System 1990-94." *Pediatr Infect Dis J* 1996;15:88-90.
70. CDC. "Update: Vaccine Side Effects, Adverse Reactions, Contraindications, and Precautions. Recommendations of the Advisory Committee on Immunization Practices (ACIP)." *MMWR* (September 6, 1996); 45(RR-12):1-35.
71. See Note 60.
72. Kazarian, EL., et al. "Optic neuritis complicating measles, mumps, and rubella vaccination." *Amer J of Ophthalmology* 1978;86:544-47.
73. Marshall, GS., et al. "Diffuse retinopathy following measles, mumps, and rubella vaccination." *Pediatrics* 1985;76:989-991.
74. Brodsky, L., et al. "Sensorineural hearing loss following live measles virus vaccination." *International Journal of Pediatric Otorhinolaryngology* 1985;10:159-63.
75. Nabe-Nielsen, J., et al. "Unilateral deafness as a complication of the mumps, measles, and rubella vaccination." *BMJ* 1988;297:489.
76. Hulbert, TV., et al. "Bilateral hearing loss after measles and rubella vaccination in an adult." *NEJM* 1991;325:134.
77. Stewart, BJA., et al. "Reports of sensorineural deafness after measles, mumps, and rubella immunisation." *Arch Dis Childhood* 1993;69:153-54.
78. Hirsch, RL., et al. "Measles virus vaccination of measles seropositive individuals suppresses lymphocyte proliferation and chemotactic factor production." *Clinical Immunology and Immunopathology* 1981;21:341-50.
79. Nicholson, JKA., et al. "The effect of measles-rubella vaccination on lymphocyte populations and subpopulations in HIV-infected and healthy individuals." *J of Acquired Immune Deficiency Syndromes* 1992;5:528-537.
80. Moskowitz, R. "The case against immunizations." *Journal of the American Institute of Homeopathy* 1983;76:7-25.
81. Moskowitz, R. "Immunizations: a dissenting view." *Dissent in Medicine—Nine Doctors Speak Out* (Contemporary Books, 1985):133-66.
82. See Note 2, pp. 33-34.
83. Thompson, NP., Wakefield, AJ, et al. "Is measles vaccination a risk factor for inflammatory bowel disease?" *Lancet* 1995;345:1071-1074.
84. Barton, JR., et al. "Incidence of inflammatory bowel disease in Scottish children between 1968 and 1983: marginal fall in ulcerative colitis; three-fold rise in Crohn's disease." *Gut* 1989;30:618-622.
85. Whelan, G. "Epidemiology of inflammatory bowel disease." *Med Clin N Am* 1990;74:1-12.

86. Ekbom, A., et al. "The role of perinatal measles infection in the aetiology of Crohn's disease: a population-based epidemiological study." *Lancet* 1994;334:508-510.
87. Miyamoto, M., et al. "Detection of immunoreactive antigen with monoclonal antibody to measles virus in tissue from patients with Crohn's disease." *J of Gastroenterology* 1995;30:28-33.
88. Scheibner, V. *Behavioural Problems in Childhood: The Link to Vaccination.* (Victoria, Australia: Scheibner Publications, 2000):170.
89. Wakefield, AJ., et al. "Evidence of persistent measles virus infection in Crohn's disease." *Journal of Medical Virology* 1993;39:345-53.
90. Wakefield, AJ., et al. "Crohn's disease: pathogenesis and persistent measles virus infection." *Gastroenterology* 1995;108:911-916.
91. Lewin, J., et al. "Confirmation of persistent measles virus infection of intestinal tissue by immunogold electron microscopy." *Gut* 1995;36:564-69.
92. See Note 85.
93. Sandler, RS. *Epidemiology of Inflammatory Bowel Disease.* Targan, S.R and Shanahan, F., eds. (Baltimore, MD: Williams and Wilkins, 1994):10.
94. See Note 83, p. 1073.
95. Wakefield, AJ., et al. "Ileal-lymphoid-nodular hyperplasia, non-specific colitis, and pervasive developmental disorder in children." *Lancet* 1998; 351:637-641.
96. Kahn, J. "Measles vaccine may be linked to bowel disease." *Medical Tribune* (May 18, 1995):2.
97. See Note 40, p. 1883.
98. See Note 1, p. 68.
99. See Note 53.
100. Aukrust, L., et al. "Severe hypersensitivity or intolerance reactions to measles vaccine in six children: clinical and immunological studies." *Allergy* 1980;35(7):581-87.
101. McEwen, J. "Early-onset reaction after measles vaccination: further Australian reports." *Medical Journal of Australia* 1983;2:503-505.
102. Koch, J., et al. "Adverse events temporally associated with immunizing agents—1987 report." *Canada Diseases Weekly Report* 1989;15:151-58.
103. See Notes 43 and 60.
104. Kelso, JM., et al. "Anaphylaxis to measles, mumps, and rubella vaccine mediated by IgE to gelatin." *J Allergy Clin Immunol* 1993;91:867-72.
105. Sakaguchi, M., et al. "IgE antibody to gelatin in children with immediate-type reactions to measles and mumps vaccines." *J Allergy Clin Immunol* 1995;96:563-65.
106. Cherry, JD. "The 'new' epidemiology of measles and rubella." *Hospital Practice* (July 1980):53-54.
107. Fulginiti, VA., et al. "Altered reactivity to measles virus: atypical measles in children previously immunized with inactivated measles virus vaccines." *JAMA* 1967;202:1075.
108. Martin, DB., et al. "Atypical measles in adolescents and young adults." *Annals of Internal Medicine* 1979;90:877.
109. See Note 106, p. 54.
110. Gold, E. "Current progress in measles eradication in the U.S." *Infect Med* 1997;14(4):297-300,310.
111. See Note 106, p. 54.
112. See Note 110.
113. Nichols, EM. "Atypical measles: a continuing problem." *American Journal of Public Health* 1979; 69(2):160-62.
114. Airola, P. "Immunization: A New Look." *Everywoman's Book* (Phoenix, AZ: Health Plus, 1979):279.
115. See Note 106, p. 53.
116. Scott, TF., et al. "Reactions to live-measles-virus vaccine in children previously inoculated with killed-virus vaccine." *New England J. of Medicine* 1967;277(5):248-251.
117. See Note 1.
118. Cherry, JD., et al. "Atypical measles in children previously immunized with attenuated measles virus vaccines." *Pediatrics* 1972;50(5).
119. St. Geme, JW., et al. "Exaggerated natural measles following attenuated virus immunization." *Pediatrics* 1976;57: 148-150.
120. "Atypical measles syndrome." *Lancet* 1979:962-963.
121. Hearings Before the Subcommittee on Health and the Environment: Vaccine Injury Compensation. 98th Congress, 2nd Session (Dec 19, 1984):110.
122. See Note 3, pp. 345-346.
123. CDC. "Summary of notifiable diseases, United States, 1993." *MMWR* 1994;42: No. 53.
124. See Note 8, p. 237.
125. Ibid.
126. Alderson, M. *International Mortality Statistics* (Washington, DC: Facts on File, 1981):182-183.
127. See Note 106, p. 50.
128. CDC. "Measles vaccination levels among selected groups of preschool-aged children—USA." *MMWR* 1991;40:36-39.
129. Schlenker, TL., et al. "Measles herd immunity: the association of attack rats with immunization rates in preschool children." *JAMA* 1992;267(6):826.
130. WHO Copenhagen. "Expanded programme on immunization—report of the meeting of national programme managers," 1989.
131. See Note 110.
132. Ibid.
133. Frank, JA., et al. "Measles elimination—final impediments." In an abstract of the *20th Immunization Conference Proceedings* 1985:22.
134. Sencer, D.J., et al. "Epidemiological basis for eradication of measles in 1967." *Public Health Report* 1967;82:253-61.
135. Hinman, AR. "The opportunity and obligation to eliminate measles from the United States." *Journal of the American Medical Association* 1979;242(11):1157-62.
136. Albonico, H., Klein, P., et al. "The immunization campaign against measles, mumps and rubella—coercion leading to a realm of uncertainty: medical objections to a continued MMR immunization campaign in Switzerland." *JAM* 1992;9(1).

137. Levy, D. "The future of measles in highly immunized populations." *American J of Epidemiology* 1984;120:39-47.
138. Neuzil, KM. "Eradication of polio, measles, and hib." *Third Annual Conference on Vaccine Research* 2000. www.id. medscape.com
139. Pan American Health Organization. "Global measles eradication: target 2010?" *EPI Newsletter* (August 1996);XVIII.
140. FDA. "FDA workshop to review warnings, use instructions, and precautionary information [on vaccines]." (Rockland, Maryland: FDA, September 18, 1992):27.
141. See Note 8, p. 238.
142. See Note 106, p. 52.
143. Ibid., pp. 52-53.
144. Faich, GA., et al. "Measles outbreak in Rhode Island." *Public Health Report* (May-June 1981); 96(3):264-266.
145. See Note 133, p. 21-23.
146. Ibid.
147. CDC. *MMWR* (Feb 1, 1985). As cited, Note 22, p. 88.
148. CDC. *MMWR* (June 1984). As cited in Note 22, pp. 87-88.
149. CDC. *MMWR* (June 6, 1987). As cited in O'Mara, P., ed., *Vaccination: Issue of Our Times* (Santa Fe, NM: *Mothering* Mag, 1997):78.
150. Gustafson, T. "Measles outbreak in a fully immunized secondary school population." *NEJM* 1987;316:771-74.
151. Markowitz, LE., et al. "Patterns of transmission in measles outbreaks in the U.S., 1985-1986." *NEJM* 1989;320:75-81.
152. Robertson, SE., et al. "A million dollar measles outbreak: epidemiology, risk factors, and a selective revaccination strategy." *Public Health Reports* (Jan-Feb 1992):24.
153. Edmonson, MB., et al. "Mild measles and secondary vaccine failure during a sustained outbreak in a highly vaccinated population." *JAMA* 1990;263:2467-71.
154. Minnesota Dept of Health. "Measles summary, 1987."
155. CDC. "Measles." *MMWR* 1989;38:329-330.
156. CDC. "Measles—Quebec." *MMWR* 1989;38:329-30.
157. Resnick, SK. "Should you get vaccinated against measles?" *Natural Health* (January/February 1992):30.
158. CDC. "Measles—United States, 1990. *MMWR* 1991; 40(2):369.
159. "Measles outbreak kills 25 children." *New Mexican* (August 25, 1993):A2.
160. See Note 110.
161. CDC. "U.S. Childhood Immunization Update: Measles." (March 1997).
162. CDC. "Measles—U.S., 1999." *MMWR* 2000;49(25):557-560.
163. See Note 110.
164. See Note 152.
165. See Note 106, p. 52.
166. Ibid.
167. See Note 110.
168. Ibid.
169. See Note 53.
170. CDC. Cited in Haney, DQ. "Wave of infant measles stems from '60s vaccinations." *Albuquerque Journal* (November 23, 1992):B3.
171. Ibid.
172. Ibid.
173. Ibid.
174. CDC. "Babies of vaccinated moms more susceptible to measles." *Pediatrics* (November 1999).
175. Klingele, M., et al. "Resistance of recent measles virus wild-type isolates to antibody-mediated neutralization by vaccinees with antibody." *J of Medical Virology* 2000;62:91-98.
176. Ibid.
177. See Note 106, p. 51.
178. Macgregor, JD., et al. "Epidemic measles in Shetland during 1977 and 1978." *BMJ* 1981;282(6262):434-436.
179. See Note 144.
180. See Note 110.
181. See Note 162.
182. Rizetto, M., et al. *J of Infectious Dis* (Jan 1982):18-22.
183. National Coalition for Adult Immunization. "Facts about measles for adults." (November 8, 2000). www.nfid.org/factsheets/measlesadult.html
184. Henderson, R.H., et al. "Immunizing the children of the world: progress and prospects." *Bull WHO* 1988;66:535-43.
185. Hayden, GF., et al. "Progress in worldwide control and elimination of disease through immunization." *Journal of Pediatrics* 1989;114:520-27.
186. See Note 110.
187. Van Ginneken, JK., et al. *Maternal and Child Health in Rural Kenya.* (London: Croom Helm, 1984).
188. Black, FL., et al. "Geographic variation in infant loss of maternal measles antibody and in prevalence of rubella antibody." *American J. of Epidemiology* 1986;124:442-52.
189. Garenne, M., et al. "Pattern of exposure and measles mortality in Senegal." *J of Infectious Disease* 1990;161:1088-94.
190. WHO-EPI. "The optimal age for measles immunization." *Weekly Epidemiology Records* 1982;57:89-91.
191. Job, JS., et al. "Successful immunization of infants at 6 months of age with high dose Edmonston-Zagreb measles vaccine." *Pediatric Infect Dis J* (April 1991);10(4):303-311.
192. Sabin, AB., et al. "Successful immunization of children with and without maternal antibody by aerosolized measles vaccine. I. Different results with undiluted human diploid cell and chick embryo fibroblast vaccines. *JAMA* 1983;249:2651-62.
193. Sabin, AB., et al. "Successful immunization of children with and without maternal antibody by aerosolized measles vaccine. II. Vaccine comparisons and evidence for multiple antibody response. *JAMA* 1984;251:2363-71.
194. Whittle, HC., et al. "Immunisation of 4-6 month old Gambian infants with Edmonston-Zagreb measles vaccine." *Lancet* 1984; ii:834-37.
195. Whittle, H., et al. "Trial of high-dose Edmonston-Zagreb measles vaccine in The Gambia: antibody response and side-effects." *Lancet* 1988;ii:811-814.
196. Aaby, P., et al. "Trial of high-dose Edmonston-Zagreb

measles vaccine in Guinea-Bissau: protective efficacy." *Lancet* 1988;i:809-811.
197. Garenne, M., et al. "Child mortality after high-titre measles vaccines: prospective study in Senegal." *Lancet* 1991;338:903-7.
198. Whittle, HC. "Effect of dose and strain of vaccine on success of measles vaccination of infants aged 4-5 months." *Lancet* 1988;i:963-66.
199. Khanum, S., et al. "Comparison of Edmonston-Zagreb and Schwartz strains of measles vaccine given by aerosol or subcutaneous injection." *Lancet* 1987;i:150-53.
200. Tidjani, O., et al. "Serological effects of Edmonston-Zagreb, Schwartz, and AIK-C measles vaccine strains given at ages 4-5 or 8-10 months." *Lancet* 1989;ii:1357-60.
201. Markowitz, LE., et al. "Immunization of six-month-old infants with different doses of Edmonston-Zagreb and Schwartz measles vaccines." *NEJM* 1990;332:580-87.
202. Awadu, KO. *Outrage! How Babies Were Used as Guinea Pigs in an L.A. County Vaccine Experiment.* (Long Beach, CA: Conscious Rastra Press, 1996).
203. See Note 197.
204. Ibid., p. 903.
205. See Notes 193-196 and Notes 198-201.
206. See Note 197, p. 903.
207. Ibid., p. 904; Table III.
208. Ibid., pp. 903-906.
209. Ibid., p. 904; Table II.
210. Ibid.
211. Ibid., p. 906.
212. Ibid., p. 903.
213. Ibid., p. 906.
214. See Note 202., p. 16.
215. Weiss, R. "Measles battle loses potent weapon." *Sci* (Oct. 23, 1992):546.
216. See Note 202., p. 20.
217. Cimons, M. "CDC says it erred in measles study." *L.A. Times* (June 17, 1996).
218. Ibid. See also Note 202, p. 6.
219. See Note 202, p. 16.
220. Ibid.
221. Ibid., pp. 13-14.
222. See Note 217.
223. See Note 202, p. 7. Data obtained from the Los Angeles County Department of Health.
224. See Note 202, p. 5.
225. Ibid., p. 7.
226. See Note 217.
227. See Note 202, p. 6.
228. See Note 217.
229. See Note 197, p. 903.
230. Ibid.
231. Ibid., p. 905.
232. Ibid., p. 903.
233. Ibid., p. 905.
234. See Note 215, p. 547.
235. Ibid.
236. See Note 202, p. 21.
237. See Note 215.
238. Ibid.
239. See Note 202, p. 21.
240. See Note 217.
241. See Note 200.
242. See Note 197., p. 906.
243. Ibid.
244. Ibid.

Mumps

1. *The World Book Encyclopedia,* Volume 13 (1994):925-926.
2. Mendelsohn, R. *How to Raise a Healthy Child...In Spite of Your Doctor.* (Ballantine Books, 1987): 234-236.
3. Ibid.
4. Ibid.
5. Fisher, BL. *The Consumer's Guide to Childhood Vaccines.* (Vienna, VA: National Vaccine Information Center, 1997):18-19.
6. CDC. "Measles, mumps, and rubella: what you need to know." *U.S. Dep't of Health and Human Serv* (Oct 15, 1991):1.
7. McKinley Health Center. "Mumps vaccine." *University of Illinois* (October 5, 1999). www.mckinley.uiuc.edu
8. CDC Fact Sheet. "Facts about mumps for adults." *National Coalition for Adult Immunization* (April 2000). www.nfid.org
9. McKinley Health Center. "Mumps vaccine." *University of Illinois* (October 5, 1998). www.mckinley.uiuc.edu (See also Note 1, pp. 925-926; Note 2, pp. 234-236; Note 5, pp. 18-19; and Note 6.)
10. Diodati, C. *Immunization: History, Ethics, Law and Health.* (Windsor, Ontario, Canada: Integral Aspects Inc., 1999):113.
11. Scheibner, V. *Vaccination: 100 Years of Orthodox Research Shows that Vaccines Represent a Medical Assault on the Immune System.* (Blackheath, NSW, Australia: Scheibner Publications, 1993):98.
12. Ibid., p. 98.
13. See Note 5, p. 19.
14. Moskowitz, R. "Immunizations: the other side." As cited in O'Mara, P., ed., *Vaccination: The Issue of Our Times* (Santa Fe, NM: *Mothering,* 1997):139.
15. Albonico, H., et al. "The immunization campaign against measles, mumps and rubella—coercion leading to a realm of uncertainty: medical objections to a continued MMR immunization campaign in Switzerland." *J of Anthroposophical Medicine* 1992;9(1).
16. West, R. "Epidemiologic study of malignancies of the ovaries." *Cancer* 1966;19:1001-1007.
17. Wynder, E., et al. "Epidemiology of cancer of the ovary." *Cancer* 1969;23:352.
18. Newhouse, M., et al. "A case control study of carcinoma of the ovary." *Brit J Prev Soc Med* 1977;31:148-53.
19. McGowan, L., et al. "The woman at risk from developing ovarian cancer." *Gynecol Oncol* 1979;7:325-344.
20. See Note 15.
21. Henle, W., et al. "Studies on the prevention of mumps. VII. Evaluation of dosage schedule for inactivated mumps vaccine." *J Immun* 1959;83:17-28.
22. Ibid.
23. Neustaedter, R. *The Vaccine Guide.* (North Atlantic Books, 1996):151.
24. World Health Organization. "Questions and answers: Is there evidence of different risks of adverse reactions with the different mumps vaccines?" (January 2004.) www.who.int
25. Merck & Co., Inc. "M-M-RII (Measles, Mumps, and Rubella Virus Vaccine Live)." Product insert.
26. Ibid.
27. Physician's Desk Reference (PDR); 55th edition. (Montvale, NJ: Medical Economics, 2001):1952.
28. See Note 25.
29. Bottiger, M., et al. "Swedish experience of two dose vaccination programme aiming at eliminating measles, mumps and rubella." *British Medical Journal* 1987;295:264-67.
30. Thomas, E. "A case of mumps meningitis: A complication of vaccination?" *J of the Canadian Med Assoc* 1988;138:135.
31. Champagne, S., et al. "A case of mumps meningitis: a post-immunization complication?" *Canadian Dis Weekly Rep* 1988;13-35:155-156.
32. Ehrengut, W. "Mumps vaccine and meningitis." *Lancet* 1989;2:751.
33. Von Muhlendahl, KE. "Mumps meningitis following measles, mumps and rubella immunisations." *Lancet* (August 12, 1989):394.
34. Cizman, M., et al. "Aseptic meningitis after vaccination against measles and mumps." *Pediatric Infectious Disease Journal* 1989;8:302-308.
35. McDonald, J., et al. "Clinical and epidemiological features of mumps meningo-encephalitis and possible vaccine-related disease." *Pediatric Infectious Dis J* (Nov 1989):751-754.
36. Gray, JA., et al. "Mumps meningitis following measles, mumps, and rubella immunisation." *Lancet* 1989;i:98.
37. Gray, JA., et al. "Mumps vaccine meningitis." *Lancet* 1989;i:927.
38. Murray, MW., et al. "Mumps meningitis after measles, mumps, and rubella immunisation." *Lancet* 1989;ii:877.
39. "Mumps meningitis and MMR vaccination." [Editorial] *Lancet* 1989;ii: 1015-1016.
40. Forsey, T., et al. "Mumps viruses and mumps, measles, and rubella vaccine." *British Medical Journal* 1989;299:1340.
41. Forsey, T., et al. "Mumps vaccines and meningitis." *Lancet* 1992; 340:980.
42. Miller, E., et al. "Risk of aseptic meningitis after measles, mumps, and rubella vaccine in U.K. children." *Lancet* 1993;341:979.
43. Sawada, et al. *Lancet* 1993;342:371.
44. Institute of Medicine. *Adverse Events Associated with Childhood Vaccines: Evidence Bearing on Causality.* (Washington, DC: National Academy Press, 1994).
45. Cizman, M., et al. "Aseptic meningitis after vaccination against measles and mumps." *Pediatric Infectious Disease Journal* 1989;8:302-308.
46. Maguire, HC., et al. "Meningoencephalitis associated with MMR vaccine." *Common Disease Report* 1991;1:R60-61.
47. Sugiura, A., et al. "Aseptic meningitis as a complication of mumps vaccination." *J of Pediatr Infect Dis* 1991;10:209-213.
48. Fujinaga, T., et al. "A prefecture-wide survey of mumps meningitis associated with measles, mumps and rubella vaccine." *Journal of Pediatric Infectious Diseases* 1991;10:204-209.
49. Colville, A., et al. "Mumps meningitis and measles, mumps, and rubella vaccine." *Lancet* 1992; 340:786.
50. Ibid.
51. Ibid.
52. "Urabe stays on." *Lancet* 1993;341:46.
53. Sultz, HA., et al. "Is mumps virus an etiologic factor in juvenile diabetes mellitus?" *J of Pediatrics* 1975;86:654-656.
54. Sinaniotis, CA., et al. "Diabetes mellitus after mumps vaccination (letter)." *Arch of Dis in Childhood* 1975;50:749-750.
55. Quast, U., et al. "Vaccine-induced mumps-like diseases." *Developments in Biological Standardization* 1979;43:269-272.
56. Otten, A., et al. "Mumps, mumps vaccination, islet cell antibodies and the first manifestation of diabetes mellitus type I." *Behring Institute Mitteilungen* 1984;75:83-88.
57. Helmke, K., et al. "Islet cell antibodies and the development of diabetes mellitus in relation to mumps infection and mumps vaccination." *Diabetologia* 1986;29:30-33.
58. Fescharek, R., et al. "Measles-mumps vaccination in the FRG: an empirical analysis after 14 years of use. II. Tolerability and analysis of spontaneously reported side effects." *Vaccine* 1990;8:446-456.
59. Pawlowski, B., et al. "Mumps vaccination and type-1 diabetes." *Deutsche Medizinische Wochenschrift* 1991;116:635.
60. Adler, JB., et al. "Pancreatitis caused by measles, mumps, and rubella vaccine." *Pancreas* 1991;6:489-490.
61. See Note 15.
62. Maclaren, N., et al. "Is insulin-dependent diabetes mellitus environmentally induced?" *NEJM* 1992;327:348-349.
63. Vaccine Adverse Event Reporting System VAERS. Rockville, MD.
64. Gunby, P. "'Atypical' mumps may occur after immunization." *JAMA* 1980;243(23):2374-75.
65. *Family Practice News* (July 15, 1980):1.
66. From an unsolicited email received by the *Thinktwice Global Vaccine Institute.* www.thinktwice.com
67. See Note 5, and Note 27, p. 1976.
68. CDC. "Summary of notifiable disease, US 1993." *MMWR* 1994;42(53).
69. Fiumara, NJ., et al. "Mumps outbreak in Westwood, Massachusetts—1981." *MMWR* 1982; 33(29):421-430.
70. Minnesota Department of Health. Figures cited by Christina Abel, of the *Minnesota Vaccine Support Group,* in a February 10, 2001 email.
71. Kaplan, KM., et al. "Further evidence of the changing

epidemiology of a childhood vaccine-preventable disease." *JAMA* 1988;260(10):1434-1438.
72. See Note 11, p. 106.
73. Briss, PA., et al. "Sustained transmission of mumps in a highly vaccinated population: assessment of vaccine failure and waning vaccine-induced immunity." *Journal of Infectious Diseases* 1994;169:77-82.
74. Sawada, et al. *Lancet* 1993;342:371.
75. See Note 27, p. 1976.
76. CDC. "Update: multistate outbreak of mumps—United States, January 1—May 2, 2006." *MMWR* (May 26, 2006);55(20):559-63.
77. Savage, E., et al. "Mumps epidemic—United Kingdom, 2004-2005." *JAMA* (April 12, 2006);295(14):1636-37.
78. Ibid.
79. See Note 76.
80. Ibid.
81. Ibid.
82. Ibid.
83. Ibid.
84. See Note 2, p. 235.
85. See Notes 2, 5, 9 and 23.
86. CDC. "Mumps—U.S., 1985-88." *MMWR* 1989;38:101-05.
87. Ibid.
88. See Note 77.
89. See Note 73.
90. See Note 76.
91. Ibid.

Rubella

1. *The World Book Encyclopedia,* Volume 16 (1994):506.
2. Mendelsohn, R. *How to Raise a Healthy Child...In Spite of Your Doctor.* (Ballantine Books, 1987):239.
3. See Notes 1 and 2.
4. Plotkin, SA. "Rubella Vaccine," *Vaccines,* edited by Plotkin, SA. and Mortimer, EA. (Philadelphia: W. B. Saunders Co., 1994):310.
5. Merck & Co., Inc. "M-M-R®II (Measles, Mumps, and Rubella Virus Vaccine Live)." Product insert. Issued: February 2006.
6. Merck & Co., Inc. "[ProQuad® (Measles, Mumps, Rubella and Varicella (Oka/Merck) Virus Vaccine Live]." Product insert from the vaccine manufacturer. Issued: July 2006.
7. Spruance, SL., et al. "Recurrent joint symptoms in children vaccinated with HPV-77DK12 rubella vaccine." *J of Pediatrics* 1972;80(3):413-17.
8. Hilleman, MR., et al. "Live attenuated rubella virus vaccines: experiences with duck embryo cell preparations." *Amer J Dis Children* 1969;118:166-171.
9. Cherry, JD. "The 'new' epidemiology of measles and rubella." *Hospital Practice* (July 1980):56.
10. Plotkin, SA., et al. "Studies of immunization with living rubella virus. Trials in children with a strain cultured from an aborted foetus." *Amer. J. Dis. Child.* 1965;110:381-389.
11. Plotkin, SA., et al. "A new attenuated rubella virus grown in human fibroblasts: evidence for reduced nasopharyngeal excretion." *Amer. J. Epidemiology* 1967;86:468-477.
12. Physician's Desk Reference (PDR); 55th edition. (Montvale, NJ: Medical Economics, 2001):1966.
13. See Notes, 5, 6, 10, 11, and 12.
14. Plotkin, SA. "Development of RA 27/3 attenuated rubella virus grown in WI-38 cells." *Wistar Institute of Anatomy and Biology.* Cited in *International Symposium on Rubella Vaccines, London 1968; Symposium Series on Immunobiol. Standards* (Karger, Basel/NY, 1969);11:249-260.
15. Hayflick, L., et al. "The serial cultivation of human diploid cell strains." *Exp. Cell Res.* 1961;25:585-621.
16. See note 10.
17. Hoskins, JM., et al. "Behaviour of rubella virus in human diploid cell strains. I. Growth of virus. II. Studies of infected cells." *Arch. ges. Virusforsch* 1967;21:283-296.
18. Hayflick, L. "The limited in vitro lifetime of human diploid cell strains." *Exp. Cell Res.* 1965;37:614-636.
19. Merck & Co., Inc. "Meruvax® (Rubella Virus Vaccine Live) Wistar RA 27/3 Strain." Product insert. Issued: September 2002.
20. See Notes 5 and 12.
21. Greene, A. "Are there dangers from hidden ingredients in vaccines? Gelatin allergies." *Dr. Greene's House Calls.* www.dr greene.com/990708.asp
22. See Note 5.
23. See Note 6.
24. Merck & Co., Inc. "Varivax® [Varicella Virus Vaccine Live (Oka/Merck)]." Product insert. Issued: April 2006.
25. See Notes 6 and 24.
26. See Note 5, 6, and 19.
27. Vaccine Adverse Event Reporting System VAERS. Rockville, MD.
28. Gold, JA. "Arthritis after rubella vaccination of women." *New England Journal of Medicine* (July 10, 1969);281(2):109.
29. Cooper, LZ., et al. "Transient arthritis after rubella vaccination." *Am J Dis Child* 1969;118:218-225.
30. Spruance, SL., et al. "Joint complications associated with derivatives of HPV-77 rubella virus vaccine." *Amer J Dis Children* 1971;122:105-111.
31. Swartz, TA., et al. "Clinical manifestations, according to age, among females given HPV-77 duck rubella vaccine." *Am J Epidem* 1971;94:246-51.
32. Weibel, RE., et al. "Influence of age on clinical response to HPV-77 duck rubella vaccine." *JAMA* 1972;222:805-807.
33. Austin, SM., et al. "Joint reactions in children vaccinated against rubella. I. Comparison of two vaccines. *Am J Epidem* (Jan 1972);95(1):53-58.
34. See Note 7.
35. Wallace, RB., et al. "Joint symptoms following an area-wide rubella immunization campaign—report of a survey." *American Journal of Public Health* (May 1972);62(5):658-61.

36. Thompson, GR., et al. "Intermittent arthritis following rubella vaccination: a three year follow-up." *American Journal of Diseases in Children* 1973;125:526-530.
37. Spruance, SL., et al. "Chronic arthropathy associated with rubella vaccination." *J. Arthritis and Rheumatism* (March 1977);20(2):741-47.
38. Gershon, A., et al. "Live attenuated rubella virus vaccine: comparison of responses to HPV-77-DE5 and RA 27/3 strains." *Am. J. Med. Sci.* 1980;279(2):95-97.
39. Weibel, RE., et al. "Clinical and laboratory studies of live attenuated RA 27/3 and HPV-77-DE rubella virus vaccines." *Proceedings of the Society for Experimental Biology and Medicine* 1980;165:44-49.
40. Unpublished data from the files of Merck Research Laboratories.
41. See Note 19.
42. Polk, BF, et al. "A controlled comparison of joint reactions among women receiving one of two rubella vaccines." *American Journal of Epidemiology* 1982 January;115(1):19-25.
43. Chantler, JK., et al. "Persistent rubella infection and rubella-associated arthritis." *Lancet* (June 12, 1982):1323-1325.
44. Tingle, AJ., et al. "Prolonged arthritis, viraemia, hypogamma-globulinaemia, and failed seroconversion following rubella immunisation." *Lancet* 1984;1:1475-1476.
45. Tingle, AJ., et al. "Postpartum rubella immunization: association with development of prolonged arthritis, neurological sequelae, and chronic rubella viremia." *Journal of Infectious Diseases* 1985;152:606-612.
46. Tingle, AJ., et al. "Rubella-associated arthritis. Comparative study of joint manifestations associated with natural rubella infection and RA 27/3 rubella immunisation." *Annals Rheumatic Diseases* 1986; 45:110-114.
47. Institute of Medicine. *Adverse Effects of Pertussis and Rubella Vaccines.* (Washington, DC: Natl Acad Press, 1991).
48. Howson, CP., et al. "Chronic arthritis after rubella vaccination." *Clin Infect Dis,* (Aug 1992);15(2):307-312.
49. Benjamin, CM., et al. "Joint and limb symptoms in children after immunisation with measles, mumps, and rubella vaccine." *British Medical Journal* 1992;304:1075-78.
50. Weibel, RE., et al. "Chronic arthropathy and musculo-skeletal symptoms associated with rubella vaccines. A review of 124 claims submitted to the National Vaccine injury Compensation Program." *J. Arthritis and Rheumatism* (September 1996);39(9):1529-34.
51. Ray, P., et al. "Risk of chronic arthropathy among women after rubella vaccination." Vaccine Safety Datalink Team. *JAMA* (August 1997);278(7):551-56.
52. Mitchell, LA., et al. "HLA-DR class II associations with rubella vaccine-induced joint manifestations." *J Infect Dis* (Jan 1998);177(1):5-12.
53. Geier, DA., et al. "A one year follow-up of chronic arthritis following rubella and hepatitis B vaccination based upon analysis of the Vaccine Adverse Event Reporting System (VAERS) database." *Clinical and Experimental Rheumatology* (Nov-Dec, 2002);20(6):767-71.
54. See Note 27.
55. Kilroy, AW., et al. "Two syndromes following rubella immunization." *JAMA* 1970;214:2287-2292.
56. Gilmarten, RC., et al. "Rubella vaccine myeloradic-uloneuritis." *Journal of Pediatrics* 1972;80:406-412.
57. Bartos, HR. "Thrombocytopenia associated with rubella vaccination." *NY State J Med* (February 15, 1972);72(4):499.
58. Schaffner, W., et al. "Polyneuropathy following rubella immunization: a follow-up study and review of the problem." *American J. of Diseases of Children* 1974;127:684-688.
59. Behan, PO. "Diffuse myelitis associated with rubella vaccination [letter]." *BMJ* (January 15, 1977);1(6054):166.
60. Kline, LB., et al. "Optic neuritis and myelitis following rubella vaccination." *Arch of Neurology,* 1982 Jul;39(7):443-44.
61. Hulbert, TV., et al. "Bilateral hearing loss after measles and rubella vaccination in an adult." *NEJM* (July 11, 1991); 325(2):134.
62. See Note 47.
63. Mühlebach-Sponer, M., et al. "Intrathecal rubella antibodies in an adolescent with Guillain-Barré syndrome after mumps-measles-rubella vaccination." *European Journal of Pediatrics* 1994;154:166.
64. See Note 27.
65. Christian, HA. *The Principles and Practice of Medicine,* 16th edition. (New York: D. Appleton-Century, 1947):582.
66. Bearn, AG. "Structural determinants of disease and their contribution to clinical and scientific progress." *SIPA Foundation Symposiums 44,* 1976: 25-40.
67. National Institutes of Health. "National Diabetes Statistics." *National Diabetes Information Clearinghouse* (NDIC); NIH Pub. No. 06-3892 (Nov 2005). www.diabetes.niddk.nih.gov
68. Ibid.
69. Ibid.
70. Menser, M., et al. "Rubella infection and diabetes mellitus." *Lancet* (January 14, 1978):57-60.
71. Ibid.
72. Rayfield, EJ., et al. "Rubella virus-induced diabetes in the hamster." *Diabetes* (December 1986);35:1278-1281.
73. Ibid.
74. Ehrengut, W. "Central nervous system sequelae of immunization against measles, mumps, rubella and poliomyelitis." *Acta Paediatrica Japonica* 1990;32:8-11.
75. Aubrey, J., et al. "Postpartum rubella immunization: association with development of prolonged arthritis, neurological sequelae, and chronic rubella viremia." *J of Infectious Diseases* (September 1985);152(3):606-612.
76. Coulter, Harris. "Childhood vaccinations and juvenile-onset (type-1) diabetes." Congressional Testimony. *Committee on Appropriations, Subcommittee on Labor, Health and Human Services, Education, and Related Agencies* (April 16, 1997).
77. Coyle, PK., et al. "Rubella-specific immune complexes after congenital infection and vaccination." *Infect. Immunity* (May 1982);36(2):498-503.

78. See Note 72.
79. Numazaki, K., et al. "Infection of cultured human fetal pancreatic islet cells by rubella virus." *Am J Clinical Pathology* 1989;91:446-451.
80. See Note 76.
81. Tobi, M., et al. "Prolonged atypical illness associated with serological evidence of persistent Epstein-Barr virus infection." *Lancet* 1982;1:61-64.
82. Bicker, U. "Some new aspects of autoimmunity." *Journal of Immuno-pharmacology* 1986;8:543-559.
83. Allen, AD. "Is RA27/3 rubella immunization a cause of chronic fatigue?" *Medical Hypotheses* 1988; 27:219.
84. Ibid., p. 217.
85. Ibid., p. 220.
86. Ibid.
87. Ibid., p. 217.
88. Lieberman, AD. "The role of the rubella virus in the chronic fatigue syndrome." *Clinical Ecology* 1991; 7(3):51-54.
89. These personal stories are typical of the emails received by the *Thinktwice Global Vaccine Institute*. www.thinktwice.com
90. See Note 2, p. 240; and Note 9, p. 55.
91. Spika, JS., et al. "Rubella vaccination: a course becomes clear." *Canadian Med Assoc J* (July 15, 1983);129(2):106-110.
92. Klock, LE., et al. "Failure of rubella herd immunity during an epidemic." *New England J of Medicine* 1973;288(2):69-72.
93. Mendelsohn, R. *But Doctor, About That Shot...The Risks of Immunizations and How to Avoid Them* (Evanston, IL: The People's Doctor Newsletter, Inc., 1988):31.
94. Allan, B. "Rubella immunisation." *Australian Journal of Medical Technology* 1973;4:26-27.
95. Lawless, M., et al. "Rubella susceptibility in sixth-graders." *Pediatrics* (June 1980);65:1086-1089.
96. See Note 9, p. 55.
97. Bart, KJ., et al. "Universal immunization to interrupt rubella." *Review of Infectious Diseases* 1985;7(1):S177-84.
98. Crowder, M., et al. "Rubella susceptibility in young women of rural East Texas: 1980 and 1985." *Texas Med* 1987;83:43-47.
99. Fulginiti, V. "Controversies in current immunization policy and practices." *Current Problems in Pediatrics* 1976;6:14.
100. Herrmann, KL., et al. "Rubella antibody persistence after immunization." *JAMA* 1982;247(2):193-196.
101. Minnesota Department of Health, Immunization Unit. "Rubella cases reported," (July 2, 1984).
102. See Note 93, p. 12.
103. See Note 99, pp. 6-16.
104. Tingle, AJ., et al. "Failed rubella immunization in adults: association with immunologic and virological abnormalities." *Journal of Infectious Diseases* 1985;151(2):330-336.
105. See Note 9, p. 55.
106. Ibid.
107. Albonico, H., Klein, P., et al. "The immunization campaign against measles, mumps and rubella—coercion leading to a realm of uncertainty: medical objections to a continued MMR immunization campaign in Switzerland." *J of Anthroposophical Medicine* 1992;9(1).
108. Fine, P. "Herd immunity: history, theory, practice." *Epidemiologic Reviews* 1993;15(2):287.
109. See Note 91, p. 106.
110. See Note 1 and Note 2, p. 240.
111. WHO Copenhagen. "Expanded programme on immunization—report of the meeting of national programme managers," 1989.
112. Schoenbaum, SC., et al. "Epidemiology of congenital rubella syndrome: the role of maternal parity." *Journal of the American Medical Association* 1975;233:151-155.
113. Ibid.
114. Diodati, C. *Immunization: History, Ethics, Law and Health.* (Windsor, Ontario, Canada: Integral Aspects Inc., 1999):17-19.
115. See Note 2, p. 240; Note 9, p. 55; and Note 91.
116. CDC. "Current trends in rubella vaccination during pregnancy —U.S., 1971-1981." *MMWR Weekly* (September 10, 1982);31(35):477-481.
117. Forrest, JM., et al. "Failure of rubella vaccination to prevent congenital rubella." *Medical J of Australia* 1977;1:77.
118. Bott, LM. "Congenital rubella after successful vaccination." *Medical Journal of Australia* 1982;1:514-515.
119. Das, BD., et al. "Congenital rubella after previous maternal immunity." *Arch of Dis in Childhood* 1990;65:545-546.
120. CDC. "Current trends increase in rubella and congenital rubella syndrome—United States, 1988-1990." *MMWR Weekly* (February 15, 1991);40(6):93-99.
121. See Note 1 and Note 2, p. 240.
122. Jonas, J. "Preventing the congenital rubella syndrome by vaccinating women at risk." *Canadian Med Assoc J* (July 15, 1983);129(2):110-112.
123. CDC. "Recommended childhood and adolescent immunization schedule—United States, 2009." *Dept of Health and Human Services.*
124. See Note 9, p. 55.
125. CDC. "Rubella and congenital rubella syndrome—United States, 1985-1988. *MMWR* 1989;38:173-178.
126. See Note 9, p. 55.
127. See Note 120.
128. Baker, B. "Rubella ready for possible worldwide eradication." *Pediatric News* 2000;34(1):18.
129. Meissner, HC., et al. "Elimination of rubella from the United States: a milestone on the road to global elimination." *Pediatrics* (March 2006); 117(3):933-35.
130. "Rubella—Public Health Information Sheet." *March of Dimes Birth Defects Foundation* (White Plains, NY: October 1984). Extracted from CDC data.
131. Victorian Government Health Information. "Rubella (German measles)." *State Government of Victoria, Australia, Department of Human Services.* www.health.vic.gov.au
132. See Note 120.
133. See Note 131.
134. Ibid.

135. Ibid.
136. CDC. "Summary of notifiable diseases, United States, 1995." *MMWR Weekly* (October 25, 1996);44(53):1-87.
137. CDC. "Notifiable diseases/deaths in selected cities weekly information." *MMWR Weekly* (Jan 5, 2001);49(51):1167-1174.
138. See Note 9, p. 55.
139. See Note 136.
140. Although the U.S. government did not begin keeping official statistics on rubella and congenital rubella syndrome until 1966 (when the CDC recorded 46,925 cases of rubella and 11 cases of CRS), some authorities assert that in 1964 and 1965 a rubella epidemic in the United States caused an *estimated* 12 million cases of rubella that resulted in "thousands of infections in pregnant women" and perhaps 20,000 cases of CRS. Estimates on the number of children who were born with some degree of deafness or blindness ranged from a low of 739 cases to a high of 10,000. [See: Meissner, HC., et al. "Elimination of rubella from the United States: a milestone on the road to global elimination." *Pediatrics* 2006; Vol. 117(3):933-935. See also: MCW Healthlink. "Rubella eliminated in the United States." www.healthlink.mcw.edu/article/1031002493.html (Last accessed: February 7, 2007.) See also: Lockett, et al. "Deaf-blind children with maternal rubella: implications for adult services." *American Annals of the Deaf* 1980, Vol. 125(8).]
141. See Note 136.
142. See Note 130.
143. See Note 136.
144. Ibid.
145. See Note 9, p. 55; and Note 122, p. 111.
146. See Note 9, p. 55.
147. See Note 122, p. 111.
148. Ibid.
149. Preblud, SR., et al. "Rubella vaccination of hospital employees (editorial)." *JAMA* (February 20, 1981);245(7):736-737.
150. McLaughlin, MC., et al. "The New York rubella incident: a case for changing hospital policy regarding rubella testing and immunization." *Amer J of Public Health* 1979;79:287-289.
151. CDC. "Rubella in hospital personnel and patients —Colorado. *MMWR Weekly Report* 1979;28:325-327.
152. Schoenbaum, SC. "Rubella policies for hospitals and health workers (editorial). *IC Infect Control* (September-October 1981);2(5):366, 416-417.
153. Mendelsohn, R. "Rubella shots for hospital employees." *The Doctor's People: A Medical Newsletter for Consumers* (Evanston, IL, Aug 1991):1-2.
154. Polk, BF., et al. "An outbreak of rubella among hospital personnel." *New England J of Medicine* 1980;303:541-545.
155. Orenstein, WA., et al. "Rubella vaccine and susceptible hospital employees: poor physician participation." *JAMA* (Feb 20, 1981):711-13.
156. Sacks, JJ., et al. "Employee rubella screening program." *J of the American Medical Association* 1983;249:2675-2678.
157. See Note 155.
158. See Note 9, p. 55.
159. See Note 149, p. 737.
160. See Note 2, p. 241.

MMR

1. Merck & Co., Inc. "M-M-R®II (Measles, Mumps, and Rubella Virus Vaccine Live)." Product insert. Issued: February 2007.
2. Plotkin, SA., et al. "Studies of immunization with living rubella virus: trials in children with a strain cultured from an aborted fetus." *Amer J of Diseases of Children* 1965;10:381-89.
3. Plotkin, SA., et al. "A new attenuated rubella virus grown in human fibroblasts: evidence for reduced nasopharyngeal excretion." *American Journal of Epidemiology* 1967;86:468-77.
4. See Note 1.
5. Ibid.
6. FDA. "Thimerosal in vaccines." www.fda.gov/cber/vaccine/thimerosal .htm (Accessed: Jan. 18, 2008.)
7. Birt, L. "MMR and mercury?" *Vaccination Liberation.* www.vaclib.org
8. See Note 1.
9. Physician's Desk Reference (PDR); 61st edition (Thompson PDR, November 30, 2006).
10. See Notes 1 and 9.
11. Vaccine Adverse Event Reporting System VAERS. Rockville, MD.
12. These unsolicited stories were received by the *Thinktwice Global Vaccine Institute.* www.thinktwice.com
13. FDA. "FDA workshop to review warnings, use instructions, and precautionary information [on vaccines]." (Rockland, Maryland: FDA, September 18, 1992):27.
14. Refer to the chapters on mumps and rubella for several examples with documentation.
15. Herrmann, KL., et al. "Rubella antibody persistence after immunization." *JAMA* 1982;247(2):193-196.
16. BBC News. "Row over MMR effectiveness," (September 3, 2001). www.news.bbc.co.uk
17. Petrovic, M., et al. "Second dose of measles, mumps, and rubella vaccine: questionnaire survey of health professionals." *British Medical Journal* 2001;322:82-85.
18. Autism Society of America. www.autism-society.org
19. Autism Society of America. "What is autism? www.autism-society.org/autism.html
20. Health with Web MD. "Autism." www.content.health.msn.com
21. Wakefield, AJ., et al. "Ileal-lymphoid-nodular hyperplasia, non-specific colitis, and pervasive developmental disorder in children." *Lancet* 1998; 351:637-641.
22. Ibid.
23. "Autism: Present Challenges, Future Needs—Why the Increased Rates?" *Government Reform Committee Hearing,* Washington, DC. (April 6, 2000.) As cited in Andrew Wakefield's testimony.
24. Deykin, EY., et al. *Am J of Epidemiology* 1979;109:628-38.
25. See Note 23.

26. Ibid.
27. See Notes 1, 11 and 12
28. See Note 9 and individual chapters on measles, mumps, and rubella.
29. Albonico, H., Klein, P., et al. "The immunization campaign against measles, mumps and rubella—coercion leading to a realm of uncertainty: medical objections to a continued MMR immunization campaign in Switzerland." *J of Anthroposophical Medicine* (Spring 1992);9(1).
30. Ibid.
31. See Note 9.
32. "Single measles jab rejected." *BBC News* (January 12, 2001).
33. See Note 12.
34. "Doctor faces ban over MMR." *BBC News* (Aug 6, 2001).
35. See Note 17.
36. See Note 12.

Autism

1. Kanner, Leo. "Autistic disturbances of affective content." *The Nervous Child II* (1942-1943):250.
2. Autism Society of America. "What is autism? www.autism-society.org/autism.html
3. Health with Web MD. "Autism." www.content.health.msn.com
4. Coulter, Harris. *Vaccination, Social Violence, and Criminality: Medical Assault on the American Brain*, (Berkeley, CA: North Atlantic, 1990):49.
5. Treffert, DA. "Epidemiology of infantile autism." *Archives of General Psychiatry* (May 1970);22(5):431-38.
6. Lotter, V. "Epidemiology of autistic conditions in young children, I. Prevalence." *Social Psychiatry* 1966; 1:24-37.
7. American Psychiatric Association. *Diagnostic and Statistical Manual of Mental Disorders*, Third Edition, Revised, (Washington, DC, 1987):36-37.
8. CDC. "Autism prevalence." www.hhs.gov
9. CDC. "Prevalence of autism spectrum disorders—ADDM Network, 14 sites, U.S., 2002. *MMWR* 2007;56(SS-01).
10. CDC. "Prevalence of autism spectrum disorders—ADDM Network, U.S. 2006." *MMWR Surveill Summ* 2009;58(SS-10).
11. Kogan, MD., et al. "Prevalence of parent-reported diagnosis of autism spectrum disorder among children in the US, 2007." *Pediatrics* 2009; 124(5):1395-1403.
12. Kim, YS., et al. "Prevalence of autism spectrum disorders in a total population sample." *American Journal of Psychiatry* (published online: May 9, 2011).
13. U.S. Autism and Asperger Association, Inc. "S. 843 Combating Autism Act passed by United States House of Representatives; landmark legislation to help scientists understand the causes and characteristics of autism." *Special Edition* (December 6, 2006).
14. Ibid.
15. Kanner, Leo. "To what extent is early infantile autism determined by constitutional inadequacies?" *Genetics and the Inheritance of Integrated Neurological and Psychiatric Patterns*, (Baltimore: Williams and Wilkins, 1954):382.
16. Kanner, Leo, et al., "Early infantile autism: 1943-1955," *Psychiatric Research Reports* 1957;7:62.
17. Kanner, Leo. "Early infantile autism," *J of Pediatrics* 1944;25:217.
18. See Note 2, "What causes autism?"
19. Gillberg, C., et al. "Social class and infantile autism," *Journal of Autism* 1982;12(3):223.
20. See Note 4, pp. 52,53.
21. Wakabayashi, S. "The Present Status of an Early Infantile Autism First Reported in Japan 30 Years Ago," *Nagoya Med J* 1984;46:35+.
22. See Note 4, p. 50.
23. Ibid.
24. "Autism: Present Challenges, Future Needs—Why the Increased Rates?" *Government Reform Committee Hearing*, Washington, DC. (April 6, 2000.) As cited in Chairman Dan Burton's opening statement.
25. Ibid. As cited in the testimony of Coleen Boyle, PhD.
26. Fisher, BL. "Autism and vaccines: a new look at an old story," (Vienna, VA: National Vaccine Information Center, 2000):3. Quoting from a CDC report released in April 2000.
27. The Hope Project. "Government must be forced to help forgotten children." www.whaleto.freeserve.co.uk/vaccines/hope.html
28. See Note 24.
29. Children's Hospital of Philadelphia. "Vaccine schedule." www.vaccine.chop.edu/schedule.shtml
30. Oleske, J. "Elevated rubeola titers in autistic children." Abstract presented by D. Zecca and Dr. Graffino at an NIH meeting (September 23, 1997). As quoted by Richard Gallup in "Autism and autoimmunity." www.chiroweb.com/archives/18/14/10.html (April 15, 2002).
31. Fudenberg, HH. "Dialysable lymphocyte extract (DlyE) in infantile onset autism: pilot study." *Biotherapy* 1996;9:143-7.
32. Gupta, S. "Immunology and immunologic treatment of autism." *Proc of Natl Autism Assoc, Chicago* 1996;455-60.
33. Statement by Bernard Rimland at the National Autism Conference in Chicago sponsored by the *Autism Research Institute* (June 1996). As quoted by Richard Gallup in "Autism and autoimmunity." www.chiroweb.com/archives/18/14/10.html (April 15, 2002).
34. Wakefield, AJ., et al. "Ileal-lymphoid-nodular hyperplasia, non-specific colitis, and pervasive developmental disorder in children." *Lancet* 1998; 351:637-641.
35. Ibid.
36. Yazbak, FE. "Autism: Is there a vaccine connection? Part I. Vaccination after delivery." 1999. www.thinktwice.com/Yazbak1.pdf
37. Yazbak, FE. "Autism: Is there a vaccine connection? Part II. Vaccination around pregnancy." 1999. www.thinktwice.com/Yazbak2.pdf

38. Yazbak, FE. "Autism: Is there a vaccine connection? Part III. Vaccination around pregnancy, the sequel." 2000. www.thinktwice.com/Yazbak3.pdf
39. An unsolicited personal story received by the *Thinktwice Global Vaccine Institute*. www.thinktwice.com
40. "Autism: Present Challenges, Future Needs—Why the Increased Rates?" *Government Reform Committee Hearing*, Washington, DC. (April 6, 2000). [Visit: www.thinktwice.com/autism.htm to read excerpts from this hearing.]
41. Mercola, J. "MMR links to 170 cases of autism." www.mercola.com
42. Peltola, et al. "No evidence for measles, mumps, and rubella vaccine-associated inflammatory bowel disease or autism in a 14-year prospective study." *Lancet* 1998;351:1327-1328.
43. See Note 40. As cited in Dr. Andrew Wakefield's testimony.
44. Taylor, et al. "Autism and MMR vaccine: no epidemiological evidence for a causal association." *Lancet* 1999;353:2026-29.
45. Miller, C. "Introduction of measles/mumps/rubella vaccine." *Health Visitor* 1988;61:116-117.
46. *Lancet* 1999; 354:949-951.
47. See Note 40. As cited in Dr. Andrew Wakefield's testimony.
48. Kawashima, K., et al. "Detection and sequencing of measles virus from peripheral mononuclear cells from patients with inflammatory bowel disease and autism." *Digestive Dis and Sciences* (April 2000); 45:723-729.
49. Reuters Medical News. "Measles persistence confirmed in some patients with IBD, autistic enterocolitis." (June 20, 2000).
50. As noted in copies of the original letters.
51. Wakefield, AJ. et al. "Enterocolitis in children with developmental disorders." *American Journal of Gastroenterology* 2000;95(9):2154-2156.
52. Wakefield, A., et al. "Measles, mumps and rubella vaccine: through a glass, darkly." *Adverse Drug Reaction and Toxicologica Reviews* 2000; 19(4):265-283.
53. Templeton, S. "MMR vaccine should not have been licensed." *Sunday Herald* (London: Dec. 10, 2000).
54. Ho, M. "Another independent scientist falls victim over findings against MMR vaccine." *Institute of Science in Society*. www.i-sis.org.uk/MMRautism.php [Accessed April 30, 2002.]
55. "Autism: why the increased rates? A one-year update." *Government Reform Committee Hearing*, Washington, DC. (April 25-26, 2001). [Visit: www.thinktwice.com/autism.htm to read excerpts from this hearing.]
56. Institute of Medicine. "Immunization safety review: measles-mumps-rubella vaccine and autism." (Washington, DC: National Academy Press, 2001).
57. "MMR: should there be a public inquiry?" *BBC News* (Sep 2, 2001).
58. Ibid.
59. Ibid.
60. Ibid.
61. Ibid.
62. BBC News. "Blair stays mum on Leo and MMR," (Dec 19, 2001).
63. Associated Press. "Tony Blair's son in vaccine debate," (December 23, 2001). www.dailynews.yahoo.com
64. BBC News. "MMR policy 'foolish' says GP," (December 24, 2001).
65. BBC News. "Wakefield stands by MMR claims." www.news.bbc.co.uk
66. BBC News. "Why Japan stopped using MMR," (February 8, 2002).
67. Fraser, L. "Anti-MMR doctor is forced out." *Telegraph. co.uk* (February 12, 2001). www.portal.telegraph.co.uk
68. Tilton, A. "Killing the messenger," *About: Autism /Pervasive Developmental Disorders*, 2002. www.autism.about.com
69. Institute of Medicine. *Immunization Safety Review: MMR Vaccine and Autism*. Stratton, K., et al. Ed. (National Acad Press: Wash, DC, 2001).
70. See Note 55. Cited in Congressman Dan Burton's opening statement.
71. Meldgaard, K., et al. "A population-based study of measles, mumps and rubella vaccination and autism." *NEJM* 2002;347(19):1477-82.
72. Bernard, S. "Denmark study on autism and MMR vaccine shows need for biological research." *Safe Minds* (November 6, 2002). In a press release. www.safeminds.org
73. Richardson, D. "Thimerosal: A missing link in Denmark MMR-autism study." *PROVE Newsletter* (November 7, 2002). Email subscriber update.
74. Jacobson, S. "Danish study: autism not linked to vaccination." *Dallas Morning News* (November 7, 2002). www.dallasnews.com
75. See Note 71, p. 1477.
76. Ioannidis, J. "Contradicted and initially stronger effects in highly cited clinical research." *JAMA* (July 13, 2005); 294(2):218-228.
77. In a copy of the Dan Burton letter to President Bush.
78. Zwillich, T. "U.S. government asks court to seal vaccine records." *Reuters Health* (November 26, 2002). www.story.news.yahoo.com
79. Gillers, S. "Why judges should make court documents public." *NY Times* (November 30, 2002). www.nytimes.com
80. "Retraction of an interpretation." *Lancet* (March 6, 2004);363:750.
81. "MMR doctor 'to face GMC charges.'" *BBC News* (June 12, 2006).
82. "Andrew Wakefield may not now face misconduct charges." *Autism Connect* (July 16, 2006). autismconnect.org
83. Ibid.
84. Ibid.
85. Sanchez, R. "Dr. Andrew Wakefield struck off medical register." *The Times* (May 25, 2010). www.timesonline.co.uk
86. Olmsted, D. "The age of autism: the Amish anomaly." *United Press International* (April 18, 2005). washtimes.com
87. Olmsted, D. "The age of autism: Julia." *United Press International* (April 19, 2005). www.washtimes.com
88. Ibid.

89. Ibid.
90. Olmsted, D. "Autism and the Homefirst® medical practice. The age of autism: a pretty big secret." *United Press International* (December 7, 2005). www.homefirst.com
91. Ibid.
92. See Note 40. As cited in Dr. Bernard Rimland' testimony.
93. Corrigan, S. "MMR fears coming true." *Mail on Sunday* (February 5, 2006). www.dailymail.co.uk
94. Ibid.
95. Palta, R. "A timeline of the thimerosal controversy." *Mother Jones* (March 1, 2004). www.motherjones.com
96. FDA. "Thimerosal as a preservative." www.fda.gov/cber/vaccine/thimerosal.htm (February 11, 2007.)
97. Legal Rights. "Thimerosal and autism symptoms resource: dangers of mercury." www.thimerosal-autism-symptoms.com/html/mercury.html (Last accessed: May 20, 2007.)
98. Ibid.
99. Wikipedia. "Thimerosal." www.en.wikipedia.org/wiki/Thimerosal
100. FDA. Vaccine Adverse Event Reporting System (VAERS).
101. See Note 40.
102. Levin, M. "'91 memo warned of mercury in vaccines." *The Los Angeles Times* (Feb 8, 2005):A-1. www.latimes.com
103. AAP/PHS. "Joint statement of the American Academy of Pediatrics (AAP) and the United States Public Health Service (PHS)," (July 7, 1999).
104. A.-Champ. "CDC failure to remove mercury from vaccines." *Advocates for Children's Health Affected by Mercury Poisoning.*" www.a-champ.org/cdcmercuryremoval.html (Last accessed: May 10, 2007.)
105. Kennedy, RF. "Time for CDC to come clean." *Huffington Post* (March 1, 2006). www.huffingtonpost.com
106. Ibid.
107. Ibid.
108. Ibid.
109. See Note 90.
110. Data accessed via the Freedom of Information Act.
111. Kennedy, RF. "Deadly immunity." *Common Dreams NewsCenter* (June 21, 2005). Originally published by *Salon.com* (June 16, 2005). Updates to the story: June 17, June 22, June 24, July 1 and July 21, 2007.
112. National Autism Association. From transcripts of the meeting (via FOIA). Received in an email dated June 28, 2006.
113. See Notes 110 and 112.
114. See Notes 110-112.
115. Ibid.
116. Ibid.
117. Ibid.
118. Ibid.
119. Ibid.
120. Ibid.
121. See Note 111.
122. Verstraeten, T., et al. "Safety of thimerosal-containing vaccines: a two-phased study of computerized health maintenance organization databases." *Pediatrics* (Nov 2003);112(5):1039-48.
123. See Note 111.
124. Ibid.
125. Ibid.
126. Ibid.
127. "Mercury in medicine: are we taking unnecessary risks?" *Government Reform Committee Hearing,* Washington, DC. (July 18, 2000). [Visit: www.thinktwice.com/autism.htm to read excerpts from this hearing.]
128. As noted in a copy of the original letter. www.altcorp.com/repburton.htm
129. Ibid.
130. Press release. "Chairman Burton requests vaccine recall," (October 26, 2000). www.house.gov/reform/press/00.10.26.htm
131. Levin, M. "Merck misled on vaccines, some say: the firm supplied shots containing a mercury compound after saying it had halted its use." *Los Angeles Times* (March 7, 2005):C-1.
132. See Note 105.
133. See Note 111.
134. "The status of research into vaccine safety and autism." *Government Reform Committee Hearing,* Washington, DC. (June 19-20, 2002).
135. Williams, V. "Congressman calls for criminal penalties at vaccine mercury hearings." *WFAA-TV News* (June 20, 2002).
136. See Note 96.
137. CDC. Childhood immunization schedules were established by health authorities under the auspices of the U.S. government. Mercury content is documented in several early editions of the *Physician's Desk Reference* (Montvale, NJ: Medical Economics).
138. FDA. "Table 3: Thimerosal and expanded list of vaccines." www.fda.gov/cber/vaccine/thimerosal.htm (Updated: March 14, 2008.)
139. FDA. "Thimerosal in vaccines: frequently asked questions." www.fda.gov/cber/vaccine/thimfaq.htm (Last accessed: Dec 22, 2008.)
140. Morgan, D. "Homeland bill rider aids drug makers: measure would block suits over vaccines." *The Washington Post* (November 15, 2002). www.washingtonpost.com
141. Pichichero, M., et al. "Mercury concentrations and metabolism in infants receiving vaccines containing thimerosal: a descriptive study." *Lancet* (Nov 30, 2002);360(9347):1737-41.
142. McNeil, D. "Study suggests mercury in vaccine was not harmful." *NY Times* (December 4, 2002). www.nytimes.com
143. Hviid, A., et al. "Association between thimerosal-containing vaccine and autism." *JAMA* 2003;290:1763-1766.
144. Rimland, B. "To the editor, re: Association between thimerosal-containing vaccine and autism." *JAMA* (Jan 14, 2004).
145. See Note 111.
146. Ibid.
147. Magos, L., et al. "The comparative toxicology of ethyl- and methylmercury. *Archives of Toxicology* 1985;57:260-67.
148. Burbacher, TM., et al. "Comparison of blood and brain levels in infant monkeys exposed to methylmercury or vaccines containing thimerosal." *Environ Health Perspect* 2005;113(8): 1015-21.
149. National Autism Association. "Senate gift to drug companies is unconstitutional." Press release: Dec 26, 2005.
150. Geier, M. and Geier, D. "Neurodevelopmental disorders after thimerosal-containing vaccines: a brief communication." *Experimental Biology and Medicine* 2003;228:660-64.
151. Geier, M. and Geier, D. "Thimerosal in childhood vaccines, neuro-developmental disorders, and heart disease in the United States." *J of Amer Phys and Surgeons* 2003;8(1):6-11.
152. Bradstreet, J., Geier, D., et al. "A case-control study of mercury burden in children with autistic spectrum disorders." *J of American Physicians and Surgeons* 2003;8(3):76-79.
153. Geier, M. and Geier, D. "Early downward trends in neuro-developmental disorders following removal of thimerosal-containing vaccines." *J of Amer Phys and Surg* 2006;11(1):8-13.
154. Geier, M. and Geier, D. "A case series of children with apparent mercury toxic encephalopathies manifesting with clinical symptoms of regressive autistic disorders." *J of Toxicology and Environ Health,* Part A: Current Issues (April 30, 2007).
155. Geier, M. and Geier, D. "A prospective study of mercury toxicity biomarkers in autistic spectrum disorders." *J of Toxicol and Environ Health,* 2007; Part A, Vol 70(20):1723-30.
156. Young, HA, Geier, M., et al. "Thimerosal exposure in infants and neurodevelopmental disorders: an assessment of computerized medical records in the Vaccine Safety Datalink." *J Neurol Sci* (August 15, 2008);271(1-2):110-18.
157. Fombonne, E., et al. "Pervasive developmental disorders in Montreal, Quebec, Canada: prevalence and links with immunizations." *Pediatrics* 2006;118(1):e139-e150.
158. Ibid.
159. National Autism Association. "Newly released Canadian data links vaccines with pervasive developmental disorder" (March 7, 2007).
160. Ibid.
161. Ibid.
162. Handley, JB. "Cal-Oregon unvaccinated survey." *Generation Rescue* (June 26, 2007). www.generationrescue.org/survey.html
163. Olmsted, D. "The age of autism: study sees vaccine risk." *Science Daily* (June 26, 2007). www.sciencedaily.com
164. See Note 111.
165. National Autism Association. "American Academy of Pediatrics (AAP) devotes little time to autism epidemic at October convention." Press release: September 19, 2005.
166. Department of Health and Human Services/CDC. "Recommended immunization schedule for ages 0-6 years, United States, 2009." The immunization schedule is approved by the Advisory Committee on Immunization Practices (ACIP) and the American Academy of Pediatrics (AAP).
167. See Note 165.
168. Ibid.
169. National Autism Association. "Autism advocacy organizations demand response from American Academy of Pediatrics (AAP) and government to autism epidemic at 'The Power of Parents Rally' Oct 7-8." Press release: Oct 3, 2005.
170. CDC. *MMWR,* 2007;56(9):193-196.
171. CDC. *MMWR* (July 28, 2006);55(10).
172. CDC. "Guidelines for vaccinating pregnant women." Updated: May 2007.
173. See Note 138.
174. National Autism Association. "Controversial vaccine preservative to be discussed at upcoming CDC meeting, says National Autism Association: parents and advocacy groups request flu shots recommended for pregnant women, infants and children be mercury-free" (February 14, 2007).
175. National Autism Association. "CDC's vaccine committee whitewashed toxic vaccine component, says National Autism Association" Feb 23, 2007.
176. Thompson, W., et al. "Early thimerosal exposure and neuropsychological outcomes at 7 to 10 years." *New England Journal of Medicine* (September 27, 2007);357:1281-92.
177. Ibid.
178. Ibid.
179. See Note 122.
180. Andrews, N., et al. "Thimerosal exposure in infants and developmental disorders: a retrospective cohort study in the United Kingdom does not support a causal association." *Pediatrics* 2004;114:584-91.
181. Heron, J., et al. "Thimerosal exposure in infants and developmental disorders: a prospective cohort study in the United Kingdom does not support a causal association." *Pediatrics* 2004;114:577-83.
182. Grandjean, P., et al. "Methymercury exposure biomarkers as indicators of neurotoxicity in children aged 7 years." *American Journal of Epidemiology* 1999;150:301-305.
183. Crump, KS., et al. "Influence of prenatal mercury exposure upon scholastic and psychological test performance: benchmark analysis of a New Zealand cohort." *Risk Anal* 1998;18 701-13.
184. See Note 176, references 22-31.
185. Schechter, R., et al. "Continuing increases in autism reported to California's Developmental Service system." *Arch Gen Psy* 2008;65(1):19-24.
186. Park, A. "How safe are vaccines?" *Time* (May 21, 2008).
187. AAP News. "Flu vaccine extended to kids 6-23 months." *American Acad. of Pediatrics* (August 2002).
188. "Childhood influenza-vaccination coverage—United States, 2002-03 influenza season." *JAMA* 2004;292: 2074-75.
189. Bettes, B., et al. "Influenza vaccination in pregnancy: practices among obstetrician-gynecologists—U.S., 2003-04 influenza season" (see editorial note). *Medscape* (Oct 28, 2005).
190. CDC. "Prevention and control of influenza: recommendations of the ACIP." *MMWR* 2005;54(1):1050-52.
191. CDC. "Preventing pneumococcal disease among infants and young children." *MMWR* 2000;49(RR09):1-38.
192. CDC. "CDC's ACIP expands hepatitis A vaccination for children." *Press Release* (October 28, 2005).
193. Prior to the mercury phaseout (pre-2000), babies received 3,925mcg of aluminum by 18 months of age. After Prevnar and

hepatitis A shots were added to the schedule, babies received 4,925mcg of aluminum by 18 months of age—a 20% increase.
194. CDC. "Recommended childhood immunization schedule for persons aged 0-6 years, United States, 2011."
195. Data on aluminum content is taken directly from the manufacturers' product inserts. See also Appendix II.
196. Zatta, P., et al. "Aluminum and health." First International Conference on Metals and the Brain: from Neurochemistry to Neurodegeneration. University of Padova, Italy (Sep 20-23, 2000). www.bio.unipd.it/zatta/ metals/document2.htm
197. Wisniewski, HM., et al. "Aluminum neurotoxicity in mammals." Environmental Geochemistry and Health (March 1990);12(1-2):115-20.
198. Ayoub, D. "Aluminum, vaccines and autism: déjà vu!" National Autism Association Annual Conference. Atlanta, GA. (November 11, 2007).
199. "Aluminum toxicity in infants and children (RE9607)," Pediatrics (March 1996); 97(3):413-416.
200. See Note 198.
201. Taylor, G. "It's not just the mercury: aluminum hydrox. in vaccines." Adventures in Autism (Mar 9, 2008). www. adventuresinautism.blogspot.com
202. Bishop, NJ., et al. "Aluminum neurotoxicity in preterm infants receiving intravenous-feeding solutions." NEJM 1997; 336(22):1557-62.
203. Rappaport, B. "Document NDA 19-626/S-019." FDA: Office of Drug Evaluation II, Center for Drug Evaluation and Research (February 13, 2004): Section 3a. www.fda.gov
204. See Notes 194 and 195.
205. See Notes 110 and 112.
206. Clements, J. "Workshop on aluminum in vaccines." Presented by National Vaccine Program Office, Dept. of Health and Human Services. San Juan, Puerto Rico (May 11-12, 2000). As noted in David Ayoub's presentation (see Note 198).
207. Holland, M., et al. "Unanswered questions from the Vaccine Injury Compensation Program: a review of compensated cases of vaccine-induced brain injury." Pace Envtl Law Rev (May 10, 2011).
208. In press releases issued by Safe Minds and the National Autism Association (May 10, 2011).
209. These unsolicited personal stories were received by the Thinktwice Global Vaccine Institute. www.thinktwice.com

Hepatitis A

1. Mayo Clinic Staff. "Hepatitis A." Mayo Clinic. www.Mayo Clinic.com (September 12, 2005).
2. U.S. Department of Health and Human Services. "Hepatitis A vaccine: what you need to know." CDC (March 21, 2006).
3. See Note 1.
4. CDC. "Prevention of hepatitis A through active or passive immunization: recommendations of the Advisory Committee on Immunization Practices (ACIP)." MMWR Weekly (October 1, 1999);48(RR12):1-37.
5. Winkler, D. "Hepatitis A facts." Concerned Parents for Vaccine Safety. www.access1.net/via/vaccine/hepafacts.htm
6. CDC. "Notifiable diseases—deaths from specified notifiable diseases, United States, 1982-1991." MMWR: Summary of Notifiable Diseases—U.S., 2003. (October 21, 1994); 42(53), Table 7.
7. See Note 1.
8. Immunization Action Coalition. "Ask the experts: hepatitis A." www.immunize.org (Last updated: January 2007).
9. Ibid.
10. See Notes 1 and 8.
11. CDC. MMWR, Morbidity and Mortality Weekly Report: Summary of Notifiable Diseases—U.S., 2005. (March 30, 2007);54(53):Table 1.
12. See Notes 1 and 2.
13. Merck Data Sheet. "Hepatitis A." www.merck.com
14. Department of Human Services, Australia. "Hepatitis A: the facts." www.hna.ffh.vic.gov.au
15. See Note 4.
16. Immunization Action Coalition. "Hepatitis A & B vaccines: be sure your patient gets the correct dose!" www.immunize.org
17. GlaxoSmithKline. "Twinrix® [hepatitis A inactivated and hepatitis B (recombinant) vaccine]." Product insert, April 2007.
18. GlaxoSmithKline. "FDA approves accelerated dosing schedule for hepatitis A and B vaccine," (April 6, 2007). www.hivandhepatitis.com
19. Merck & Co., Inc. "(Hepatitis A Vaccine, Inactivated) Vaqta®." Product insert from the vaccine manufacturer. Issued June 2006.
20. Ibid.
21. SmithKline Beecham Biologicals, unpublished data, 1995. As cited in Note 4.
22. GlaxoSmithKline Biologicals. "Havrix® (Hepatitis A Vaccine, Inactivated)." Prescribing information (December 2006).
23. See Note 19.
24. Vaccine Adverse Event Reporting System VAERS. Rockville, MD.
25. See Note 4.
26. This personal story is typical of the vaccine queries and comments received by the Thinktwice Global Vaccine Institute. www.thinktwice.com
27. See Note 4.
28. See Note 6, Tables 1 and 4.
29. See Note 19.
30. Ibid.
31. See Notes 4 and 19.
32. Ibid.
33. See Note 4.
34. CDC. MMWR: Summary of Notifiable Diseases—United States, 2003 (April 22, 2005);52(54).
35. CDC. MMWR: Summary of Notifiable Diseases—United States, 2004 (June 16, 2006);53(53).

Hepatitis B

1. U.S. Department of Health and Human Services. "Hepatitis B vaccine: what you need to know." CDC (July 11, 2001).
2. Braunwald, E., et al. Harrison's Principles of Internal Medicine (McGraw-Hill, 1994).
3. Immunization Action Coalition. "Vaccine Information for the public and health professionals: hepatitis B disease." www.vaccineinformation.org (Reviewed by the CDC, Aug 2005.)
4. See Notes 1 and 3.
5. Ibid.
6. CDC. MMWR: Summary of Notifiable Diseases—United States, 2004 (June 16, 2006);53(53).
7. CDC. MMWR: Summary of Notifiable Diseases—U.S., 2005 (March 30, 2007);54(53): Table 1.
8. See Notes 1 and 3.
9. Scheibner, V. Vaccination: 100 Years of Orthodox Research. (Blackheath, Australia: Scheibner Pub, 1993):3.
10. See Notes 1 and 3.
11. Neustaedter, R. The Vaccine Guide. (Berkeley, California: North Atlantic Books, 1996):171.
12. Alter, MJ., et al. "The changing epidemiology of hepatitis B in the United States." JAMA 1990;263:1218-1222.
13. CDC. MMWR: Summary of Notifiable Diseases—U.S., 2003 (April 22, 2005);Vol. 52, No. 54.
14. See Note 6.
15. See Note 7, Table 3.
16. See Notes 6 and 13.
17. CDC. MMWR: Summary of Notifiable Diseases—U.S., 2003 (April 30, 2004);Vol. 51, No. 53.
18. Dienstag, JL., et al. "Occupational exposure to hepatitis B virus in hospital personnel: infection or immunization?" American Journal of Epidemiology 1982;115(1):26-39.
19. Merck & Co., Inc. "Recombivax HB Hepatitis B Vaccine (Recombinant)." Product insert. Issued: June 2005.
20. GlaxoSmithKline Biologicals. "Engerix-B [Hepatitis B Vaccine (Recombinant)]." Product insert (December 2005).
21. Jacobson, IM., et al. "Lack of effect of hepatitis B vaccine of T-cell phenotypes." NEJM 1984;311(16):1030-1032.
22. Institute of Medicine, Adverse Events Associated with Childhood Vaccines: Evidence Bearing on Causality (Washington, DC: National Academy Press, 1994).
23. See Note 19.
24. Ibid.
25. Ibid.
26. See Notes 19 and 20.
27. See Note 1.
28. Tan, LJ. "The hepatitis B vaccine." American Medical Association; AMA helping doctors help patients. www.ama-assn.org (Dec 9, 2004).
29. See Notes 31-133.
30. Vaccine Adverse Event Reporting System VAERS. Rockville, MD.
31. Rogerston, SJ., et al. "Hepatitis B vaccine associated with erythema nodosum and polyarthritis." BMJ 1990;301:345.
32. Hachulla, E., et al. "Reactive arthritis after hepatitis B vaccination." Journal of Rheumatology 1990; 17:1250-1251.
33. Vautier, G., et al. "Acute sero-positive rheumatoid arthritis occurring after hepatitis vaccination." Br J Rheumatol (October 1994);33(10):991.
34. Hassan, W., et al. "Reiter's syndrome and reactive arthritis in health care workers after vaccination." BMJ (July 9, 1994);309(6967):94.
35. Fraser, PA., et al. "Reiter's syndrome attributed to hepatitis B immunisation." BMJ 1994 Dec;309(6967):1513.
36. Birley, HD., et al. "Hepatitis B immunisation and reactive arthritis." BMJ 1994 Dec;309(6967):1514.
37. Gross, K., et al. "Arthritis after hepatitis B vaccination. Report of three cases." Scand J Rheumatol 1995;24(1):50-2.
38. Biasi, D., et al. "Rheumatological manifestations following hepatitis B vaccination. Report of three cases." Scand J Rheumatol 1995;24:50-2.
39. Aherne, P., et al. "Psoriatic arthropathy." Irish Medical Journal (March-April, 1995);88(2):72.
40. Harrison, BJ., et al. "Patients who develop inflammatory polyarthritis (IP) after immunization are clinically indistinguishable from other patients with IP." Br J Rheum (Mar 1997);36(3): 366-9.
41. Bracci, M., et al. "Polyarthritis associated with hepatitis B vaccination." Br J Rheumatol (February 1997);36(2):300-1.
42. Pope, JE., et al. "The development of rheumatoid arthritis after recombinant hepatitis B vaccination." J Rheum (Sep 1998);25(9):1687-93.
43. Grasland, A., et al. "Adult-onset Still's disease after hepatitis A and B vaccination?" Rev Med Interne (February 1998); 19(2):134-6.
44. Maillefert, JF., et al. "Rheumatic disorders developed after hepatitis B vaccination." Rheumatol (Oxford), (October 1999);38(10):978-83.
45. Toussirot, E., et al. "Sjogren's syndrome occurring after hepatitis B vaccination." Arthritis Rheuma (September 2000); 43(9):2139-40.
46. Ribera, ER., et al. "Polyneuropathy associated with administration of hepatitis B vaccine." N Engl J Med (September 8, 1983);309(10):614-5.
47. Shaw, FE Jr., et al. "Postmarketing surveillance for neurologic adverse events reported after hepatitis B vaccination. Experience of the first three years." Am J Epidemiol (February 1988);27(s):337-52.
48. Biron, P., et al. "Myasthenia gravis after general anesthesia and hepatitis B vaccine." Arch Intern Med. (December 1988); 148(12):2685.
49. Herroelen, L., et al. "Central nervous system demyelination after immunization with recombinant hepatitis B vaccine." Lancet (November 9, 1991);338(8776):1174-75.
50. Tudela, P., et al. "Systemic lupus erythematosus and vaccination against hepatitis B." Nephron 1992 62(2):236.
51. Martinez, E., et al. "Evan's syndrome triggered by

recombinant hepatitis B vaccine." *Clin Infect Dis*. 1992;15:1051.
52. Ganry, O., et al. "Peripheral facial paralysis following vaccination against hepatitis B. Apropos of a case." *Therapie* 1992;47:437-438.
53. Waisbren, BA. "Other side of the coin (letter)." *Inf Dis News* 1992;5:2.
54. Trevisani, F., et al. "Transverse myelitis following hepatitis B vaccination." *J of Hepatology* (Sep 1993);19(2):317-8.
55. Mahassin, F., et al. "Acute myelitis after vaccination against hepatitis B." *Presse Med* (Dec 1993); 22(40):1997-1998.
56. Nadler, JP. "Multiple sclerosis and hepatitis B vaccination." *Clin Infect Dis* (Nov 1993);17(5):928-9.
57. Mamoux, V., et al. "Lupus erythymatosus disseminatus and vaccination against hepatitis B virus." *Arch Pediatr* 1994; 1:307-309.
58. Deisenhammer, F., et al. "Acute cerebellar ataxia after immunisation with recombinant hepatitis B vaccine." *Acta Neurol Scand* (June 1994);89(6):462-3.
59. Kaplanski, G., et al. "Central nervous system demyelination after vaccination against hepatitis B and HLA haplotype." *J Neurol Neurosurg Psychiatry* (June 1995);58(6):758-9.
60. Tartaglino, LM., et al. "MR imaging in a case of postvaccination myelitis." *Am J Neuroradiol* 1995;16(3):581-2.
61. Guiserix, J. "Systemic lupus erythematosus following hepatitis B vaccine." *Nephron* 1996;74(2):441.
62. Grezard, P., et al. "Cutaneous lupus erythematosus and buccal aphthosis after hepatitis B vaccination in a 6-year old child." *Ann Dermatol Venereol* 1996;123(10):657-9.
63. Manna, R., et al. "Leukoencephalitis after recombinant hepatitis B vaccine." *J of Hepatology* (June 1996);24(6):764-5.
64. Mathieu, E., et al. "Cryoglobulinemia after hepatitis B vaccination." *New England J Med* (Aug 1996); 335(5):335.
65. Cohen, AD., et al. "Vaccine-induced autoimmunity." *J Autoimmunity* (Dec 1996);9(6):699-703.
66. Kakar, A., et al. "Guillain Barre syndrome associated with hepatitis B vaccination." *Ind J Ped* (Sep-Oct 1997); 64(5):710-2.
67. Song, M., et al. "Acute Myelitis after hepatitis B vaccination." *J Korean Med Sci* (Jun 1997);12(3):249-51.
68. Maillefert, JF., et al. "Mental nerve neuropathy as a result of hepatitis B vaccination." *Oral Surgery, Oral Medicine, Oral Pathology, Oral Radiology and Endodontology* (June 1997);83(6):663-4.
69. Wise, RP., et al. "Hair loss after routine immunizations." *JAMA* (Oct 8, 1997);278(14):1176-8.
70. Finielz, P., et al. "Systemic lupus erythematosus and thrombocytopenic purpura in two members of the same family following hepatitis B vaccine." *Nephrol Dial Transplant* 1998;13(9):2420-1.
71. Flemmer, M., et al. "The bald truth." *Am J Gastroenterol* (April 1999);94(4):1104.
72. Creange, A., et al. "Lumbosacral acute demyelinating polyneuropathy following hepatitis B vaccination." *Autoimmunity* 1999;30:143-6.
73. Tourbah, A., et al. "Encephalitis after hepatitis B vaccination: recurrent disseminated encephalitis or MS?" *Neurology* (July 22, 1999);53(2):396-401.
74. Renard, JL., et al. "Acute transverse cervical myelitis following hepatitis B vaccination. Evolution of anti-HBs antibodies." *Presse Med* (Jul 3-10, 1999);28(24):1290-2.
75. Gran, B., et al. "Martin R. Development of multiple sclerosis after hepatitis B vaccination." *Neurol* 2000;54(suppl 3):A164.
76. Sinsawaiwong, S., et al. "Guillain-Barré syndrome following recombinant hepatitis B vaccine and literature review." *J Med Assoc Thai*. (Sept 2000);83(9):1124-6.
77. Konstantinou, D., et al. "Two episodes of leukoencephalitis associated with recombinant hepatitis B vaccination in a single patient." *Clin Inf Dis* (November 15, 2001);33:1772-3.
78. Hernán, MA., et al. "Recombinant hepatitis B vaccine and the risk of multiple sclerosis: a prospective study." *Neurology* 2004;63:838-842.
79. Terney, D., et al. "Multiple sclerosis after hepatitis B vaccination in a 16-year-old patient." *Chinese Medical Journal* 2006;119(1):77-79.
80. Yann, M., et al. "Hepatitis B vaccine and the risk of CNS inflammatory demyelination in childhood." *Neurology* (Oct 8, 2008). [published online]
81. Ness, JM., et al. "Hepatitis vaccines and pediatric multiple sclerosis. Does timing or type matter?" *Neurology* (Dec 17, 2008). [published online]
82. Fried, M., et al. "Uveitis after hepatitis B vaccination." *Lancet* (September 12, 1987):631-2.
83. Brezin, A., et al. "Visual loss and eosinophilia after recombinant hepatitis B vaccine." *Lancet* (August 28, 1993);342(8870):563-4.
84. Achiron, LR., et al. "Postinfectious hepatitis B optic neuritis." *Optom Vis Sci* 1994;71:53-6.
85. Brezin, AP., et al. "Acute posterior multifocal placoid pigment epitheliopathy after hepatitis B vaccine." *Arch Ophthalmol* (March 1995);113(3):297-300.
86. Devin, F., et al. "Occlusion of central retinal vein after hepatitis B vaccination." *Lancet* (June 1996); 347(9015):1626.
87. Baglivo, E, et al. "Multiple evanescent white dot syndrome after hepatitis B vaccine." *Am J Ophthalmol* (September 1996);122(3):431-2.
88. Berkman, N., et al. "Bilateral neuro-papillitis after hepatitis B vaccination." *Presse Med* (Sep 28, 1996);25(28):1301. [French.]
89. Bonfils, P., et al. "Fluctuant perception hearing loss after hepatitis B vaccine." *Ann Otolaryngol Chir Cervicofac* 1996; 113(6):359-61. [French.]
90. Granel, B., et al. "Occlusion of central retinal vein after vaccination against viral hepatitis B with recombinant vaccines. 4 cases." *Presse Med* (February 1, 1997);26(2):62-5. [French.]
91. Berkman, N. "A case of segmentary unilateral occlusion of the central retinal vein following hepatitis B vaccination." *Presse Med* (April 26, 1997);26(14):670. [French.]
92. Albitar, S., et al. "Bilateral retrobulbar optic neuritis with hepatitis B vaccination." *Nephrol Dial Transplant* (October 1997);12(10):2169-70.

93. Arya, SC. "Ophthalmic complications of vaccines against hepatitis B virus." *Int Ophth* 1997;21(3):177-8.
94. Orlando, MP., et al. "Sudden hearing loss consequent to hepatitis B vaccination: a case report." *Annals of the New York Academy of Sciences* (December 29, 1997);830:319-321
95. Biacabe, B., et al. "A case report of fluctuant sensorineural hearing loss after hepatitis B vaccination." *Auris, Nasus, Larynx* (October1997);24(4):357-60.
96. Bourges, JL., et al. "Multifocal placoid epitheliopathy and anti-hepatitis B vaccination." *J Fr Ophtalmol* (November 1998);21(9):696-700. [French.]
97. Stewart, O., et al. "Simultaneous administration of hepatitis B and polio vaccines associated with bilateral optic neuritis." *Br J Ophthalmol* (October 1999);83(10):1200-1.
98. Fledelius, HC. "Unilateral papilledema after hepatitis B vaccination in a migraine patient. A case report including forensic aspects."*Acta Ophthalmol Scand* (December 1999);77(6):722-4.
99. Voigt, U., et al. "Neuritis of the optic nerve after vaccinations against hepatitis A, hepatitis B and yellow fever." *Klin Monatsbl Augenheilkd* (Oct 2001);218(10):688-90. [German.]
100. Cockwell, P., et al. "Vasculitis related to hepatitis B vaccine." *BMJ* (Dec 1, 1990);301(6763):1281.
101. Allen, MB., et al. "Pulmonary and cutaneous vasculitis following hep B vaccination." *Thorax* (May 1993); 48(5):580-1.
102. Nagafuchi, S., et al. "Eosinophilia after intradermal hepatitis B vaccination." *Lancet* 1993;342:998.
103. Poullin, P., et al. "Thrombocytopenic purpura after recombinant hepatitis B vaccine." *Lancet* (November 1994); 344(8932):1293.
104. Meyboom, RH., et al. "Thrombocytopenia reported in association with hepatitis B and A vaccines." *Lancet* (June 1995);345(8965):1638.
105. Neau, D., et al. "Immune thrombocytopenic purpura after recombinant hepatitis B vaccine: retrospective study of seven cases." *Scan J. Infect Dis* 1998;30(2):115-8.
106. Ronchi, F., et al. "Thrombocytopenic purpura as adverse reaction to recombinant hepatitis B vaccine." *Arch Dis Child* (Mar 1998);78(3):273-4.
107. Muller, A., et al. "Thrombocytopenic purpura: adverse reaction to a combined immunisation (recombinant hepatitis B and measles-mumps-rubella-vaccine) and after therapy with Co-trimoxazole." *Eur J Pediatr* (Dec 1999);158 Suppl 3:S209-10.
108. Le Hello, C., et al. "Suspected hepatitis B vaccination related vasculitis."*J of Rheumatology* (Jan 1999);26(1):191-4.
109. Rabaud, C., et al "First case of erythermalgia related to hepatitis B vaccination." *J of Rheum* (Jan 1999);26(1):233-4.
110. De Keyser, F., et al. "Immune-mediated pathology following hepatitis B vaccination. Two cases of polyarteritis nodosa and one case of pityriasis rosea-like drug eruption." *Clin Exp Rheumatol* (Jan-Feb 2000);18(1):81-5.
111. Viallard, JF., et al. "Severe pancytopenia triggered by recombinant hepatitis B vaccine." *Br J Haematol* (July 2000); 110(1):230-3.
112. Zaas, A., et al. "Large artery vasculitis following recombinant hepatitis B vaccination. 2 cases." *J Rheumatol* (May 2001);28(5):1116-20.
113. Conesa, A., et al. "Thrombocytopenic Purpura after Recombinant Hepatitis B Vaccine. A rare association." *Haematologica* (March 2001);86(3):E09. [Italian.]
114. Goolsby, PL. "Erythema nodosum after Recombivax HB hepatitis B vaccine." *N Engl J Med* (Oct 1989);321:1198-9.
115. Castresana-Isla, CJ., et al. "Erythema nodosum and Takayasu's arteritis after immunization with plasma derived hepatitis B vaccine." *J Rheumatol* (August 1993);20(8):1417-8.
116. Trevisian, G., et al. "Lichen ruber planus following HBV vaccination." *Acta Dermato-Venereologica* (February 1993);73(1):73.
117. Aubin, F., et al. "Lichen planus following hepatitis B vaccination." *Archives of Dermatology* (October 1994);130(10): 1329-30.
118. Di Lernia, V., et al. "Bisighini G. Erythema multiforme following hepatitis B vaccine." *Ped Derma* (December 1994);11(4):363-4.
119. Saywell, CA., et al. "Kossard S. Lichenoid reaction to hepatitis B vaccination." *Australasian J Derm* (August 1997);38(3):152-4.
120. Dauod, M., et al. "Anetoderma after hepatitis B immunization in two siblings." *J Amer Acad Dermatol* (May 1997);36(5 Pt 1):779-80.
121. Ferrando, MF., et al. "Lichen planus following hepatitis B vaccination." *Br J Dermatol* (Aug 1998);23(2):350.
122. Barbaud, A., et al. "Allergic mechanisms and urticaria/angioedema after hepatitis B immunization." *Br J Dermatol* (Nov 1998);139(5):925-6.
123. Schupp, P., et al. "Lichen planus following hepatitis B vaccination." *Inter J of Dermat* (Oct 1999);38(10):799-800.
124. Loche, F., et al. "Erythema multiforme associated with hepatitis B immunization." *Clin Exp Dermatol* (March 2000); 25(2):167-8.
125. Agrawal, S., et al. "Lichen planus after HBV vaccination in a child: a case report from Nepal." *J Dermatol* (September 2000);27(9):618-20.
126. Al-Khenaizan, S. "Lichen planus occurring after hepatitis B vaccination: a new case." *J Am Acad Dermatol* (October 2001);45(4):614-5.
127. Usman, A., et al. "Lichenoid eruption following hepatitis B vaccination: first North American case report."*Pediatr Dermatol* (Mar-Apr 2001);18(2):123-6.
128. Lilic, D., et al. "Liver dysfunction and DNA antibodies after hepatitis B vaccination." *Lancet* (November 1994); 344(8932):1292-3.
129. Macario, F., et al. "Nephrotic syndrome after recombinant hepatitis B vaccine." *Clin Nephrol* (May 1995);43(5):349.
130. Classen, John Barthelow. "Childhood immunisation and diabetes mellitus," *New Zealand Med J* (May 24, 1996):195.
131. Classen, John Barthelow. "The diabetes epidemic and the hepatitis B vaccine." *New Z Med J* (May 24, 1996):366.
132. Ranieri, VM., et al. "Liver inflammation and acute

respiratory distress syndrome in a patient receiving hepatitis B vaccine: a possible relationship?" *Intensive Care Medicine* (January 1997);23(1):119-21.

133. Islek, I., et al. "Nephrotic syndrome following hepatitis B vaccination." *Pediatr Nephrol* (Jan 2000);14:89-90.

134. Snider, GB., et al. "A possible systemic reaction to hepatitis B vaccine." *JAMA* (March 1, 1985);253(9):1260-1.

135. AADRAC. "Australian Adverse Drug Reactions Advisory Committee: Reactions to hepatitis B vaccines." *Australian Adverse Drug Reactions Bulletin* (August 1990).

136. Morris, K., et al. "Nature and frequency of adverse reactions following hepatitis B vaccine...in children in New Zealand, 1985-1988." Presented at the Vaccine Safety Committee, IOM. Wash, DC, (May 4, 1992).

137. Germanaud, J., et al. "A case of severe cytolysis after hepatitis B vaccination." *Amer J Med* (June 1995);98(6):595-6.

138. Fisher, BL, Ed. "Hepatitis B vaccine: the untold story." *The Vaccine Reaction: National Vaccine Information Center* (September 1998).

139. Belkin, Michael. "Government-mandated thalidomide for babies." *WorldNetDaily* (Jan 25, 1999). worldnetdaily.com

140. Howd, A. "Ounce of Prevention, Pound of Misery." *Insight Magazine* (Mar 12, 1999). www.insightmag.com

141. Bethell, T. "Shots in the Dark." *American Spectator* (May 1999).

142. Wallstin, B. "Immune to Reason." *The Houston Press* (June 3, 1999). www.houstonpress.com

143. Shaw, FE. "Uproar over a little known preservative, thimerosal, jostles U.S. hepatitis B vaccine policy." *Hepatitis Control Report* (Summer 1999); Vol. 4, no. 2. www.hepatitis controlreport.com/v4n2.html

144. Spalding, B J. "Miracle or murder? The hepatitis B vaccine controversy." *Biospace.com* (Nov 11, 1999). www.biospace.com

145. These personal stories are typical of the hundreds of unsolicited hepatitis B vaccine queries and comments received by the *Thinktwice Global Vaccine Institute*. www.thinktwice.com

146. Reported in an NVIC press release on hepatitis B (Jan 27, 1999).

147. National Vaccine Information Center. "MedAlert: Online access to the U.S. government's Vaccine Adverse Event Reporting System (VAERS)." www.medalerts.org

148. CDC. "Summary of notifiable diseases, United States, 1996." *MMWR* (Oct 31, 1997); Vol. 45, No. 53:39.

149. See Note 146.

150. Ibid.

151. *Science* (July 31, 1998).

152. "France suspends use of hepatitis B vaccine." As reported in an NVIC public notice. www.909shot.com/hepbfrance.htm

153. Mica, John L. "Hepatitis B vaccine: helping or hurting public health?" Opening Statement Before Congress. *Subcommittee on Criminal Justice, Drug Policy and Human Resources; Committee on Government Reform.* (Wash., DC: May 18, 1999).

154. Belkin, Michael. "Hepatitis B vaccine: helping or hurting public health?" Congressional Testimony. *Subcommittee on Criminal Justice, Drug Policy and Human Resources; Committee on Government Reform.* (Washington, DC: May 18, 1999).

155. Ibid., Classen, J. Barthelow.

156. Cantwell, A. "The gay experiment that started AIDS in America." *Not Aids* (Jan 13, 2006.) www.notaids.com/en/node/84

157. See Notes 19 and 20.

158. See Note 19.

159. Wainwright, RB., et al. "Duration of immunogenicity and efficacy of hepatitis B vaccine in a Yupik Eskimo population, preliminary results of an 8-year study," in "Viral hepatitis and liver disease," Hollinger, FB., et al (eds.), (Williams & Wilkins, 1990:762-66).

160. Hadler, SC., et al. "Evaluation of long-term protection by hepatitis B vaccine for 7 to 9 years in homosexual men," in "Viral hepatitis and liver disease," Hollinger, FB., et al (eds.), (Williams & Wilkins, 1990:766-68).

161. Hadler, SC., et al. "Long-term immunogenicity and efficacy of hepatitis B vaccine in homosexual men." *NEJM* (July 24, 1986);315:209-14.

162. Stevens, CE., et al. "Prospects for control of hepatitis B virus infection: implications of childhood vaccination and long-term protection." *Pediatrics* 1992;90:170-173.

163. Street, AC., et al. "Persistence of antibody in healthcare workers vaccinated against hepatitis B." *Infec Control Hosp Epidem* 1990;11:525-530.

164. Pasko, MT., et al. "Persistence of anti-HBs among health care personnel immunized with hepatitis B vaccine." *American Journal of Public Health* 1990;80:590-593.

165. World Health Organization. "Hepatitis B vaccines: immunogenicity reappraised." *WHO Drug Infor* 1994;8(2).

166. Ballinger, AB., et al. "Severe acute hepatitis B infection after vaccination." *Lancet* 1994;344:1292-1293

167. Goffin, E., et al. "Acute hepatitis B infection after vaccination." *Lancet* 1995;345:263.

168. Freed, GL., et al. "Reactions of pediatricians to a new Centers for Disease Control recommendation for universal immunization of infants with hepatitis B vaccine." *Pediatrics* 1993;91:699-702.

169. Freed, GL., et al. "Family physician acceptance of universal hepatitis B immunization of infants." *Journal of Family Practice* 1993;36:153-157.

170. See Notes 19 and 20.

Meningitis

1. CDC. "Disease listing, meningococcal disease, general information." www.cdc.gov (October 12, 2005).

2. "Viral meningitis." *Directors of Health Promotion and Education.* www.dhpe.org/infect/vmenin.html (Jan 30, 2007).

3. Ibid.

4. "Bacterial meningitis." *Directors of Health Prom & Educ.* www.dhpe.org/infect/bacmeningitis.html (Jan 30, 2007).

5. See Note 1.

6. See Notes 1 and 4.

7. See Note 1.

8. Waggoner-Fountain, LA., et al. "The emergence of haemophilus influenzae types e and f as significant pathogens." *Clinical Infectious Disease* (November 1995);21(5):1322-24.

9. Physician's Desk Reference; 53rd Edition. (Montvale, NJ: Medical Economics, 1999);1524 and 1861.

10. Sanofi Pasteur, Inc. "Meningococcal (Groups A, C, Y and W-135) polysaccharide diphtheria toxoid conjugate vaccine: Menactra." Product insert from the manufacturer. Product information as of Sept. 2006.

11. See Note 1.

12. See Note 9, p. 3072.

13. Wyeth Pharmaceuticals, Inc. "Pneumococcal 7-valent Conjugate Vaccine (Diphtheria CRM$_{197}$ Protein)." Product insert from the vaccine manufacturer. Revised: May 2006.

14. See Note 10.

Hib

1. Centers for Disease Control and Prevention. "Frequently asked questions about Haemophilus influenzae type b (Hib) and Hib vaccine." www.cdc.gov

2. Ibid.

3. Adams, WG., et al. "Decline of childhood haemophilus influenzae type b (Hib) disease." *JAMA* 1993;269:221-226.

4. Kaplan, SL., et al. "Update on bacterial meningitis." *Journal of Child Neurology* 1988;3:82-93.

5. See Note 1.

6. See Notes 1 and 3

7. Sell, SH. "Haemophilus influenzae type b meningitis: manifestations and long-term sequelae." *Pediatric Infectious Disease J* 1987;6:775-778.

8. See Note 1.

9. National Institutes of Health. "The haemophilus influenzae type b (Hib) vaccine—long-term research pays off." www.niaid.nih.gov

10. See Note 1.

11. Fisher, BL. *The Consumer's Guide to Childhood Vaccines.* (Vienna, VA: NVIC, 1997):21.

12. Zwillich, Todd. "Hib rates in U.S. children higher among minorities than whites." *Reuters Medical News* (August 18, 2000).

13. Centers for Disease Control and Prevention. "Haemophilus Influenzae Type b." www.cdc.gov/nip/publications/pink/hib.pdf (January 8, 2007).

14. Smith, E., et al. "Changing incidence of haemophilus influenzae meningitis." *Pediatrics* 1972;50(5):723-727.

15. See Note 11, p. 21.

16. Bjune, G., et al. "Effect of outer membrane vesicle vaccine against group b meningococcal disease, Norway." *Lancet* 1991;338(8775):1093-96.

17. See Note 1.

18. See Note 16.

19. Craighead, J E. "Report of a workshop: disease accentuation after immunization with inactivated...vaccines." *J Inf Dis* 1975;1312(6):749-54.

20. Sutter, R., et al. "Attributable risk of DTP injection in provoking paralytic poliomyelitis during a large outbreak in Oman." *Journal of Infectious Diseases* 1992;165:444-449.

21. American Academy of Pediatrics. "Acellular DTP Vaccine." *AAP News Release* (September 5, 1988).

22. Hinman, A., et al. "Immunization practices in developed countries." *Lancet* 1990;335:707-710.

23. Kimura, M., et al. "Acellular pertussis vaccines and fatal infections." *Lancet* (April 16, 1988):881-882.

24. Ibid.

25. Ibid.

26. Scheibner, V. *Vaccination: 100 Years of Orthodox Research.* (Blackheath, Australia: Scheibner Pub, 1993):133.

27. See Note 1.

28. Physician's Desk Reference (PDR); 53rd Edition. (Montvale, NJ: Medical Economics, 1999):3072.

29. See Note 12.

30. See Note 13, p. 116.

31. See Note 12.

32. Petersen, GM., et al. "Genetic factors in Haemophilus influenzae type b disease susceptibility and antibody acquisition." *Journal of Pediatrics* 1987;110:228-33.

33. Granoff, DM., et al. "Response to immunization with Haemophilus influenzae type b polysaccharide-pertussis vaccine and risk of Haemophilus meningitis in children with the Km(1) immunoglobulin allotype." *J. Clin. Invest.* 1984;74:1708-14.

34. See Note 12.

35. Harrison, LH., et al. "Haemophilus influenzae type b polysaccharide vaccine: an efficacy study." *Pediatrics* 1989;84:255-61.

36. Black, S., et al. "Efficacy of Haemophilus influenzae type b capsular polysaccharide vaccine," *Pediatric Infectious Disease J* 1988;7:149-156.

37. Cochi, SL., et al. "Primary invasive Haemophilus influenzae type b disease: a population-based assessment of risk factors." *Journal of Pediatrics* 1986;108:887-96.

38. Istre, GR., et al. "Risk factors for primary invasive Haemophilus influenzae disease: increased risk from day-care attendance and school-aged household members." *Journal of Pediatrics* 1985;106:190-95.

39. Makintubee, S., et al. "Transmission of invasive Haemophilus influenzae type b disease in daycare settings." *J Pediatrics* 1987;111:180-86.

40. Osterholm, MT., et al. "The risk of subsequent transmission of Haemophilus influenzae type b disease among children in day care." *NEJM* 1987;316:1-5.

41. Murphy, MT., et al. "Risk of subsequent disease among day-care contacts of patients with systemic Haemophilus influenzae type b disease." *NEJM* 1987;316:5-10.

42. Redmond, SR., et al. "Haemophilus influenzae type b disease: an epidemiologic study with special reference to day-care centers." *JAMA* 1984;252:2581-84.

43. Vadheim, CM., et al. "Risk factors for invasive Haemophilus influenzae type b in Los Angeles County children 18-60 months of age." *Amer J Epid* 1992; Vol 136, No.2:221-22.
44. Cochi, SL., et al. "Primary invasive Haemophilus influenzae type b disease: a population-based assessment of risk factors. *Journal of Pediatrics* 1986;108:887-96.
45. Takala, AK., et al. "Risk factors of invasive Haemophilus influenzae type b disease among children in Finland." *National Public Health Institute;* Helsinki, Finland. (Supported by Connaught Laboratories as a part of the Hib vaccination project: May 24, 1989):694-5.
46. Broome, CV. "Epidemiology of Haemophilus influenzae type b infection in the United States." *Pediatric Infectious Dis J* 1987;6:779-82.
47. Nesheim, SR., et al. "Systemic Haemophilus influenzae disease in children: a 10-year retrospective study of an urban hospital population." *Clin. Pediatr* 1986;25:605-609.
48. Bjilmer, HA., et al. The epidemiology of Haemophilus influenzae meningitis in children under five years of age in The Gambia, West Africa." *J of Infect Dis* 1990;161:12f0-15.
49. See Note 43.
50. Harrison, LH., et al. "Haemophilus influenzae type b polysaccharide vaccine: an efficacy study." *Pediatrics* 1989; 84:255-61.
51. Istre, GR., et al. "Risk factors for primary invasive Haemophilus influenzae disease: increased risk from day-care attendance and school-aged household members." *Journal of Pediatrics* 1985;106:190-95.
52. See Notes 43-45.
53. *New England J of Medicine* (December 18, 1986):315.
54. Emery, CE. "In the public health." *Providence Journal Bulletin* (December 1986).
55. Mosby's Medical and Nursing Dictionary, 1983:483.
56. Gellis, S. "Pediatric notes: the weekly commentary," (January 15, 1987); Vol. 11:2.
57. Mendelsohn, RS. "New vaccine to combat day care infections," *The People's Doctor Newsletter*, Vol. 9(11):5. [Figures reported by Dr. Stephen L. Coeni of the CDC.]
58. Eskola, J. "Combined vaccination of Haemophilus influenzae type b conjugate and diphtheria-tetanus-pertussis containing acellular pertussis." *The Lancet Interactive* (Dec 11, 1999). www.findarticles.com
59. See Notes 9 and 46.
60. "Updates: vaccine use extended to infants," *FDA Consumer* (January-February 1991):2.
61. See Notes 1 and 9.
62. Wyeth Pharmaceuticals, Inc. "Haemophilus b Conjugate Vaccine (Diphtheria CRM $_{197}$ Protein Conjugate) HibTITER." Product insert from the vaccine manufacturer (Revised: Feb 2005).
63. Sanofi Pasteur SA. "Haemophilus b Conjugate Vaccine (Tetanus Toxoid Conjugate) ActHIB." Product insert (Dec 2005).
64. Merck & Co., Inc. "Liquid PedvaxHIB [Haemophilus b Conjugate Vaccine (Meningococcal Protein Conjugate)]" Product insert: Jan 2001.
65. See Note 13, p. 120.
66. See Note 64.
67. Ibid.
68. See Note 28, pp. 1520, 2316, and 3072.
69. See Notes 62-64.
70. Institute of Medicine. *Adverse Events Associated with Childhood Vaccines: Evidence Bearing on Causality*. Washington, DC: National Academy Press, 1994.
71. Gervaix, M., et al. "Guillain-Barre syndrome following immunization with Haemophilus influenzae type b conjugate vaccine." *European Journal of Pediatrics* 1993;152:613-14.
72. D'Cruz, OF., et al. "Acute inflammatory demyelinating polyradiculoneuropathy (Guillain-Barre syndrome) after immunization with Haemophilus influenzae type b conjugate vaccine." *J of Pediatrics* 1989;115:743-46.
73. Vadheim, CM., et al. "Effectiveness and safety of an Haemophilus influenzae type b conjugate vaccine (PRP-T) in young infants." *Pediatrics* 1993;92:272-79.
74. Ward, J., et al. "Efficacy of a Haemophilus influenzae type b conjugate vaccine in Alaska native infants." *New England Journal of Medicine* 1990;323(2):1393-1401.
75. Milstien, JB., et al. "Adverse reactions reported following receipt of Haemophilus influenzae type b vaccine: an analysis after one year of marketing." *Pediatrics* 1987;80:270-74.
76. Granoff, DM., et al. "Response to immunization with Haemophilus influenzae type b polysaccharide-pertussis vaccine and risk of haemophilus meningitis in children with the km(1) immunoglobulin allotype." *J Clin Investigation* 1984;74:1708-14.
77. Vaccine Adverse Event Reporting System VAERS. Rockville, MD.
78. See Note 28, pp. 1521.
79. See Notes 62-64.
80. Dokheel, TM. "An epidemic of childhood diabetes in the United States." *Diabetes Care* 1993;16:1601-1611.
81. Gardner, S., et al. "Rising incidence of insulin dependent diabetes in children under 5 years in Oxford region: time trend analysis." *British Medical Journal* 1997;315:713-716.
82. Karvonen, M., et al. "Association between type 1 diabetes and Haemophilus influenzae type b vaccination: birth cohort study." *British Medical Journal* 1999;318:1169-1172.
83. Classen, JB., et al. "Clustering of Cases of Insulin Dependent Diabetes (IDDM) Occurring Three Years After Haemophilus Influenza B (HiB) Immunization Support Causal Relationship Between Immunization and IDDM." *Autoimmunity* 2002;35(4):247-53.
84. Classen, JB., et al. "Association between type 1 diabetes and Hib vaccine." *British Medical Journal* 1999;319:1133.
85. PRNewswire. "Hemophilus meningitis vaccine linked to diabetes increase; many diabetics may be eligible for compensation" (May 7, 1999).
86. See Note 84.
87. See Note 85.
88. Ibid.
89. See Notes 84 and 85.
90. See Note 84.
91. Classen, JB. "Public should be told that vaccines may have long term adverse effects." *BMJ* 1999;318:193.
92. See Note 84.
93. Electronic responses to the data in Note 84. www.bmj.com/cgi/eletters/319/7217/1133 [This reference applies to the first three adverse reaction reports; the following reference applies to the remaining reports.]
94. These personal stories are typical of the unsolicited Hib vaccine queries and comments sent via email to the *Thinktwice Global Vaccine Institute.* www.thinktwice.com
95. Mendelsohn, Robert. *But Doctor, About That Shot...The Risks of Immunizations and How to Avoid Them.* (Evanston, IL: The People's Doctor Newsletter, Inc., 1988):88.
96. See Notes 62-64.
97. Weiss, R. "Meningitis Vaccine Stirs Controversy," *Science News* (Oct 24, 1987);132:260.
98. American Academy of Pediatrics. "Policy Statement: Haemophilus b polysaccharide vaccine (HbPV)," *AAP News* (November 1987):7.
99. See Note 36.
100. Harrison, LH., et al. "A day care-based study of the efficacy of Haemophilus influenzae type b polysaccharide vaccine." *J of the American Med Assoc* 1988;260:1413-1418.
101. Osterholm, MT., et al. "Lack of efficacy of Haemophilus b polysaccharide vaccine in Minnesota." *J of the American Medical Association* 1988;260:1423-1428.
102. Shapiro, ED., et al. "The protective efficacy of Haemophilus influenzae polysaccharide vaccine." *J of the American Medical Association* 1988;260:1419-1422.
103. Hiner, EE., et al. "Spectrum of disease due to Haemophilus influenzae type b occurring in vaccinated children." *Journal of Infectious Disease* 1988;158(2):343-48.
104. Daum, RS. et al. "Decline in serum antibody to the capsule of Haemophilus influenzae type b in the immediate post immunization period." *J of Pediatrics* 1989;1114:742-47.
105. Marchant, DD., et al. "Depression of anticapsular antibody after immunization with Haemophilus influenzae type b polysaccharide-diphtheria conjugate vaccine." *Pediatric Infectious Disease Journal* 1989;320:75-81.
106. Sood, SK., et al. "Disease caused by Haemophilus influenzae type b in the immediate period after homologous immunization: immunologic investigation." *Pediatrics* 1990;85 (4 Pt 2):698-704.
107. See Note 13, p. 116.
108. Gellis, SS. "Pediatric notes: the weekly pediatric commentary," (January 15, 1987);11:2.
109. See Notes 12 and 28.
110. See Note 74.
111. See Note 58.
112. See Note 62.
113. Wyeth Pharmaceuticals, Data on File: Prevnar Study D118-P7.
114. CDC. "Disease listing, meningococcal disease, general information," (October 12, 2005). www.cdc.gov
115. Urwin, G., et al. "Invasive disease due to haemophilus influenzae serotype f: clinical and epidemiologic characteristics in the H. Influenzae serotype b vaccine era. The haemophilus influenzae study group." *Clinical Infectious Disease* (June 1996);22(6):1069-76.
116. Ibid.
117. Waggoner-Fountain, LA., et al. "The emergence of haemophilus influenzae types e and f as significant pathogens." *Clinical Infectious Disease* (November 1995);21(5):1322-24.
118. Sarangi, J., et al. "Invasive haemophilus influenzae disease in adults." *Epidem and Infection,* (June 2000); 124(3):441-447.
119. Gonzalez Lopez, M., et al. "Meningitis due to haemophilus influenzae type f." *Anales Españoles Pediatria,* (October 2000);53(4):369-71. [Spanish.]
120. Lipsitch, M. "Vaccination against colonizing bacteria with multiple serotypes." *Proceedings of the National Academy of Sciences* (June 10, 1997);94(12):6571-76.
121. See Note 118.
122. Ibid.
123. Dworkin, MS., et al. "The changing epidemiology of invasive haemophilus influenzae disease, especially in persons ≥65 years old." *Clinical Infectious Diseases* 2007;44:810-816.
124. Boggs, W. "Invasive H. influenzae disease in adults may require new vaccine." *Reuters Health Info* (March 8, 2007).
125. "Frequently asked questions about Haemophilus influenzae type b (Hib) and Hib vaccine." *CDC.* www.cdc.gov/nip/Q&A/clinqa.htm
126. See Note 114.
127. Ibid.
128. Replacement chapter for "Immunisation against infectious disease" 1996: Chapter 23, Meningococcal. [British] Department of Health. (Published by the NHS Executive.) www./doh.gov.uk/meningitis-vaccine/chapter23.htm

Pneumococcal

1. Inserts from the vaccine manufacturer: clinical pharmacology. www.pneumo.com/vaccine/PI.html
2. Physician's Desk Reference; 53rd Edition. (Montvale, NJ: Medical Economics, 1999):1524 and 1861.
3. Wyeth Pharmaceuticals, Inc. "Pneumococcal 7-valent Conjugate Vaccine (Diphtheria CRM $_{197}$ Protein)." Product insert from the vaccine manufacturer (Revised: May 2006).
4. Maugh II, Thomas H. (Los Angeles Times). "Meningitis vaccine for children touted." *Houston Chron* (Sep 26, 1998).
5. American Academy of Family Physicians. "Pneumococcal conjugate vaccine: what a parent needs to know." www.familydoctor.org (Updated: November 2006.)
6. "Meningococcal disease." *CDC* (Reproduced by the McKinley Health Center.) www.mckinley.uiuc.edu/health-info/discond/commdis/meningit.html
7. Beattie, G. *Vaccination: A Parent's Dilemma*. (Australia: Bunya Books, 1997).

8. Beattie, G. "What is Hib disease?" www.whaleto.freeserve.co.uk/v/beattie.html

9. Ibid.

10. Red Book report of the Committee on Infectious Diseases, 23rd edition. *American Academy of Pediatrics* 1994:371.

11. Merck & Co., Inc. "Pneumovax 23 (pneumococcal vaccine polyvalent)." Product insert (Issued: March 2007).

12. Drugs.com. "Pneumococcal vaccine polyvalent (systemic)." www.drugs.com (Accessed: July 5, 2007.)

13. Dooren, JC. "FDA approves new version of Pfizer's Prevnar vaccine." *Wall Street Journal* (February 24, 2010).

14. Wyeth Pharmaceuticals, Inc. "Prevnar 13 (Pneumococcal 13-valent Conjugate Vaccine (Diphtheria CRM$_{197}$ Protein)." Product insert from the vaccine manufacturer (Revised: Feb 2010).

15. Ibid.

16. Ibid.

17. Overturf, G. "Technical report: prevention of pneumococcal infections, including the use of pneumococcal conjugate and polysaccharide vaccines and antibiotic prophylaxix (RE9960)." *American Academy of Pediatrics and the Committee on Infectious Diseases.* www.aap.org/policy/re9960t.html

18. Black, S., Shinefield, H., et al. "Efficacy, safety and immunogenicity of heptavalent pneumococcal conjugate vaccine in children." Northern California Kaiser Permanente Vaccine Study Center Group. *Pediatric Infectious Disease Journal* (March 2000);19(3):187-95.

19. Black, S., Shinefield, H., et al. "Efficacy of heptavalent conjugate pneumococcal vaccine (Lederle Laboratories) in 37,000 infants and children." Results of the Northern California Kaiser Permanente Efficacy Trial. 36th ICAAC, San Diego, CA. (September 24-27, 1998).

20. See Notes 3 and 14.

21. See Note 3.

22. See Note 14.

23. See Note 3.

24. Ibid.

25. Ibid.

26. See Note 14.

27. "Role of aluminum sensitivity in delayed persistent immunization reactions." *J Clinical Pathology* 1991;44:876-77.

28. "Aluminum toxicity in infants and children (RE9607)." *Pediatrics* (March 1996); 97(3):413-416.

29. Woolley, P. "Vaccines show sinister side." *Vancouver Free Press* (March 23, 2006). www.straight.com/article/vaccines-show-sinister-side

30. Press release. "FDA told pneumococcal vaccine likely to cause epidemic of diabetes." (Nov. 8, 1999).

31. Classen, JB., et al. "Association between type 1 diabetes and Hib vaccine." *British Medical Journal* 1999;319:1133.

32. Classen, JB., et al. "Clustering of cases of insulin dependent diabetes (IDDM) occurring three years after haemophilus influenza B (HiB) immunization support causal relationship between Immunization and IDDM." *Autoimmunity* 2002;35(4):247-53.

33. See Note 30.

34. Ibid.

35. Classen, B. "New 'Tuskegee-Like Experiment' planned with pneumococcal vaccine." www.vaccines.net/pneumoco.htm

36. See Note 30.

37. Unsolicited emails sent to the *Thinktwice Global Vaccine Institute.* www.thinktwice.com [Reference applies to the 3rd, 6th and 7th adverse reaction reports.]

38. Williams, Valeri. "News 8 investigates: Prevnar, Part 1." (Feb 23, 2001) www.wfaa.com [Reference applies to the 1st adverse reaction report.]

39. Pneumo.com Online Forum. www.pneumo.com/msgboard/messages/parent-messages.html [Reference applies to the 2nd, 4th and 5th adverse reaction reports.]

40. See Notes 3 and 14.

41. See Note 14.

42. Ibid.

43. Coffey, TJ., et al. "Recombinational exchanges at the capsular polysaccharide biosynthetic locus lead to frequent serotype changes among natural isolates of Streptococcus pneumoniae." *Journal of Molecular Microbiology* (January 1998);27(1):73-83.

44. Lipsitch, M. "Bacterial vaccines and serotype replacement: lessons from haemophilus influenzae and prospects for streptococcus pneumoniae." *Emerging Infectious Diseases* (May-Jun 1999);5(3):336-45.

45. Lipsitch, M. "Vaccination against colonizing bacteria with multiple serotypes." *Proceedings of the National Academy of Sciences* (June 1997);94(12):6571-76.

46. See Note 43.

47. Farrell, DJ., et al. "Increased antimicrobial resistance among nonvaccine serotypes of *streptococcus pneumoniae* in the pediatric population after the introduction of 7-valent pneumococcal vaccine in the United States." *Pedia Infec Dis J* 2007;26(2):123-28.

48. Ibid.

49. Ibid.

50. Ibid.

51. Singleton, RJ., et al. "Invasive pneumococcal disease caused by nonvaccine serotypes among Alaska native children with high levels of 7-valent pneumococcal conjugate vaccine coverage." *JAMA* (April 25, 2007);297:1784-92.

52. Ibid.

53. See Notes 3 and 14.

54. See Note 1.

55. See Notes 3 and 14.

56. Ibid.

57. Ibid.

58. Ibid.

59. Inserts from the vaccine manufacturer: simultaneous administration with other vaccines. www.pneumo.com/vaccine/PI.html

60. Harvard Medical School Office of Public Affairs. "Researchers find use of pneumococcal conjugate vaccine for children could reduce disease-related costs." News release: March 14, 2000. www.hms.harvard.edu

61. Associated Press. "New vaccine reduces risk of severe pneumonia in children" (October 1, 1999). www.idahonews.com

62. Horwin, M. "Prevnar: a critical review of a new childhood vaccine: potential conflicts of interest in testing, promotion and approval" (Sep 19, 2000). www.vaccineinfo.net/issues/Pneumococcal/prevnar.htm (See also: www.whale.to/v/prevnar2.html)

63. American Home Products: 1997 Annual Report. www.ahp.com/annrpt97/sreport3.htm

64. Conflicts of Interest in Vaccine Policy Making (Majority Staff Report). Committee on Government Reform, U.S. House of Representatives (August 21, 2000):17.

65. Mercola, J. "Prevnar." www.mercola.com/2001/mar/3/prevnar.htm

66. See Note 62.

67. See Notes 62, 64 and 65.

68. See Notes 62 and 65.

69. Leary, V. Secretary of the Department of Health and Human Services. 1994 WL 43395 (Fed. Cl.).

70. www.pneumo.com

71. See Notes 62 and 65.

72. See Notes 62, 65 and 70.

73. University of Maryland School of Medicine Faculty. www.medschool.umaryland.edu/cvd/faculty.htm

74. Rennels, MB., et al. "Lack of an apparent association between intussusception and wild or vaccine rotavirus infection." *Pediatric Infectious Disease J* (October 1998);17(10):924-5.

75. FACA: Conflicts of Interest and Vaccine Development: Preserving the Integrity of the Process. Committee on Government Reform, U.S. House of Representatives (June 15, 2000):2.

76. Doctor's guide to medical and other news. "Experimental vaccine shows promise against pneumococcal disease in kids" (April 7, 1998). www.pslsgroup.com/dg/6B37A.htm

77. University of Maryland School of Medicine Donors and Medical System Donors. www.umm.edu/annualreport/9798ar/site/main.htm

78. See Notes 62 and 65.

79. Rennels, MB., et al. "Safety and immunogenicity of heptavalent pneumococcal vaccine conjugated to CRM$_{197}$ in US infants." *Pediatrics* (Apr 1998);101(4 Pt 1):604-611.

80. See Notes 20, 62 and 65.

81. Pfizer. "Change in price for Prevnar 13." *Cumberland Pediatric Foundation* (March 10, 2011).

82. Wilson, D. "Vaccine approved for child infections." *New York Times* (February 24, 2010).

Meningococcal

1. CDC. "Disease listing, meningococcal disease, general information." www.cdc.gov/ncidod/dbmd/diseaseinfo/meningococcal_g.htm (October 12, 2005).

2. Ibid.

3. British Department of Health. "What about other strains of meningococcal disease?" Immunisation fact sheet. *NHS* 2006.

4. Iannelli, Vincent. "Menactra, new vaccine for meningococcal disease." *About Pediatrics.* www.pediatrics.about.com (May 17, 2005).

5. CDC. "Prevention and control of meningococcal disease: recommendations of the Advisory Committee on Immunization Practices (ACIP)." *MMWR* May 27, 2005 / 54(RR07);1-21.

6. "Immunization program: meningococcal conjugate (Menactra) vaccine supply update." *King County Public Health:* Seattle, WA. www.metrokc.gov (Updated: Dec 4, 2006).

7. Hincapie, M., et al. "Neisseria Meningitidis." *Brown University:* Providence, RI. www.brown.edu/Courses/Bio_160/Projects1999/bmenin/nmenin.html (Last accessed: Jan 28, 2007).

8. See Note 1.

9. Ibid.

10. Sanofi Pasteur, Inc. "Meningococcal (Groups A, C, Y and W-135) polysaccharide diphtheria toxoid conjugate vaccine: Menactra." Product insert from the manufacturer. Product information as of Sept 2006.

11. Ibid.

12. Communicable Disease Surveillance and Response. Meningococcal Disease Update: 1998 Cases and Deaths of Meningococcal Disease, Reported to WHO. WHO/OMS, 1998. (Last updated: July 11, 2000). www.who.int

13. Meningococcal C vaccine (Meningitis C) factsheet. *Dept of Health and the Health Education Authority* 1999:1. [British.]

14. Office for National Statistics. "Mortality statistics: childhood, infant and perinatal, England and Wales," 1997; Series DH3, no.30, p. 37.

15. Sanofi Pasteur, Inc. "Meningococcal polysaccharide vaccine, groups A, C, Y and W-135 combined: Menomune." Product insert from the vaccine manufacturer (December 2005).

16. Beattie, G. *Vaccination: A Parent's Dilemma* (Australia: Bunya Books, 1997).

17. Beattie, G. "What is Hib disease?" www.whaleto.freeserve.co.uk

18. *Sydney Morning Herald* (April 24, 1997).

19. Replacement chapter for "Immunisation against infectious disease" 1996: Chapter 23, Meningococcal. See Graph 1. [British] Department of Health. (Published by the NHS Executive.) www./doh.gov.uk/meningitis-vaccine/chapter23.htm

20. Replacement chapter for "Immunisation against infectious disease" 1996: Chapter 23, Meningococcal. [British] Department of Health. (Published by the NHS Executive.) www./doh.gov.uk/meningitis-vaccine/chapter23.htm

21. Ibid.

22. Ibid.

23. Chiu, Cheng-Hsun. "A typical chryseobacterium meningosepticum and meningitis and sepsis in newborns and the Immunocompromised, Taiwan." *Emerging Infect Dis* 2000;6(5).

24. Bloch, KC., et al. "Chryseobacterium meningosepticum: an emerging pathogen among immunocompromised adults." *Medicine* 1997;76:30-41.

25. Gold, Eli. "Current progress in measles eradication in the United States." *Infect Med* 14(4):297+.

26. See Note 23.
27. Ibid.
28. See Notes 5 and 7.
29. Raghunathan, PL., et al. "Opportunities for control of meningococcal disease in the United States." *Annual Review of Medicine, CDC.* (February 2004); Vol. 55:333-353.
30. See Note 1.
31. See Note 5.
32. Ibid.
33. See Note 1.
34. CDC. "Guillain-Barré syndrome among recipients of Menactra meningococcal conjugate vaccine: U.S., June-July 2005." *MMWR* (Oct 6, 2005);54(Disp.):1-3. See also Note 10.
35. Barclay, L. "CDC issues new guidelines for meningococcal vaccination." *Medscape Medical News* (July 13, 2007).
36. Medical News Today. "Menactra, Meningococcal Vaccine For Infants From 9 Months Approved By FDA" (April 23, 2011).
37. Novartis Media Release. "FDA approves the Novartis quadrivalent meningococcal conjugate vaccine, Menveo®, for use in children from 2 years of age" (January 31, 2011).
38. See Note 15.
39. See Note 10.
40. Woodman, R. "Meningitis C vaccine not responsible for deaths." *Reuters Medical News* (Sept 5, 2000).
41. Ibid.
42. Vaccine Adverse Event Reporting System VAERS. Rockville, MD.
43. See Note 5.
44. "Meningococcal polysaccharide vaccine: side effects." Unpublished data available from Aventis Pasteur, Inc. *RxList.* www.rxlist.com (Last updated: June 8, 2006).
45. See Notes 5 and 10.
46. See Note 10.
47. See Note 5.
48. Ibid.
49. Ibid.
50. See Note 34.
51. Ibid.
52. Ibid.
53. "FDA and CDC update information on Menactra meningococcal vaccine and GBS." www.yourlawyer.com/articles/read/12212 (Oct 20, 2006). Extracted from: www.fda.gov
54. "Rare disorder reported with Menactra drug recall alerts." James Scott Farrin, North Carolina Personal Injury Lawyers. www.farrin.com (October 20, 2006).
55. See Note 53.
56. See Note 34.
57. See Note 53.
58. See Note 6.
59. See Note 4.
60. See notes 5 and 15.
61. Ibid.
62. Ibid.
63. See Note 5.
64. See Notes 5 and 10.
65. Ibid.
66. See Notes, 5, 10 and 15.
67. See Note 7.
68. See Note 6.
69. "Serogroup B." *Brown University:* Providence, RI. www.brown.edu/Courses/Bio_160/Projects2005/meningitis/vaccines.htm (January 28, 2007).
70. See Note 7.
71. "Enhanced surveillance of meningococcal disease: national annual report, July 2002— June 2003." *British Health Protection Agency.* www.hpa.org.uk/infections (January 28, 2007).
72. Antignac, A., et al. "Neisseria meningitidis strains isolated from invasive infections in France (1999-2002): phenotypes and antibiotic susceptibility patterns." *Clin Infec Dis* 2003;37:912+.
73. See note 5.
74. National Institutes of Health. "Safety and immunogenicity study of group B meningococcal vaccine to prevent meningitis." *Walter Reed Army Institute of Research.* www.clinicaltrials.gov/ct/show/NCT00248833 (Last updated: October 27, 2006).
75. Law, D., et al. "Invasive meningococcal disease in Québec, Canada, due to an emerging clone of ST-269 serogroup B meningococci with serotype antigen 17 and serosubtype antigen P1.19(B:17:P1.19)." *J Clin Micro* (Aug 2006);44(8):2743-49.
76. Ibid.
77. Diermayer, M., et al. "Epidemics of serogroup B meningococcal disease in Oregon: the evolving epidemiology of the ET-5 strain." *JAMA* 1999; Vol. 281, no.16:1493-97.
78. Ibid.
79. Manchanda, V., et al. "Meningococcal disease: history, epidemiology, pathogenesis, clinical manifestations, diagnosis, antimicrobial susceptibility and prevention." *Indian J of Medical Microbiology* 2006;24, Issue 1:7-19.
80. Ibid.
81. See Note 72.
82. See Notes 5, 10 and 15.
83. An unsolicited email received by the *Thinktwice Global Vaccine Institute.* www.thinktwice.com
84. See Note 7.
85. National Institutes of Health. "Safety and immunogenicity study of group B meningococcal vaccine to prevent meningitis." *Walter Reed Army Institute of Research.* www.clinicaltrials.gov/ct/show/NCT00248833 (Last updated: October 27, 2006).
86. Burstyn, BS. and Law, R. "The meningococcal gold rush—second edition." *Scoop Independent News* (May 30 2005). www.scoop.co.nz
87. Ibid.
88. "New meningitis C vaccine for school children and young babies." [British] Department of Health. (Published by the NHS Executive: November 1, 1999). www.doh.gov.uk/meningitis-vaccine/pressmo.htm
89. See Note 15, p. 4.
90. "Meningitis C vaccine: the immunisation campaign." [British] Department of Health. (Published by the NHS Executive:

November 1, 1999). www.doh.gov.uk/meningitis-vaccine/immunisation.htm
91. Steele, RW. "Pediatric ID update: the HUS-Antibiotic connection, and vaccine news." (Meningococcal Vaccine for College Students.) *Medscape Infectious Diseases* 2000.
92. CDC. "Meningococcal disease and college students." *MMWR* (June 30, 2000);49(RR07):11-20.
93. See note 5.
94. Ibid.
95. Ibid.
96. See Note 92.
97. See Note 5.
98. See Note 35.

Chickenpox

1. Merck & Co., Inc. "Varivax [Varicella Virus Vaccine Live (Oka/Merck)]." Product insert (Issued: February 2007).
2. National Foundation for Infectious Diseases. *What Parents Need to Know About Chickenpox (informational pamphlet).* Bethesda, MD.
3. Preblud, SR. "Varicella: complications and costs." *Pediatrics* 1986; 78:728-735.
4. Ibid.
5. See Note 2.
6. Neustaedter, R. *The Vaccine Guide.* (Berkeley, California: North Atlantic Books, 1996):180.
7. Gorman, Christine. "Chickenpox Conundrum." *Time* (July 19, 1993):53.
8. Phillip, A. "What you should consider before taking the chickenpox vaccine." *Informed Parents Vaccination Home Page.* www.unc.edu ~aphillip/www/vaccine/varivax.htm
9. See Notes 2 and 7.
10. National Vaccine Information Center. "The Vaccine Reaction" (May 1995). Reprinted online: www.909shot.com/cpnlrarticle.htm
11. Wessel, D. "Long incubation: A vaccine to prevent chickenpox is near; now, will it be used?" *Wall Street Journal* (January 16, 1985):1.
12. See Note 7.
13. Lieu, TA., et al. *JAMA* 1994;271:375-81.
14. Medical Sciences Bulletin. "Chickenpox vaccine approved" (April 1995):2. Reprinted: www.pharminfo.com/pubs/msb/chipox.html See also Note 7.
15. Sullivan-Bolyai, JZ., et al. "Impact of chickenpox on households of healthy children." *Pediatric Infectious Disease Journal* 1987;6:33-35.
16. American Academy of Pediatrics. "The chickenpox vaccine: what parents need to know" (public education brochure). Reprinted online: www.aap.org/family/chckpox.htm
17. Rozenbaum, MH., et al. "Cost-effectiveness of varicella vaccination programs: an update of the literature." *Expert Rev Vaccines* 2008;7(6):753-782.
18. Goldman, GS. "Cost–benefit analysis of universal varicella vaccination in the U.S. taking into account the closely related herpes–zoster epidemiology." *Vaccine* 2005;23:3349-55.
19. Physician's Desk Reference (PDR);53rd Edition. (Montvale, NJ: Medical Economics, 1999):1908. See also Note 1.
20. Ibid.
21. Vaccine Adverse Event Reporting System VAERS. Rockville, MD.
22. Wise, RP., et al. "Postlicensure safety surveillance for varicella vaccine." *JAMA* (September 13, 2000):1271-79.
23. Ibid.
24. Ibid., p. 1272.
25. CDC. "Biologics surveillance, 1991-1995," 1997. Dept. of Health and Human Services Report 94.
26. See Note 22, p. 1271.
27. Cliggott Publishing Co. *Infec Med* 2000; 17(3):150.
28. Estrada, B. "What's new in varicella vaccine?" *Pediatric Bulletin* 2000:1. www.id.medscape.com
29. See Note 22, p. 1273: Table 1.
30. See Note 22, pp. 1274 and 1278.
31. Klinman, D., et al. *Nature Med* 2000;6:381-82, 451-54.
32. McKinney, M. "Varicella zoster vaccine reactivates when immunity declines." *Reuters Health.* www.id.medscape.com
33. Plotkin, S. "Hell's fire and varicella-vaccine safety." *New England Journal of Medicine* 1988;318:573-75.
34. Kohl, S., et al. "Natural varicella-zoster virus reactivation shortly after varicella immunization in a child." *Ped Infect Dis J.* 1999;18:1112-13.
35. Roan, S. "Stubborn chickenpox fighting back." *New Mexican* (April 28, 2007): D-2. Reprinted from *The Los Angeles Times.*
36. Goldman, Gary. "Universal varicella vaccination: efficacy trends and effect on herpes zoster." *Internat J of Toxicology* 2005;24:205-213.
37. Goldman, Gary. "International journal of toxicology release: chickenpox vaccine associated with shingles epidemic." *PRNewswire* (September 1, 2005).
38. Ibid.
39. Goldman, Gary. "Cost-benefit analysis of universal varicella vaccination in the U.S. taking into account the closely related herpes zoster epidemiology." *Vaccine* (May 9, 2005): 3349-3355.
40. LookSmart. "Trading chickenpox for shingles?" *Mothering* (Nov-Dec 2005). www.findarticles.com
41. See Notes 36 and 37.
42. Goldman, Gary. "Chickenpox vaccine associated with shingles epidemic." *Press Release:* August 2005.
43. See Note 37.
44. Merck & Co., Inc. "Patient information about Zostavax" (Issued: May 2006).
45. These personal stories are typical of the unsolicited chickenpox vaccine queries and comments sent via email to the *Thinktwice Global Vaccine Institute.* www.thinktwice.com
46. Goldman, G. "Chickenpox vaccine: a cycle of disease. Appendix 3. Clinical descriptions of five different serious adverse affects that followed varicella vaccination." *Nexus New Times Magazine* (July-August 2007).

47. Fisher, BL. *The Consumer's Guide to Childhood Vaccines* (Vienna, VA: NVIC, 1997):45.
48. Salzman, MB., et al. "Transmission of varicella-vaccine virus from a healthy 12-month-old child to his pregnant mother." *Journal of Pediatrics* (July 1997);131(1 Pt 1):151-54.
49. See Note 22, p. 1277.
50. As reported in an NVIC press release chickenpox vaccine (Sep 13, 2000). www.909shot.com/chickenpoxvaers91300.htm
51. See Note 1.
52. Halloran, ME., et al. *Am. J Epidemiology* 1994;140:81-104.
53. See Note 14.
54. See Note 2.
55. See Note 8, p. 2.
56. Patten-Hitt, E. "Varicella outbreak occurs among adults in Alabama." *Reuters Medical News* (August 18, 2000). www.id.medscape.com
57. Haney, D Q. "Wave of infant measles stems from '60s vaccinations." *Albuquerque Journal* (November 23, 1992):B3. (Data in this article was taken from CDC statistics.)
58. See Note 19, p. 1910.
59. See Note 22, p. 1278.
60. Esmaeli-Gutstein, B. et al. "Uveitis associated with varicella virus vaccine." *Am J Ophthalmol* (June 1999); 127(6):733-34.
61. Singer, S., et al. "Urticaria following varicella vaccine associated with gelatin allergy." *Vaccine* (January 28, 1999);17(4):327-29.
62. Sakaguchi, M., et al. "IgE-mediated systemic reactions to gelatin included in the varicella vaccine." *J Allergy Clin. Immunol.* (February 1997);99(2):263-64.
63. See Notes 1, 21 and 47.
64. Merck Press Release. "Chickenpox complications" (May 21, 1997). Reprinted by *Kidsource*. www.kidsource.com
65. See Notes 1 and 21.
66. See Notes 21 and 22.
67. Gilden, DH., et al. "Neurologic complications of the reactivation of varicella-zoster virus." *NEJM* 2000;342:635-45.
68. Hosseinipour, MC., et al. "Middle cerebral artery vasculitis and stroke after varicella in a young adult." *South Med J.* 1998;91:1070-72.
69. Lee, MS., et al. "Varicella zoster virus retrobulbar optic neuritis preceding retinitis in patients with acquired immune deficiency syndrome." *Ophthalmology* 1998;105:467-71.
70. Furuta, Y., et al. "Detection of varicella-zoster virus DNA in patients with acute peripheral facial palsy by the polymerase chain reaction, and its use for early diagnosis of zoster sine herpete." *Journal of Med Virol.* 1997;52: 316-19.
71. Arvin, AM., et al. "Live attenuated varicella vaccine." Annu Rev Microbiol. 1996;50:59-100.
72. Kleinschmidt-DeMasters, BK., et al. "Patterns of varicella zoster virus encephalitis." *Hum Pathol.,* 1996;27:927-38.
73. Mayer, JL., et al. "Varicella-associated thrombocytopenia." *Pediatr Res.* 1996;40:615-19.
74. Wright, JF., et al. "Characterization of platelet-reactive antibodies in children with varicella-associated acute immune thrombocytopenic purpura (ITP)." *Br J Haematol* 1996;95:145-52.
75. Morgan, M., et al. "Is Bell's palsy a reactivation of varicella zoster virus?" *J Infect.* 1995;30:29-36.
76. Taub, JW., et al. "Characterization of autoantibodies against the platelet glycoprotein antigens IIb/IIIa in childhood idiopathic thrombocytopenic purpura." *Am J Hematol.* 1995; 48:104-107.
77. Winiarski, J., et al. "Platelet antigens in varicella associated thrombocytopenia." *Arch Dis Child.* 1990; 65:137-39.
78. Miller, OH., et al. "Optic neuritis following chickenpox in adults." *J Neurol.* 1986;233:182-84.
79. Robillard, RB., et al. "Ramsay Hunt facial paralysis." *Otolaryngol Head Neck Surg.* 1986;95:292-97.
80. Heng, MC. "Henoch-Schonlein purpura." *Br Journal Dermatol.* 1985;112:235-240.
81. Kahane, S., et al. "Detection of anti-platelet antibodies in patients with idiopathic thrombocytopenic purpura (ITP) and in patients with rubella and herpes group viral infections." *Clin Exp Immunol.* 1981;44:49-56.
82. Tovi, F., et al. "Viral infection and acute peripheral facial palsy." *Isr J Med Sci.* 1980;16:576-80.
83. Feusner, JH., et al. "Mechanisms of thrombocytopenia in varicella." *Am J Hematol.* 1979;7:255-64.
84. See Note 22, p. 1277.
85. See Note 45.
86. National Vaccine Information Center. "MedAlert: Online access to the U.S. government's Vaccine Adverse Event Reporting System (VAERS)." www.medalerts.org (Database last accessed: July 31, 2007.)
87. See Note 22, p. 1272.
88. This unsolicited personal story is typical of the correspondence received by the *Thinktwice Global Vaccine Institute.* www.thinktwice.com
89. See Note 50.
90. Ibid.
91. See Note 22, p. 1276.
92. Ibid.
93. CDC Office of Communications Media Relations. "Facts about chickenpox (varicella)" (May 16, 1997):2. www.cdc.gov
94. Ibid.
95. Watson, BM., et al. "Modified chickenpox in children immunized with Oka-Merck varicella vaccine." *Pediatrics* 1993;91:17-22.
96. Naruse, H., et al. "Varicella infection complicated with meningitis after immunization." *Acta Paediatrica Japonica* 1993;35:345-47.
97. See Note 1.
98. Ibid.
99. Ibid.
100. See Notes 1, 95 and 96.
101. See Note 1.
102. See Notes 16, 21 and 22.
103. See Note 22, p. 1278.
104. Chaves, SA., et al. "Loss of vaccine-induced immunity to varicella over time." *NEJM* (March 15, 2007);356:1121-29.

105. Ibid.
106. Marwick, Charles. "Varicella vaccine expected to be ready by 1993." *JAMA* (Aug. 19, 1992):852.
107. See Note 1.
108. Buttram, H. As quoted in the Preface of *Vaccines: Are They Really Safe and Effective?* by Miller, NZ. (Santa Fe, NM: New Atlantean Press, 2008):10.
109. Ahmady, AS., et al. *Indian Pediatrics* 1981:49-52.
110. American Academy of Pediatrics Committee on Infectious Diseases. "Recommendations for the use of live attenuated varicella vaccine." *Pediatrics* 1995;95:791-96.
111. See Note 14.
112. See Notes 27 and 28.
113. Close, John. *Kern Valley Sun* (Oct 20, 1999):2. Reprinted online: www.kvsun.com/health/stories/99102001h.html
114. See Note 47.
115. See Note 113.
116. Barclay, L. "Guidelines updates for varicella prevention in children, teens, adults." *Medscape Medical News* (June 26, 2007). www.medscape.com
117. Ibid.
118. Ibid.

Rotavirus

1. Iannelli, Vincent. "RotaTeq Rotavirus vaccine." *About Pediatrics.* www.pediatrics.about.com (Accessed: September 11, 2006).
2. Russell, Sabin. "FDA okays safer vaccine for children: second treatment to fight rotavirus also in the works." *San Francisco Chronicle* (February 4, 2006). www.sfgate.com
3. Rotavirus Vaccine Program: A PATH Affiliate. "Rotavirus Facts." PATH. www.rotavirusvaccine.org (Accessed: September 22, 2006).
4. Centers for Disease Control and Prevention. "Rotavirus and drinking water from private wells." *CDC Fact Sheet* (Summer 2006). www.cdc.gov
5. Mitchell, Ellen. "New rotavirus vaccine urged for babies: oral dose offers protection against diarrhea, vomiting." *Newsday* (September 5, 2006).
6. Tucker, AW., et al. "Cost-effectiveness analysis of a rotavirus immunization program for the United States." *JAMA* 1998;279:1371-1376.
7. Weijer, Charles. "The future of research into rotavirus vaccine." *British Medical Journal* 2000;321:525-526.
8. Greene, A. "Rotavirus vaccine and intussusception." *Pediatric Update* (September 16, 1999). www.drgreene.org
9. See Notes 3 and 5.
10. CDC. "Withdrawal of rotavirus vaccine recommendation." *MMWR Weekly* (November 5, 1999);48(43):1007.
11. See Notes 7 and 8.
12. "Conflicts of Interest and Vaccine Development: Preserving the Integrity of the Process." *Govt. Reform Committee Hearing,* Washington, DC. (June 15, 2000.) As cited in Chairman Dan Burton's opening statement.
13. "Conflicts of Interest in Vaccine Policy Making Majority Staff Report." *Committee on Government Reform,* U.S. House of Representatives (June 15, 2000). As cited in section IV, FDA, VRBPAC; B. Conflict of Interest Review, Waivers by the FDA.
14. Congressional Press Release. "Burton critical of vaccine approval process: staff report details FDA and CDC conflicts in approval of controversial rotavirus vaccine." *Committee on Government Reform* (Aug 23, 2000).
15. See Notes 12-14.
16. Ibid.
17. See Note 12.
18. Mitchell, S. "Congressional report slams FDA, CDC policies on disclosing financial conflicts." *Reuters Medical News* (August 24, 2000).
19. Ibid.
20. Vesikari, T., Matson, D., Offit, P., Clark, HF., et al. "Safety and efficacy of a pentavalent human-bovine (WC3) reassortment rotavirus vaccine." *NEJM* (January 5, 2006);354:23-33.
21. Ibid.
22. Biology News. "New rotavirus vaccine joins routine infant immunization schedule." www.biologynews.net/archives (Feb 22, 2006).
23. See Note 20.
24. Gillis, J. "Rotavirus vaccine urged for babies." *Washington Post* (February 22, 2006). www.washingtonpost.com
25. Ibid.
26. Rotavirus Vaccine Program: A PATH Affiliate. "Vaccine Facts." PATH. www.rotavirusvaccine.org (Accessed: September 22, 2006).
27. Reuters. "FDA approves Rotarix® [Rotavirus vaccine, live, oral]..." (April 3, 2008). www.reuters.com
28. Merck & Co., Inc. "RotaTeq [Rotavirus Vaccine, Live, Oral, Pentavalent]." Product insert (Issued: February 2006).
29. See Note 2.
30. Manning, Anita. "Rotavirus vaccines pass trials." *USA Today* (January 5, 2006). www.usatoday.com
31. Greene, Alan. "A-Z Guide: Intussusception." *DrGreene Content* (September 30, 2002). www.drgreene.org
32. Merck & Co., Inc. "Patient Information: RotaTeq, rotavirus vaccine, live, oral, pentavalent" (Feb. 2006).
33. See Note 20.
34. Ibid.
35. Wikipedia. www.wikipedia.org/wiki/hematoschezia
36. National Vaccine Information Center. "MedAlert: Online access to the U.S. government's Vaccine Adverse Event Reporting System (VAERS)." www.medalerts.org (Database last accessed: July 27, 2007.)
37. Grossman, Rami. "Seizures." *Pediatric Neurology Site* 2006. www.childbrain.com/shtml
38. See Note 28.
39. Ibid.
40. Ibid.
41. See Note 20.

42. See Note 28.
43. Barclay, L. and Murata, P. "New guidelines for pediatric use of rotavirus vaccine." *Medscape Medical News* (September 5, 2006).
44. National Institutes of Health. "Otitis Media (Ear Infection)." *National Institute on Deafness and Other Communication Disorders*. www.nidcd.nih.gov (Accessed: September 18, 2006).
45. See Note 28.
46. Ibid.
47. Ibid.
48. Ibid.
49. Ibid.
50. Strebel, Peter M., et al. "Epidemiology of poliomyelitis in U.S. one decade after the last reported case of indigenous wild virus associated disease," *Clinical Infectious Diseases* (CDC: February 1992):568-79.
51. Gorman, Christine. "When the vaccine causes polio." *Time* (October 30, 1995):83.
52. Shaw, Donna. "Unintended casualties in war on polio." *Philadelphia Inquirer* (June 6, 1993):A1.
53. U.S. Department of Health and Human Services. "Rotavirus vaccine: what you need to know." *CDC*. (April 12, 2006).
54. CDC. "Recommended childhood immunization schedule for persons aged 0-6 years, United States, 2011."
55. Ibid.
56. GlaxoSmithKline. "Rotarix® (Rotavirus Vaccine, Live, Oral) Oral Suspension." Product insert from the manufacturer. (Revised: April 2008.)
57. Ibid.
58. Ruiz-Palacios, GM, et al. "Safety and efficacy of an attenuated vaccine against severe rotavirus gastroenteritis." *NEJM* (January 5, 2006);354:11-22. See also Table 2.
59. Linker, A. "Study: GSK vaccine may increase risk of convulsion, death." *Triangle Business Journal* (Feb 15, 2008).
60. Friedland, L. "GSK's human rotavirus vaccine Rotarix®: presentation to the ACIP." *GlaxoSmithKline* (June 25, 2008).
61. Fisher, BL. "FDA panel approves Rotarix safety 11-1." *Vaccine Awakening* (February 21, 2008).
62. FDA. Center for biologics evaluation and research: product approval information—STN: BL 125122 (March 14, 2008).
63. Parrillo, SJ. "Pediatrics, Kawasaki disease." eMedicine, WebMD (April 15, 2008).
64. Health Canada. "Summary basis of decision (SBD) Rotarix™." (July 23, 2008):16. www.hc-sc.gc.ca
65. See Note 56.
66. See Note 27.
67. See Note 58.
68. FDA. Center for biologics evaluation and research, vaccines and related biological products advisory committee meeting (February 20, 2008):44-46.
69. Ibid.
70. Ibid.
71. Ibid, pp. 127-128.
72. See Note 58.
73. See Note 20.
74. Ibid.
75. See Note 56
76. See Note 28.
77. Sander, DM. "Diarrhoea viruses: astroviruses; caliciviruses; reoviruses (rotaviruses)." *Tulane University* (February16,1999). www.tulane.edu
78. See Note 3.
79. See Note 32.
80. Roderick, et al. *Epidem and Infection* 1995;114:277-288.
81. See Note 76.
82. See Notes 20 and 28.
83. See Note 43.
84. See Notes 3 and 43.
85. See Note 28.
86. See Note 30.
87. See Note 76.
88. This unsolicited personal story was received by the *Thinktwice Global Vaccine Institute*. www.thinktwice.com
89. See Notes 3 and 5.
90. Victora, CG., et al. "Reducing deaths from diarrhoea through oral rehydration therapy." *Bull WHO* 2000;78(10):1246-55.

Human Papilloma Virus (HPV)

1. National Cancer Institute. "Vaccine Protects Against Virus Linked to Half of All Cervical Cancers." *U.S. National Institutes of Health* (November 26, 2002). www.cancer.gov
2. FDA. "HPV (Human Papillomavirus)" (August 25, 2006). www.fda.gov/womens/getthefacts/hpv.html
3. Ibid.
4. Reuters. "Cervical cancer rates fall" (Feb 4, 2007). www.msnbc.com
5. American Cancer Society. "Estimated new cancer cases and deaths by sex for all sites, U.S., 2007." *Cancer Facts and Figures 2007*.
6. National Cancer Institute. "Cervix uteri cancer (invasive): Age adjusted SEER incidence rates by year, race and age, Table V-2." *Surveillance Epidemiology and End Results (SEER) Cancer Statistics Review*, 1975-2004. National Institutes of Health. www.seer.cancer.gov (July 10, 2007).
7. National Cancer Institute. "Cervix uteri cancer (invasive): Age adjusted U.S. death rates by year, race and age, Table V-3." *SEER Cancer Statistics Review*, 1975-2004. National Institutes of Health. www.seer.cancer.gov (Last accessed: July 10, 2007.)
8. See Notes 6 and 7.
9. American Cancer Society. "What are the key statistics about cervical cancer?" www.cancer.org (Last accessed: July 20, 2007.)
10. American Cancer Society. *Cancer Facts and Figures 2007*, p. 21.
11. CDC. "Cancer—cervical cancer statistics." www.apps.nccd.cdc.gov
12. National Cancer Institute. "Median age of cancer patients at diagnosis, 2000-2004; Table I-11." *SEER Cancer Statistics Review*, 1975-2004. National Institutes of Health. www.seer.cancer.gov (Last accessed: July 10, 2007.)
13. National Cancer Institute. "Age distribution (%) of incidence cases by site, 2000-2004; Table I-10." *SEER Cancer Statistics Review*, 1975-2004. National Institutes of Health. www.seer.cancer.gov (July 10, 2007).
14. National Cancer Institute. "Age distribution (%) of deaths by site, 2000-2004; Table I-12." *SEER Cancer Statistics Review*, 1975-2004. National Institutes of Health. www.seer.cancer.gov (Last accessed: July 10, 2007.)
15. National Cancer Institute. "SEER incidence and U.S. death rates, age-adjusted and age-specific rates, by race; Table V-4." *SEER Cancer Statistics Review*, 1975-2004. NIH. www.seer.cancer.gov (July 10, 2007).
16. National Cancer Institute. "U.S. complete prevalence counts, invasive cancers only, January 1, 2004; Table I-22." *SEER Cancer Statistics Review*, 1975-2004. NIH. www.seer.cancer.gov (Last accessed: July 10, 2007.)
17. CDC. "Age-adjusted invasive cancer incidence rates... United States, Females 2003; Table 1.1.1.1F. *United States Cancer Statistics: 2003 Incidence and Mortality*.
18. U.S. Food and Drug Administration. "FDA licenses new vaccine for prevention of cervical cancer and other diseases in females caused by human papillomavirus" (June 8, 2006). www.fda.gov/bbs/topics/NEWS/2006/NEW01385.html
19. Medical News Today. "CDC panel recommends HPV vaccine Gardasil for all girls ages 11, 12, recommends coverage by federal program" (July 4, 2006). www.medicalnewstoday.com
20. WebMD. "Sexual health glossary: human papillomavirus (HPV)" (Aug 6, 2006). www.climodien.com/glossary/glossary.htm
21. Merck & Co., Inc. "Patient Information About Gardasil" (June 2006).
22. Merck & Co., Inc. "Product news: FDA approves Merck's Gardasil, the world's first and only cervical cancer vaccine." Merck Press Release: June 8, 2006. www.merck.com
23. Medical News Today. GSK does not expect FDA approval of HPV vaccine Cervarix until end of 2009" (July 3, 2008).
24. Merck & Co., Inc. "Gardasil [Quadrivalent Human Papillomavirus (Types 6, 11, 6, 18) Recombinant Vaccine)]." Product insert from the vaccine manufacturer (Issued: June 2006).
25. Inserts from manufacturer: Description. www.pneumo.com
26. "Role of aluminum sensitivity in delayed persistent immunization reactions." *J Clinical Pathology* 1991;44:876-77.
27. Kawahara, M., et al. "Effects of Aluminum on the Neurotoxicity of Primary Cultured Neurons and on the Aggregation of Betamyloid Protein." *Brain Res. Bulletin* 2001;55:211-217.
28. Redhead, K., et al. "Aluminum-adjuvanted vaccines transiently increase aluminum levels in murine brain tissue." *Pharmacol. Toxico* 1992;70:278-280.
29. Sahin, G., et al. "Determination of aluminum levels in the kidney, liver and brain of mice treated with aluminum hydroxide." *Biol. Trace. Elem. Res.* (April-May 1994):129-135.
30. Gherardi, M., et al. "Macrophagic myofastitis lesions assess long-term persistence of vaccine-derived aluminum hydroxide in muscle." *Brain* 2001; Vol 124, No. 9:1821-1831.
31. Shingde, M., et al. "Macrophagic myofastitis associated with vaccine derived aluminum. *MJA* 2005; 183(03):145-146.
32. "Aluminum toxicity in infants and children (RE9607)," *Pediatrics* (Mar 1996) 97, No. 3.;413-416. www.aap.org/policy
33. See Note 24, Table 6.
34. Koutsky, LA., et al. "A Controlled Trial of a Human Papillomavirus Type 16 Vaccine." *NEJM* (Nov. 21, 2002);347 (21):1650, Table 4.
35. Ibid, p. 1650.
36. FDA. "Gardasil™ HPV Quadrivalent Vaccine, May 18, 2006 VRBPAC Meeting." Vaccines and Related Biological Products Advisory Committee Background Document.
37. HealthDay. "FDA Documents Reveal Concerns About HPV Vaccine." *Health Highlights* (May 17, 2006). www.health info.cedars-sinai.edu
38. See Note 24, Pregnancy.
39. Ibid.
40. Ibid.
41. See Note 36.
42. See Note 24, Adverse Reactions and Table 10.
43. National Vaccine Information Center. "MedAlert: Online access to the U.S. government's Vaccine Adverse Event Reporting System (VAERS)." www.medalerts.org
44. Vaccine Adverse Event Reporting System VAERS. Rockville, MD.
45. Judicial Watch. "Examining the FDA's HPV vaccine records: detailing the approval process, side-effects, safety concerns, and marketing practices of a large-scale public health experiment." (June 30, 2008.) www.judicialwatch.org/gardasil
46. Hall, R. "HPV vaccine distribution stalled by adverse reactions.'" *Cybercast News Service* (Jun 1, 2007). www.cnsnews.com
47. See Notes 43-45.
48. Institute of Medicine. "Vaccine safety committee proceedings." (*National Academy of Sciences*: Washington, DC, May 11, 1992):40-41.
49. See Notes 43 and 44.
50. Hurwitz, ES., et al. "Guillain-Barré syndrome and the 1978-79 influenza vaccine." *NEJM* 1981;304:1557-61.
51. Kaplan, JE., et al. "Guillain-Barré syndrome in the United States, 1978-1981: Additional observation from the national surveillance system." *Neurology* 33:633-37.
52. Scheibner, V. "Flu vaccination: Is it safe?" *Natural Health* (June/July 1993):19-21.
53. See Note 24, Adverse reactions: safety in concomitant use with other vaccines.
54. See Notes 43 and 44.
55. Collier, K., et al. "Vaccine linked to sickness." *News.com* (May 22, 2007). www.news.com.au
56. "Parents urged not to panic over Gardasil." *The Age Company* (May 22, 2007).
57. Collier, K., et al. "Call for cancer vaccine calm." *Adelaide Now* (May 22, 2007).

58. See Note 34, pp. 1645-1646.
59. See Note 34, pp. 1646-1647.
60. Ibid.
61. See Note 34, p. 1649.
62. Bosch, FX., et al. "Prevalence of human papillomavirus in cervical cancer: a worldwide perspective." *J National Cancer Inst* 1995;87:796-802.
63. See Note 34, Table 1.
64. See Note 34, p. 1648.
65. The Henry J. Kaiser Family Foundation. "FDA Announces Approval of HPV Vaccine Gardasil" (June 9, 2006). www.kaiser network.org
66. See Note 24, Clinical Studies.
67. Medical News Today. "Merck's HPV Vaccine in Phase III Trial 100% Effective for Two Strains Causing 70% of Cervical Cancer Cases" (October 9, 2005). www.medicalnewstoday.com
68. See Note 22.
69. See Note 67.
70. See Note 24, Table 1.
71. Carreyrou, J. "Questions on efficacy cloud a cancer vaccine." *The Wall Street Journal* (Apr 16, 2007): A1 and A11.
72. See Note 24, Clinical Studies.
73. See Note 24, Precautions.
74. See Note 18.
75. See Note 24, Clinical Studies; Table 1; Table 2.
76. See Note 18.
77. See Note 71.
78. Ibid.
79. Ibid.
80. See Note 21, Bridging the Efficacy of Gardasil from Young Adults to Young Adolescents.
81. See Note 24, Bridging the Efficacy of Gardasil from Young Adult Women to Adolescent Girls.
82. Ibid., Table 5.
83. Garenne, M., et al. "Child mortality after high-titre measles vaccines: prospective study in Senegal." *Lancet* 1991;338:903-7.
84. See Note 81.
85. See note 18.
86. Fisher, BL. "Merck's Gardasil Vaccine Not Proven Safe for Little Girls: National Vaccine Information Center Criticizes FDA for Fast-Tracking Licensure." *National Vaccine Information Center*. Press Release: June 27, 2006. www.909shot.com
87. Ibid.
88. See Notes 43-45..
89. Dunne, EF., et al. "Prevalence of HPV infection among females in the United States." *JAMA* 2007;297:813-19.
90. Ibid.
91. American Social Health Association. "Learn about HPV myths and misconceptions." *National HPV and Cervical Cancer Resource Center*. www.ashastd.org/hpv/hpv_learn_myths.cfm (Accessed: July 23, 2007.)
92. See Note 89.
93. See Note 24.
94. See Notes 24 and 36.
95. Koutsky, MA., et al. (The Future II Study Group.) "Quadrivalent vaccine against human papillomavirus to prevent high-grade cervical lesions." *New England Journal of Medicine* (May 10, 2007);356:1915-27.
96. Maugh II, TH., et al. "Study raises questions about HPV vaccine." *The New Mexican* (May 10, 2007): A1 and A4.
97. Saslow, D. "American Cancer Society guideline for human papillomavirus (HPV) vaccine use to prevent cervical cancer and its precursors." *CA: A Cancer Journal for Clinicians* 2007; 57:7-28.
98. See Notes 24 and 36.
99. See note 36.
100. See Note 36.
101. Roehr, R. "HPV vaccine provides cross-protection against other strains." *Medscape Medical News* (Sep 20, 2007). www.medscape.com [Data was presented in Chicago at the 47th Annual Interscience Conference on Antimicrobial Agents and Chemotherapy. Not yet published in a peer-reviewed journal.]
102. Susman, E. "ICAAC: Gardasil provides cross protection against wide array of HPV types." *Medpage Today* (Sep 20, 2007). www.medpagetoday.com [Data had not yet been published.]
103. See Note 24.
104. ASCUS-LSIL Triage Study (ALTS) Group. "Results of a randomized trial on the management of cytology interpretations of atypical squamous cells of undetermined significance." *Amer J Obstet and Gynecology* 2003;188:1383-92.
105. Sawaya, GF., et al. "HPV vaccination—more answers, more questions." *NEJM* (May 10, 2007);356:1991-93.
106. See Notes 104 and 105.
107. Ibid.
108. See Note 105.
109. Ibid.
110. Ibid.
111. See Notes 1 and 2.
112. See Notes 24 and 36.
113. Abma, JC., et al. "Teenagers in the United States: sexual activity, contraceptive use, and childbearing, 2002." *Vital Health Statistics 23*, 2004:1-48.
114. See Note 71.
115. Ibid.
116. Jit, M., et al. "Prevalence of HPV antibodies in young female subjects in England." *Br J of Cancer* 2007;97:989-991.
117. Maugh II, TH., et al. "Doubts arise about cancer vaccine: benefits of HPV shots are called 'modest'; young women, parents are urged to be cautious." *Baltimore Sun* (May 10, 2007). www.baltimoresun.com
118. See Note 36.
119. Ibid.
120. See Notes 43 and 44.
121. Urwin, G., et al. "Invasive disease due to haemophilus influenzae serotype f: clinical and epidemiologic characteristics in the H. Influenzae serotype b vaccine era. The haemophilus influenzae study group." *Clinical Infectious Disease* (June 1996);22(6):1069-76.

122. Lipsitch, M. "Bacterial vaccines and serotype replacement: lessons from haemophilus influenzae and prospects for streptococcus pneumoniae." *Emerging Infectious Diseases* (May-June 1999);5(3):336-45.
123. Lipsitch, M. "Vaccination against colonizing bacteria with multiple serotypes." *Proceedings of the National Academy of Sciences* (June 10, 1997);94(12):6571-76.
124. Farrell, DJ., et al. "Increased antimicrobial resistance among nonvaccine serotypes of *streptococcus pneumoniae* in the pediatric population after the introduction of 7-valent pneumococcal vaccine in the United States." *Pediatric Infectious Disease Journal* 2007;26(2):123-28.
125. See Note 105.
126. See Note 36.
127. See Note 105.
128. See Notes 36 and 105.
129. Peterson, LA. "Texas governor orders anti-cancer vaccine for schoolgirls." *Examiner* (Feb 2, 2007). www.examiner.com
130. See Note 71.
131. Hoppe, C. "Perry orders HPV vaccine: surprise move mandates shots for schoolgirls to prevent sex virus that leads to cancer." *Dallas News* (Feb. 3, 2007). www.dallasnews.com
132. See Notes 71, 129 and 131.
133. Peterson, LA. "Merck lobbies states over cancer vaccine." *The Associated Press* (January 30, 2007). www.chron.com
134. See Note 131.
135. See Note 71.
136. See Note 133.
137. Gardner, A. "Merck to stop pushing to require shots." *Wash. Post* (Feb. 21, 2007). www.washingtonpost.com
138. Sturgeon, J. "Merck speaker muddies decision." *The Roanoke Times* (March 3, 2007). www.roanoke.com
139. Ibid.
140. Reuters. "Texas governor backs down on HPV vaccine effort." *Scientific American* (May 8, 2007). www.sciam.com
141. Laine, N. "Life with big brother: California on track to mandate STD vaccine." *World Net Daily* (July 5, 2007). www.wnd.com
142. This unsolicited personal story was received by the *Thinktwice Global Vaccine Institute*. www.thinktwice.com
143. Stewart, AM., et al. "Mandating HPV vaccination— private rights, public good." *NEJM* (May 10, 2007);356:1998-99.
144. Ibid.
145. Gostin, LO., et al. "Mandatory HPV vaccination: public health vs private wealth." *JAMA* (May 2, 2007);297:1921-23.
146. Ibid.
147. Stewart, N., et al. "DC bill would mandate vaccine." *Washington Post* (January 10, 2007):A1.
148. See Note 141.
149. See Note 105.
150. Fisher, BF. "Going for the throat: hyping HPV vaccine for boys." *Vaccine Awakening* (Sep 12, 2007). www.vaccine awakening.blogspot.com
151. Ibid.
152. Adams, M. "Absurd vaccine marketing calls for cervical cancer vaccinations for young boys!" *News Target* (August 29, 2007). www.newstarget.com
153. Stein, Rob. "Cervical cancer vaccine gets injected with a social issue: some fear a shot for teens could encourage sex." *Washington Post* (October 31, 2005). www.washingtonpost.com
154. Ibid.
155. Ibid.
156. Ibid.
157. Block, G., et al. "Fruit, vegetables, and cancer prevention: a review of the epidemiological evidence." *Nutrition and Cancer* 1992;18:1-29.
158. Steinmetz, K., et al. "A review of vegetables, fruit and cancer. I. Epid." *Cancer Causes, Control* 1991;2:325-357.
159. Steinmetz, K., et al. "A review of vegetables, fruit and cancer. II. Mechanism." *Cancer Causes, Control* 1991;2:427-442.
160. Hernandez, BY., et al. "Diet and premalignant lesions of the cervix: Evidence of a protective role for folate, riboflavin, thiamin, and vitamin B12." *Cancer Causes and Control* (Nov. 2003);14(9):859–70.
161. Butterworth CE Jr, Hatch KD, et al. "Oral folic acid supplementation for cervical dysplasia: A clinical intervention trial." *Am J Obstet Gynecol*. (March 1992);166(3):803–9.
162. Butterworth, CE, et al. "Folate deficiency and cervical dysplasia." *JAMA* 1992;267:528-533.
163. Butterworth, CE Jr, Hatch, KD., et al. "Improvement in cervical dysplasia associated with folic acid therapy in users of oral contraceptives." *Am J Clin Nutr*. (Jan 1982);35(1):73–82.
164. Kwanbunjan, K., Saengkar, P., et al. "Folate status of Thai women cervical dysplasia." *Asia Pac J Clin Nutr*. 2004;13(Suppl):S171.
165. Sedjo, RL., Fowler, BM., et al. "Folate, vitamin B12, and homocysteine status: Findings of no relation between human papillomavirus persistence and cervical dysplasia." *Nutrition* (June 2003);19(6):839–46.
166. Goodman, MT., et al. "Association of methylenetetrahydrofolate reductase polymorphism C677T and dietary folate with the risk of cervical dysplasia." *Cancer Epidemiol Biomarkers Prev*. (Dec 2001); 10(12):1275–80.
167. Weinstein, SJ., et al. "Low serum and red blood cell folate are moderately, but nonsignificantly associated with increased risk of invasive cervical cancer in U.S. women." *J Nutr*. (July 2001);131(7):2040–8.
168. Piyathilake, CJ., et al. "Methylenetetrahydrofolate reductase (MTHFR) polymorphism increases the risk of cervical intraepithelial neoplasia." *Anticancer Res*. (May-June 2000); 20(3A):1751–7.
169. Fowler, BM., et al. "Hypomethylation in cervical tissue: Is there a correlation with folate status?" *Cancer Epidemiol Biomarkers Prev*. (October 1998);7(10):901–906.
170. Kwasniewska, A., et al. "Folate deficiency and cervical intraepithelial neoplasia." *Eur J Gynaecol Oncol*. 1997; 18(6):526–30.
171. Zarcone, R,. Et al. "Folic acid and cervix dysplasia."

Minerva Ginecol. (Oct 1996);48(10):397–400.
172. Christensen, B. "Folate deficiency, cancer and congenital abnormalities. Is there a connection?" *Tidsskr Nor Laegeforen.* (January 20, 1996);116(2):250–4.
173. Childers, JM., et al. "Chemoprevention of cervical cancer with folic acid: a phase III SWOG intergroup study." *Cancer Epidemiol Biomarkers Prev.* 1995;4:155-9.
174. Grio, R., et al. "Antineoblastic activity of antioxidant vitamins: The role of folic acid in the prevention of cervical dysplasia." *Panminerva Med.* (December 1993);35(4):193–6.
175. Potischman, N., et al. "A case-control study of serum folate levels and invasive cervical cancer." *Cancer Res.* (September 1991);51(18):4785–9.
176. Whitehead, N., et al. "Megaloblastic changes in the cervical epithelium: association with oral contraceptive therapy and reversal with folic acid." *JAMA* 1973;226:1421-1424.
177. Linden, Ann. "Folic Acid: An important way to prevent birth defects." *Baby Center* (March 2004). www.babycenter.com
178. Ibid.
179. Baby Hopes. "Why is Folic Acid important for conception and pregnancy?" www.babyhopes.com/articles/folic-acid.html
180. Meschino, James. "The reversal of cervical dysplasia with vitamin therapy." www.tidesoflife.com/cervical_dysplasia. htm (Sep 10, 2006).
181. See Notes 172 and 174.
182. French, AL., et al. "Association of vitamin A deficiency with cervical squamous intraepithelial lesions in human-immunodeficiency virus-infected women." *J Infect Dis.* (October 2000);182(4):1084–9.
183. Romney, SL., et al. "Effects of beta-carotene and other factors on outcome of cervical dysplasia and human papillomavirus infection." *Gynecol Oncol.* (June 1997);65(3): 483–92.
184. Comerci, JT. Jr., et al. "Induction of transforming growth factor beta-1 in cervical intraepithelial neoplasia in vivo after treatment with beta-carotene." *Clin Cancer Res.* (February 1997);3(2):157–60.
185. Volz, J., et al. "Changes in the vitamin A status in dysplastic epithelium of the cervix." *Zentralbl Gynakol.* 1995; 117(9):472-5.
186. Meyskens, FL. Jr., et al. "Enhancement of regression of cervical intraepithelial neoplasia II (moderate dysplasia) with topical applied all-trans-retinoic acid: a randomized trial." *J Natl Cancer Inst* 1994;86:539-43.
187. De Vet, HC., et al. "Risk factors for cervical dysplasia: implications for prevention." *Am J Pub Health* 1994;108:241-9.
188. De Vet, HC., et al. "The role of beta-carotene and other dietary factors in the aetiology of cervical dysplasia: Results of a case-control study." *Int J Epid* (Sep 1991); 20(3):603–10.
189. Winkelstein, W. Jr. "Smoking and cervical cancer - current status." *Am J Epid* 1990;131:945-57; (discussion:958-60).
190. Palan, PR., et al. "Decreased plasma beta-carotene levels in women with uterine cervical dysplasia and cancer (letter)." *J Natl Cancer Inst* 1988;80:454-5.
191. Lippman, S., et al. "Retinoids as preventive and therapeutic anticancer agents. Part I." *Cancer Treat Rep* 1987; 71:391-405.
192. Graham, V., et al. "Phase II trial of beta-all-trans-retinoic acid for intraepithelial cervical neoplasia delivered via a collagen sponge and cervical cap." *West J Med* 1986;145:192-5.
193. Wylie-Rosett, JA., et al. "Influence of vitamin A on cervical dysplasia and carcinoma in situ." *Nutr Cancer* 1984; 6(1):49–57.
194. Meyskens, FL. Jr., et al. "A phase I trial of beta-all-trans-retinoic acid for mild or moderate intraepithelial cervical neoplasia delivered via a collagen sponge and cervical cap." *J Natl Cancer Inst* 1983;71:921-5.
195. Romney, SL., et al. "Retinoids and the prevention of cervical dysplasias." *Am J Obstet Gynecol.* (December 15, 1981);141(8):890–4.
196. Yeo, AS., et al. "Serum micronutrients and cervical dysplasia in Southwestern American Indian women." *Nutr Cancer* 2000;38(2):141–50.
197. Kanetsky, PA., et al. "Dietary intake and blood levels of lycopene: association with cervical dysplasia among non-hispanic, black women." *Nutr Cancer* 1998;31:31-40.
198. Goodman, MT., et al. "The association of plasma micronutrients with the risk of cervical dysplasia in Hawaii." *Cancer Epidemiol Biomarkers Prev.* (June 1998);7(6):537–44.
299. Buckley, DI., et al. "Dietary micronutrients and cervical dysplasia in southwestern American Indian women." *Nutr Cancer* 1992;17(2):179–85.
200. Van Eenwyk, J., et al. "Dietary and serum carotenoids and cervical intraepithelial neoplasia." *Int J Canc* 1991;48:34-38.
201. Rybnikov, VI. "Trace element content in the blood and tissues of patients with precancerous and precursor diseases of the female genitalia." *Vopr Onkol.* 1985;31(3):18–21.
202. Liu, T., et al. "A case control study of nutritional factors and cervical dysplasia." *Cancer Epidemiol Biomarkers Prev.* (Nov-Dec 1993);2(6): 525–30.
203. Ramaswamy, PJ., "Vitamin B6 status in patients with cancer of the uterine cervix." *Nutr Cancer* 1984;6(3):176–80.
204. Kwasniewska, A., et al. "Frequency of HPV infection and the level of ascorbic acid in serum of women with cervix dysplasia." *Med Dosw Mikrobiol.* 1996;48(3–4):183–8.
205. Basu, J., et al. "Plasma ascorbic acid and beta-carotene levels in women evaluated for HPV infection, smoking, and cervix dysplasia." *Cancer Detect Prev.* 1991;15:165-70.
206. Romney, SL., et al. "Plasma reduced and total ascorbic acid in human uterine cervix dysplasias, cancer." *Ann N Y Acad Sci* 1987;498:132-43.
207. Romney, SL., et al. "Plasma vitamin C and uterine cervical dysplasia." *Am J Obstet Gynecol* (April 1, 1985); 151(7):976–80.
208. Wassertheil-Smoller, S., et al. "Dietary vitamin C and uterine cervical dysplasia." *Am J Epidemiol* (November 1981);114(5):714–24.
209. Friedman, M., et al. "Anticarcinogenic effects of glycoalkaloids from potatoes against human cervical, liver, lymphoma, and stomach cancer cells." *J Agric Food Chem.* (July 27, 2005);53(15):6162–9.
210. Greenlee, H., et al. "Supplement use among cancer

survivors in the Vitamins and Lifestyle (VITAL) study cohort." *J Altern Complement Med.* (August 2004);10(4):660–6.
211. Shannon, J., et al. "Dietary risk factors for invasive and in-situ cervical carcinomas in Bangkok, Thailand." *Cancer Causes Control* (October 2002);13(8):691–9.
212. Sedjo, RL., et al. "Human papillomavirus persistence and nutrients involved in the methylation pathway among a cohort of young women." *Cancer Epidemiol Biomarkers Prev.* (April 2002);11(4):353–9.
213. Kwasniewska, A., et al. "Dietary factors in women with dysplasia colli uteri associated with human papillomavirus infection." *Nutr Cancer* 1998;30(1):39–45.
214. Potischman, N., et al. "Nutrition and cervical neoplasia." *Cancer Causes Control* (January 1996);7(1):113–26.
215. Meyskens, FL., et al. "Prevention of cervical intraepithelial neoplasia and cervical cancer." *Am J Clin Nutr* 1995; 62(suppl):1417S-9S.
216. Liu, T., et al. "A longitudinal analysis of human papillomavirus 16 infection, nutritional status, and cervical dysplasia progression." *Cancer Epidemiol Biomarkers Prev.* (June 1995);4(4):373–80.
217. Amburgey, CF., et al. "Undernutrition as a risk factor for cervical intraepithelial neoplasia: case-control." *Nutr Cancer* 1993;20(1):51–60.
218. Batieha, AM., et al. "Serum micronutrients and the subsequent risk of cervical cancer in a population-based nested case-control study." *Cancer Epidemiol Biomarkers Prev.* 1993; 2:335-9.
219. Schneider, A., et al. "The role of vitamins in the etiology of cervical neoplasia: an epidemiological review." *Arch Gynecol Obstet* 1989;246:1-13.
220. Brock, KE., et al. "Nutrients in diet and plasma and risk of in situ cervical cancer." *J Natl Cancer Inst* 1988;80:580-5.
221. Grail, A., et al. "Copper and zinc levels in serum from patients with abnormalities of the uterine cervix." *Acta Obstet Gynecol Scand.* 1986;65(5):443–7.
222. Ziegler, RG. "Epidemiological studies of vitamins and cancer of the lung, esophagus, and cervix." *Adv Exp Med Biol.* 1986;206:11–26.
223. Lee, GJ., et al. "Antioxidant vitamins and lipid peroxidation in patients with cervical intraepithelial neoplasia." *J Korean Med Sci.* (April 2005);20(2):267–72.
224. Palan, PR., et al. "Alpha-tocopherol and alpha-tocopherol quinone levels in cervical intraepithelial neoplasia and cervical cancer." *Am J Obstet Gynecol.* (May 2004);190(5):1407–10.
225. Palan, PR., et al. "Plasma concentrations of coenzyme Q10 and tocopherols in cervical intraepithelial neoplasia and cervical cancer." *Eur J Cancer Prev.* (August 2003);12(4):321–6.
226. Kim, SY., et al. "Changes in lipid peroxidation and antioxidant trace elements in serum of women with cervical intraepithelial neoplasia and invasive cancer." *Nutr Cancer* 2003;47(2):126–30.
227. Ho, GY., et al. "Viral characteristics of human papillomavirus infection and antioxidant levels as risk factors for cervical dysplasia." *Int J Canc* (Nov 23, 1998);78(5):594–9.
228. Giuliano, AR., et al. "Can cervical dysplasia and cancer be prevented with nutrients?" *Nutr Rev.* (Jan 1998);56(1 Pt 1): 9–16.
229. Giuliano, AR., et al. "Antioxidant nutrients: Associations with persistent human papillomavirus infection." *Cancer Epidemiol Biomarkers Prev.* (November 1997);6(11):917–23.
230. Palan, PR., et al. "Plasma levels of beta-carotene, lycopene, canthaxanthin, retinol, and alpha- and tau-tocopherol in cervical intraepithelial neoplasia and cancer." *Clin Cancer Res.* (January 1996);2(1):181–5.
231. Palan, PR., et al. "Plasma levels of antioxidant beta-carotene and alpha-tocopherol in uterine cervix dysplasias and cancer." *Nutr Cancer* 1991;15(1):13–20.
232. Weber, WM., et al. "Anti-oxidant activities of curcumin and related enomes." *Bioorg Med Chem.* (June 1, 2005); 13(11):3811–20.
233. Ahn, WS., et al. "Protective effects of green tea extracts (polyphenon E and EGCG) on human cervical lesions." *Eur J Cancer Prev.* (October 2003);12(5):383–90.
234. Gagandeep, DS., et al. "Chemopreventive effects of Cuminum cyminum in chemically induced forestomach and uterine cervix tumors in murine model systems." *Nutr Cancer* 2003;47(2):171–80.
235. See Notes 187, 193 and 195.
236. See Note 200.
237. See Note 197.
238. See Note 208.

RSV

1. CDC. "Respiratory syncytial virus." *National Center for Infectious Disease* 1999. www.cdc.gov/ncidod/dvrd/nrevss/ rsvfeat.htm
2. Public Health Laboratory Service, United Kingdom. "Seasonal diseases: RSV infections." www.phls.co.uk/seasonal/rsv/ RSV13.htm (Mar 16, 2000).
3. Baltimore, JG. "RSV—a serious subject." *The Triplet Connection* 2000. www.tripletconnection.com
4. See Note 1.
5. Ibid.
6. Travel and Health. "Questions and answers on Synagis." www.travelandhealth.com/synagis.htm
7. See Note 3.
8. Morris, JA. "Recovery of cytopathogenic agent from chimpanzees with coryza (22538)." *Proc Soc Exp Biol Med* 1956;92:544-49.
9. Scheibner, Viera. *Vaccination: 100 Years of Orthodox Research Shows that Vaccines Represent a Medical Assault on the Immune System.* (Blackheath, NSW, Australia: Scheibner Publications, 1993):153.
10. Parrot, RH., et al. "II. Serological studies over a 34-month period in children with bronchiolitis, pneumonia and minor respiratory diseases." *JAMA* 1961;176(8):653-57.

11. Chanock, RM., et al. "Respiratory syncytial virus." *J of the American Medical Association* 1961; 176(8):647-53.
12. Ibid.
13. Hamparian, V., et al. "Recovery of new viruses (coryza) from cases of common cold in human adults." *Proc Soc Exp Med Biol* 1961;108:444-453.
14. Keep Kids Healthy. "Preventing RSV." www.keepkidshealthy.com
15. Applied Genetic News. "Eat your vaccine, dear." *Business Communications Company* (August 2000). www.findarticles.com
16. Initiative for Vaccine Research. "Respiratory syncytial virus (RSV)." *World Health Org* 2007. www.who.int
17. See Note 3.
18. FDA. "FDA licenses biotech product to prevent serious RSV disease." *U.S. Department of Health and Human Services* (June 19, 1998). www.fda.gov/bbs/topics/answers/ans00878.html
19. Medimmune, Inc. "Synagis® (Palivizumab) for intramuscular administration." Manufacturer's product insert (October 2007).
20. See Note 14.
21. "More on cost of synagis..." (Posted March 26, 1999 on an internet forum.) www.home.vicnet.net.au
22. See Note 19.
23. The Impact-RSV Study Group. "Palivizumab, a humanized respiratory syncytial virus monoclonal antibody, reduces hospitalization from respiratory syncytial virus infection in high-risk infants." *Pediatrics* 1998;102:531-537.
24. See Note 19.
25. Ibid.
26. National Cancer Institute. "SGOT." *U.S. National Institutes of Health.* www.cancer.gov (Nov. 24, 2007).
27. See Notes 19 and 23.
28. Ibid.
29. Ibid.

Anthrax

1. Turkington, CA. "Anthrax." *Gale Encyclopedia of Medicine* 1999. www.findarticles.com
2. "Anthrax." Encarta Encyclopedia. www.encarta.msn.com (Accessed: October 2001).
3. CDC. "Anthrax." www.cdc.gov/ncidod/dbmd/diseaseinfo /anthrax_g.htm (Accessed: October 2001).
4. Ibid.
5. Ritter, M. "Precautions on ranches and in factories have helped keep the disease rare in the U.S." *Albuquerque Journal* (October 21, 2001):B8.
6. See Note 1.
7. Ibid.
8. See Note 5.
9. Stolberg, SG., et al. "After a week of reassurances, Ridge's anthrax message is grim." *The New York Times* (Oct 26, 2001). www.nytimes.com
10. See Notes 1 and 3.
11. Ibid.
12. Flegel, DE. "FDA oks use of doxycycline after anthrax exposure." WebMD (October 22, 2001). www.content.health.msn.com
13. CDC. *MMWR Morb Mortal Wkly Rep* 2001;50:1031-1034.
14. "Cipro." *Drug InfoNet* 2000. www.druginfonet.com/ cipro.htm
15. Ibid.
16. Park, A. "Cipro to Doxy: Why the Switch?" *Time.com* (November 5, 2001). www.time.com
17. Reuters Medical News. "Postal workers report high rate of adverse events from anthrax prophylaxis." *Medscape* (November 29, 2001).
18. Health Square. "Doryx (Doxycycline hyclate)." *The PDR Family Guide to Prescription Drugs.* www.healthsquare.com (November 1, 2001).
19. See Note 14.
20. Begley, S., et al. "Anthrax: what you need to know." *Newsweek* (October 29, 2001):39.
21. See Notes 1 and 3.
22. Ibid.
23. Ibid.
24. See Note 20
25. See Notes 1 and 3.
26. See Note 2.
27. Ibid.
28. Nass, M. "New vaccines and new vaccine technology: anthrax vaccine— model of a response to the biologic warfare threat." *Infectious Disease Clinics of North America* (W.B. Saunders Company, 1999);13(1):188.
29. Shlyakov, EN., et al. "Human live anthrax vaccine in the former USSR." *Vaccine* 1994;12:727.
30. Turnbull, PCB. "Anthrax vaccines; past, present and future." *Vaccine* 1991;9:533.
31. Ibid.
32. Anthony, BF., et al. "The role of te FDA in vaccine testing and licensure." In Lelvine, MM., et al., (eds.): *New Generation Vaccins,* ed. 2. (NY: Marcel Dekker, 1997):1185.
33. Oppliger, D. "Congressional memorandum (about the Sept 24, 1998 hearing on the sale of MBPI)." *House Majority Counsel* (Sept 23, 1998).
34. Wright, GG., et al. "Studies on immunity in anthrax. V. Immunizing activity of alum-precipitated protective antigen." *J Immun* 1954;73:387-391.
35. Ibid.
36. Darlow, HM., et al. "The use of anthrax antigen to immunise man and monkey." *Lancet* 1956;2:476-479.
37. Brachman, PS., et al. "Field evaluation of a human anthrax vaccine." *American Journal of Public Health* 1962;52:632-645.
38. Ibid.
39. Ibid.
40. See Note 28, p. 189.
41. Institute of Medicine. "An Assessment of the Safety of the Anthrax Vaccine." (March 30, 2000):3-4.
42. Official Document. "Anthrax vaccine chronology." *JFSorg*
2001. www.enter.net/~jfsorg/timeline.pdf
43. Ibid.
44. See Note 41.
45. Peeler, RN., et al. "Intensive immunization of man: evaluation of possible adverse consequences." *Annals of Internal Med* 1965;63(1):44-57.
46. White, CS., et al. "Repeated immunization: possible adverse effects." *Annals of Internal Med* 1974; 81(5):594-600.
47. See Note 41, p. 5.
48. Ivins, BE., et al. "Immunization studies with attenuated strains of Bacillus anthracis." *Infect Immun* 1986; 52:454.
49. Little, SF., et al. "Comparative efficacy of Bacillus anthracis live spore vaccine and protective antigen vaccine against anthrax in the guinea pig." *Infect Immun* 1986;52:509-512
50. Ivins, BE., et al. "Recent advances in the development of an improved, human anthrax vaccine." *European Journal of Epidemiology* 1988;4:12.
51. Turnbull, PCB., et al. "Antibodies to anthrax toxin in humans and guinea pigs and their relevance to protective immunity." *Med Microbiol Immunol* 1988;177:293.
52. Ivins, BE., et al. "Immunization against anthrax with aromatic compound-dependent (Aro-)mutants of Bacillus anthracis and with recombinant strains of Bacillus subtilis that produce anthrax protective antigen." *Infect Immun* 1990;58:303.
53. Ivins, BE., et al. "Immunization against anthrax with Bacillus anthracis protective antigen combined with adjuvants." *Infect Immun* 1992;60:662.
54. Ivins, BE., et al. "Efficacy of a standard human anthrax vaccine against Bacillus anthracis spore challenge in guinea pigs." *Vaccine* 1994;12:872.
55. Ivins, BE., et al. "Experimental anthrax vaccines: efficacy of adjuvants combined with protective antigen against aerosol Bacillus anthracis spore challenge in guinea pigs." *Vaccine* 1995;13:1779.
56. Welkos, SL., et al. "Comparative safety and efficacy against Bacillus anthracis of protective antigen and live vaccines in mice." *Microb Pathog* 1988;5:127.
57. Welkos, SL., et al. "Pathogenesis and host resistance to Bacillus anthracis: a mouse model." *Salisbury Medical Bulletin* 1990;68:49.
58. See Notes 52 and 53.
59. See Notes 49-57.
60. Broster, MG., et al. "Protective efficacy of anthrax vaccines against aerosol challenge." *Salisbury Med Bulletin* 1990;68:91.
61. Turnbull, PCB., et al. "Protection conferred by microbially supplemented UK and purified PA vaccines." *Salisbury Medical Bulletin* 1990;68:89.
62. Jones, MN., et al. "Efficacy of the UK human anthrax vaccine in guinea pigs against aerosolized spores of Bacillus anthracis." *Salisbury Medical Bulletin* 1996:87:123.
63. Friedlander, AM., et al. "Postexposure prophylaxis against experimental inhalation anthrax." *Journal of Infectious Diseases* 1993;167:1239.
64. Ivins, BE., et al. "Efficacy of a standard human anthrax vaccine against Bacillus anthracis aerosol spore challenge in rhesus monkeys." *Salisbury Medical Bulletin* (Special Supplement) 1996;87:125-126.
65. Enserink, M. "This time it was real: knowledge of anthrax put to the test." *Science* 2001;294:490-91.
66. See Note 64.
67. See Notes 45, 46; 48-57 and 60-63.
68. See Note 64.
69. Ivins, BE., et al. "Comparative efficacy of experimental anthrax vaccine candidates against inhalation anthrax in rhesus macaques." *Vaccine* 1998;16, No. 11/12:1141-1148.
70. Ibid.
71. Fellows, P., et al. "Anthrax vaccine efficacy against B. anthracis strains of diverse geographic origin." Presented at the International Anthrax Conference (September 1998). As noted in the Congressional testimony of Dr. Meryl Nass: *Subcommittee on National Security, Veterans Affairs and International Relations* (April 29, 1999).
72. See Note 37.
73. As noted in the FDA's Anthrax product information leaflet.
74. Avila, J. "Anthrax vaccine limitations." *MSNBC Nightly News* (October 9, 2001). www.msnbc.com/news/640484.asp (Quoting Dr. Meryl Nass.)
75. Brachman, PS., et al. "Anthrax." In Plotkin, SA., et al. (eds.): *Vaccines,* ed. 2. (Philadelphia, PA: W.B. Saunders, 1994):729.
76. See Note 28, p. 189.
77. See Note 73.
78. See Note 74.
79. See Note 28, p. 190.
80. Ibid., p. 189.
81. See Note 73.
82. Ibid.
83. Ibid.
84. National Institutes of Health. "HHS announces contracts for developing a new anthrax vaccine." www.3.niaid.nih.gov (October 3, 2002).
85. Ibid.
86. Associated Press. "New anthrax vaccine shows promise." MSNBC.www.msnbc.msn.com (September 27, 2006).
87. See Notes 74 and 86.
88. Medical News Today. "VaxGen awarded anthrax vaccine contract worth $877.5 million." www.medicalnewstoday.com (November 7, 2004).
89. Medical News Today. "Next clinical trial of VaxGen's anthrax vaccine delayed." www.medicalnewstoday.com (Nov 4, 2006).
90. Merle, R. "VaxGen wins extension on anthrax vaccine." Washington Post (Nov 17, 2006). www.washingtonpost.com
91. See Notes 89 and 90.
92. See Note 90.
93. See Note 86.
94. France, D. "The families who are dying for our country." *Redbook* (September 1994):116.

95. "Experts find link to war illness." *The Albuquerque Tribune* (April 10, 1995):A1+.
96. Geoffrey, C., et al. "Tracking the Second Storm." *Newsweek* (May 16, 1994):56.
97. Brown, D. "Diagnosis Unknown: Gulf War Syndrome." *The Washington Post* (July 26, 1994):A1+.
98. Senator John D. Rockefeller IV, Chair, "Is military research hazardous to veterans' health? Lessons from the cold war, the Persian Gulf, and today: Opening Statement," *United States Senate, Committee on Veterans' Affairs* (May 6, 1994).
99. Diana Zuckerman, PhD., and Patricia Olson, D.V.M., Ph.D., "Is military research hazardous to veterans' health? Lessons from the Persian Gulf: preliminary staff findings," *US Senate, Committee on Veterans' Affairs* (May 6, 1994).
100. Ibid.
101. Ibid.
102. Majority Staff. "Unproven Force Protection." *Subcommittee on National Security, Veterans Affairs and International relations, House Committee on Government Reform* (February 17, 2000):6.
103. These letters are typical of the unsolicited emails received by the *Thinktwice Global Vaccine Institute*. www.thinktwice.com
104. United States District Court for the District of Columbia. John Doe #1, et al, Plaintiffs v. Donald H. Rumsfeld, et al, Defendants; Civil Action No. 03-707. www.dcd.uscourts.gov/03-707.pdf
105. Ibid., www.dcd.uscourts.gov/03-707c.pdf
106. Global Research. "Anthrax vaccine for soldiers serving in Iraq, Afghanistan and South Korea." www.globalresearch.ca (October 17, 2006).
107. "Gulf War illnesses, anthrax vaccine, and steps toward improving DVA healthcare and research for Gulf War veterans." *Hearing, House Committee on Veterans' Affairs, Subcommittee on Health,* Washington, DC. (July 26, 2007).
108. See Note 107; verbal testimony of Meryl Nass, MD.
109. See Note 107; written testimony of Meryl Nass, MD.
110. Ibid.
111. Unwin, S., et al. "Health of U.K. servicemen who served in Persian Gulf War." *Lancet* (Jan 16, 1999);353(9148):169-78.
112. Goss-Gilroy. "Study of Canadian Gulf War Veterans: NR-98.050." Study contracted by the *Canadian Department of National Defense* (Released: June 29, 1998).
113. See Note 107; written testimony of Meryl Nass, MD.
114. Vaccine Adverse Event Reporting System. Rockville, MD.
115. See Note 107; verbal testimony of Meryl Nass, MD.
116. Richardson, D. "Feds designate dubious anthrax "emergency," immunizing themselves from liability." *Prove Newsletter* (October 16, 2008).

Shingles

1. Moon, JE., et al. "Herpes Zoster." *eMedicine.* www.emedicine.com
2. U.S. Department of Health and Human Services. "Shingles vaccine: what you need to know." *CDC.* (September 11, 2006).
3. Zwillich, T. "FDA approves first shingles vaccine—some experts express concerns over cost of vaccine called Zostavax." *WebMD Medical News* (May 25, 2006). www.webmd.com
4. U.S. Department of Health and Human Services. "Shingles (Herpes Zoster)." *CDC.* www.cdc.gov (Sep 13, 2006).
5. See Note 1.
6. See Notes 2 and 4.
7. See Note 4.
8. Ibid.
9. Goldman, Gary. "Universal varicella vaccination: efficacy trends and effect on herpes zoster." *International Journal of Toxicology* 2005;24:205-213.
10. Goldman, Gary. "International journal of toxicology release: chickenpox vaccine associated with shingles epidemic." *PRNewswire* (September 1, 2005).
11. Fisher, Barbara. "Shingles vaccine targets baby boomers." *Vaccine Awakening* (May 1, 2006). www.vaccineawakening.blogspot.com
12. Simpson, Hope. "The nature of herpes zoster" a long-term study and new hypothesis." *Proc. R. Soc. Med.* 1965:58:9-20.
13. See Notes 10-12.
14. See Note 4.
15. See Notes 1 and 2.
16. Yih, WK., et al. "The incidence of varicella and herpes zoster in Massachusetts as measured by the Behavioral Risk Factor Surveillance System (BRFSS) during a period of increasing varicella vaccine coverage, 1998-2003." *BioMed Central, Ltd.* (June 16, 2005).
17. Civen, RH., et al. "2004: Annual report of the active varicella surveillance and epidemiologic studies cooperative agreement No. U66/CCU911165-10." *County of Los Angeles Department of Health Services, Acute Communicable Disease Control and CDC* (Sep 30, 2003 through Sep 29, 2004).
18. See Notes 9 and 10.
19. Goldman, Gary. "Cost-benefit analysis of universal varicella vaccination in the U.S. taking into account the closely related herpes zoster epidemiology." *Vaccine* (May 9, 2005); 3349-3355.
20. LookSmart. "Trading chickenpox for shingles?" *Mothering* (Nov-Dec 2005). www.findarticles.com
21. See Notes 9 and 10.
22. Goldman, Gary. "Chickenpox vaccine associated with shingles epidemic." Press Release: August 2005.
23. See Note 10.
24. In a personal email communication with the author.
25. See Note 10.
26. Ibid.
27. See Notes 10, 11, 20 and 22.
28. See Note 10.
29. Merck & Co., Inc. "Patient Information about Zostavax" (Issued: May 2006).
30. See Notes 9, 10, 11, 20, 22 and 24.
31. See Note 24.
32. See Note 22.
33. Merck & Co., Inc. "Zostavax [Zoster vaccine live (Oka/Merck)]." Product insert from the vaccine manufacturer (Issued: May 2006).
34. Oxman, MN., et al. "A vaccine to prevent herpes zoster and postherpetic neuralgia in older adults." *New England Journal of Medicine* (June 2, 2005); Vol. 352, No. 22:2271-2284.
35. See Notes 33 and 34.
36. Ibid.
37. Ibid.
38. Ibid.
39. See Note 33.
40. Ibid.
41. Ibid.
42. Ibid.
43. Ibid.
44. National Vaccine Information Center. "MedAlert: Online access to the U.S. government's Vaccine Adverse Event Reporting System (VAERS)." www.medalerts.org (Database last accessed: August 6, 2007).
45. See Note 33.
46. FDA. "Product approval information—licensing action: Zostavax questions and answers." www.fda.gov (Updated: May 26, 2006).
47. See Note 33.
48. See Note 34.
49. See Note 3.
50. See Note 34.
51. See Note 33.
52. See Note 34.
53. Ibid.
54. Barclay, L., et al. "Herpes zoster vaccine may be effective in older adults." *Medscape Medical News* (June 2, 2005).
55. See Notes 34 and 54.
56. Ibid.
57. Ibid.
58. The Associated Press. "FDA approves new shingles vaccine: shots will be for older adults who have had chickenpox." *MSNBC* (May 26, 2006). www.msnbc.com
59. FDA. "FDA licenses new vaccine to reduce older Americans' risk of shingles." *FDA News* (News Release: May 26, 2006). www.fda.gov
60. Pollack, Andrew. "Vaccine curbs shingles cases and severity." *The New York Times* (June 2, 2005). www.nytimes.com
61. See Note 3.

Pneumonia

1. University of Michigan Health System. "Pneumococcal pneumonia shot." www.med.umich.edu (July 5, 2007).
2. Ibid.
3. Ibid.
4. Ibid.
5. CDC. "Pneumococcal polysaccharide vaccine: what you need to know." Vaccine information statement (July 29, 1997).
6. See Note 1.
7. See Note 5.
8. Merck & Co., Inc. "Pneumovax® 23 (pneumococcal vaccine polyvalent)." Product insert (Issued: March 2007).
9. Drugs.com. "Pneumococcal vaccine polyvalent (systemic)." www.drugs.com (Accessed: July 5, 2007).
10. See Notes 8 and 9.
11. See Note 8.
12. Ibid.
13. Ibid.
14. CDC. "Recommendation of the Advisory Committee on Immunization Practices—prevention of pneumococcal disease." *MMWR* (April 4, 1997);46(RR-8):1-25.
15. An unsolicited email received by the *Thinktwice Global Vaccine Institute.* www.thinktwice.com
16. Jackson, LA., et al. "Effectiveness of pneumococcal polysaccharide vaccine in older adults." *NEJM* 2003;348:1747-55.
17. Watson, L., et al. "Pneumococcal polysaccharide vaccine: a systemic review of clinical effectiveness in adults." *Vaccine* 2002;20:2166-73.
18. Christenson, B., et al. "Effects of a large-scale intervention with influenza and 23-valent pneumococcal vaccines in adults aged 65 years or older: a prospective study." *Lancet* 2001;357:1008-1011.
19. Cornu, C., et al. "Efficacy of pneumococcal polysaccharide vaccine in immuno-competent adults: a meta-analysis of randomized trials." *Vaccine* 2001;19:4780-90.
20. French, N., et al. "23-valent pneumococcal polysaccharide vaccine in HIV-1-infected Ugandan adults: double blind, randomized, placebo controlled trial." *Lancet* 2000;355:2106-11.
21. "Pneumococcal vaccines ineffective." *Utah Vaccine Awareness Coalition* (December 2000); 2(3):6.
22. Fine, MJ., et al. "Efficacy of pneumococcal vaccine in adults: a meta-analysis of randomized controlled trials." *Archives of Internal Medicine* 1994;154:2666-77.
23. Forrester, HL., et al. "Inefficacy of pneumococcal vaccine in a high-risk population." *Amer J of Med* 1987;83:425-30.
24. Simberkoff, MS., et al. "Efficacy of pneumococcal vaccine in high-risk patients: results of a Veterans Administration cooperative study." *NEJM* 1986;315:1318-27.
25. Broome, CV. "Efficacy of pneumococcal polysaccharide vaccines." *Rev. Infect. Dis.* 1981;3(suppl): S82-S96.
26. De Roux, A., et al. "Pneumococcal vaccination." *European Respiratory Journal* 2005;26(6):982-83.
27. Ibid.
28. Dear, KB., et al. "Vaccines for preventing pneumococcal infection in adults." *The Cochrane Collaboration: Cochrane Database of Systematic Reviews* (John Wiley & Sons, Ltd.), 2007(2). Art. No. CD000422.
29. Ibid.
30. See Note 8.
31. Ibid.

Tuberculosis

1. Buchwald, G. *The Decline of Tuberculosis Despite 'Protective' Vaccination.* (Germany: F. Hirthammer Verlag GmbH, 2004):14.
2. Directors of Health Promotion and Education. "Tuberculosis." www.dhpe.org/infect/tb.html (Last accessed: March 22, 2007).
3. See Note 1.
4. Donegan, JLM. "Tuberculosis: is the BCG vaccine any good?" www.whale.to/v/donegan.html (March 22,2007).
5. Colston, J. "Tuberculosis: the return of the great white plague." *National Institute for Medical Research, Mill Hill Essays* 1995. www.nimr.mrc.ac.uk
6. Finnish National Public Health Institute. "Tuberculosis (or BCG) vaccination." www.ktl.fi (Last accessed: March 27, 2007).
7. See Note 2.
8. Ibid.
9. See Note 5.
10. See Note 1, pp. 53-63.
11. See Note 2.
12. Cheng, M. "TB cases ease, but resistant varieties a concern." *Assoc Pr* (Mar 23, 2007). www.the globeandmail.com
13. Stobbe, M. "U.S. TB cases at an all-time low." *Washington Post* (March 22, 2007). www.washingtonpost.com
14. See Note 2.
15. See Notes 2 and 6.
16. See Note 1, p. 108.
17. CDC. "TB elimination: BCG vaccine." www.cdc.gov/tb (April 2006).
18. Medical News Today. "Cooperation to create a new tuberculosis vaccine." (October 9, 2004).
19. BBC News. "New TB vaccine shown to be safe: the first TB vaccine to be developed in 80 years has passed safety trials in the UK." www.news.bbc.co.uk (October 24, 2004).
20. See Note 1, p. 109.
21. See Note 6.
22. Starke, J., et al. "The role of BCG vaccine in the prevention and control of tuberculosis in the United States—a joint statement: Table 1." *MMWR; CDC* (Apr 26, 1996);45(RRr-4):1-18.
23. Constock, GW., et al. "Long-term results of BCG in the southern United States." *American Review of Respiratory Disease* 1966;93(2):171-83.
24. Hart, RDA., et al. "BCG and vole bacillus vaccines in the prevention of tuberculosis in adolescence and early adult life." *British Medical Journal* 1977;ii:293-95.
25. World Health Organization. "Trial of BCG vaccines in South India for tuberculosis prevention." *Bulletin of the World Health Organization* 1979;57:819-827.
26. See Note 1, pp. 112-113.
27. "BCG: Bad news from India." *Lancet* (January 12, 1980):73-74.
28. Germanaud, J. "BCG vaccination and healthcare workers." *British Medical Journal* 1993;306:651-652.
29. Karonga Prevention Trial Group. "Randomized controlled trial of single BCG, repeated BCG, or combined BCG and killed Mycobacterium leprae vaccine for prevention of leprosy and tuberculosis in Malawi." *Lancet* (July 6, 1996);348(9019);17-24.
30. Ibid.
31. See Note 1, pp. 114-116.
32. Tuberculosis Research Centre. "Fifteen year follow-up trial of BCG vaccines in South India for tuberculosis prevention." *Indian Journal of Medical Research* 1999;110:56-69.
33. Brosch, R., et al. "Genome plasticity of BCG and impact on vaccine efficacy." *Proceedings of the National Academy of Sciences* (March 27, 2007);104(13):5596-5601.

TB Test

1. Nissi, J. "Tuberculin skin tests." WebMD. www.webmd.com (Last updated: May 25, 2005).
2. Wikipedia. "Mantoux test." www.en.wikipedia.org/wiki/Mantoux_test (Last modified: March 6, 2007).
3. Aventis Pasteur Limited. "Tuberculin purified protein derivative (Mantoux) Tubersol®." Product insert from the vaccine manufacturer. Product information as of September 2001.
4. Lifekind. "Chemical glossary." www.lifekind.com/catalog//chemical_glossary.php (Last accessed: March 18, 2007.)
5. U.S. Environmental Protection Agency. "Pollution prevention and Toxics: OPPT chemical fact sheets—1,4-dioxane fact sheet: support document." www.epa.gov/chemfact/dioxa-sd.txt (Feb 1995).
6. Lakes Environmental Software. "Phenol." Data extracted from: the EPA's Integrated Risk Information System (IRIS); the Agency for Toxic Substances and Disease Registry's (ATSDR's) *Toxicological Profile for Phenol*; Hazardous Substances Data Bank (HSDB); and Registry of Toxic Effects of Chemical Substances.
7. Associated Press. "Westchester to pay woman in false TB scare." *NY Times* (May 13, 2007). www.nytimes.com
8. See Notes 1-3.
9. Ibid.
10. Cassel, I. "Alternatives to TB testing: reasons to avoid the Mantoux skin test." *Vaccination Liberation; Idaho Observer* (July 2005). www.proliberty.com/observer/20050717.htm
11. Ayoub, D. "The rationale for TB screening of healthcare workers and other low-risk populations: a critical review of CDC policy." www.vaclib.org/basic/tbtest.htm
12. See Notes 1-3.
13. Herb Allure. "The Herb Allure Forum Complex." www.herballure.com
14. This personal letter is typical of the unsolicited queries and comments received by the *Thinktwice Global Vaccine Institute.* www.thinktwice.com
15. BioMeridian. "MSAS Professional." www.biomeridian.com
16. Carrillo, D. "Non-invasive TB test alternatives." *Vaccination Liberation.* www.vaclib. org (Posted on the "Herb Allure Forum Complex" (July 14, 2005); see Note 12.

Yellow Fever

1. Yellow Fever Online. "About yellow fever." www.yellowfever.com.au
2. U.S. Department of Health and Human Services. "Yellow fever vaccine: what you need to know." *CDC.* (Nov 9, 2004).
3. World Health Organization. "Yellow fever." www.who.int
4. See Notes 1 and 2.
5. Sanofi Pasteur. "Preventable diseases: yellow fever"
6. See Note 3.
7. World Health Organization. "Epidemic and pandemic alert and response: [yellow fever] trends since 1950." www.who.int (June 12, 2007).
8. See Notes 3 and 5.
9. CDC. "Traveler's health: yellow book—health information for international travel, 2005-2006. Chapter 4—prevention of specific infectious diseases: yellow fever."
10. World Health Organization. "Epidemic and pandemic alert and response: country profiles for yellow fever: Nigeria." www.who.int (Last updated: September 21, 2005).
11. World Health Organization. "Epidemic and pandemic alert and response: country profiles for yellow fever: Ghana (West Africa)." www.who.int (Updated: September 21, 2005).
12. See Note 9.
13. Ibid.
14. Sanofi Pasteur, Inc. "Yellow fever vaccine, YF-VAX®." Product insert from the vaccine manufacturer. Product information 2005.
15. See Note 2.
16. Martin, M., et al. "Fever and multisystem organ failure associated with 17D-204 yellow fever vaccination: a report of four cases." *Lancet* 2001;358(9276):98-104.
17. CDC. "Recommendations of the Advisory Committee on Immunization Practices (ACIP), yellow fever vaccine." *MMWR* 2002;51(RR17):1-10.
18. See Notes 9 and 14.
19. Ibid.
20. See Notes 2, 9 and 14.
21. Monath, TP., et al. "Comparative safety and immunogenicity of two yellow fever 17D vaccines (ARILVAX and YF-VAX) in a phase III multicenter, double-blind clinical trial." *Amer J of Tropical Med and Hygiene* 2002;66(5):533-41.
22. Fitel, M. "Encephalitis after yellow fever vaccination." *Pediatrics* 1960;25(6):956-58.
23. Vogt, D., et al. "Chromosomal changes following yellow fever vaccination." *Monatsschr Kinderheilkd* 1970;118(6):316-317. [German.]
24. Schoub, BD., et al. "Encephalitis in a 13-year-old boy following 17D yellow fever vaccine." *Journal of Infection* 1990;21(1):105-106.
25. Oyelami, SA., et al. "Severe post-vaccination reaction to 17D yellow fever vaccine in Nigeria. *Revue Roumaine de Virologie* 1995;45(1-2):25-30. [Romanian.]
26. Receveur, MC., et al. "Ketoacidotic coma four days after yellow fever vaccination." *La Presse Médicale* 1995;24(1):41. [French.]
27. Guzman, JR., et al. "Threat of dengue haemorrhagic fever after yellow fever vaccination." *Lancet* 1997;349 (9068):1841.
28. Kelso, JM., et al. "Anaphylaxis from yellow fever vaccine." *J of Allergy and Clinical Immunology* 1999;103(4):698-701.
29. Weir, E. "Yellow fever vaccination: be sure the patient needs it." *Canadian Medical Assoc J* 2001;165, pt. 7:941.
30. CDC. "Vaccine safety datalink project: safety of yellow fever vaccine." www.cdc.gov/od/science/iso/research_activities/vsd_studies.htm (Last accessed: June 11, 2007).
31. Vasconcelos, PF., et al. "Serious adverse events associated with yellow fever 17DD vaccine in Brazil: a report of two cases." *Lancet* 2001;358(9276):91-97.
32. Chan, RC., et al. "Hepatitis and death following vaccination with 17D-204 yellow f. vaccine." *Lancet* 2001;358 (9276):121-22.
33. See Note 16.
34. Pedro, FC., et al. "Serious adverse events associated with yellow fever 17DD vaccine in Brazil: a report of two cases." *Lancet* 2001; 358(9276):91-97.
35. "Adverse events following yellow fever vaccination." *Weekly Epidemiological Record* 2001;76(29):217-18.
36. Martin, M. "Advanced age a risk factor for illness temporally associated with yellow fever vaccination." *Emerging Infectious Disease* 2001; I(6).
37. Galler, R., et al. "Phenotypic and molecular analyses of yellow fever 17DD vaccine viruses associated with serious adverse events in Brazil." *Virology* 2001;290(2):309-19.
38. Kengsakul, K., et al. "Fatal myeloencephalitis following yellow fever vaccination in a case with HIV infection." *J of the Medical Association of Thailand* 2002;85(1):131-134.
39. See Note 17.
40. See Note 9.
41. Struchiner, CJ., et al. "Risk of fatal adverse events associated with 17DD yellow fever vaccine." *Epidemiology and Infection* 2004;132:939-46.
42. Lawrence, GL., et al. "Age-related risk of adverse events following yellow fever vaccination in Australia." *Communicable Diseases Intelligence* 2004;28(2):244-48.
43. Ibid.
44. Kitchener, S. "Viscerotropic and neurotropic disease following vaccination with the 17D yellow fever vaccine, Arilvax." *Vaccine* 2004;22(17-18):2103-05.
45. Gerasimon, et al. "Rare case of fatal yellow fever vaccine-associated viscerotropic disease." *Southern Medical Journal* 2005;98(6):653-56.
46. Doblas, A., et al. "Yellow fever vaccine-associated viscerotropic disease and death in Spain." *Journal of Clinical Virology* 2006;36(2):156-158.
47. Vellozzi, C., et al. "Yellow fever vaccine-associated viscerotropic disease and corticosteroid therapy: eleven United States cases, 1996-2004." *American Journal of Tropical Medicine and Hygiene* 2006;75(2):333-36.
48. Bayas, JM., et al. "Herpes zoster after yellow fever

vaccination." *Journal of Travel Medicine* 2007;14(1):65-66.
49. McMahon, AW., et al. "Neurologic disease associated with 17D-204 yellow fever vaccination: a report of 15 cases." *Vaccine* 2007;25(10):1727-34.
50. Fernandez, GC., et al. "Neurological adverse events temporally associated to mass vaccination against yellow fever in Juiz de Fora, Brazil, 1999-05." *Vaccine* 2007;25(16):3124-28.
51. See Note 14.
52. Ibid.
53. See Notes 9 and 14.
54. See Notes 2 and 9.

Typhoid Fever

1. CDC. "Typhoid fever." *Department of Health and Human Services* (October 24, 2005).
2. New York Department of Health. "Typhoid fever," (November 2006).
3. Sanofi Pasteur. "Typhoid fever." www.sanofipasteur.us (Last updated: April 4, 2005).
4. Wikipedia. "Typhoid fever." www.en.wikipedia.org (Last accessed: September 12, 2007).
5. See Notes 1-4.
6. See Notes 2 and 4.
7. See Note 1.
8. See Note 3.
9. DeRoeck, D., et al. "Putting typhoid vaccination on the global health agenda." *NEJM* (Sep 13, 2007);357(11):1069-71.
10. National Network for Immunization Information. "Immunization Science: typhoid fever in travelers." www.immunizationinfo.org.
11. See Notes 1 and 10.
12. See Note 1.
13. Chisholm, H. *The Encyclopedia Britannica: A Dictionary of Arts, Sci, Lit and Gen Information,* 11ᵗʰ ed. Vol. XXVIII, p. 162. (NY, 1911).
14. Wikipedia. "Frederick F. Russell." www.en.wikipedia.org
15. Ibid.
16. See Notes 3 and 10.
17. Avant Immunotherapeutics, Inc. "Typhoid vaccine demonstrates excellent clinical potential." Company Press Release (Issued: May 18, 2007).
18. Begier, EM., et al. "Postmarketing safety surveillance for typhoid fever vaccines from the Vaccine Adverse Event Reporting System, July 1990 through 2002." *Clin Infec Dis* (Feb 26, 2004);38:771-9.
19. Ibid.
20. See Note 1.
21. National Network for Immunization Information. "Vaccine information: typhoid fever." www.immunization info.org (Last accessed: Sep 12, 2007).
22. See Note 2.
23. See Note 18.

Cholera

1. CDC. "Cholera." *Department of Health and Human Services.* www.cdc.gov (Last reviewed: June 20, 2007).
2. CDC: Division of Bacterial and Mycotic Diseases. "Cholera." *Dept of Health and Human Serv* (Oct 6, 2005).
3. See Notes 1 and 2.
4. Ibid.
5. Ibid.
6. Ibid.
7. Ibid.
8. Barlow, K. "Researchers create cholera rice vaccine." *ABC Online: The World Today* (June 12, 2007). www.abc.net.au
9. Wills, H. "Cholera vaccination." *EMIS, Patient Plus* (May 8, 2006). www.patient.co.uk/showdoc/40025006
10. Eisinger, AJ., et al. "Acute renal failure after TAB and cholera vaccination." *BMJ* (February 10, 1979);1(6160):381-2.
11. Driehorst, J., et al. "Acute myocarditis after cholera vaccination." *Dtsch Med Wochenschr* (February 3, 1984);109(5):197-8. [German.]
12. Gavrilesco, S., et al. "Associated ventricular tachycardia and auricular fibrillation after anticholera vaccination." *Acta Cardiol.* 1973;28(1):89-94. [French.]
13. Marton, K., et al. "Anti-cholera vaccination and its secondary effects. Cutaneous lesions observed in mass vaccination." *Int J Dermatol.* (Apr-Jun, 1972);11(2):112-5.
14. Gentile, A., et al. "Case of leuko-encephalomyelitis due to anticholera vaccine." *Acta Neurol* (Sep-Oct, 1974);29(5):516-19. [Italian.]
15. D'Costa, DF., et al. "Transverse myelitis following cholera, typhoid and polio vaccination." *J R Soc Med.* (October 1990); 83(10):653.
16. Patil, SN., et al. "Sixth nerve paralysis following cholera inoculation." *Indian J Ophthalmol* (January 1977);24(4):37.
17. Spina, A. "Neuropsychiatric syndromes subsequent to cholera vaccination in Puglia during a recent epidemic." *Acta Neurol* (Jan-Feb 1974);29(1):58-65. [Italian.]
18. See Note 1.
19. See Note 9.
20. See Notes 1 and 2.

Japanese Encephalitis

1. CDC. "Japanese encephalitis vaccine: what you need to know." *Dept of Health and Human Services* (May 11, 2005).
2. Health Promotion and Education. "Japanese encephalitis." www.dhpe.org/infect/jpenceph.html (September 13, 2007).
3. Wikipedia. "Japanese encephalitis." www.en.wikipedia.org (Last accessed: September 13, 2007).
4. See Notes 1-3.
5. See Note 2.
6. CDC. "Inactivated Japanese encephalitis virus vaccine recommendations of the Advisory Committee on Immunization

Practices (ACIP)." *MMWR* (January 8, 1993);42(RR-01).
7. See Notes 2 and 3.
8. See Note 2.
9. Aventis Pasteur. "Japanese encephalitis virus vaccine inactivated, JE-VAX®." Product insert from the vaccine manufacturer. (Last accessed from website: Sep 13, 2007).
10. Ibid.
11. See Note 3.
12. Ibid.
13. See Note 9.
14. See Notes 6 and 9.
15. See Note 9.
16. Ibid.
17. Ibid.
18. MyDr. "Japanese encephalitis." www.MyDr.com.au
19. CDC. "Questions and answers about Japanese encephalitis." www.cdc.gov/ncidod/dvbid/jencepjalitis/qa.htm
20. See Note 1.
21. See Notes 1 and 2.
22. Medline Plus. "Japanese encephalitis vaccine." www.nlm.nih.gov (Last revised: April 1, 2007).

Rabies

1. Wikipedia. "Rabies." www.en.wikipedia.org (Last accessed: September 11, 2007).
2. Aventis Pasteur. "Rabies information and prevention." www.rabies.com (Accessed: September 11, 2007).
3. Health Central Network. "Health encyclopedia: diseases and conditions—rabies." www.healthscout.com (Sep 11, 2007).
4. Sanofi Pasteur. "Preventable diseases: rabies." www.sanofipasteur.us (Last updated: April 4, 2005).
5. Ibid.
6. CDC. "Rabies vaccine: what you need to know." *U.S. Department of Health and Human Services* (January 12, 2006).
7. Vaccine Education Center. "A look at each vaccine: rabies vaccine." *The Children's Hospital of Philadelphia.* www.chop.edu (Sep 11, 2007).
8. See Notes 3 and 4.
9. See Note 4.
10. See Note 6.
11. Ibid.
12. See Note 1.
13. Ibid.
14. Ibid.
15. See Notes 4 and 7.
16. Chiron Corporation. "Rabies vaccine Rabvert®—rabies vaccine for human use." Product insert (Revised: April 2004).
17. Ibid.
18. The Centre for Cancer Education. "Propiolactone." *University of Newcastle upon Tyne.* www.cancerweb.ncl.ac.uk (September 11, 2007).
19. Immunization Action Coalition. "Rabies vaccine." www.vaccine information.org (Last reviewed by CDC: Oct 2005).
20. See Notes 6 and 16.
21. See Notes 6, 16 and 19.
22. See Note 16, Table 2.
23. See Notes 4, 6 and 16.
24. See Note 6.
25. See Note 16.
26. Ibid.
27. Ibid.
28. Lakes Environmental Air Toxic Index. "b-propiolactone." *Lakes Environmental Software.* www.lakes-environmental.com/toxic/propiolacton .html (Last accessed: September 11, 2007.) [Data extracted from the Hazardous Substances Databank, the International Agency for Research on Cancer, the Registry of Toxic Effects of Chemical Substances, The Merck Index, and EPA's Integrated Risk Information System.]
29. CDC. "Notice to readers: manufacturer's recall of human rabies vaccine—April 2, 2004." *MMWR* (April 2, 2004); 53(Dispatch):1-2.
30. See Note 16.
31. Ibid.
32. Ibid.

Rhogam

1. Ortho-Clinical Diagnostics. "What does it mean to be Rh-negative?" www.rhogam.com/English/Patients/rh_meaning.aspx (December 27, 2006).
2. Hart, K. "Prenatal Pregnancy." *Vegan Pregnancy.* www.vegfamily.com
3. See Note 1.
4. Ibid.
5. Tenpenny, S. "Ask the Experts." *Mothering Magazine Forum.* www.mothering.com (Last accessed: March 21, 2007).
6. Ibid.
7. Reagan, L. "Vaccine conference exclusive report." *Holistic Pediatric Association* (Oct 18, 2005). www.hpakids.org
8. Ibid.
9. Miles, JH., et al. "Lack of association between Rh status, Rh immune globulin in pregnancy and autism." *American J of Medical Genetics* (July 1, 2007);143(13):1397-1407.
10. Miles, JH., et al. "Thimerosal exposure again not linked to autism." *Reuters Health* (May 18, 2007). www.medscape.com
11. Ortho-Clinical Diagnostics. "Information to review with your doctor." www.rhogam.com/English/Patients/rh_meaning .aspx (Last updated: December 27, 2006).
12. Tracie. "How easily medical personnel threaten people." *À La Carte.* www.lacarte.org/health/rhogam/index.html
13. Ortho-Clinical Diagnostics. "Rhₒ(D) Immune Globulin (Human) RhoGAM®." Product insert from manufacturer, 2001.
14. Ibid.
15. Lifekind. "Chemical glossary." www.lifekind.com/catalog//chemical_glossary.php (Last accessed: March 18, 2007).
16. U.S. Environmental Protection Agency. "Pollution prevention and Toxics: OPPT chemical fact sheets— 1,4-dioxane

fact sheet: support document." www.epa.gov/chemfact/dioxa-sd.txt (February 1995).
17. See Note 13.
18. Ortho-Clinical Diagnostics. "Frequently asked questions: does Rhogam Ultra-filtered have side effects?" www.rhogam .com (December 27, 2006).
19. See Note 12.
20. See Notes 2 and 12.
21. See Note 2.
22. Ibid.
23. See Notes 1, 2 and 12.
24. See Note 2.

Vitamin K

1. Better Health Fact Sheet. "Vitamin K and newborn babies." www.betterhealth.vic.gov.au (2004).
2. Tenpenny, S. "Ask the Experts." *Mothering Magazine Forum.* www.mothering.com (Last accessed: March 19, 2007).
3. Ibid.
4. Sutor, AH. et al. "Late form of vitamin K deficiency bleeding in Germany." *Klin Pediatr* (May-Jun 1995); 207, No. 3:89-97. [German.]
5. American Acad of Pediatrics. *Pediatric Nutrition Handbook,* 2004.
6. Palmer, LF. "Vitamin K at birth: to inject or not." *International Chiropractic Pediatric Association Newsletter* (Sept/Oct 2002; updated May 19, 2004). www.babyreference.com
7. Hogenbirk, K., et al. "The effect of formula versus breast feeding and exogenous vitamin K_1 supplementation on circulating levels of vitamin K_1 and vitamin K-dependent clotting factors in newborns." *Euro J of Pediatrics* (Jan 1993);152, No. 1:72-4.
8. See Note 2.
9. Van Droom, J., et al. "Vitamin K deficiency in the newborn (letter). *Lancet* 1977;ii:708-09.
10. Merck & Co., Inc. "Injection, AquaMephyton® (Phytonadione) Aqueous Colloidal Solution of Vitamin K_1." Product insert from the vaccine manufacturer (Issued: Feb. 2002).
11. Drug Information Online. "AquaMephyton advanced consumer information: vitamin K (systemic)." www.drugs.com
12. Roche Products Pty Ltd. "Konakion MM paediatric." Consumer medicine information (July 7, 2006.)
13. See Note 10.
14. See Note 12.
15. See Note 2.
16. Falcao, R. "General discussion of oral vitamin K instead of injected vitamin K." *Gentle Birth.* As quoted in *Natural Health* (September/October 1995). www.gentlebirth.org (Last accessed: March 19, 2007.)
17. Hancock, B. "Vitamin K: is this really safe and necessary?" *Vaccination Information Service* (Oct 2003). www.vaccination. inoz.com/vitaminK.html
18. See Note 16.
19. See Notes 10 and 11.
20. Golding, J., et al. "Factors associated with childhood cancer in a national cohort study." *British Journal of Cancer* 1990;62:304-308.
21. Golding, J., et al. "Childhood cancer, intramuscular vitamin K, and pethidine given during labour." *British Medical Journal* 1992;305:341-346.
22. Vitamin K Ad Hoc Tash Force. "Controversies concerning vitamin K and the newborn." *Pediatrics* 1993; 91:1001-1002.
23. Passmore, SJ., et al. "Case-control studies of relation between childhood cancer and neonatal vitamin K administration." *British Medical Journal* 1998;316(7126):178-84.
24. Ibid.
25. Parker, L., et al. "Neonatal vitamin K administration and childhood cancer in the north of England: retrospective case-control study." *BMJ* 1998;316(7126):189-93.
26. See Note 2.
27. Ibid.
28. Neustaedter, R. "Are vitamin K shots necessary?" *Mothering Magazine Forum.* www.mothering.com (Mar 19, 2007).
29. See Note 6.
30. See Notes 1, 6, 12, 16, and 22.
31. Stanford School of Medicine. "Guidelines for vitamin K prophylaxis" (2007). www.newborns.stanford.edu/vitaminK .html
32. Harkins, D. "National standard mandates newborn vitamin K injection." *Idaho Observer* (July 1999). www.proliberty .com/observer/19990710.htm

Multiple Vaccines

1. CDC. "Recommended immunization schedule for persons ages 0-6 Years — United States, 2011."
2. Ibid.
3. Vaccine Adverse Event Reporting System (VAERS), Rockville, MD.
4. Ibid.
5. Ibid.
6. Blaylock, R. "Vaccinations: the hidden dangers." *The Blaylock Wellness Report* (May 2004):1-9.
7. Ottaviani G., et al. "Sudden infant death syndrome (SIDS) shortly after hexavalent vaccination: another pathology in suspected SIDS?" *Virchows Archiv* 2006;448:100–104.
8. Zinka, B., et al. "Unexplained cases of sudden infant death shortly after hexavalent vaccination." *Vaccine* 2006 Jul 26;24(31-32):5779-80.
9. "Autism: Present Challenges, Future Needs—Why the Increased Rates?" *Govt Reform Committee Hearing,* Washington, DC. (April 6, 2000.) As cited in Andrew Wakefield's testimony.
10. Sears, RW. *The Vaccine Book* (NY: Little, Brown and Company, 2007):236-237.
11. Cave, S. *What your Doctor May Not Tell You About Children's Vaccinations* (NY: Warner Books, 2001):196.
12. Miller, NZ., et al. "Infant mortality rates regressed against number of vaccine doses routinely given: is there a biochemical

or synergistic toxicity?" *Hum Exp Toxicol* (May 4, 2011). Published online: www.het.sagepub.com
13. Miller, NZ. *Vaccines: Are They Really Safe and Effective?* (Santa Fe, NM: New Atlantean Press, 2010), p. 98 ("Reporting Vaccine Reactions") and p. 102 ("Claims for Compensation").
14. See Note 3.
15. Ibid.
16. These unsolicited stories were received by the *Thinktwice Global Vaccine Institute.* www.thinktwice.com

New Vaccines

1. Tant, C. *Awesome Green* (Angleton, TX: Biotech Pub, 1994):108-115.
2. See Congressional Bill, H.R. 78, 103rd Congress, 1st Session (Jan 5, 1993).
3. *New England J of Medicine* (June 7, 2007);356:2421-22.
4. Moskowitz, R. "Vaccination: A Sacrament of Modern Medicine," *Mothering* (Spring 1992):53.
5. Leviton, R. "A Shot in the Dark," *Yoga Journal* (May/June, 1992):128.
6. Johnson, LA. "Merck's experimental AIDS vaccine fails." *Associated Press* (September 22, 2007).
7. Ibid.
8. Zhang, H., et al. "Possible origin of current influenza A H1N1 viruses." *The Lancet H1N1 Resource Centre* (August 2009).
9. Sullivan, MG. "U.S. CDC chief: most pandemic flu patients won't be seriously ill." *The Lancet H1N1 Resource Centre* (September 3, 2009).
10. Sullivan, MG. "Pediatric pandemic flu deaths concentrated in high-risk groups." *The Lancet H1N1 Resource Centre* (September 3, 2009).
11. Brown, D. "Flu vaccine panel creates priority list: pregnant women, caregivers are first." *Washington Post* (July 30, 2009).
12. Hurwitz, ES., et al. "Guillain-Barré syndrome and the 1978-79 influenza vaccine." *New England Journal of Medicine* 1981;304:1557-61.
13. Kaplan, JE., et al. "Guillain-Barré syndrome in the U.S., 1978-1981: Additional observations from the national surveillance system." *Neurology* (May 1983);33(5):633-37.
14. Edemariam, A. "Swine flu will be biggest pandemic ever, warns world health chief." *The Guardian* (July 16, 2009). www.guardian.co.uk
15. In a private email exchange between Dr. Tedd Koren and Barbara Mulach, PhD.
16. Singer, S. "CDC: school kids may have to get up to 4 flu shots in the fall." *Palm Beach Post* (July 15, 2009).
17. Mercola, J. "Squalene: the swine flu vaccine's dirty little secret exposed." *Organic Consumers Assoc.* (Aug. 4, 2009).
18. Asa, PB., et al. "Antibodies to squalene in recipients of anthrax vaccine." *Experimental and Molecular Pathology* (August 2002);73:19-27.
19. Campbell, C. "Swine flu science update." *Science and Development Network* (June 30, 2009). www.scidev.net
20. Sullivan, M. "Legal immunity set for swine flu vaccine makers." *Now Public* (August 21, 2009). www.nowpublic.com
21. See Notes 11 and 16.
22. Lamb, E. "Swine flu vaccine required for all military personnel." *Norfolk Health Care Examiner* (September 8, 2009). www.examiner.com
23. Bortnick, CJ. "Local nurse won't comply with state vaccination order." *YNN Rochester* (September 6, 2009). www.rochester.ynn.com
24. Fisher, BL. "Pandemic H1N1 swine flu: what about you and your family?" *NVIC* (September 9, 2009). www.nvic.org
25. Corbett, J. "FDA approves Sanofi-Aventis H5N1 bird-flu vaccine." *Marketwatch* (April 17, 2007). www.marketwatch.com
26. Reuters. "Indonesia announces plans to use human bird flu vaccine." *Medscape* (June 22, 2007). www.medscape.com
27. Barclay, L., et al. "Low-dose avian-flu vaccine may be safe, immunogenic." *Medscape* (Sep 5, 2006). www.medscape.com
28. "New vaccine for middle-ear infection." *Medical Progress* (March 3, 2006). www.medicalprogress.org
29. "Ear infection vaccine developed." *BBC News* (March 3, 2006). www.newsvote.bbc.co.uk
30. Ibid.
31. Reuters. "Vaccine aims to wipe out ear, sinus infections." *CNN.com* (September 26, 2006). www.cnn.health
32. Diodati, C. *Vaccine Guide for Dogs and Cats: What Every Pet Lover Should Know.* (Santa Fe, NM: New Atlantean Press, 2003).
33. Pollock, RVH., et al. "Maternally derived immunity to canine parvovirus infection: transfer, decline and interference with vaccination." *Journal of the American Veterinary Medical Association* (January 1, 1982):42.
34. See Note 32, p. 83.

Laws, Options and More

1. As confirmed in numerous unsolicited personal accounts received by the *Thinktwice Global Vaccine Institute.* www.thinktwice.com
2. Ibid.
3. Strebel PM., et al. Epidemiology of poliomyelitis in U.S. one decade after the last reported case of indigenous wild virus associated disease, *Clin Infect Dis* CDC (Feb 1992):568–79.
4. Associated Press. "Vaccine blamed in polio outbreak." *The New Mexican* (October 6, 2006):A-8.
5. Mendelsohn R. *How to Raise a Healthy Child...In Spite of Your Doctor.* (Ballantine Books, 1987.)

Index